Readings in
Gerontological
Nursing

Readings in Gerontological Nursing

Edited by

Judith Ann Allender, EdD, RN,C

Professor
Department of Nursing
School of Health and Human Services
California State University
Fresno, California

Cherie L. Rector, PhD, RN,C

Associate Professor
Coordinator for School Nurse Credential Program
Department of Nursing
School of Health and Human Services
California State University
Fresno, California

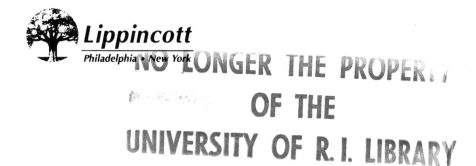

Lippincott
Philadelphia • New York

Sponsoring Editor: Susan M. Keneally
Project Editor: Sandra Cherrey Scheinin
Production Manager: Helen Ewan
Production Coordinator: Patricia McCloskey
Assistant Art Director: Kathy Kelley-Luedtke

9 8 7 6 5 4 3 2 1

Library of Congress Cataloging-in-Publications Data

Readings in gerontological nursing / edited by Judith Ann Allender,
    Cherie L. Rector.
        p.   cm.
    Includes bibliographical references and index.
    ISBN 0-7817-9201-0 (alk. paper)
    1. Geriatric nursing.   I. Allender, Judith Ann.   II. Rector.
Cherie L.
    [DNLM: 1. Geriatric Nursing—collected works.   WY 152 R2871 1998]
RC954.R43   1998
610.73'65—dc21
DNLM/DLC
for Library of Congress   97-33646
                                                                        CIP

Care has been taken to confirm the accuracy of the information presented and to describe generally accepted practices. However, the authors, editors, and publisher are not responsible for errors or omissions or for any consequences from application of the information in this book and make no warranty, express or implied, with respect to the contents of the publication.

The authors, editors and publisher have exerted every effort to ensure that drug selection and dosage set forth in this text are in accordance with current recommendations and practice at the time of publication. However, in view of ongoing research, changes in government regulations, and the constant flow of information relating to drug therapy and drug reactions, the reader is urged to check the package insert for each drug for any change in indications and dosage and for added warnings and precautions. This is particularly important when the recommended agent is a new or infrequently employed drug.

Some drugs and medical devices presented in this publication have Food and Drug Administration (FDA) clearance for limited use in restricted research settings. It is the responsibility of the health care provider to ascertain the FDA status of each drug or device planned for use in their clinical practice.

⊗ This Paper Meets the Requirements of ANSI/NISO Z39.48-1992
    (Permanence of Paper).

To
grandmothers, especially our fondly remembered
hardy, resilient, indefatigable role models:

Elizabeth Anna Lutz (1890–1982)
Maria Schuepp (1887–1972)
and
Lula Mae Martin (1893–1983)
Myrtle Maria Beckstead Egbert (1895–1970)

Contributors

Dolores M. Alford, PhD, RN, FAAN
Gerontic Nursing Consultant
Dallas, Texas

Robert Atchley, PhD
Director, Scripps Gerontology
    Center
Miami University
Oxford, Ohio

Sally Ax, RNC, BSN
Medical Supervisor, Cardiac
    Program
TGC Home Health Care
Lakeland, Florida

Nellie C. Bailey, MS, MA, RN, CS
Assistant Professor and Community
    Health Nurse
SUNY-Health Science Center
Brooklyn College of Nursing
Brooklyn, New York

Susan J. Barnes, RN, MSN
Doctoral Student
University of Texas Health Science
    Center
San Antonio School of Nursing
San Antonio, Texas

Amanda Smith Barusch, MSW, PhD
Professor and Director
Social Research Institute
Graduate School of Social Work
University of Utah
Salt Lake City, Utah

Margaret Berrio
Coordinator
Quality Management and
    Management Information Systems
Nursing Service
Boston Veterans Affairs Medical
    Center
Boston, Massachusetts

Gloria Black, RN, CS, MS
Clinical Nurse Specialist for Home
    Health
South Carolina Department of
    Health and Environmental
    Control
Appalachia II District
Greenville, South Carolina

Sandra Black, PhD
Assistant Professor
Department of Internal Medicine
Center on Aging
University of Texas Medical Branch
Galveston, Texas

Elizabeth Bondy, PhD
Assistant Professor
College of Education
University of Florida
Gainesville, Florida

Lois M. Brandriet, RN, PhD
Assistant Professor
College of Nursing
Brigham Young University
Provo, Utah

Luanne Brogna, RN, MS, CETN
Clinical Nurse Specialist
Enterostomal Therapy
Hackensack Medical Center Home
  Health Agency
Hackensack, New Jersey

Margaret J. Bull, RN, PhD
Associate Professor
University of Minnesota
School of Nursing
St. Paul, Minnesota

Margaret Burney-Puckett, MSN, RN
Vanderbilt University
School of Nursing
Nashville, Tennessee

Marybeth Tank Buschman, RN, PhD
Professor, College of Nursing
The University of Illinois
Chicago, Illinois

Marylea Benware Carr, MS
Women's Studies
Mankato State University
Mankato, Minnesota

Fen-Lei Chang, PhD, MD
Director of the UCSF
Fresno Alzheimer's Disease Center
Chief of Neurology and
  Rehabilitation Service
Veterans' Administration Medical
  Center
Fresno, California

Yeou-Lan Duh Chen, PhD, RN
Associate Professor
School of Nursing
Westminster College
Salt Lake City, Utah

Eileen R. Chichin, DSW, RN
Department of Geriatrics and Adult
  Development
Mount Sinai School of Medicine
New York, New York

Phillip G. Clark, ScD
Professor and Acting Director
Program in Gerontology
University of Rhode Island
Kingston, Rhode Island

Ruby M. Van Croft, RN, MS
Director of Community Affairs
Visiting Nurse Association
President, Capital Home Health
  Association
Washington, DC

Neal Cutler, PhD
Director, Boettner Center of
  Financial Gerontology
School of Social Work
University of Pennsylvania
Philadelphia, Pennsylvania

Daniel Detzner, PhD
Associate Professor, Family Social
  Science Department
Director, Refugee Studies Center
University of Minnesota
St. Paul, Minnesota

Steven Devlin, PhD
Associate Director
Boettner Center of Financial
  Gerontology
School of Social Work
University of Pennsylvania
Philadelphia, Pennsylvania

Marguerite Dixon, RN, PhD
Retired Dean
Chicago State University
School of Nursing
Chicago, Illinois

Preface

The United States has seen dramatic increases in the number and percentage of older adults. It is anticipated that this trend will continue and, within 30 years, the present large number of elderly will double. Life expectancy continues to rise, with some experts in aging professing that humans have a lifespan potential of 120 years. We presently recognize that the population over the age of 85 is the fastest growing age group in America. These demographics have significant implications for the nation, the health care delivery system, and the professionals in health care.

This anthology of readings was developed to enhance the beginning professional's understanding of elders in today's world. The choices made represent the most current and innovative developments in the field and are designed to assist the nurse in understanding the broad field of aging and what caring for elders involves.

The chapters come from over twenty different nursing and interprofessional sources, primarily from the years 1994, 1995, and 1996. One of the chapters was written in 1997 especially for this edition by experts in the field. The 52 chapters included make this text a rich resource for the undergraduate and graduate nursing student. In some courses this text can be used with beginning nursing or medical-surgical nursing texts. It could also be the primary text in a gerontological nursing course. The text can be a handy reference tool to enhance the practice of experienced nurses or nurses new to the field of gerontology. Although it is extensive it does not represent a complete look at aging. The readings selected represent the latest ideas from policy makers, innovative practice models, research methodologies, and situations unique to the aging client, family members, and caregivers. We conclude each unit with a selected bibliography useful to the reader as a supplement to the readings in the text.

Readings in Gerontological Nursing contains 8 units, each covering a major category of concern in gerontological nursing. Unit 1, The Elders Are Coming! The Elders Are Coming! Social Policy Issues and Aging, presents timely pieces that deliberate the future of health care and nursing practice with the elderly. Leaders in gerontology discuss trends in policy formation, financing reform affecting elders, and health care delivery for our aging population. This unit touches on ethical and moral issues surrounding care for elders, especially in the areas of Medicare, Medicaid, family financial responsibility, advance directives, and managed care. It also examines ageist beliefs and practices that lead to ineffective health care.

Unit 2, Promoting Quality of Life and Longevity, presents selected approaches to enhance wellness and quality of life in the elderly, including use of humor, basing teaching on the elder's life experiences, promoting sexual health, elders' perceptions of being strong and surviving, and looking at menopause holistically as a transitional phase to a healthy last third of one's life.

Unit 3, Age Segregation, Grandparenting, and Ethnicity: Sociocultural Issues in an Aging America, focuses on social and cultural forces that shape the roles of elders in our society. It begins with an examination of age as a segregating factor and the need for greater age integration. It goes on to examine the dynamic role of grandparents and the importance of ethnicity and cultural beliefs in the development of health behaviors. The health beliefs and behaviors of Mexican American and Chinese American elders are described, and the effect that poverty plays in access to health care.

Unit 4, Innovative Programs in Gerontological Nursing, explores selected programs that affect the lives of elders. Chapters on preventative nursing care and a community-based nursing center present ways to provide elder care and focus on wellness. The Omaha Information System, geriatric rehabilitation, and a cardiac rehabilitation model demonstrate organizational systems for ill elders. Older adults in long-term care have their lives enhanced by workshops for women residents and a center on ethics in long-term care.

Unit 5, If I Live to Be 102, Will I Be Able to Tie My Shoes? Theory Development and Research With Older Adults, presents theories on aging and the application of theoretical frameworks to problems or issues of aging, specifically the process of life review and the progression of cognitive decline in dementia patients. Qualitative research methods and validity threats are described, and current research studies that demonstrate these grounded theory and ethnographic approaches are presented. The unit ends with a quantitative evaluation research study on discharge planning.

Unit 6, From Malnutrition to Sleep Problems: Assessing Older Adults, emphasizes the importance of careful assessment and examination of our own thoughts and biases regarding the definition of "quality of life." Additional chapters on the assessment of nutritional status, sleep disturbances, elder abuse, adverse drug reactions, and cognitive functioning in the elderly complete this unit.

Unit 7, Managing Elders With Selected Health Care Issues, presents several common issues that affect the elderly and consequently influence the role of the health care professional. Selections include dealing with elders who have controlling dispositions, the depressed elder, preventing falls in the frail elderly, managing postoperative pain and congestive heart failure effectively, sundown syndrome, acquired immunodeficiency syndrome (AIDS) in the elderly, and written for this edition is a chapter on the latest research and therapeutic modalities used with Alzheimer's disease victims and their families.

Finally, Unit 8, Older Adults and Caregivers: Changing Needs and Settings, concludes the contributions in this text and focuses on the transitional needs of elders and their caregivers as the aging process places more demands on family systems and the human body. The chapters focus on daughter and mother relationships and changing roles, caring for the caregiver, restraint-free care, pressure ulcer management, communicating with the confused old-old client, and the role of hospice nurses who help elders confront death.

The selection of readings flows from the broad view of aging agendas at the national level to promoting wellness and longevity and using innovative programs to enhance the lives of elders at the local level. We then share the need for developing theory and conducting research to continue to expand the knowledge base in gerontological nursing. Tools and specific health issues follow with assessment tools and managing selected health care problems. The text concludes with the changing needs of elders as they are managed in changing settings. This organization follows the broad to specific and wellness to illness approaches, making it useful in nursing programs or nursing courses that use a similar organizational structure.

We are thankful for the individuals who have contributed to the birth of this book. Their willingness to have faith in the need for this publication through their support, suggestions, assistance, and contributions have been invaluable. We especially want to thank Linda Hewett and Fen-Lei Chang for their original work; our many photo subjects—especially the late Elizabeth Schuepp, Gil Allender, John R. Van Doren, Sam Allender, Mike Raphael, Jack and Jewell Egbert, and Tobey and Kelly Wosnik; those who helped with our photographs and manuscript preparation—Zachary Couch, Paul L. Firth, A and V Custom Photo Lab in Fresno, CA., and Benjamin Rector, Darrell Lakey, and Susan Wilson.

Our special thanks go to our supportive editor at Lippincott-Raven Publishers, the late Mary Gyetvan, who's love for and commitment to the field of gerontology facilitated the development of this book. Thanks is also extended to her excellent assistant Susan Keneally, associate editor, for her timely assistance. Finally, we thank our families, especially our husbands, Gilbert F. Allender and John J. "Jerry" Rector for being patient with wives who always take on more than we know we should!

Judith Ann Allender, EdD, RN,C
Cherie L. Rector, PhD, RN,C

Contents

Unit 1
The Elders Are Coming!
The Elders Are Coming!
Social Policy Issues and Aging

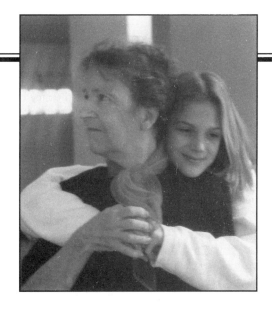

With the explosion in the elderly population expected early in the 21st century caused by the aging of the baby boom generation, many policy makers are concerned that the already stiff competition for limited government dollars may escalate into an intergenerational war. Already, many link the increasing numbers of children living in poverty to the gains our elderly have made in financial security. Although this either/or association is tenuous at best, this type of intergenerational finger pointing demonstrates the need for careful consideration and planning in policy making areas so that all of our citizens can enjoy health, security, safety, and a beneficial quality of life.

It is to our advantage, as a nation, to promote and protect the health and well being of all of our citizens and to keep in mind that we will all be traveling the same path of life. However, many important decisions may be made simply on

1

the merits of their cost-effectiveness and the realities of budget constraints. It will be especially important for those of us working with the elderly to understand the social policies that affect our clients' access to health care and their rights to direct that care.

This unit consists of chapters that outline the need for a clear social policy on aging, and covers some of the most important issues facing policy makers today — Medicare, Medicaid, Social Security, managed care, projected demographic trends, predjudice toward the elderly, and the rights of aging patients to direct which life support measures they want used. It moves from broad, "big picture" issues surrounding financing and social programs to more immediate, narrow concerns, such as educating patients in health care facilities about their rights to have a living will. Intermediate issues, such as methods health maintenance organizations (HMOs) can use to provide quality care to elders, and how stereotypical perceptions of elderly can shape our caregiving behaviors also are addressed.

The unit begins with a chapter examining the most pressing crises in the area of gerontology and the need to place these issues in a broad, contextual framework while opening up the debate to a wide variety of professionals. It continues with chapters discussing the growing number of families who are straining to care both for their children and their aging parents; the restructuring of Medicare; the potential effects on the elderly of proposed policy changes in Medicaid; the needs of the elderly population in managed care systems; how ageism affects programs for the elderly, health care providers' perceptions of elderly, as well as elders' self-perceptions; and how health care facilities can improve compliance with the patient notification requirements surrounding advance directives.

This unit provides gerontological nurses with the basics of a social policy background necessary to enable them to be more effective client advocates, program planners, and caregivers.

Chapter 1

Mainstreaming Gerontology in the Policy Arena

FERNANDO M. TORRES-GIL   MICHELE A. PUCCINELLI

America is at a crossroads. By the end of this century, one in five Americans will be age 55 or older, and in the year 2010, the first baby boomers will turn 65. As policymakers debate the converging issues of an aging population, an expensive and mutating health care system, and public pressure for balanced budgets, it is important that nurses join in this discussion. Fernando Torres-Gil, a well-known gerontologist and Assistant Secretary for Aging, and Michele Puccinelli propose a broad, contextual framework for examining policy issues related to aging. The many inconsistencies in policies and politics that affect the aging population must be addressed, and the increasing numbers of interested parties joining in the debate every day should be welcomed. How we address these crucial issues, and who is included in framing the debate will have long-range implications for our society into the next century. The authors suggest that viewing the issues across generations and within a broader context can help us better plan for the future.

Public policies concerning older persons are increasingly shaping the domestic agenda. Recent developments on the aging policy front illustrate this phenomenon — public and congressional scrutiny about entitlements to middle-income and older persons, attempts to make the Social Security Administration an independent agency, using Medicare "savings" to pay for health care and budgetary reforms. Policy proposals to raise the eligibility age for receipt of some public benefits illustrate the shifting sands of public attitudes toward the elderly population.

The increasing public debates about paying for benefits to the elderly and political concerns about preparing for the retirement of baby boomers reflect the growing importance of aging issues in domestic affairs. However, as these issues permeate the political debate, they are too often based on misperceptions about demographic trends and their effects on economic and budgetary politics. Proposals that respond to population aging are too often couched in the language of winners and losers: What one group

From *The Gerontologist* 34(60):749–752, 1994. Reprinted with permission.

receives, another group loses. The media, in particular, portray political options in the context of generational competition and interest group politics.

The purpose of this discussion is not to assess the merits and demerits of specific policy issues confronting an aging society, but to promote a broader framework within which the policy options and decisions can be addressed. This goal necessarily requires a sense of urgency for gerontologists to be more vested in these debates.

▰ THE EMERGENT ISSUES

The central domestic policy issues of the next 20 years may hinge on the intersection of aging, financing, and eligibility. Political choices may center around who receives, who pays, and under what conditions. These new circumstances go beyond the traditional confines of interest group struggles and a politics of aging, whereby our analysis focuses on the interplay of persons, institutions, and groups concerned primarily with older persons.

Today, and into the foreseeable future, gerontologists will find that their interests have become "mainstream," attracting the attention of the wider professional and political circles of economics, political science, public policy, and government. In many respects, the early warnings about these new circumstances and the need to develop a broader contextual framework are a validation of the work of early pioneers in gerontology (Binstock, 1983; Hudson & Strate, 1985; Neugarten, 1979) who argued that the political and policy consequences of aging and gerontology would attract — and should attract — the broader society, and that the debates within gerontology about who receives and who pays for public benefits to the elderly would, in fact, be a central issue for government and society. Long after those pioneers prodded us to broaden our intellectual and analytical horizons, we find an even greater need to engage our policy analysis and research into mainstream concerns about the direction of government and how it responds to a society getting older and more diverse.

The evidence for a more urgent involvement in the macro policy debates around aging is compelling. In recent years, for example, congressional proposals to balance the budget have focused on a dramatic restructuring of entitlements to older persons. Proposals to means-test the Medicare program, lifting the Social Security age even further, and raising the age at which federal workers can retire are symptomatic of such macro concerns. The growing attention to paying for the retirement of future cohorts has led to the use of "generational accounting" techniques, which focus on the financial burdens placed on future generations through tax policy made today.

The restructuring of today's old-age systems of benefits and services, a system evolving over the last 60 years, is now undergoing dramatic changes. The health care reform debates have generally relied on phasing out the Medicaid program and an integration of the Medicare program into a more universal and comprehensive health care system. Long-term care proposals to create a universal system of home- and community-based services are now predicated on Activities of Daily Living (ADLs), rather than on age, thus broadening eligibility to all persons with a disability, regardless of age. Continuing controversy over the targeting provisions of the Older Americans Act (a delicate approach in a non-means-tested program for older adults without the resources to be a true entitlement program for all senior citizens) illustrates the shifting debates about public policies for older persons.

These examples point out the inconsistencies of our current approach to old-age policies, and also indicate that we may be in the midst of a transition from the legacy of a modern aging period (1930–1990), when there was widespread support for age-based criteria, to a new aging period in which old age alone may not be sufficient grounds for certain public benefits (Torres-Gil, 1992). This transition is fraught with uncertainties and insecurities.

We vacillate, for example, about how to respond to longevity and a healthier and more productive work force of older persons and retirees. Do we rapidly raise the age at which persons can leave the work force with unreduced retirement benefits beyond what is scheduled to take place under current law (e.g., as some would suggest with the Social Security program)? Do we develop an all-encompassing approach to population aging and prepare for twice as many retirees in the next century, assuming we use the existing definition of being old? Or do we continue our current categorical approach, whereby older persons and retirees are handled through discrete agencies and policies within government and the Congress — for example, private pension regulation in the Department of Labor, Social Security and Older Americans Act policies in the Department of Health and Human Services, tax policies in the Treasury Department, and multiple congressional committees with multiple jurisdictions?

In sorting out how we can best address the increasing effect of aging policies on the domestic agenda of the federal government, we are also handicapped by a lack of public and societal consensus about who is responsible, and to what extent, for aging concerns. To what extent, for example, should individuals be held responsible for their own aging and for preparing for a long life span, for example, with savings and thrift policies? In what ways should government ensure a social safety net to older persons, and how should the level of income and assets be factored into eligibility criteria? Do we focus scarce resources on the most vulnerable of the elderly, for instance, those with low incomes or disabilities, and thereby risk losing broader political support for programs for older persons? And to what extent should the private sector be held accountable for ensuring that employees have health, long-term care, pensions, and other social protection such as that provided by the Family and Medical Leave Act?

■ GERONTOLOGY AND THE BROADER ARENA

Those issues point out the link between gerontological interests in the political and policy dimensions of aging and the larger societal concerns about an aging society. The current approach in responding to these issues appears to be couched in narrow economic and fiscal terms? Do we means-test Medicare? Should deficit reduction policies keep Social Security trust funds on budget? Do we make it easier for retirees to work and keep pension and Social Security benefits?

On the other hand, gerontologists, as well as those who are engaged in the politics and policy dimensions of aging, have much to contribute to those narrow political and economic debates about an aging society. They cannot allow themselves to be left out of the macro policy debates about aging and public policy. They must now compete with other disciplines and interest groups outside of gerontology if they are to continue to influence the public debate and be "players" in the political arena.

As we move toward a new and greatly expanding playing field in which the entire society addresses aging-related issues, we should consider the following.

First, there is a tremendous lack of factual information about the true aspects of an aging society. On one front, both the public and decision makers are not fully informed about the value of public benefits and services to older persons that have evolved over the last 30 to 60 years. The fact that Social Security has not only reduced poverty but enabled the growth of a middle class is not widely celebrated. The recognition of social insurance as a policy approach and a set of principles in benefiting wide segments of society and promoting a sense of community is crucial. Confusing and misleading statements about demographic trends distort our ability to conduct rational policy analyses. For example, using straight-line projections to decide whether we can afford the current level of public benefits to the elderly (e.g., increases in longevity and their effects on health care costs, and the declining worker-to-retiree ratio) ignores a whole set of other mitigating factors (e.g., increases in worker productivity, employment opportunities for retirees, decreases in mortality and morbidity rates). The need to inform and educate the public about the true circumstances of population aging calls for a concerted marketing strategy tied to policy analysis and research and the dissemination of information.

Second, there is need to recognize the new players who will have an increasingly crucial role in influencing public policy decisions around aging. Along with the traditional role of the Department of Health and Human Services and its key operating divisions in this area — Social Security Administration, Administration on Aging, Health Care Financing Administration, Public Health Service — other cabinet agencies, the Departments of Labor, Treasury, Veterans Affairs, as well as the Corporation for Public Service, are recognizing the need to be involved in policy and political decisions affecting an aging society and older persons. In the policy arena are yet additional key players with a stake in these issues: the Advisory Council on Social Security and Medicare, the National Academy on Aging, the National Academy on Social Insurance. Depending on any given policy issue, a wide array of groups will have a stake in aging-related issues.

Third, there is a need to avoid a narrow paradigm of economic and fiscal analysis in assessing the short- and long-term implications of aging. Immediate fiscal pressures are helping to focus many policy makers to discuss the implications of an aging society almost exclusively in terms of deficit and budgetary factors, such as the solvency of private pensions, and ways to address the entitlement nature of Social Security and the Medicare program vis-a-vis their influence on public budgeting. These economic analyses will likely (or threaten to) frame policies affecting public benefits and services to older persons in a narrow fashion. While recognizing that the issues surrounding entitlement, deficits, and retirement age have an important bearing on planning ahead for an aging society, it is equally important to make sure that a broad array of social policy issues is included in this discussion. A narrow focus on fiscal and economic analysis may well ignore a host of critical social issues that will also have an important bearing on how we should plan ahead. These issues include:

- long-term care and increasing the availability of home- and community-based services to maximize the independence of older persons;
- employment of older persons who wish to remain in the work force, and worker productivity;
- affordable and accessible transportation for aging persons who can no longer operate their own vehicles;
- housing and home modifications;
- demographic changes affecting family and social structures, such as fewer children, and more elderly living alone;
- federal and state tax policies;
- life-style choices and individual responsibility;
- special needs of older women who have lacked traditional employment benefits such as pensions;
- life expectancies and what those mean for various subpopulations of an aging society;
- the effect of biomedical research on longevity and morbidity;
- welfare for poor and disabled older adults; and
- diversity and the phenomenon of a largely minority/immigrant/female work force supporting a largely white retiree population.

By looking at a broader agenda, we will be in a better position to tackle sensitive subjects of financing and benefit programs within a framework of economic and social concerns.

▬LOOKING TO THE FUTURE

Finally, in promoting greater information and education about the true nature of aging, while recognizing a growing set of players interested in our traditional concerns, and while promoting a broader conceptual framework for public analysis and formulation, we cannot forget that the visceral political agenda may be driven by a quest for retirement security among the soon-to-be-elderly. Those approaching retirement, baby boomers in their forties, and even twenty-something-year-olds will react to aging on a very personal level: Will I be better off as I get old, and will the decisions made today hinder or help my future retirement? On the one hand, this reaction demonstrates a growing recognition about how aging affects everyone, young or old. On the other hand, it means that elected officials will be very sensitive to how their constituents react to any policy proposals, however well thought out.

A hearing held by the House Ways and Means Subcommittee on Social Security on the retirement security concerns of baby boomers certainly dramatized the growing congressional and public interest in this area (Tor-res-Gil, 1993). At that hearing, the Congressional Budget Office released a report asserting that baby boomers would do well in their retirement because their level of pension coverage was greater today than it was for their parents when they were young. The ensuing dialogue about whether or not that report's conclusions reflected an accurate picture of baby boomers' relative security in their old age illustrated the confusion and contradictions about how younger groups will view political decisions that affect their later retirement.

Through all this we cannot forget that the even larger issues facing the United States — its economic status and geopolitical relationships — will also influence how we respond to the economic and social aspects of an aging society. Debates and decisions that affect the economic prosperity of the United States will influence our ability to afford public benefits and services to older persons. The success of the North American Free Trade Agreement (NAFTA) will have a direct bearing on the economic and trade fortunes of the United States, as well as on the impact of immigration on the growing diversity of the U.S. population. Our ability to understand and learn from the experiences of other nations that are aging, such as Japan, Western Europe, and how they address similar issues of aging, fiscal and economic pressures, and public benefits to retirees, can help us adapt to our own aging population.

The next 20 years promise to be a very exciting time for the field of gerontology and the United States. Aging has come of age and is now one of the important domestic issues facing the United States. What we do or don't do in the 1990s will determine what type of aging society we will have in the next century. The challenge we face as gerontologists is to think about new ways to help broaden the debate about preparing for an aging society in a comprehensive manner that takes into account the many diverse disciplines and interest groups that will increasingly shape aging-related issues. Those who have labored in the field of aging when it was a relatively cloistered profession should delight in the new-found respect and recognition of their work by the larger society. On the other hand, this main-streaming of aging will create new challenges and opportunities, as we look ahead to the new aging.

■ REFERENCES

Binstock, R. H. (1983). The aged as a scapegoat. *The Gerontologist 23*, 2, 136–143.

Hudson, R. B., & Strate, J. (1985). Aging and political systems. In R. H. Binstock & E. Shanas (Eds.), *Handbook of aging and social sciences* (2nd ed.) (pp. 544–588). New York: Van Nostrand Reinhold.

Neugarten, B. L. (1979). Policy for the 1980's: Age or need entitlement? In J. P. Hubbard (Ed.), *Aging: Agenda for the eighties* (pp. 48–52). Washington, DC: The Government Research Corporation.

Torres-Gil, F. M. (1992). *The new aging: Politics and change in America.* New York: Auburn House.

Torres-Gil, F. M. (1993). Can baby-boomers afford to retire? Statement before the U.S. House of Representatives Committee on Ways and Means, Subcommittee on Social Security, September 21, 1993.

Chapter 2

A Framework for Understanding Financial Responsibilities Among Generations

NEAL E. CUTTER   STEVEN J. DEVLIN

Famiiy networks have changed during the 20th century, moving from large, interdependent, intergenerational extended families who lived and worked together on family farms to much smaller, discrete, nuclear families living great distances from grandparents and other extended family members. However, increased longevity forces us to reexamine the financial interdependence between generations and our ever-evolving family structures. There are increasing numbers of "middle-agers" who are simultaneously caring for their own children and their aging parents. This continuing demographic trend is shifting middle-agers' financial burden from their adolescent children to their aging parents. As greater responsibility for aging parents falls on growing families, will they be ready to cope?

The impact of increased longevity beyond age 65 on individual aging and population aging is a well-documented demographic trend. Over the next twenty-five years the number of people over age 65 will increase by 54 percent, and the number of people over age 80 will increase by 45 percent. Yet "older aging," like all demographic trends, is not a simple or unidimensional phenomenon, and the consequences of this trend must be studied within the context of both society and families.

The societal impact of older-aging has been the focus of extensive research from a variety of disciplinary perspectives. For example, some economists argue that population aging will increase the strain on our already overworked healthcare system and place the future of both Medicare and Social Security in doubt. However, less well studied is the economic impact of older-aging within the context of the family. What happens to the financial status of a family as the grandparent generation becomes elderly and their "children" become middle-aged? How does the older-aging of the grandparents affect the intergenerational financial relationships among

From *Generations* 24–28, 1996, Spring. Reprinted with permission.

grandparents, their middle-aged children, and their grandchildren? This article provides a framework for understanding the financial impact of the aging of grandparents within a family context, with particular attention to the intergenerational transfers that can affect the financial status of a multigenerational family.

▬ THE MULTIGENERATIONAL FAMILY AND THE HUMAN 'WEALTH SPAN'

The financial implications of older-aging within a multigenerational context must address the interrelationships among three distinct age groups as they represent interacting stages of the life cycle, or as it is known in the vocabulary of financial gerontology, stages of the human "wealth span" (Gregg, 1992; Cutler, 1995). The human wealth span model — developed by Davis Gregg, founding director of the Boettner Center — divided the life span into two basic stages of financial behavior: the accumulation stage and the expenditure stage. For most people, the financial accumulation stage begins with employment and ends, roughly speaking, with retirement. The expenditure stage begins at retirement and continues until the end of one's life. Of course, real life is much more complex than this heuristic model would suggest, and the accumulation and expenditure of wealth is dynamically influenced by employment patterns, pension participation, health status, financial literacy and behavior, and family structure.

Between grandparents, who are typically in the expenditure stage, and grandchildren, who are beginning their accumulation stage, are middle-agers. They are simultaneously children and parents and — because of both their developmental age in the wealth span and their middle position in family structure — are thus straddling the transition from the accumulation to the expenditure stages of the wealth span.

Since gerontology is the study of the process of aging over the life course, and not just the study of "old people," understanding the dynamics of middle-aging and middle-agers is a central part of gerontology. Indeed, the "onset" of middle-age is a time in the life cycle, in one's wealth span, when a variety of emotional, biological, social, and financial changes begin to emerge and are likely to form the basis of new sets of expectations and concerns and therefore of plans and financial decisions within the family unit (Cutler, 1991; George, 1993; Karp, 1988; Schaie and Willis, 1991). In terms of historical dynamics, today's middle-agers are a generation whose wealth span is much different from that of their parents. Today's middle-agers are extending their education, entering work later in life, and planning to retire earlier, and they will live longer than their parents. As a result, the time they have to accumulate assets before retirement is getting shorter, and the expenditure/retirement stage will be longer.

These social and cultural reasons for focusing on middle-aging are magnified by the gerontological demographics of middle-aging. January 1, 1996, marked an important real as well as symbolic milestone in American social history, as the first baby boomers celebrate their fiftieth birthday. These "very young-old" Americans represent the oldest segment or "leading edge" of the baby boom, and these "babies" are now stampeding into middle age. Thus, in addition to the developmental and gerontological reasons for understanding middle age, from a practice and policy perspective the sheer number of middle-generation men and women (middle-aging boomers) focuses our attention on the growing importance of intergenerational financial relationships within the family.

■ THE EFFECT OF INCREASED LONGEVITY ON FAMILY STRUCTURES

To better illustrate the growing importance of the relationships among these three generations, consider the impact of increasing old-age longevity on family structure. Improved longevity is typically discussed in terms of either the individual or the population as a whole. That is, lengthening life expectancy is usually identified as having an impact on such things as chronic illness or faltering pensions and savings accounts (individual aging), or on national financial security and healthcare-financing policies and programs (population aging). Much less often considered is the impact of increased longevity on the multigenerational structure of the family.

The impact of increasing life expectancy on family structure was estimated by Uhlenberg (1980), who asked, What is the probability that a family structure with certain characteristics would be found in 1900 as compared to 1976, given what we know about trends in old-age longevity then as compared to now? Among the family structures and characteristics examined were two questions of central importance to our present concerns: (1) What is the probability that a teenager will have three or four living grandparents? and (2) What is the probability that a middle-aged couple will have at least two living parents? The results of Uhlenberg's analysis suggest that increased longevity has dramatically altered the intergenerational structure of families (Table 2-1). In 1900, when old-age life expectancy was significantly lower, less than 20 percent of families could expect to have three living generations. However, by 1976, 55 percent of teenagers had three or four living grandparents, and 47 percent of middle-

TABLE 2-1   The Intergenerational Effects of Greater Longevity

	Year	
	1900	1976
The probability that		
a 15-year-old would have three or four living grandparents	17%	55%
a middle-aged couple would have at least two of their parents still alive	10%	47%

Source: Boettner Center of Financial Gerontology

aged couples had at least two parents still alive. Increased longevity within the older generations has caused these odds to increase even more since this study was completed.

■TRENDS IN MULTIGENERATIONAL RESPONSIBILITIES

The most direct consequence of these demographic dynamics is that there is increased financial stress on the family and growing pressure on middle-agers to care for both their own children and their aging parents. In order to better understand these dynamics, we constructed an Older Parent Support Ratio and a Teenage Support Ratio, both of which measure burdens on middle-agers and focus on the *relationships* that create the responsibilities felt by middle-agers (Fig. 2-1). The goal is to identify the historical trends in these burdens of support and to see how they are changing as a means of better understanding intergenerational financial relationships.

We examined the relationships among three age groups: younger middle-agers (age 40–49), their demographic "parents" (age 60–74), and their demographic "teenage children" (age 10–19). The Older Parent Support Ratio measures the aggregate impact of increasing old-age life expectancy on the family as a social and financial organization. Most analyses of the impact of demographic trends on financial issues use the traditional ratio of older (age 65-plus) "dependent" persons to younger, working-age (20–64) people. Not only is this so-called dependency ratio flawed as a measure of financial dependency (Crown, 1985; Gibson, 1989), but it is not the appropriate variable to use in the evaluation of multigenerational families.

The Older Parent Support Ratio — the ratio of the size of the middle-age group to the size of their older parent group — focuses on one facet of the intergenerational caregiving relationships. It directs attention to the potential caregiving relationship between middle-agers and their older parents. To directly examine the demographic basis of changing intergenerational burdens on middle-agers, we computed a second measure, the Teenage Support Ratio, reflecting the population ratio of middle-aged parents to their children. We use this pair of support ratios to assess the proposition that the responsibilities and burdens of middle-agers in America are shifting *toward* their aging parents and *away* from their maturing offspring.[1]

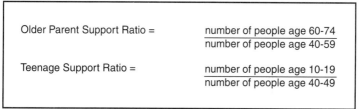

$$\text{Older Parent Support Ratio} = \frac{\text{number of people age 60-74}}{\text{number of people age 40-59}}$$

$$\text{Teenage Support Ratio} = \frac{\text{number of people age 10-19}}{\text{number of people age 40-49}}$$

FIGURE 2-1 Support ratios. (From Boettner Center of Financial Gerontology)

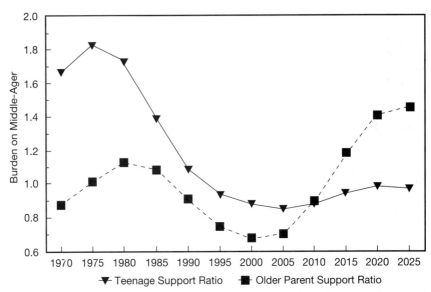

FIGURE 2-2   The changing burden on middle-agers. (From Boettner Center of Financial Gerontology)

The middle-agers are the focus because this age group faces increasingly intense multigenerational burdens of support and responsibility. In both ratios the middle-agers are in the denominator,[2] with the ratios identifying the number of older parents or the number of teenagers per one middle-aged person. The higher the number, the greater the burden. For example, if a community had 200 older parents and 200 middle-agers, the older parent ratio would be 1.0, but if there were 200 older parents and only 100 middle-agers, then the aggregate burden on those middle-agers doubles, and the ratio rises to 2.0.

Analysis of the trends within the United States for the Older Parent Support Ratio and the Teen-Age Support Ratio indicate that the aggregate burden placed on middle-agers will shift from responsibilities for their children to responsibilities to their aging parents during the next quarter century. From 1970 until 1995, the number of teenagers decreased 11.5 percent, from 40.2 million to 35.6 million, and the number of older parents increased 35.5 percent, from 21.2 million to 28.7 million. During this same period the number of middle-agers increased 56.9 percent, from 24.1 million to 37.9 million. The impact of these demographic changes on the burden placed on middle-agers is evident in the changes in the support ratios as evidenced in Fig. 2-2.

That is, during the past quarter century, teenaged children have been the dominant burden felt by middle-agers, and the burden placed on middle-agers by their older parents has been relatively low. Consequently, between 1970 and 1995, the Teenage Support Ratio decreased 43.4 percent, from 1.66 to .94, while the Older Parent Support Ratio decreased, albeit minimally, from .88 to .76.

This historical pattern, however, is in contrast with that of the next quarter century — 1995 to 2020 — during which the Teenage Support Ratio stabilizes, indicating that middle-agers will not experience an increase in the aggregate burden placed on them by their own children. But the most important trend during the next twenty-five years will be the intergenerational burden placed on middle-agers by their older parents. The Older Parent Support Ratio will increase dramatically. Today there are .76 older parents requiring support from each middle-ager. Within twenty-five years there will be 1.42 older parents potentially requiring support by each middle-ager, an increase of 86.8 percent.

In sum, the changing nature of these intergenerational burdens will have direct impact on the financial relationships among the three generations because it represents a fundamental shift in the social and financial demands placed on families. During the past quarter century, the primary financial focus of families has been on the children of middle-agers. The demographic conditions that define the burdens placed on a family are changing, and a new gerontological demography is emerging in which the financial focus of the family is changing away from teenage grandchildren and toward elders and grandparents. However, what is unknown is the extent to which families are prepared for the financial transitions that will be crucial to mature families during the next quarter century.

Unfortunately, there is some evidence to suggest that a gap already exists within many families, and especially among middle-agers, between expectations about the future and the realities of how changing generational burdens will influence a family's financial status. Where such a gap exists — between expectations and reality — there also exists an opportunity for gerontological professionals to work with multigenerational families. Recent research by the Boettner Center has begun to identify those domains in which families lack crucial information about their changing financial focus. We refer to this crucial knowledge about finances as *financial literacy*. Our concluding comments discuss three examples in which the changing financial focus of families suggests the potential of a gap between expectations and realities and therefore increases the need for financial literacy among multigenerational families of the future.

▬GRANDPARENTS AND FAMILY CARE: FINANCIAL OVERCONFIDENCE AND THE NEED FOR FINANCIAL LITERACY

Over the past several years, several studies of the financial preparedness of younger Americans for their old age have focused on the knowledge and behavior of the now-middle-aging baby boomers. Most studies have documented that the general level of financial preparations within this middle generation is fairly meager — relatively low levels of savings for retirement and even less systematic financial planning.

One recent study in particular provides important clues about the role that family and intergenerational issues play in this picture — and where the solution to the problem may be found. The fourth annual Fiscal Fitness Survey, carried out by the Yankelovich survey organization and sponsored by the Phoenix Home Life Insurance company (Fiondella, 1994), polled a national sample of middle-class boomers (households with at least $40,000 annual income). The survey found that even though most respondents were not saving much for their retirement, they expressed high levels of confidence about their financial future and their retirement preparation. It is apparent that this confidence is more appropriately labeled as "over-confidence."

In searching for the sources of this overconfidence, the survey documented what might be called problems of intergenerational misunderstanding. In particular, the responses to three of the survey's questions provide substantial evidence of the need for increased information and higher levels of financial literacy: (1) Are you currently providing any financial support to your (or your spouse's) parents and do you expect to provide financial support in the future? (2) How likely is it that you (or your spouse) or your children will inherit any money, real estate, or other valuables from your parents, parents-in-law, grandparents, or someone else? (3) Do you expect your employer to provide you with health insurance after you retire?

The responses to these questions offer an emerging profile of a misinformed generation with substantial misconceptions about how their own aging and the aging of their parents will create new burdens on their family financial resources. Consider the response data and the realities:

- Only 9 percent said they were currently providing any support to their parents, and only 13 percent said they anticipate doing so in the future. No doubt the parents of these boomers are, in the aggregate, still relatively healthy. Trends in longevity, however, clearly suggest that their parents are likely to live into their eighties and nineties, and probably much more likely to do so than their middle-age children and grandchildren currently expect. Furthermore, as studies of aging and activities of daily living document (e.g., Cutler, 1993), living longer does not necessarily mean living healthier, and as is well-documented, family members are the most prevalent sources of care for dependent elders.
- Sixty-six percent of these respondents anticipate receiving an inheritance, and 51 percent anticipate inheriting at least $100,000, a perception perhaps fueled by macroeconomic studies that suggest that the baby boom in the aggregate may inherit billions and billions of dollars (e.g., Avery and Rendall, 1993). Apart from the econometric difficulties of such estimates, any distribution of such bequests will, of course, be highly selective and uneven, and most boomers will not receive a substantial inheritance. More to the point, for many families the increased longevity of grandparents — with or without the health problems, medical costs, and modifications of living arrangements that often accompany

advanced age — is likely to require the spending of resources that might otherwise constitute modest bequests to children and grandchildren.

▪ Fifty-five percent expect to receive employer-provided retiree health insurance. If your employer pays for any health insurance you need over and above what Medicare may provide in the future, this would constitute a major savings to your retirement budget, enabling substantial funds to pay for other things. *However,* while this may have been a realistic scenario in the past, the situation has dramatically changed in the last couple of years. Corporate accounting rules recently enacted by the Financial Accounting Standards Board now require companies to include the cost of future health benefits as a current business liability. As a consequence, many companies are cutting back on this employee benefit, and some are eliminating it altogether. The news may not have fully reached middle-aged boomers yet, and when it does it should serve as a substantial reality check on the financial confidence they now have in their future retirement.

No one study can completely and unerringly describe the true state of national knowledge about financial, and especially future financial, complexities. But this 1994 poll identifies important warnings about the overconfidence of this large middle generation now moving into middle age. The solutions are to be found in public policy, in gerontological demography, and in the future state of the economy. But the appropriate responses must also be found in increased attention to financial literacy. A major piece of the answer to the basic question "Who's responsible for my family's financial future?" (Cutler, 1994) is that the family and the individual are increasingly responsible. While governments, employers, and unions will continue to play their parts, the fundamental challenge is to gerontologists, educators, and service providers to provide more, more complete, and earlier financial literacy for grandparents and grandchildren alike.

▰NOTES

1. This U.S. analysis is part of more comprehensive cross-national comparative research. For a fuller description on the basic concepts and the international analyses, see Devlin and Cutler (1995) (copies are available from the authors).

2. There is substantial research in the United States indicating that middle-aged caregiving to older parents is parimarily a female burden (e.g., Brody, 1981; Brody and Schoonover, 1986; Lewis and Meredith, 1988). Indeed, the Boettner Center's earlier research focusing on projected estimates of care-providing in the United States uses middle-aged women (rather than men and women) as the denominator of the support ratios (Cutler, 1993). In the present analysis, however, we use the total number of men and women in the middle-age group in each year because the focus here is not on the "hands-on" provision of elder care by family members, but on the financial responsibilities of and burden on the family unit.

■ **REFERENCES**

Avery, R. B., and Rendall, M. S. 1993. "Inheritance and Wealth." Paper presented at the Philanthropy Roundtable.

Brody, E. M. 1981. "Women in the Middle and Family Help to Older People." *Gerontologist* 21:471–80.

Brody, E. M., and Schoonover, C. B. 1986. "Patterns of Parent Care When Adult Daughters Work and When They Do Not." *Gerontologist* 26:372–81.

Crown, W. H. 1985. "Some Thoughts on Reformulating the Dependency Ratio." *Gerontologist* 25:166–71.

Cutler, N. E. 1991. "Financial Services and the Middle-Aging of America." *Journal of the American Society of CLU & ChFC* 65(1):16–19.

Cutler, N. E. 1993. "Population Aging and Dependency: Caregiving in the 21st Century." In S. B. Goldsmith, ed., *Long-Term Care Administration Handbook*. Gaithersburg, Md.: Aspen.

Cutler, N. E. 1994. "Who's Responsible for My Pension Now? The Need for More Financial Literacy at Younger Ages." *Journal of the American Society of CLU & ChFC* 68(1):31–36.

Cutler, N. E. 1995. "Davis Gregg's Model of the Human Wealth Span: Defining the Theory and Practice of Financial Gerontology Over a Lifetime and Across Historical Time." In L. A. Vitt and J. K. Siegenthaler, eds., *Encyclopedia of Financial Gerontology*. Westport, Conn.: Greenwood.

Devlin, S. J., and Cutler, N. E. 1995. "Assessing the Real Implications of Aging on Insurance and Financial Services: Cross-National Trends (and Projections) in the Demographic Burden on Middle-Agers." Paper presented at the Annual Meeting of the International Insurance Society, Washington, D.C.

Fiondella, R. W. 1994. "Many Americans Need a Fiscal Wake-Up Call" *Best's Review/(Life/Health edition)* 9(6):82–84.

George, L. K. 1993. *Financial Security in Later Life: The Subjective Side*. [The 1993 Boettner Lecture]. Philadelphia: Boettner Center of Financial Gerontology, University of Pennsylvania.

Gibson, D. E. 1989. "Advancing the Dependency Ratio Concept and Avoiding the Malthusian Trap." *Research on Aging* 11:147–57.

Gregg, D. W. 1992. "Human Wealth Span: The Financial Dimensions of Successful Aging." In N. E. Cutler, D. W. Gregg, and M. P. Lawton, eds., *Aging, Money, and Life Satisfaction: Aspects of Financial Gerontology*. New York: Springer.

Karp, D. A. 1988. "A Decade of Reminders: Changing Age Consciousness Between Fifty and Sixty Years Old." *Gerontologist* 28:727–38.

Lewis, J., and Meredith, B. 1988. "Daughters caring for Mothers: The Experience of Caring and its Implications for Professional Helpers." *Aging and Society* 8:1–20.

Schaie, K. W., and Willis, S. L. 1991. *Adult Development and Aging*, 3d ed. New York: Harper Collins.

Uhlenberg, P. 1980. "Death and the Family." *Journal of Family History* 5:313–20.

Chapter 3

Rethinking Medicare

JUDITH R. LAVE

> Few people disagree that Medicare has met its initial goal of
> providing greater access to quality health care for the nation's elderly.
> However, the problems of current costs, artificial structural barriers,
> as well as the projected shifts in retiree-to-worker ratio are critical
> concerns. Many proposals for Medicare reform have been proposed,
> almost since its inception. Which one is best? Judith Lave proposes
> that deliberations for Medicare reform should be linked with an
> evolving health care system, and suggests ideas to move it toward a
> choice-based system and restructure its financing, thus better ensuring
> its ultimate survival.

In 1995, the Congress passed the Medicare Preservation Act, which proposed major changes to the Medicare program. One justification for this act, which was vetoed by the president, was a call for action by the Board of Trustees of the Federal Health Insurance Trust Fund, which oversees Medicare, urging Congress to begin a careful evaluation of the program because the trust fund faced significant financial problems in both the short and the long term (Board of Trustees, 1995). Such urging is not rare. For instance, in 1991 I chaired a health technical panel for the 1991 Advisory Council on Social Security that reached the following conclusion: "the current state of the Medicare program is precarious, and the status quo cannot be maintained. . . . policy makers will have to make a number of difficult choices about how to bring the HI Trust Fund into balance and how to control the increasing costs of the SMI program" (Advisory Council on Social Security, 1991).[1]

In fact, ever since the implementation of Medicare, the research and policy community has not been reluctant to recommend changes in the program. The professional journals have been filled with recommendations — both large and small. For instance, among the many suggested changes in benefits are the following: (1) to expand Medicare by adding long-term-care benefits and prescription drugs, (2) to restructure the cost-sharing provisions under fee-for-service and include a limit on out-of-pocket payments, or even (3) to change Medicare from a defined benefit to a

From *Generations* 19–23, 1996, Summer. Reprinted with permission.

defined contribution (voucher) program. In other words, people have been "rethinking" Medicare since its inception.

The purpose of this paper is to consider what types of changes the Medicare program should undergo in the near term. First is a brief discussion of some of Medicare's successes; second, some of the major problems; and last, issues related to the restructuring and financing of the Medicare program.

■ MEDICARE'S SUCCESSES

Medicare has been a successful program in many respects. It dramatically increased access to high-quality medical care for America's older people. It has facilitated the development and spread of modern medical techniques and technology in such areas as cardiac surgery, ophthalmology, and prosthesis and joint replacement that have contributed to the quality and length of life. Furthermore, under Medicare, most older people are treated equally; that is, providers receive the same payments for providing a specific service to the rich or the poor. As a group, Medicare beneficiaries are more satisfied with their health plan than are other large identified groups (employed people, Medicaid recipients, unemployed people) (Davis, 1995). Finally, the program has relatively low administrative costs compared to private sector insurance programs.

■ MEDICARE'S PROBLEMS

A number of problems are also associated with Medicare and have resulted in calls for change. The principal factor precipitating congressional proposals to change Medicare is cost. At the present time, Hospital Insurance (HI) disbursements exceed revenues (primarily payroll taxes) and, unless changes are made, the Hospital Insurance Trust Fund will be bankrupt by 2002. Furthermore, the increase in the costs of the Supplementary Insurance program (SMI), which is funded through general revenues and beneficiary premiums, is not sustainable. In 1995, the Medicare program consumed 13 percent of the federal budget; by 2000, according to projections, it will consume 16 percent. The long-term financial issues are even more pressing. As the baby boom generation begins to retire in 2010, the number of workers relative to retirees will decrease significantly.

The main factor driving the increase in Medicare cost has been technological change (Newhouse, 1992), which will no doubt continue to be a major force (Aaron, 1995). Still, several features of the Medicare program itself have contributed to inefficiencies in the provision of healthcare services and to the increase in Medicare outlays.

First, the structure of the program, with its distinction between HI (primarily inpatient) and SMI (primarily outpatient) services is a relic — a holdover from the healthcare system of the 1960s. The Medicare program is designed to cover short-term acute care services or acute exacerbations of chronic conditions, thus many preventive services and long-term-care services are not covered. (Even so, in recent years a major factor contributing to cost increases has been the rapid expansion in long-term-care services — specifically home health services and nursing home care [Prospective Payment Assessment Commission, 1995].) What is more, the cost-sharing provisions, which could be seen as a major tool for reshaping healthcare utilization patterns into a more efficient and cost-effective form, are ineffective. The SMI deductible is too low, the skilled nursing facility co-insurance is too high, the "episode of illness" concept is obsolete, and there is no limit on beneficiary liability. The majority of Medicare beneficiaries have Medigap policies, so, while the cost-sharing provisions have an impact on the allocation of the costs of Medicare-covered services between the government and the beneficiaries, these provisions are unlikely to have any significant impact on the utilization of healthcare services.

Rather than controlling costs by changing utilization patterns, Medicare uses price controls as its prime cost-containment instrument. And, because the American healthcare system itself is fluid, with little government control over growth in the number and variety of service providers or settings in which services are provided, there is continuous pressure to expand the types of providers, settings, and services covered under Medicare. While the Medicare program has been innovative, its administrators at the Health Care Financing Administration have not been handed the tools to manage the fee-for-service program efficiently. To contain costs, Medicare has implemented a fee schedule for physicians, a prospective payment system for hospitals, and payment limits for nursing home and home health services. While these payment systems are improvements over the ones they replaced, they are incomplete control mechanisms, since they do not control volume of use. Increases in use, particularly in home health and skilled nursing home services as noted above, have been a major factor contributing to the growth in Medicare costs. In addition, since Medicare prices have sometimes been set below the cost of care, the result has been some shifting of costs from the Medicare program to the private sector (Prospective Payment Assessment Commission, 1995).

As an alternative to the traditional fee-for-service system, the Congress has implemented the Medicare risk program, which pays for beneficiaries who enroll in health maintenance organizations. The number of beneficiaries enrolling in HMOs has been increasing rapidly. By 1995, 2.9 million, or 8 percent of beneficiaries, were enrolled in some kind of risk program. However, the structure of the Medicare risk program has many problems (Prospective Payment Assessment Commission, 1995; Physician Payment Review Commission, 1996). The method that Medicare uses to pay HMOs to deeply flawed. Most (e.g., Physician Payment Review Commission, 1996; Brown et al., 1993), although not all (Rogers and Smith, 1996), believe that there is biased selection into HMOs; that is, that the HMO beneficiaries are healthier than the Medicare population in general. In this case, payment rates to HMOs are seen as too high and the risk program is seen as more costly to Medicare than the fee-for-service system. Medicare beneficiaries receive relatively little information about the HMOs they could join from the Health Care Financing Administration or other public organizations. Furthermore, the program is designed so that most savings result in new health benefits for HMO enrollees rather than in savings to Medicare.

The current structure of the Medicare program is inconsistent with the restructuring of the healthcare system that is taking place for younger people. As the economist Henry Aaron (1995) described it in testimony before the Senate Budget Committee: "Most working Americans and the health care providers who serve them are experiencing revolutionary changes in the organization of health care financing arrangements and the delivery of health care services. Managed Care in its countless manifestations is forcing individuals into health arrangements in which the third parties oversee, supervise and manage the traditional direct relationships between providers and patients." These new systems are designed to encourage providers to act efficiently and to provide incentives for the insured to select low-cost plans (ideally, those in which providers are acting efficiently).

▰SOME MODEST PROPOSALS

Two years ago, this country was in the middle of a debate over healthcare reform. There was considerable discussion about how to extend access to health insurance to all Americans. Now, there seems to be little public interest in extending access. Furthermore, current commitments to disadvantaged members of the society are being threatened. Consequently, it is difficult to propose a "rethinking" of Medicare that would involve a major expansion of publicly financed services to that population given that they enjoy a relatively favored position in the healthcare arena.

In the long term, there will need to be a fundamental reevaluation of the nature of the contract between the federal government and its older citizens. The aims here are much more modest. I discuss four proposals for change: merging the Hospital Insurance and Supplementary Medical Insurance programs, improving the Medicare risk program, "modernizing" traditional fee-for-service Medicare, and changing the distribution of financing between beneficiaries and the government.

Merging HI and SMI

When the Medicare program was first implemented, the hospital played the critical role in the healthcare system. All major and most minor procedures were done in hospitals, and a hospital stay was often a self-contained episode. Since 1965, the role of the hospital has changed as more and more care is provided in outpatient settings. With the development of managed care, in which one entity is responsible for providing all needed services in exchange for a single, fixed amount, the separation of medical care services into two separate funding sources makes little sense. Therefore, the Congress should consider merging these two programs. The funding sources for the merged programs should be a defined combination of payroll tax, income tax, and beneficiary premiums.

Improving the Medicare Risk Program
Medicare beneficiaries should have access to quality healthcare services. They should have choices among a number of health plans. They should have incentives to select efficient plans, and plans should have incentives to manage care efficiently. There is a need to bring Medicare beneficiaries into the types of managed care systems that are evolving in the private sector. This will not be easy to do; indeed, it is not obvious that it can be done without putting many Medicare beneficiaries at risk.

Researchers and policy analysts have offered a number of plans for moving Medicare into a "managed choice" model (Dowd et al., 1992; Butler and Moffitt, 1995; Aaron and Reischauer, 1995; Medicare Work Group, 1995). The proposed plans differ in a number of ways: 1. In the range of choices that beneficiaries should be allowed to make (e.g., HMOs, HMOs plus point of service, other fee-for-service plans, and catastrophic insurance plus Medical Savings Accounts). 2. In the proposed methods for paying health plans (e.g., administered prices, negotiated prices, or competitive prices). 3. In whether Medicare should be a competitive option; that is, whether, depending on the prices of the other plans, Medicare beneficiaries should pay more or less to enroll in traditional Medicare.

The choices that one makes across this range of possibilities depends upon the answers to questions such as the following: How important is risk selection? Can Medicare adjust for health status in setting payment rates? How relevant is the experience of the private employed sector to the Medicare population? And how will the most vulnerable beneficiaries fare?

The Medicare population is different from the employed population in significant ways. It is older, sicker, poorer, and more demented. Current Medicare beneficiaries have much less experience in making the kinds of decisions that are being made by the employed population. Furthermore, risk selection is an important factor. It would be easy for a health plan to target its advertising to attract relatively healthy beneficiaries, and the consequences of having disproportionately healthy people join risk plans are serious. If Medicare cannot adjust its rates appropriately, the overall cost of the program will rise. This event, in turn, will put pressure on the Congress to reduce the prices paid under the fee-for-service system, a practice that could lead to problems of access for those beneficiaries who remain in that system. In addition, the Medicare risk pool will be broken up. The Medigap premiums will rise, reflecting the poorer health of those beneficiaries remaining in traditional Medicare.

Therefore, it is necessary to develop the appropriate infrastructure for a choice-based system for Medicare. This development involves identifying an organization at the local level that would manage the choice-based system and be responsible for gathering information and hearing complaints. This organization could be a government or government-contracted private agency. There should be an annual open enrollment period in which all competing plans would offer one standardized health plan or one of a set of standardized plans. (This feature could be modeled on the current system used to market Medigap policies.) Medigap plans should be included in this open enrollment period. Catastrophic plans or Medical Savings

Accounts should not be included as an option because I believe that they would break up the Medicare risk pool in a detrimental way. A standard set of information should be made available. It would include price, outcome, and beneficiary satisfaction data. There should be an annual lock-in, but with an allowable disenrollment period the first time an individual enrolls in a specific plan. Lock-ins are desirable because they lead a decrease in risk-selection problems.

Medicare payments to HMOs should be based on a revised adjusted average per capita cost (the name given to the method the Health Care Financing Administration uses to set the capitation rates paid, based on the cost of traditional Medicare in the same county). This system would base the prices paid to the local plans on a blended cost of local, regional, and national fee-for-service costs. The costs associated with the payments that Medicare pays to disproportionate-share hospitals (which serve a high volume of indigent patients) and teaching hospitals for the direct and indirect costs of graduate medical education should not be included in these prices. The best available risk adjustors should be used in making payments to the health plans. As is currently the case, the Health Care Financing Administration (HCFA) should continue to sponsor research and demonstrations to evaluate payment methods, risk adjustment methods, and methods for moving toward a more competitive system.

These suggestions are not unique. They are close to those proposed by Congress's Prospective Payment Review Commission in 1995 and Aaron and Reischauer (1995) among others. They differ from the recommendations of more conservative analysts, since they would limit the types of plans that Medicare would sponsor. They also suggest a more gradual approach to encouraging Medicare beneficiaries to enroll in risk plans.

It should be pointed out that a substantial number of researchers have received funds to work on these issues, and various panels of experts have been assembled to examine the findings and push the research forward. In addition to the projects funded by HCFA, three activities are worth noting. In early 1996, the Institute of Medicine sponsored a conference to address informational needs of a Medicare choice-based system. The Kaiser Family Foundation has awarded a grant to monitor advertising and other marketing tools used by Medicare risk plans, and the National Academy of Social Insurance has established a panel on Medicare capitation and choice under its Restructuring Medicare for the Long Term project.

Modernizing Traditional Medicare

Under most projections, the traditional Medicare program will continue to be the predominant program for Medicare services for some time to come. Therefore, it is important to strengthen the fee-for-service system and to let it evolve into a managed indemnity system (Ethridge, 1995). Medicare needs to be given the necessary tools to accomplish this task — in spite of the public's current distrust of government. There needs to be a careful evaluation of the administrative procedures system to see how it can be changed to enable HCFA to operate more like a private business. There needs to be a careful evaluation of those areas where HCFA can move into selective contracting. In addition, HCFA needs to continue to work on improving its price-setting methods.

I believe it would be useful to reevaluate the cost-sharing structure of Medicare in order to make it consistent with current practice. Furthermore, I would recommend that consideration be given to letting HCFA offer a catastrophic benefit package — which, if designed correctly, could lead to a decrease in the demand for supplemental insurance to cover front-end cost sharing. It surely is more efficient for Medicare to market a linked catastrophic plan than for the private market to do so.

Once again, it is worthwhile noting that recommendations to improve traditional Medicare are legion (e.g., Moon, 1993; Moon and Davis, 1995). In addition, groups of experts are being assembled to assess methods for modernizing Medicare. For example, under its long-term project on Medicare, the National Academy has established a panel to explore ways to strengthen traditional Medicare.

Changing the Financing of Medicare

Under current law, the HI trust fund is financed primarily by the payroll tax and secondarily from interest on the government securities held by the fund. The SMI trust fund is financed by general revenues and from beneficiary-paid premiums. When the Medicare program was first established, beneficiary premiums covered 50 percent of SMI funding; they now cover about 25 percent. The share of SMI costs covered by premiums was a contentious issue during the recent debate over Medicare: the Congress wanted to keep the share at just over 30 percent, while the president wanted to revert to the permanent limit of 25 percent. However, the share of the Medicare premium to be paid by Medicare beneficiaries, particularly those with incomes considerably above the poverty level, needs to be reevaluated.

▬OTHER ISSUES

Unlike private health plans, Medicare has several obligations and responsibilities that go beyond providing healthcare services for an enrolled population. For example, the Medicare program is a major source of funding for graduate medical education in the country. It has become an important source of funds for rural hospitals and hospitals that serve a disproportionate number of low-income people. These responsibilities increase the cost of Medicare. If Medicare is to be compared with private health plans, these responsibilities have to be taken into consideration. If Medicare is to be competitive with private health plans, alternative approaches to providing these services will have to be examined.

In conclusion, the Medicare program must change, and the structure of the Medicare program has to be consistent with the healthcare system that is evolving for the majority of Americans. Furthermore, it will be necessary to reevaluate the relative roles of the federal government, the states, and beneficiaries in financing care for the elderly. None of this will be easy. However, the current system is not tenable for the long term, and a restructured system will need to be in place when the baby boomers start to retire.

▬ NOTE

1. The Medicare program is divided into two parts: The Hospital Insurance program (HI) and the Supplementary Medicare Insurance program (SMI), sometimes known as Part A and Part B, respectively.

▬ REFERENCES

Aaron, H. J. 1995. Testimony Before the U.S. Senate Budget Committee. Washington, D.C.

Aaron, H. J., and Reischauer, R. D. 1995. "The Medicare Reform Debate: What is the Next Step?" *Health Affairs* 14(4):253–64.

Advisory Council on Social Security, Health Technical Panel. 1991. *Report on Medicare Projections.* Washington, D.C.

Board of Trustees of the Federal Health Insurance Trust Fund. 1995. *1995 Annual Report.* Washington, D.C.

Brown, R. S., et al. 1993. *Does Managed Care Work for Medicare? An Evaluation of the Medicare Risk Program for HMOs.* Princeton, N.J.: Mathematic Policy Research.

Butler, S. M., and Moffitt, R. E. 1995. "The FEHBP as a Model for a New Medicare Program." *Health Affairs* 14(4):276–80.

David, K. 1995. "Medicare Turns 30." Testimony Before the U.S. Senate Finance Committee. Washington, D.C.

Dowd, B., et al. 1992. "Issues Regarding Health Plan Payments Under Medicare and Recommendations for Reform." *Milbank Quarterly* 70(3):423–53.

Ethridge, L. 1995. *Reengineering Medicare: From Bill-Paying Insurance to Accountable Purchases.* Brief prepared for Health Insurance Reform Project, George Washington University, Washington, D.C.

Medicare Work Group. 1995. *Comments and Recommendations on Medicare Reform.* Washington, D.C.: American Academy of Actuaries.

Moon, M. 1993. *Medicare Now and in the Future.* Washington, D.C.: Urban Institute Press.

Moon, M., and Davis, K. 1995. "Preserving and Strengthening Medicare." *Health Affairs* 14(4):202–13.

Newhouse, J. P. 1992. "Medical Care Costs: How Much Welfare Loss?" *Journal of Economic Perspectives* 6(3):127–32.

Physician Payment Review Commission. 1996. *Annual Report to Congress.* Washington, D.C.

Prospective Payment Assessment Commission. 1995. *Medicare and the American Health Care System.* Report to the Congress. Washington, D.C.

Prospective Payment Assessment Commission and Physician Payment Review Commission. 1995. *Joint Report to the Congress on Managed Care for Medicaid.* Washington, D.C.

Rodgers, J., and Smith, K. E. 1996. *Is There Biased Selection in Medicare HMOs?* Washington, D.C.: Price Waterhouse.

Chapter 4

Another Look at Medicaid

BARBARA LYONS   DIANE ROWLAND   KRISTINA HANSON

Medicaid is used by the elderly as a supplement to their Medicare coverage, mostly in circumstances related to long-term care. Elders receiving Medicaid use a disproportionately larger percentage of the total expenditures of this program than other age groups. To work effectively with their aging clients, especially those with lower incomes, nurses must be knowledgeable about the eligibility requirements for Medicaid. This chapter discusses Medicaid eligibility, as well as the current dilemma facing federal and state governments who are trying to balance budgets at a time when demand for Medicaid funds is increasing. The authors review possible policy changes regarding Medicaid, and evaluate their potential effects on this vulnerable population.

Medicaid is the healthcare financing program that complements Medicare coverage for the elderly population, providing assistance to more than one in ten Americans age 65 or older (Chulis et al., 1993). Nearly four million low-income elderly people receive Medicaid assistance with medical and long-term care expenses, accounting for over one-quarter of total Medicaid spending (Kaiser Commission, 1995). Medicaid plays three essential roles for elderly people. First, Medicaid makes Medicare affordable for low-income beneficiaries by paying Medicare's premiums, deductibles, and other cost-sharing requirements. Second, Medicaid provides coverage of medical benefits that Medicare does not cover, such as prescription drugs. Third, Medicaid stands alone as virtually the only public source of financial assistance for long-term care in both institutional and community settings.

Today, Medicaid is a means-tested entitlement program that is jointly financed by the federal and state governments and run by the states within federal guidelines. The debate over federal and state responsibilities for Medicaid and restructuring the financing and operation of the program could have substantial implications for elderly Americans, especially those with low incomes and longterm-care needs. This article provides an overview of Medicaid's current role for elderly people, describes Medicaid expenditures on the elderly population, and highlights policy issues affecting the

From *Generations* 24–30, 1996, Summer. Reprinted with permission.

elderly population and the future of Medicaid coverage as the debate over restructuring the financing and operation of the Medicaid program continues.

▬ MEDICAID COVERAGE OF ELDERS

Initially designed to provide health benefits for welfare recipients, Medicaid now plays a role for vulnerable population groups that has steadily expanded over the past three decades as policy makers have increasingly turned to Medicaid to fill gaps in Medicare and private-sector coverage. Providing coverage for over 36 million Americans at a cost of $156 billion in 1995, Medicaid now serves as this nation's primary health insurance program for low-income families and finances acute and long-term care for low-income elderly and disabled people (Congressional Budget Office, 1996).

In 1993, Medicaid covered 32 million people, including 3.7 million elderly people, 4.9 million blind and disabled people, 16.1 million low-income children, and 7.4 million low-income adults (Liska et al., 1995). Because the health needs of the various populations served by Medicaid are quite different, there is substantial variation in use of services and Medicaid spending across groups. The elderly account for 12 percent of Medicaid's beneficiaries and 28 percent of total expenditures (Fig. 4-1) (Liska et al., 1995). In contrast, low-income families account for the majority (73 percent) of beneficiaries, but for only about one-quarter (27 percent) of overall spending. The disabled constitute the remaining 15 percent of Medicaid beneficiaries and the largest share (31 percent) of Medicaid spending. Disproportionate-share hospital (DSH) payments, contributions directed to hospitals that serve a high volume of indigent patients, account for 14 percent of Medicaid spending.

The higher level of Medicaid spending per beneficiary that is associated with the elderly ($9,293) — about eight times greater than spending for children ($1,191) and five times greater than spending for low-income adults ($2,067) — is primarily related to their more intensive use of services, particularly nursing home care (Fig. 4-2) (Liska et al., 1995). About three-quarters of Medicaid spending on the elderly goes toward long-term-care services. Because virtually all elderly people have Medicare for coverage of medical services, Medicaid's acute care spending for the elderly acts as a supplement by covering services that Medicare does not cover and by helping with Medicare's premiums and cost-sharing. Most important for the elderly population with physical and cognitive disabilities, Medicaid offers assistance with the high cost of long-term care in institutions and in the community.

Low-income elderly people can receive assistance from Medicaid through several alternative pathways. The benefits covered for elderly beneficiaries vary depending on how they qualify for assistance. Medicaid is a means-tested program, however, and, unlike insurance, provides assistance only for individuals with low incomes or for those whose financial resources are

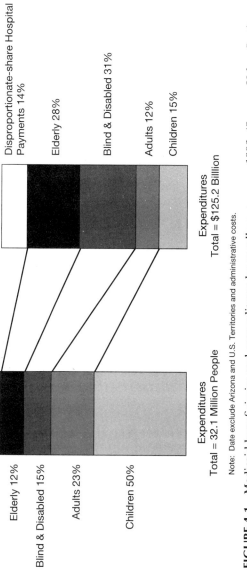

FIGURE 4-1 Medicaid beneficiaries and expenditures by enrollment group, 1993. (Source: Urban Institute analysis of Health Care Financing Administration data, 1994.)

29

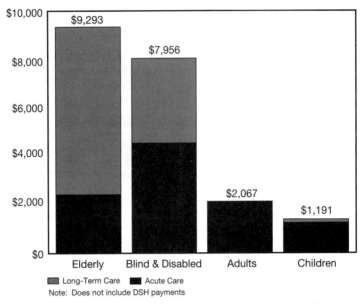

FIGURE 4-2   Medicaid spending per beneficiary, 1993. (Source: Urban Institute analysis of Health Care Financing Administration data, 1995.)

exhausted. Elderly people may qualify for Medicaid if they meet the following requirements:

1. *Qualify for Supplemental Security Income cash benefits.* Elderly people who are poor enough to qualify for cash assistance under the federal Supplemental Security Income (SSI) program are generally eligible for Medicaid as "categorically eligible" beneficiaries. These beneficiaries must have incomes at or below the SSI benefit level (in 1995, $5,640 for an individual, $8,460 for a couple), and assets are generally limited to $2,000 for an individual and $3,000 for a couple.

    In 1993, 2.1 million elderly people received Medicaid coverage of acute care and long-term-care services because of their "categorical" eligibility for SSI, although about one-third of these did not actually receive SSI payments (U.S. Department of Health and Human Services, 1994). Medicaid beneficiaries who qualify for cash assistance are provided the broadest coverage under Medicaid, including payment of Medicare premiums, cost-sharing, and payment for additional services such as prescription drugs, vision care, and dental care covered under state Medicaid programs.

2. *Have such high medical or long-term-care expenses that they "spend down" to Medicaid eligibility requirements.* Individuals defined as "medically needy" have incomes above welfare cash assistance levels but incur expenses for healthcare services that exceed a defined level of income and assets. In the 36 states that offer medically needy programs,

elderly people who require nursing home assistance are able to qualify for Medicaid because the high cost of nursing home care depletes their financial resources. In 1993, about 800,000 elderly beneficiaries received Medicaid assistance through the medically needy provisions (U.S. Department of Health and Human Services, 1994). Institutionalized elderly people with incomes up to 300 percent of the SSI level can qualify for nursing home coverage in states without a medically needy program.

Before Medicaid will pay for services, an elderly person must deplete almost all personal assets and apply all monthly income, except for a small personal allowance, toward the cost of nursing home care. The spouse of a nursing home resident is permitted to keep higher levels of income and assets. Spousal protections do not provide Medicaid coverage for the spouse at home, but they do allow the spouse of a nursing home resident to retain sufficient resources on which to live.

3. *Are low-income Medicare beneficiaries.* A third group of Medicaid beneficiaries is eligible through the Qualified Medicare Beneficiary (QMB) program. Enacted as part of the Medicare Catastrophic Coverage Act of 1988, the QMB program requires states to pay for Medicare premium and cost-sharing requirements for elderly and disabled Medicare beneficiaries with incomes below the poverty level. They are not required to provide the full range of Medicaid benefits. Asset restrictions are set at twice the SSI levels for these beneficiaries. Medicare beneficiaries with incomes between 100 and 120 percent of poverty are eligible for payment of Medicare premiums only. About two million Medicare beneficiaries are estimated to receive assistance through the QMB program (O'Sullivan, 1995). However, many others who meet income requirements appear to be unaware of these provisions or do not apply (Neumann et al., 1995).

Medicaid spending on behalf of elderly beneficiaries largely reflects gaps in Medicare's coverage of various services, particularly long-term care. Of the $34 billion Medicaid spent in 1993 for low-income elderly beneficiaries, acute care services and Medicare payments accounted for one quarter of spending, while long-term care accounted for three-quarters of spending (Fig. 4-3) (Liska, 1995).

▬MEDICAID SPENDING TO SUPPLEMENT MEDICARE ACUTE CARE

In 1993, Medicaid spent $8.7 billion on acute care to supplement Medicare's coverage for low-income elderly people. Of this amount, Medicaid paid $2.7 billion to the Medicare program on behalf of low-income Medicare beneficiaries for premiums and $6 billion to augment Medicare's coverage of hospital and physician care and to cover other services, such as prescription drugs, not covered by Medicare (Fig. 4-4) (Liska, 1995).

Prescription drugs account for a major part of the Medicaid money spent on acute care for the elderly. Medicare's Part B premium (which

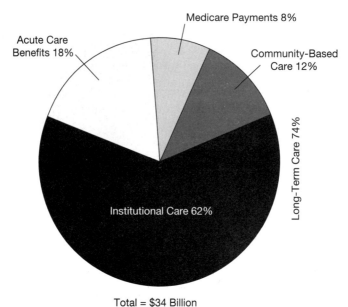

Acute Care
Benefits 18%

Medicare Payments 8%

Community-Based
Care 12%

Long-Term Care 74%

Institutional Care 62%

Total = $34 Billion

FIGURE 4-3   Medicaid expenditures for the elderly, 1993. (Source: Urban Institute analysis of Health Care Financing Administration data, 1994.)

recipients must pay) for 1996 is $510 per year, and required cost-sharing and deductibles add substantially to the overall cost of care for those with health expenses (Federal Hospital Insurance Trust Fund, 1995). Medicare's cost-sharing requirements include a hospital deductible of $736 per stay, a deductible of $100 per year for Part B services, and 20 percent cost-sharing for physician and other medical services. Medicaid pays these copayments for low-income Medicare recipients and provides coverage of additional services.

Because low-income elderly people are likely to have fewer retiree health benefits and less access to and ability to pay for private "Medigap" coverage compared to higher-income elderly, they are more vulnerable to Medicare's gaps in coverage (Rowland et al., 1992). Research has shown that the financial obligations of Medicare can in fact create significant burdens on low-income elderly people. Such findings were used to support expansions of federal eligibility enabling elderly people to receive Medicaid assistance for Medicare premiums and cost-sharing (Rowland, 1990).

In addition, low-income elderly people are more likely than their higher-income counterparts to have poorer health status and to suffer from chronic conditions such as diabetes and hypertension that often require ongoing medical treatment, including prescription drugs and regular monitoring (Rowland, 1990). Medicaid's coverage of Medicare's cost-sharing requirements and additional medical services helps ensure that low-income elderly people have access to the healthcare they need.

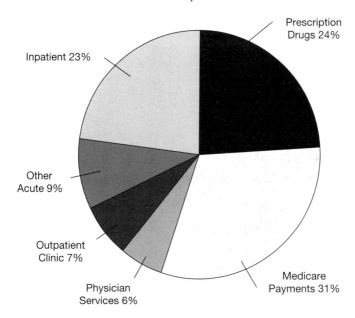

Note: Does not include DSH payments.

FIGURE 4-4 Medicaid acute care spending for the elderly to supplement Medicare, 1993. (Source: Urban Institute analysis of Health Care Financing Administration data, 1995.)

▬MEDICAID SPENDING FOR LONG-TERM CARE

As noted, Medicaid is virtually the only source of public financing of long-term-care services for the elderly. In 1993, Medicaid spent $25.5 billion for long-term-care services for elderly beneficiaries. This amount represents 58 percent of the $44 billion Medicaid spent on long-term-care services for all population groups. The majority of spending was for care delivered in nursing facilities (84 percent). Community-based care, including mental health services and home health and personal care services accounted for 14 percent of spending (Fig. 4-5).

Medicaid provided nursing home payments on behalf of 1.6 million elderly people in 1993 (U.S. Department of Health and Human Services, 1994). Often in nursing homes because of severe physical and cognitive limitations, nursing home residents tend to be over age 80, female, and without a spouse in the community. Most have few choices available to them, and the need for continuous care and monitoring makes remaining in the community unaffordable and impractical.

Medicaid has also played an important role in covering community-based services for the elderly population with disabilities. Medicaid pays for skilled home healthcare in all states; 28 states and the District of Colum-

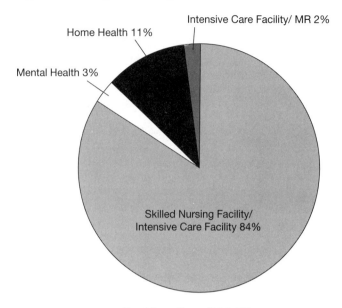

Total Spending = $25.5 Billion

Note: Does not include DSH payments

FIGURE 4-5 Long-term care medicaid expenditures for the elderly, by type of service, 1993. (Source: Urban Institute analysis of Health Care Financing Administration data, 1995.)

bia have elected to cover the optional benefit of personal care in the home. Through home- and community-based waivers, states have been able to design programs to provide services, such as personal care, homemaker services, and adult daycare to specific populations. Many states have implemented innovative programs to deliver coordinated community services to foster independence and provide an alternative to nursing home care, but most programs are small in scope and serve only a small number of frail elderly people. In 1993, Medicaid spent $2.8 billion for home- and community-based services for 300,000 people under long-term-care demonstration programs (Winterbottom, Liska, and Obermaier, 1995). Medicaid long-term-care spending, however, remains heavily skewed toward institutional care. Only six states — New Hampshire, New York, Oregon, Vermont, West Virginia, and Wyoming — spend 25 percent or more of Medicaid long-term-care dollars on community-based services (Liska et al., 1995).

■ THE MAJOR ISSUE
The major issue facing Medicaid is how to continue to provide coverage for acute and long-term care for low-income and vulnerable populations in the face of intense pressure to limit public spending. Because Medicaid

provides coverage to those with severe health problems and costly medical needs — including people who cannot obtain private insurance coverage — it has become a major budgetary commitment for both the federal and state governments. Federal Medicaid expenditures of $90 billion account for 6 percent of the federal budget, while state expenditures for their share of Medicaid spending account for 13 percent of state spending (Kaiser Commission, 1995).

As part of the Balanced Budget Act of 1995, Congress sent the president legislation that would have replaced the Medicaid program and its entitlement for low-income people with a block grant to the states. This would have provided broad discretion over program structure in return for a cap on federal spending that would have reduced federal Medicaid expenditures by $163 billion over the next seven years. President Clinton vetoed that legislation in December 1995 and offered an alternative plan for Medicaid reform as part of his balanced budget plan. The president's plan would retain the Medicaid entitlement, place limits on federal spending, and provide more flexibility for the states. This plan would reduce projected federal Medicaid spending by $55 billion over the next seven years.

Whatever the outcome of the ongoing struggle between the president and the Congress, and between the states and the federal government, over an approach for Medicaid reform and restructuring, it is clear that the Medicaid program is under intense fiscal and programmatic pressure at both the federal and state level. With or without restructuring legislation, states are looking to trim costs and have greater control over how the program operates. Shifting the delivery of medical care from fee-for-service to managed care for a monthly capitation fee, changing provider payment methods and levels, gaining more control over long-term-care spending, and reviewing priorities for coverage and services are on virtually all states' Medicaid agendas.

Because the elderly low-income population depends on Medicaid to supplement Medicare and provide long-term care, these uses of Medicaid are costly components of Medicaid spending in most states. In 33 states, spending on the elderly accounts for 25 percent or more of overall Medicaid spending. Thus, the elderly will undoubtedly feel the effects of the efforts to revamp Medicaid occurring in the states. Some of the policy changes that could affect Medicaid's coverage for elderly people are reviewed below.

POSSIBLE CHANGES IN MEDICAID'S ROLE IN ACUTE CARE

Because Medicaid's coverage of Medicare premium payments and other acute-care services for the elderly accounts for a relatively small proportion of total Medicaid spending, there is limited potential for substantial program savings through reform of this aspect of Medicaid. Still, policy changes are being considered, and there are several areas in which they could alter the way Medicaid works today to supplement Medicare for provision of acute care.

Enrollment in Managed Care

Although managed care has been viewed as holding the potential for cost savings, the potential for states to realize large savings from enrolling their elderly population in managed care is limited because Medicare pays for most acute care. To date, most state-managed care programs are focused primarily on women and children in low-income families, a population group that is relatively healthy and for whom care is relatively low-cost. Although a few states, including Arizona, Tennessee, Oregon, and Minnesota, are enrolling their elderly Medicaid beneficiaries into managed care on a statewide basis, most states have limited experience with managed care for this population (Saucier, 1995). Managed care plans have limited experience providing care to these populations, and setting appropriate capitation rates is difficult because little is known about risk adjustment for older people with high rates of chronic illness and disability.

Cost-Shifting to Medicare

The separate financing streams for acute and long-term care create stumbling blocks for efforts to improve care coordination and delivery for elderly people (Saucier and Riley, 1994). Increased budget pressure is likely to exacerbate cost-shifting between the Medicare and Medicaid programs. Financial incentives to churn frail elderly patients back and forth between hospitals, where Medicare is the primary source of financing, and nursing homes, where Medicaid is the dominant payer, could be intensified and adversely affect the delivery of appropriate levels of care.

Coverage of Medical Benefits Not Covered by Medicare

Medicaid plays an important role for low-income elderly people by providing coverage of services that Medicare does not cover. Many of these are optional services that states can provide and for which they then receive federal matching payments. Prescription drugs, case management, dental services, and vision care fall under this category. Under fiscal pressure, a state could cut back on prescription drug coverage, for example. Eliminating coverage of prescription drugs or placing stringent limits on the number of prescriptions covered could have serious health consequences for elderly people with health conditions that require drug treatment. This in turn could lead to greater costs overall if hospital or institutional care is required.

Coverage of Medicare's Premium and Cost-Sharing Requirements

Medicaid makes Medicare work for the low-income elderly by paying Medicare premiums and cost-sharing requirements, but this coverage imposes financial obligations on state Medicaid programs. States maintain they have no control over the level of these obligations and that it should be the federal government's role to assume these responsibilities. If the federal requirement to provide this coverage were eliminated, states would be unlikely to make Medicare premium and cost-sharing assistance a first priority for state spending. Poor and near-poor elderly would not be protected from financial obligations incurred through use of Medicare. Alternatively, states may seek to provide coverage of Medicare's cost-sharing at the Medicaid payment rate or prescription drugs only if a beneficiary enrolls in managed care. These alternatives could limit access to care for low-income Medicare beneficiaries.

▬POSSIBLE CHANGES IN MEDICAID LONG-TERM-CARE COVERAGE AND SPENDING

Because long-term care constitutes such a large part of Medicaid spending, long-term care will undoubtedly be an area where states will look hard for savings. Significant reductions in the growth of Medicaid spending could alter the scope of long-term-care benefits offered, as well as eligibility for assistance, payment levels, and the quality of care. Given the prominent role of Medicaid in long-term care, financing half of all long-term-care services in the United States, these changes could have far-reaching effects for people with disabilities and their families.

Eligibility and Coverage for Long-Term-Care Services

Tightening eligibility requirements for nursing home care is often viewed as an alternative to limit Medicaid spending. Under the current Medicaid program, states could tighten eligibility requirements for nursing home care by reducing financial eligibility levels, increasing disability requirements, or eliminating the optional medically needy program. These policy changes would shift more of the cost of long-term-care services to elderly people and their families. Today, private payments, primarily out-of-pocket spending, account for a major share of long-term-care financing. Medicare was not designed to be a long-term-care program and provides only minimal long-term-care services, generally limited to skilled, rehabilitation-oriented care. In the absence of adequate private financing alternatives, setting appropriate limits on Medicaid's ability to help individuals and families with long-term care will continue to be a source of tension in program policy and spending.

Confronted with tight fiscal constraints, states may face difficulty continuing coverage of home- and community-based services, even though these sites are often the most apporpriate sites of care, are preferred by the elderly and their families, and in some cases are a cost-effective alternative to nursing home care. This is an area where today states need waivers from the federal government to expand services; if greater flexibility to design community-based alternatives were provided to states, states could better target these services while controlling spending.

Payment and Standards for Long-Term-Care Services

State payments to nursing homes are now required to be reasonably related to the cost of care, under the so-called Boren Amendment to the federal Medicaid statute. In recent years, providers have used the Boren Amendment provisions to sue state Medicaid agencies, arguing that Medicaid payment rates are inadequate to meet the cost of operating nursing facilities and to accommodate the changes being implemented as part of nursing home reform. Repealing the Boren Amendment provisions would give states greater leeway to reduce payments to nursing homes. However, this could result in payments that do not provide adequate resources to cover quality care in some states.

Moreover, the nursing home reforms effective in 1990 established requirements for providing care to Medicare and Medicaid beneficiaries related to scope of services, staffing levels and qualifications, residents' rights, and the physical environment. Under current law, nursing facilities must comply with these requirements in order to receive reimbursement from Medicare and Medicaid, and research has shown improvements in the quality of nursing home care since passage of these reforms (Hawes, 1995). Although elimination of nursing home quality standards is unlikely, the current guarantees to care could be modified, and primary responsibility for enforcement of standards could be shifted from the federal government to the states. Moreover, reductions in nursing home payments to very low levels could compromise maintenance of these standards in some states.

■ SUMMARY

Medicaid's coverage helps low-income elderly people gain access to health-care services, eases financial burdens for medical expenses, and provides a safety net for long-term-care coverage. Cuts in Medicaid spending, program restructuring, and changes to Medicare could affect coverage and benefits for millions of elderly Americans. The full impact of proposals to restructure Medicaid is dependent on the level of cuts in federal funding, the degree of flexibility given to individual states, and ultimately, the decisions made by individual states.

Although it is difficult to predict how restructuring Medicaid and cutting the growth in spending would affect the vulnerable populations served by the program, the role and scope of the program for the elderly population could change substantially. Medicaid is not one uniform program, but rather plays different roles for the different population groups it serves. For the elderly population, we need to more fully understand where the Medicaid program works well and where deficiencies in financing and care delivery result in delayed and fragmented care. Moreover, we need to proceed slowly and carefully with reform because many of the people served by Medicaid are in poor health, have disabilities, and have few other sources of assistance.

Pressure to restrain spending growth and to find new ways of providing care under the Medicaid program is unlikely to diminish. The aging of the population is likely to place increased scrutiny over the role of public programs serving the elderly population. As the federal and state governments reexamine their roles and responsibilities in financing and delivering care for vulnerable populations and search for solutions to constrain spending, it is important to ensure that the health and well-being of low-income and vulnerable population groups who rely on Medicaid for assistance with acute and long-term care are not endangered.

■REFERENCES

Chulis, G., et al. 1993. "Health Insurance and the Elderly: Data from the Medicare Current Beneficiary Survey." *Health Care Financing Review* 14(3):163–81.

Congressional Budget Office. 1996. Congressional Budget Office Baseline Data for 1995–2006 (March). Washington, D.C.

Federal Hospital Insurance Trust Fund. 1995. *1995 Annual Report of the Board of Trustees of the Federal Hospital Insurance Trust Fund.* Washington, D.C.

Hawes, C. 1995. Memorandum to Mary Harahan, Sept. 26. Durham, N.C.: Research Triangle Park.

Kaiser Commission on the Future of Medicaid, 1995. *Medicaid and the Elderly.* A Policy Brief. Washington, D.C.

Kaiser Commission on the Future of Medicaid. 1995. *Medicaid and Federal, State, and Local Budgets.* A Policy Brief. Washington, D.C.

Liska, D., et al. 1995. *Medicaid Expenditures and Beneficiaries: National and State Profiles and Trends, 1984–1993.* Washington, D.C.: Kaiser Commission on the Future of Medicaid.

Neumann, P., et al. 1995. "Participation in the Qualified Medicare Beneficiary Program." *Health Care Financing Review* 17(2):169–78.

O'Sullivan, J. 1995. *The Qualified Medicare Beneficiary Program.* CRS Issue Brief. Washington, D.C.: Congressional Research Service.

Rowland, D., et al. 1992. *Medicaid at the Crossroads.* Baltimore, Md.: Kaiser Commission on the Future of Medicaid.

Saucier, P. 1995. *Public Managed Care for Older Persons and Persons with Disabilities: Major Issues and Selected Initiatives.* Waltham, Mass.: Center for Vulnerable Populations.

Saucier, P., and Riley, T. 1994. *Managing Care for Older Beneficiaries of Medicaid and Medicare: Prospects and Pitfalls.* Portland, Me.: National Academy of State Health Policy.

U.S. Department of Health and Human Services, Health Care Financing Administration. 1994. Medicaid Statistics: Program and Financial Statistics, Fiscal Year 1993 [incomplete].

Winterbottom, C., Liska, D., Obermaier, K. 1995. *State-Level Databook on Health Care Access and Financing.* Washington, D.C.: Urban Institute.

Chapter 5

The Promise and Performance of HMOs in Improving Outcomes in Older Adults

EDWARD H. WAGNER

Health maintenance organizations (HMOs) are rapidly proliferating across this country; however, benefits to elderly clients under managed systems of health care have been largely undocumented. Is managed care a good alternative for elderly clients? Dr. Wagner illustrates three basic approaches to case management used by HMOs, and delineates the current best practices of managed geriatric care. The use of expert teams (comprised of professionals with gerontological or geriatric training), effective patient education programs, as well as patient registries and computer data systems, are cited as critical components of this new model of care. Nurses can participate in these teams in many ways, and must use every opportunity to promote quality health care for older adults within these cost-constraining systems.

What is a managed care organization? Today it means little more than corporate or organizational involvement in the financing or delivery of health care. The term now encompasses a broad continuum of organizational forms that have at one end insurance companies that do little more than contract with doctors to provide care to a list of enrollees. These managed care companies generally try to influence the practices of those physicians through financial incentives and restrictions on paying for care. Physician involvement is minimal, and the commitment of the professionals to the managed care company is as deep and abiding as one's commitment to one's auto insurance company.

At the other end of the continuum are traditional group/staff model health maintenance organizations. These are very different organizations indeed. They are generally non-profit, integrated delivery systems with their own staff, their own facilities, and with long-term involvements in their local communities. Physicians are salaried, full-time employees of the orga-

From *Journal of the American Geriatrics Society* 44(10):1251–1257. Reprinted with permission.

TABLE 5-1 Characteristics of Traditional HMOs Supportive of Care Management

- Defined population
- Accountable primary care provider
- Comprehensive services
- Data systems

- Balance between generalists and specialists
- Shared clinical culture
- Preventive orientation
- Centralized resources

---

nization or of a medical group that does all or most of its business with the organization. The physicians and other health professionals are heavily involved in decision-making that affects their practices and patients. Although not all physicians love their HMO or feel that it listens to them, it is nonetheless their HMO.

Traditional HMOs have structural characteristics that could, if exploited, enhance the care of older people (Table 5-1). These begin with a clearly defined population, each member of which has an accountable primary care provider. This structure provides the essential foundation on which to plan and deliver care to every member of that population. This opportunity is enhanced by the presence in the same organization of the full complement of professionals and services needed to care for older enrollees with various needs. Integrated data systems facilitate planning and evaluating care. Because of the central role of primary care, professional power is more evenly balanced between primary and specialty care. This balance is critical, in my view, to offset the tendency of specialists to rely on expert opinion and underestimate the ability of generalists *and* the tendency of generalists to overestimate their ability to manage complex problems without assistance. Organized efforts to improve care are greatly enhanced by a shared organizational identity and clinical culture among providers, a preventive orientation, and centralized resources like patient education or home care.

Managed care organizations have used three very different approaches to influencing care (Table 5-2). Traditional HMOs achieved their cost savings decades ago by selecting conservative physicians, limiting the acquisition of specialists, new technologies and hospital beds, and fostering a

---

TABLE 5-2 Managing Care

- Macromanagement
  Managing capacity and culture
- Micromanagement
  Regulating individual patient care
- Population-based management
  Collaborative effort to maximize outcomes and reduce costs for a defined population by assuring delivery of effective services and elimination of ineffective ones

---

conservative culture — that is, by managing supply or macromanagement.[2] Managing care meant managing resources, not involvement in the details of patient care. Hire well trained, conservative physicians, put them in a nice building, and leave them alone. A variety of studies from the 1960s and 1970s confirmed that this approach provided care that was 20 to 25% less expensive than fee-for-service care, because of substantially reduced hospital use, but of quality comparable to fee-for-service care.[3-5] However, by the late 1980s and early 1990s this cost advantage had largely dissipated because of the impacts of DRGs and of competition on hospital use in the non-HMO sector.[5]

What about the elderly? Managed care experience with older adults is relatively new. As recently as 1980 there were only a handful of HMOs contracting with HCFA to provide Medicare services. This number grew rapidly through the 1980s, but growth slowed as many MCOs with Medicare risk contracts saw profit margins shrink and ultimately turn from black to red. The HCFA Medicare Demonstration[6] and the Medical Outcomes Study[7] showed that again the quality of care in HMOs was similar to that of fee-for-service care, allaying the concern that HMOs would be hazardous to the health of older people. But some began to question why HMO care was not *better* given the structural advantages mentioned above.

Friedman and Kane surveyed the medical directors of 64 (75% of all) HMOs with Medicare risk contracts in 1991.[8] They found that most did not have a formally trained geriatrician or generalist with a Certificate of Added Qualifications in Geriatrics on staff, and the large majority were not systematically assessing functional status or other important social or health characteristics. Systematic approaches to major geriatric syndromes such as polypharmacy or inactivity and deconditioning were rare. Without special expertise or plans, it is not surprising that the structural advantages of HMOs were not being exploited.

But, the failure to control costs and the increasing scrutiny of their quality of care by purchasers and regulators has stimulated many HMOs in recent years to try to manage care delivery. Organizations have generally taken one of two approaches (Table 5-2). The first approach attempts to regulate or micromanage clinical decisions affecting specific patients. Such approaches have proliferated. The growth of micromanagement parallels the rapid growth of newer, looser managed care organizations consisting largely of capitated contractual arrangements with private practices to care for the small percentage of the practice's patients covered by that particular plan. Such insurance companies must rely on micromanagement and financial incentives rather than clinical culture to influence clinical behavior. Early evidence suggests that the impact of these techniques on physician stress levels far exceeds their impacts on costs.[5] This trend toward micromanagement has been resisted by many traditional HMOs because of its inflammatory effects on physicians.

Micromanagement generally assumes that problems in care emanate from excessive utilization. Older people are indeed very high utilizers of medical service, but that doesn't mean that their critical health care needs are being met. For example, Hirsch and Winograd[9] have documented that only a small minority of randomly selected practices in California provide such needed services for frail older people as functional assessment, interdisciplinary evaluation, or visits of sufficient length. These deficiencies, found equally within and without managed care, reflect barriers to good geriatric care in practice and the absence of planned, organized approaches to overcoming those barriers. These problems are highly unlikely to be affected by bed cops or 800 numbers.

To meet the needs of older patients, practices and systems must alter the basic orientation and reflexes of primary care, which are oriented and organized to respond to the acute and urgent needs of its patients.[10] The emphasis is on ameliorating today's symptoms and physiological abnormalities. Because primary care is so oriented to acute illness, it tends to respond similarly to patients with acute and chronic illness, irrespective of age. Kottke and colleagues[11] suggest that this reactivity encourages physicians to be respondents, not "initiators."

The dominance of symptoms and signs, and concerns over their import, in the thinking of physicians tends to have two adverse effects on the care of older patients:

1. It leaves little time or intellectual energy for addressing the preventive and psychosocial needs of older patients, and
2. It diminishes attention to the patient's role in the management of chronic illness and the prevention of disability.

Much of good geriatric care is devoted to the prevention of disability and dependence through attention to risk factors for decline. Epidemiological and clinical evidence accumulating over the past decade has begun to clarify those risk factors, such as inactivity, poor muscle strength, psychoactive medication use, sensory deprivation, and psychological distress, that are associated with declines in function. In fact, Tinetti et al. recently pointed out that the same set of four risk factors — chair stands, arm strength, vision and hearing, and anxiety — conveyed a significantly increased risk of falls, incontinence, and functional dependence.[12] Tested interventions are available for these factors if they are assessed and the practice has the capacity to implement them.

Medical care's inclination to swat at symptoms and signs accentuates the physician's primacy and diminishes the patient's role in her clinical course. The prevention of functional decline and other complications of aging and chronic illness requires the active participation of the patient. This view is not just politically correct; it is supported by good evidence that active patients have better outcomes. For example, Greenfield and colleagues[13,14] examined the impact on disease outcomes on an intervention that gives patients information, skills, and encouragement to discuss important questions and concerns with their physician. The intervention not only increased patient involvement in the interaction but improved disease outcomes like glycohemoglobin levels in diabetics as well.

This should come as no surprise since patients' ability to alter their behavior, manage their regimen, and grapple with the emotional impacts of their losses and declines is fundamental to successful therapy.[15] Older patients and those with chronic illness must:

- Engage in activities that build physiological reserve, e.g., exercise, nutrition, social activity, and sleep.
- Interact with health care providers and systems to develop a management plan, and adhere to that plan.
- Monitor physical and emotional status and make appropriate management decisions on the basis of symptoms and signs.
- Manage the impacts of illness, aging, and loss on ability to function in important roles, on emotions and self-esteem, and on relations with others.

This is very hard work, indeed. Most patients, especially older patients, defer to their doctors, and medical care must actively encourage patient participation in self-management to overcome this tendency to deference. The literature suggests that medical care take the following steps:

1. *Identify common threats to independence and quality of life* such as the risk factors mentioned above.
2. *Collaboratively define problems of significance to both patients and doctors,* including barriers to behavior change, emotional distress, interference with daily functioning, and difficulties carrying out treatments.
3. *Collaboratively target, set goals, and create an action plan* for management of illness and prevention of loss of function and quality of life based on scientific evidence.
4. *Continuously provide patient education and support for self-management* that supplies the information, mentoring, and support structures needed to execute the care plan.
5. *Sustain follow-up* that monitors, structures, and rewards self-management.

Developing consistent approaches to meeting these requirements for all older patients at risk of disability will be essential to improving geriatric outcomes in primary care. In a busy practice day with a mixture of acute and chronically ill patients, it is difficult for even the most motivated providers to assure these elements of care. Office staff and systems are also geared to react to acute illness, and practice teams have neither the time nor inclination to meet and organize themselves for geriatric care. Non-physician staff are occupied with managing access and patient flow so that responsibilities for assessments, care planning, counseling and follow-up, by default, fall to the already overburdened physician. The information necessary for organizing or planning care is buried in a paper medical record, which for geriatric patients may require a forklift. The lack of organization and information reinforces the focus on today's symptoms, which only encourages the addition of more drugs to the regimen.

Reorienting and redesigning primary care to better meet the needs of the older patient requires a different approach to planning and managing care. From the inception of the HMO movement, the potential for HMOs to use the resources available to a large, integrated health care organization, and the public health perspectives and methods to optimize care for its defined population, have been there. Patients with particular clinical needs could be identified, their care planned according to formal clinical policies, and they could be supported by organizational efforts to assure that their needs were met.[16–18] Perhaps because of the historic success of traditional HMOs, this potential was often not exploited. To remedy this and help make traditional HMOs more competitive, a new form of care management has evolved, which we call population-based management (Table 5-2). Its roots are in community medicine and the application of epidemiology to care.

This new form of care management uses the medical literature, modern provider and patient behavior change techniques, as well as organizational interventions, to maximize patient health status. The means are the implementation of programs that identify patients with specific health problems (frail older people, for example), define the outcomes to be improved, and assure that they receive services proven to be effective in improving those outcomes. To reduce costs and iatrogenicity, efforts are also made to eliminate ineffective services. However, even the most elegant population-based management plan will fail unless there are the resources and a practice environment capable of assuring the systematic delivery of effective services.

▅ A MODEL OF MANAGED GERIATRIC CARE

To design population-based strategies for older patients based on science rather than intuition, we reviewed the literature to identify those interventions that have been shown to deliver effective services and improve outcomes in chronically ill populations.[10] This review revealed many studies that evaluated specific interventions such as reminder systems or patient education programs, but few examples of comprehensive efforts to improve care were found. Based on this review, we have proposed a model for improving the care of the chronically ill (Fig. 5-1).

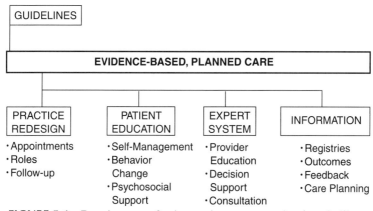

FIGURE 5-1 Requirements for improving outcomes in chronic illness.

The implementation of such a model forces systems to consider their basic clinical strategy. Who will provide routine care for older adults? Will it be generalists, specialists, case managers, etc? Our model assumes that the vast majority of care will be provided by generalists and that the broadest improvements in outcomes will result from enhancing primary care. These enhancements to primary care tend to fall into five areas: evidence-based guidelines, practice redesign, patient education and self-management support, expert systems, and clinical information.

Guidelines

Successful clinical programs operate from a protocol or plan that provides an explicit statement of what needs to be done for patients, at what intervals, and by whom. In contrast to acute care, population-based care is planned and requires that doctors make the intellectual leap from worrying about the specific patient to considering all patients with specific clinical needs and how those needs might be met. This leap is much easier if there are clinical policies and priorities at the organizational level to assist practices in their efforts to meet the needs of older patients.

In our work to improve care for frail older people in primary care, the most common question we receive is, "Where do I begin?" The geriatric literature is confusing on this point. Major geriatric interventions, like geriatric evaluation and management units (GEMS), exhibit remarkable variability in staffing and goals, much less clinical priorities.[19] In fact, very few of the now dozens of published GEM trials have explicated their clinical priorities or specific patient management strategies, which may help explain the wide variability in results.

To guide our work to improve geriatric primary care at Group Health, we have had to generate our own list of clinical priorities in the absence of comprehensive national guidelines. To no one's surprise, we have focused on risk factors for dependence, including functional deficits, inactivity, incontinence, falls, overmedication, and depression. These will be summarized and codified in evidence-based clinical policies or guidelines. Guidelines based on clinical epidemiological evidence of effectiveness (evidence-based) rather than on expert opinion have been an important advance.[20] Opinion-based guidelines tend to be written by specialists for generalists, and too often they give greater emphasis to making desirable referrals than to guiding management. Guidelines relying on randomized trial evidence tend to be much leaner because few diagnostic maneuvers or treatments have been shown to improve outcomes in rigorous studies and favor older treatments, which have been subjected to more testing.

Guidelines will end up in the trash bin unless the organization considers how guidelines will be implemented in practice.[21] Regular practice team meetings in which the team reviews the guideline and their own practices, and formulates its plan for implementing the guideline, may be an essential element.[18] The plan must include the definition of the roles and responsibilities of each team member. Regular team meetings have significantly predicted better care and outcomes in British studies of primary care for diabetes[22] and in VA hypertension clinics.[23] Clinical team meetings and clinical planning are not familiar activities in most practices; they will need time and help to develop.

Practice Redesign

Busy primary care teams cannot provide high quality, planned geriatric care unless they have the time and resources to assess their patients, develop and implement treatment plans, meet educational and psychosocial needs, and maintain adequate follow-up. To accomplish these things, health care providers must rethink and redesign the basic ways they deliver care — make appointments, allot clinic time, delegate tasks, allocate special resources, manage clinical data, etc. Wholesale changes in the way a practice organizes itself and allocates roles seem to be necessary. The need for such comprehensive change in geriatrics is exemplified by the GEMs, which reorganize care for frail elders to allot more time and a broader array of resources to their care. We are currently testing two different strategies for bringing the advantages of geriatric assessment units into primary care.

The "chronic care mini-clinic,"[24] a British primary care innovation, changes the orientation and design of primary care practice for chronically ill patients, but it does so *periodically, not permanently*. The key features of the innovation include:

1. The invitation of a group of patients with a given condition to participate in specially designed visits with the primary care practice team at regular intervals.
2. Each visit characterized by a planned set of assessments, individual visits with the doctor and nurse, and visits with other health professionals such as a pharmacist or social worker.
3. A group meeting.
4. Systematic follow-up.

Mini-clinics by general practitioners in Great Britain have been associated with better glycemic control,[25,26] reduced hospitalizations,[27] and improved process measures among diabetic patients.[28] We are currently conducting a randomized trial of mini-clinics for frail older people and Type II diabetics at Group Health. The clinics for frail older people address the clinical priorities mentioned above. Assessments include, but are not limited to, functional status, depression, falls, incontinence, behaviors such as exercise, and a medication review by the clinic pharmacist. The group sessions, led by a social worker, address problems in self-management identified by the group. John Scott at Kaiser-Permanente's Colorado region is testing a related practice redesign innovation in which older patients receive assessments, education, and support in groups of 20 or more led by a physician.

A second approach is to complement primary care with a coordinated set of more specialized services rendered outside the practice, but with close communication with the primary care physician. We have randomized 200 chronically ill patients age 70 and older, referred by their primary physician, who are not regular attenders of their local senior center to either a senior center-based program or usual care. The program at the senior center, managed by a geriatric nurse practitioner (GNP), focuses on the same clinical priorities as the mini-clinic but with additional attention paid to self-management, supervised exercise, and involvement in social activities. The efforts to involve patients in the exercise and social activities of the senior center include the use of volunteer mentors, motivated older adults who are regular users of the center. Chronic disease self-management skills taught by the GNP are reinforced by group sessions developed by Dr. Kate Lorig and colleagues at Stanford.[29]

Regular follow-up is an essential ingredient of effective programs. Telephone follow-up may have important advantages that are only beginning to be appreciated. Several studies have shown that practice-initiated phone calls improve health status and patient satisfaction and reduce costs for chronically ill patients.[30,31] We are trying to incorporate practice-initiated phone calling in all of our interventions.

Patient Education and Self-Management Support

Reducing complications and symptoms of most chronic diseases requires changes in lifestyle and the development of self-management competencies by the patient and family. Interventions that facilitate behavioral change and acquisition of self-management skills are conventionally subsumed under the rubric of patient education. Essentially all successful chronic illness programs provide some sort of psychoeducational programming to meet these needs. Modern self-management programs have improved important outcomes in chronic diseases. The key features appear to be the program's ability to identify and respond to the individual needs and priorities of patients consistently over time, not its method of delivery. Approaches that systematically assess the patient's behaviors, readiness to change, and self-efficacy; develop a personalized improvement plan and provide feedback on progress; teach specific skills; and address some of the psychosocial demands of these illnesses are more likely to be successful.[32,33] Such personalized strategies need not be incompatible with system-wide interventions.

The literature also suggests that personal physicians are important motivators whose involvement enhances the effectiveness of behavioral programs. But physicians are generally neither well trained nor confident behavioral counselors. The most effective self-management support programs will likely be delivered in primary care practice by non-physician staff, even trained lay persons, and/or computers and incorporated into day-to-day medical care. Such an approach to patient education for diabetes and hypertension is now a subsidized element of the German health care system.[34,35]

Most chronic disease patient education programs target the specific knowledge and behaviors associated with that disease and its treatment. Many older persons have multiple chronic diseases, which, if treated with separate patient education approaches, might have them in class all day. Kate Lorig and colleagues[36] have concluded that patients with chronic illnesses and disability face common challenges. They have modified their successful arthritis program to meet the needs of patients with a variety of chronic illnesses. This intervention differs from conventional patient education programs in its use of lay leaders rather than health professionals and its emphasis on patient empowerment and psychological status. If it proves to be as effective as the arthritis program, this low cost intervention will provide a general model for the design of managed care programs for chronic illness.

Clinical Expertise

It is unlikely that geriatricians or other specialists receive more training or devote more attention to practice organization, the use of guidelines, counseling, or the other aspects of care associated with better outcomes in chronic illness. Therefore, any debate about generalist versus geriatrician care is really about the importance to outcomes of specialized clinical knowledge or expertise. The positive results of several GEM trials suggest that geriatric expertise may be important to outcomes.

Certainly the most common approach for increasing expertise has been continuing education courses. The literature suggests strongly that conventional, didactic, lecture approaches generally have no enduring effects on practice style.[37] More personalized physician education through tutorials,[38] academic detailing,[39] and related interventions does seem to have some impact, although several of the more successful studies involved residents and faculty. Some training of providers, preferably using more personalized, hands-on methods, would seem to be an important initial step. However, these educational strategies cannot meet the ongoing needs for expertise in the management of specific patients. Conventional referral/consultation remains the dominant source of expert assistance in managed care as well as fee-for-service practice. Referrals, however, run the potential risk of further fragmenting care, may not increase the skills of the referring physician, and contribute to increased costs. Alternatives to referral have been tried, the most interesting of which include innovations in generalist/specialist interactions. For example, a diabetes program used a "hotline" to increase access of residents to diabetes expert advice.[40]

Most promising are collaborative care strategies whereby specialists and generalists manage patients together in the primary care setting. At the Group Health Cooperative of Puget Sound (GHC), a key feature of our diabetes improvement program is an expert team (diabetologist and nurse specialist) who spend most of their time in primary care practices seeing difficult patients with the primary care teams and conducting educational sessions.[16,41] These population-based specialists also work on guidelines and other interventions to improve diabetes care system-wide. Similar models of distributed geriatric expertise may prove to be far more cost-effective for older patients than the more conventional specialty referral models.

Information

Information about patients, their care, and their outcomes is an essential ingredient of all population-based strategies to improve chronic illness care. Without a list of all patients with a given condition — a registry — providers are forced to be responsive, waiting for patients to present for care. Successful strategies must be proactive, inviting or reminding patients to participate in care in accord with an explicit plan of care. The presence of a defined practice population, as in capitated care, greatly facilitates the creation of registries.

At GHC, Medicare recipients comprise 12% of our enrollees. This translates into 200 or more older patients in the average primary care panel. Some form of stratification of this large group is necessary for clinical planning. As one example of risk stratification, we have borrowed from the work of Boult and colleagues at the University of Minnesota.[42] They developed a set of criteria to predict repeated hospitalizations, their indicator of frailty. We adapted their criteria so that we could rely exclusively on data already available in GHC computer systems. The criteria are listed in Table 5-3. Chronic disease score is a weighted sum of medications taken for chronic illness.[43] These characteristics were tested in multiple regression models, and the best criteria were selected and tested again on an independent sample. These criteria were then used to create a frailty score (the probability of being hospitalized two or more times in the next 4 years) for each of GHC's more than 40,000 Medicare patients.

We evaluated the validity of the score by comparing the mortality and the average annual health care costs over the next 5 years among deciles ranked by frailty score. Figure 5-2 shows that mortality among GHC seniors increased eightfold to more than 40% and annual costs increased fourfold to more than $8000 per year across deciles. Our interventions for frail older adults target the top one or two deciles.

The availability of a list of all patients and a few other key data elements present opportunities to remind patients and physicians of needed follow-up or preventive interventions. At GHC, we successfully used paper and pencil diabetes registries for 3 years. We have now automated the registry. Automation allows practices to see important results, enter key data like foot care and behavior change activities, and plan care for individual patients as well as the practice as a whole more efficiently. An essential element of

---

TABLE 5-3   Variables Used to Predict Compute Frailty Score (Probability of 2+ Hospitalizations in 4 Years)*

- Age
- In Coronary Heart Disease Registry†
- In Diabetes Registry‡
- 6+ visits in last year
- Hospitalized in last year
- Male
- Chronic Disease Score

* Adapted from Boult et al.
† From inpatient diagnoses and/or receipt of a nitrate prescription.
‡ From inpatient diagnosis, receipt of hypoglycemic drugs, or presence of elevated glucose or HbA1C values.

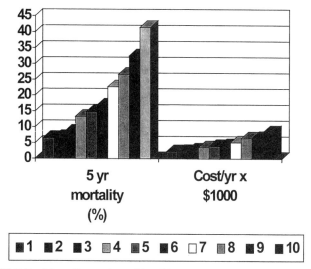

FIGURE 5-2 Mortality and total health care costs by frailty score decile.

effective geriatric care appears to be development of a shared treatment plan, providing structure and coherence as the patient negotiates the string of care episodes that characterize his/her care. The availability of computerized clinical information systems, even limited ones like our registry, greatly facilitate care planning.

▬INTEGRATED SYSTEMS OF CHRONIC ILLNESS CARE

Managed care is increasingly recognizing the importance of developing organized systems of care for chronic illness that reach the bulk of their patient populations. Large purchasers are demanding evidence of an effect on outcomes, and most organizations realize that this will not be achieved by their historical tendency to offer a smattering of programs (a class here or a care manager there) that reach only a small percentage of patients. Many large managed care systems have begun to construct integrated care management strategies for older, chronically ill patients. Our review of such strategies indicates that there is real uncertainty as to whether to build integrated systems, based in and supportive of primary care, or to develop specialized geriatrician/case manager systems for frail older people. I worry about the latter, as a recent study of geriatric case management in HMOs found that most were focused on utilization reduction not health improvement.[44]

I believe we are at a crossroads, uncertain about the basic care model for older patients. Specialized programs using medical specialists or case managers offer some obvious advantages — increased expertise and less complicated implementation. Integrated primary care models, on the other hand, can reach all older adults, not just a targeted subset, while maintaining patients' crucial relationships with their doctor as well as continuity of care.

▄ SUMMARY

In summary, the promise of HMOs in caring for older adults far exceeds their performance to date. Until recently they had neither the motivation nor the knowledge to revamp their delivery systems to better meet the needs of older, chronically ill patients. Market pressures and skyrocketing costs have provided the motivation. Physicians and researchers trained in epidemiology and health services research from programs such as that at UCLA are providing the knowledge. Based on the literature and experience described above, HMOs with the characteristics supportive of population-based care can put into place an approach to geriatric care likely to improve outcomes if they heed their patients and professionals rather than their accountants. These organizations will give hghest priority to preserving function and will be guided by explicit clinical guidelines. Care will be rendered by organized primary care teams supported by systematic self-management approaches, standardized interventions for key risk factors, clinically useful computer systems, and available geriatric expertise. It will require a small revolution as old approaches, roles, and relationships will not go quietly. We are in the early phases of this revolution, and it's not too late to join us on the barricades.

▄ REFERENCES

1. Fillit H. Geriatrics and health care reform: Opportunities in managed care for preserving excellence in the care of the elderly. Ann NY Acad Sci 1994;729:178–181.
2. Wagner EH. Managing medical practice: The potential in HMOs. In: Gelijns AC, ed. IOM Workshop Proceedings. The Changing Health Care Economy: Impact on Physicians, Patients, and Innovators. Washington DC: National Academy Press, 1992, pp 51–61.
3. Luft HS. Health Maintenance Organizations: Dimensions of Performance. New York: John Wiley and Sons, 1981.
4. Manning WG, Leibowitz A, Goldberg GA et al. A controlled trial of the effect of a prepaid group practice on use of services. N Engl J Med 1984;310:1505.
5. Miller RH, Luft HS. Managed Care: Past evidence and potential trends. Front Health Serv Manage 1993;9:3–37.
6. Retchin SM, Preston J. Effects of cost containment on the care of elderly diabetics. Arch Intern Med 1991;151:2244–2248.
7. Greenfield SM, Rogers W, Mangotich M et al. Outcomes of patients with hypertension and non-insulin-dependent diabetes mellitus treated by different systems and specialities. JAMA 1995;274:1436–1444.
8. Friedman B, Kane RL. HMO medical directors' perceptions of geriatric practice in medicare HMOs. J Am Geriatr Soc 1993;41:1144–1149.
9. Hirsch CH, Winogard CH. Clinic-based primary care of frail older patients in California. West J Med 1992;156:385–391.
10. Wagner EH, Austin B, Von Korff M. Improving outcomes in chronic illness. Manag Care Q 1996;4:12–25.
11. Kottke TE, Brekke ML, Solberg LI. Making "time" for preventive services. Mayo Clin Proc. 1993;68:785–791.
12. Tinnetti ME, Inouye SK, Gill TM, Doucette JT. Shared risk factors for falls, incontinence, and functional dependence. JAMA 1995;273:1348–1353.

13. Greenfield S, Kaplan SH, Ware JE et al. Patients' participation in medical care: Effects on blood sugar control and quality of life in diabetes. J Gen Intern Med 1988;3: 448–457.
14. Greenfield S, Kaplan SW, Ware JE. Expanding patient involvement in care. Effects on patient outcomes. Ann Intern Med 1985;102:520–528.
15. Clark NM, Becker MH, Janz NK et al. Self-management of chronic disease by older adults: A review and questions for research. J Aging Health 1991;3:3–27.
16. Wagner EH. Population-based management of diabetes care. Patient Educ Coun 1995;26:225–230.
17. Thompson RS, Taplin SH, McAfee TA et al. Primary and secondary prevention services in clinical practice. JAMA 1995;273:1130–1135.
18. Payne TH, Galvin MS, Taplin SH et al. Practicing population-based care in a HMO: Evaluation after 18 months. HMO Pract 1995;9:101–106.
19. Wieland D, Hedrick SC, Rubenstein LZ et al. Inpatient geriatric evaluation and management units: Organization and care patterns in the Department of Veterans Affairs. Gerontologist 1994;34:652–657.
20. Eddy DM. A manual for assessing health practices and designing practice policies. In: The Explicit Approach. Philadelphia, PA: American College of Physicians, 1992.
21. Gottlieb LK, Margolis CZ, Schoenbaum SC. Clinical practice guidelines at an HMO: Development and implementation in a quality improvement model. Qual Rev Bull 1990;16:80–86.
22. Farmer A, Coulter A. Organization of care for diabetic patients in general practice: Influence on hospital admission. Br J Gen Pract 1990;40:56–58.
23. Stason WB, Shepard DS, Perry, Jr HM et al. Effectiveness and costs of veterans affairs hypertension clinic. Med Care 1995;32:1197–1215.
24. Thorn PA, Watkins P. Organization of diabetic care. Br Med J 1982;285:787–789.
25. Bradshaw C, Eccles MP, Steen IN, Choi HY. Work-load and outcomes of diabetes care in general practice. Diabetic Med 1992;9:275–278.
26. Pringle M, Stewart-Evans C, Coupland C et al. Influences on control in diabetes mellitus: Patient, doctor, practice, or delivery of care? Br Med J 1993;306:630–634.
27. Farmer A, Coulter A. Organization of care for diabetic patients in general practice: Influence on hospital admission. Br J Gen Pract 1990;40:56–58.
28. Koperski M. Systematic care of diabetic patients in one general practice: How much does it cost? Br J Gen Pract 1992;42:370–372.
29. Lorig KL, Holman H. Arthritis self-management studies: A twelve-year review. Health Educ Q 1993;20:17–28.
30. Wasson J, Gaudette C, Whaley F et al. Telephone care as a substitute for routine clinic follow-up. JAMA 1992;267:1788–1793.
31. Weinberger M, Kirkman MS, Samsa GP et al. A nurse-coordinated intervention for primary care patients with non-insulin-dependent diabetes mellitus: Impact on glycemic control and health-related quality of life. J Gen Intern Med 1995;10:59–66.
32. Glasgow RE, Toobert DJ, Hampson SE, Noell JW. A brief office-based intervention to facilitate diabetes self-management. Health Educ Res 1996;10:467–478.
33. Strecher VJ, Kreuter M, Den-Boer DJ et al. The effects of computer-tailored smoking cessation messages in family practice settings. J Fam Pract 1994;39:290–291.
34. Muhlhauser I, Sawicki PT, Didjurgeit U et al. Evaluation of a structured treatment and teaching programme on hypertension in general practice. Clin Exp Hypertens 1993; 15:125–142.
35. Gruesser M, Bott U, Ellermann P et al. Evaluation of a structured treatment and teaching program for non-insulin-treated Type II diabetic outpatients in Germany after the nationwide introduction of reimbursement policy for physicians. Diabetes Care 1993;16:1268–1275.
36. Lorig KR, Mazonson PD, Holman HR. Evidence suggesting that health education for self-management in patients with chronic arthritis has sustained health benefits while reducing health care costs. Arthritis Rheum 1993;36:439–446.
37. Davis DA, Thomson MA, Oxman AD, Haynes B. Evidence for the effectiveness of CME: A review of 50 randomized controlled trials. JAMA 1992;268:1111–1117.
38. Inui TS, Yourtee EL, Williamson JW. Improved outcomes in hypertension after physician tutorials: A controlled trial. Ann Intern Med 1976;84:646–651.

39. Soumerai SB, Avorn J. Principles of educational outreach (academic detailing) to improve clinical decision making. JAMA 1990;263:549–555.
40. Vinicor F, Cohen SJ, Mazzuca SA et al. DIABEDS. A randomized trial of the effects of physician and/or patient education on diabetes patient outcomes. J Chronic Dis 1987;40:345–356.
41. McCullouch D, Glasgow RE, Hampson SE, Wagner E. A systematic approach to diabetes management in the post-DCCT era. Diabetes Care 1994;17:1–5.
42. Boult C, Dowd B, McCaffrey D et al. Screening elders for risk of hospital admission. J Am Geriatr Soc 1993;41:811–817.
43. Von Korff M, Wagner E, Saunders K. A chronic disease score from automated pharmacy data. J Clin Epidemiol 1992;45:197–203.
44. Pacala JT, Boult C, Hepburn KW et al. Case management of older adults in health maintenance organizations. J Am Geriatr Soc 1995;43:538–542.

Chapter 6

The Effects of Ageism on Individual and Health Care Providers' Responses to Healthy Aging

LYNDA D. GRANT

Stereotypes about the elderly can affect policy decisions for our aging clients and, ultimately, the programs that are created to serve them. However, ageism's circular causality is also reflected in how elders view themselves — are they "healthy and vital" or "debilitated and useless?" Consequently, their perceptions are implemented in their health behaviors — do they simply "manage" their illnesses or do they "work toward" a healthy lifestyle? Societal perceptions of the elderly, as well as their individual physical, cognitive, and emotional factors, all play a crucial role. Could programs that include input from elderly clients in their design and management be the key to overcoming entrenched ageist practices? This author posits that nurses and other health care professionals, must confront their own attitudes, values, and beliefs about aging in order to become more effective caregivers and client advocates.

Ageism has been described as "thinking or believing in a negative manner about the process of becoming old or about old people" (Doty, 1987, p. 213). Society's attitudes and beliefs about aging are culturally embedded and can have a profound effect on how people view themselves and others who are aging. Unfortunately, negative stereotypes about aging are still quite prevalent (Rowe & Kahn, 1987). Health care providers are not immune to these insidious stereotypes. This article reviews a number of ageism stereotypes in society generally and in the health care field. The aim is to demonstrate that ageism can negatively affect health care providers' professional training and service delivery and, ultimately, their clients' behavior and health outcomes.

For many years service providers used the World Health Organization (WHO, 1947) definition of health: "Health is a state of complete physical, mental, and social well-being, and not merely the absence of disease"

From *Health & Social Work* 21(1):9–15. Reprinted with permission.

(p. 16). This concept of health was a radical departure from the traditional model that saw health only as the absence of disease. WHO recognized that psychosocial well-being is an important component of health. However, health remained an abstract concept and, therefore, an ideal difficult to achieve. More recently, *Achieving Health for All* (Health and Welfare Canada, 1986) defined health in terms of "quality of life" and included in the definition the opportunity to make choices and to gain satisfaction from living despite functional limitations. This document suggested that health is a dynamic process of interaction between communities and individuals. Health involves freedom of choice: Communities (including health care providers) and individuals choose to take deliberate action to make the changes necessary for healthy aging.

Unfortunately, ageism can often affect the choices people are presented with and the decisions they make about those choices. If people believe that some of the "inevitable deterioration" of aging is preventable, they are likely to be more active in their own self-care. If health care providers believe that elderly people are valuable, equal members of society, then this belief should be reflected in professional training and service provision. Consequently, confronting ageism by enhancing positive beliefs about aging is a vital component of health promotion training and programming.

◼ EFFECT OF AGEISM ON FACTORS IN AGING
Sociological Factors

Traditionally, aging has been viewed as a continual process of decline. Unfortunately, this stereotyping results in systematic discrimination that devalues senior citizens and frequently denies them equality (Butler, 1987).

In his review of the attitudes toward aging shown by humor, Palmore (1986) found that elderly people were often portrayed negatively. The humor tended to focus on physical and mental losses, as well as on decreases in sexual attractiveness and drive. Jokes about older women tended to be more negative than those about older men.

In North American culture, employability is often viewed as a primary measure of one's ability to contribute meaningfully to society and as a source of self-identity and self-esteem (Moody, 1988). Botwinck (1984) reviewed the literature on the effects of ageism on employment. He found that although age was not an important factor in the evaluation of work competence, older age was given as one of the reasons for poor applicant quality if the person was not hired. When a younger applicant was not hired, lack of effort or inability was given as the reason.

Snyder and Barrett (1988) reviewed 272 federal court cases dealing with age discrimination and employment filed between 1970 and 1986. Sixty-five percent were decided in favor of the employer. The researchers found a number of problems with how these cases were decided. First, there was frequent use of generalities about the differences between older and younger workers' abilities, despite the fact that there was no documented evidence of consistent group differences in actual job performance. Often neither the employers nor the expert witnesses were asked for specific evidence concerning the plaintiff's actual physical capabilities and the specific job requirements. Second, the variability of decreased physical strength and fitness with age was frequently not addressed. Third, the possible effects of redesigning the workplace to accommodate older workers was often not considered.

These societal attitudes can affect not only how elderly people are perceived but also how they view themselves. Bodily (1991) surveyed inactive nurses to find out why they were not working. She was surprised to find that many respondents cited their age as the reason for not working without giving any other qualifiers. As Bodily stated,

> *What concerned me the most about the ways respondents were using "age" was that its meaning was being taken for granted; that is, as if the implications of phrases like "because of my age" or "I'm too old" were sufficiently obvious to require nothing more than a sympathetic nod on the part of the reader. While I was sympathetic, it was not because respondents were in fact too old, but because they were using "age" to disqualify themselves or ortherwise limit their range of choices. (p. 248)*

The quotation demonstrates the reciprocal nature of ageism. Negative stereotyping in society can lead to viewing elderly people in a depreciatory manner and as less valuable members of society. Elderly people who adopt these aging myths may see decline as inevitable and becoming more passive members of society as the only option available (Rodin & Langer, 1980). Unfortunately, when elderly people act according to these stereotypes, society's misperceptions about the aging process can be reinforced (Butler, 1987).

Physical Factors

Long-held beliefs in the health care field about the aging process are now being seriously questioned. Rowe and Kahn (1987) pointed out that much of what was considered to be inevitable deterioration is the result of individual behavior and environmental conditioning. They criticized researchers for perpetuating a narrow view of aging by concentrating on the central tendencies within a group and ignoring the substantial differences in functional aging (Troll, 1989).

Although changes in physiology are a part of aging, accumulated evidence indicates that many so-called usual disease processes can be modified and minimized (Rowe & Kahn, 1987). Diet and exercise have significant effects on carbohydrate metabolism, osteoporosis, cholesterol levels, diabetes, blood pressure, respiratory functioning, and hydration (Rowe & Kahn, 1987). Other studies have found that chronic pain can be greatly reduced through increased exercise and decreased medication use (Fordyce, 1976). Because musculoskeletal diseases account for 37 percent of all disabilities in the aged population (National Advisory Council on Aging, 1989b), increased mobility can have a significant effect on functional abilities and quality of life.

The lack of understanding about the aging process or the belief that continual decline is inevitable can lead to disease management as opposed to proactive intervention. Elderly people receive more medication prescriptions than younger people for equivalent symptoms (Rodin & Langer, 1980). Anxiolytic use more than doubles from 65 years of age on, and hypnotic medication use more than triples (Health and Welfare Canada, 1989). These statistics are quite disturbing given that 40 percent of all emergency department visits by elders are medication related.

Emotional Factors

It is well established that psychological well-being plays a significant role in the preservation of physical health and functional capacity (Zautra, Maxwell, & Reich, 1989). However, it has only recently been recognized that many of the variables that put elderly people at risk emotionally are responsive to intervention. In their review of the literature, Rowe and Kahn (1987) showed that lack of or decrease in social support increases elderly people's mortality and morbidity rates and decreases adherence to health-promoting regimens. As an example, they cited studies showing that moving from familiar surroundings to a nursing home or institution increased mortality rates. Longitudinal studies in Sweden revealed that death rates increased by 48 percent for men and 26 percent for women within the first three months after losing a spouse (Svanborg, 1990). Other risk factors include the stress of managing on a fixed income, elder abuse, isolation, perceived health limitations, and the strain of being a caregiver (National Advisory Council on Aging, 1989a).

Unfortunately, psychological problems in older people can go untreated for a number of reasons. Emotional difficulties in elderly people can be difficult to diagnose because they are often masked by physical symptoms that can lead to further isolation and decreased activities. These important symptoms may be misdiagnosed and written off as part of the "normal aging process" (Katz, Curlick, & Nemetz, 1988). Compared to younger adults presenting with the same symptoms, elderly patients are referred less frequently for psychiatric assessments (Hillerbrand & Shaw, 1990). Elderly people themselves are often reluctant to seek assistance for emotional difficulties, even though there are many ways of relieving psychological distress and helping elderly individuals achieve a greater sense of well-being. Whether they attach a stigma to such help or lack knowledge about what type of help is available is unclear.

Cognitive Factors

There is strong evidence to suggest that a sense of well-being is in large part determined by a person's belief systems (Beck, 1991; Persons, 1989). Although a system involves a number of beliefs, two are seen as crucial: belief about control and belief about self-worth (that is, self-esteem). Although discussed separately, they are very much interrelated.

SENSE OF CONTROL.   The belief in the ability to exert control over an event influences how that event is appraised and subsequent coping activity (Lazarus & Folkman, 1984). A sense of control results from the belief that certain actions will lead to certain results and the conviction that one has the capacity to take the action necessary to produce those results (Bandura, 1977, 1982). This is an important concept when considering the aging process because sense of control can often be compromised in elderly people. If they see physical and mental deterioration as uncontrollable, the perceived lack of control is likely to reduce active coping behaviors (Rodin & Langer, 1980). A sense of helplessness in elderly people has been shown to decrease responsiveness, motivation, and self-esteem and eventually to increase illness, mortality rates, and memory problems (Parnham, 1987). Unfortunately, research has shown that increased contact with helping professionals can reinforce this sense of helplessness (Rodin, 1986).

Providing elderly people with the opportunity to increase perceived control over the environment leads to improved memory, alertness, activity, and physical health and decreased morbidity and mortality (Rodin, 1986). In one noteworthy study, alterations that increased residents' control of the environment in a nursing home demonstrated that even small changes can have a profound effect (Langer & Rodin, 1976). When the researchers returned 18 months after the intervention, they found that the experimental group (with increased control) had a 48 percent increase in subjective happiness; were increasingly active, alert, and social; and, perhaps most surprisingly, had a 50 percent lower mortality rate than the control group.

Successful aging cannot be equated with total independence and lack of reliance on others. Everyone maintains a balance between dependence and independence. The need for self-determination encompasses the right to choose not to exercise control. Therefore, service providers must be sensitive to the fact that it is the individual who chooses his or her level of dependence (Clark, 1988).

SELF-ESTEEM. *Self-esteem* is a basic feeling of self-worth and a belief that one is fundamentally a person of value. In George's (1987) review of the literature on self-esteem and older adults, she suggested that the same factors that predict self-esteem in younger adults apply to elderly people: measures of personal achievement, success in interpersonal relationships, and meaningful leisure activities. However, correlates of self-esteem that were unique to older adults were health status and attitudes toward aging.

If aging is seen only in terms of the negative side of growing old and not as another stage of development, self-esteem can be seriously compromised. Rodin and Langer (1980) studied actions commonly seen as characteristic of older people. The young and middle-aged participants saw elderly people as primarily involved in nonsocial behavior and passive activities and attributed to them unpleasant personal characteristics to a much greater extent than positive ones. They also found that all respondents, including the older ones, appeared to have a stereotype of elderly people that included the idea of senility. Ninety percent of the elderly respondents believed that there was a strong possibility they would become senile. However, medical estimates indicate that only 4 percent of people over 64 years of age suffer from a severe form of senility, and only another 10 percent suffer from a milder version (Katzman & Carasu, 1975).

Purpose and meaning in life influence self-esteem (George, 1987). For elderly people, this component is related to whether growing older is viewed as a time for continued contribution, goal setting, and purpose (Baltes, 1990). A perceived meaningless existence can lead to anxiety, depression, hopelessness, and physical decline, whereas meaning and purpose in life are associated with positive mental and physical health (Reker, Peacock, & Wong, 1987). Although meaning in life changes with each developmental phase, the need to be challenged and valued remains the same (Troll, 1989).

■ EFFECTS OF AGEISM ON HEALTH CARE TRAINING AND SERVICE DELIVERY

Gatz and Pearson (1988) stated that although global negative attitudes of aging may not exist in the health care field, specific biases may. Part of the responsibility for health care professionals' biases belongs to the educational institutions. Santos and VandenBos (1982) pointed out that few graduate programs in the social sciences offered training in gerontology. Whitbourne and Hulicka (1990) analyzed 139 psychology textbooks written over 40 years for evidence of ageism. They found that aging issues received little attention even in the later editions. When aging was addressed the texts tended to focus on problems rather than successes and described older adults as suffering from multiple deficits and handicaps that were attributed entirely to the aging process. The texts also only infrequently mentioned intellectual plasticity, the difference between normal aging and disease processes, and the ways in which individuals can compensate for losses associated with aging. The authors concluded that these texts exposed students to a narrow and permanently fixed view of the aging process.

Researchers argue that when others believe that an older person's range of physical and cognitive abilities is narrowing, there is a tendency to restrict individual freedom even further (Clark, 1989). These restrictions can lead to reinforcement of dependent rather than independent behavior by the helping professions (Baltes & Barton, 1979) and to symptom management rather than health promotion (Rodin & Langer, 1980). This behavior may best be conceptualized as "disabling support" versus "enabling support" (Rowe & Kahn, 1987).

One study exemplifies the impact of the two approaches. Avorn and Langer (1982) divided residents in a nursing home into three groups and gave them a jigsaw puzzle to complete. One group was actively assisted by the staff to complete the puzzle (helped group), one was encouraged but received only minimal assistance (encouraged group), and one was left to complete the puzzle on its own (control group). All three groups were tested before and after puzzle assembly on ability to complete the task and on self-confidence ratings. The "helped" group's performance deteriorated posttest and they rated the task as more difficult, compared with the "encouraged" group, who improved their performance and felt more confident in their abilities. Even the control group, who received no help at all, increased their speed of performance slightly. It may be that the expectation of disability becomes disabling in and of itself. It could be argued that what has been termed "helpless behavior" in elderly people is an active attempt to cope with a system that reinforces adherence to stereotypes and dependent behavior.

Clarfield (1989) also pointed out that established practice defines physical diseases and psychological difficulties according to the way they typically present in 20- to 40-year-old individuals. Diagnosis and treatment of a more complex presentation in older people generally has received only minimal attention. Behavior that would warrant further investigation in a younger person may be less rigorously investigated in an elderly person. Elderly people are also more likely to receive less long-term therapy and to be institutionalized for the same symptoms that would be treated more aggressively in a younger population (Rodin & Langer, 1980). A study of age bias in a general hospital (Hillerbrand & Shaw, 1990) found that compared to younger patients, geriatric patients were less likely to be referred for psychiatric consultation. The study also found that the suicidal ideation and past psychiatric history evaluations were not as complete for older patients. The authors found this oversight disturbing because the suicide rate for the elderly population is 50 percent higher than for younger populations.

Schaie (1988) criticized psychological research for having ageism undertones. He listed a number of methodological mistakes, including failing to operationalize the concept of the aging variable (that is, grouping everyone over 60 together as if they were a homogeneous group), not providing reasonable estimates of effect size in age comparisons, confounding findings with other concomitant age changes (for example, uncorrected peripheral sensory deficits), using test materials that are normed on young adults, and not considering the range of individual differences that result in overlapping distributions. He concluded that to avoid being accused of inadvertently supporting ageist biases, researchers in psychology need to address the above concerns and be as sensitive to these issues as they would to issues of race and gender.

▬ EFFECTS OF AGEISM ON HEALTH CARE POLICY

Subtle ageism may be partly to blame for the deficits in service delivery to the elderly population. In his review of the effects of ageism on public policy, Kimmel (1988) stated that 45 percent of U.S. community mental health centers reported having no specific programs for elderly people and that 41 percent did not have any clinical staff members trained to deliver geriatric services. Roybal (1988) called for an expansion of the federal response to mental health and aging. He pointed out that even though elderly people make up 12 percent of the U.S. population, only 6 percent of people served by mental health centers are older Americans.

The American Psychological Association and the American Psychological Society were cosponsors of a recent report entitled *Vitality for Life: Psychological Research for Productive Aging* (Adler, 1993). This report recognized that elderly people have been poorly represented in research and funding priorities. It lists four priorities in the area of aging: (1) learning how best to maximize elderly people's productivity at work, (2) developing mental health assessment and treatment strategies to enhance vitality, (3) learning how to change older people's health behavior, and (4) increasing research on how to optimize the functioning of those over 75. The report's sponsors will use the report to demonstrate to Congress the importance of providing more funding to agencies that support behavioral science research on aging.

▬ DISCUSSION

The recent acknowledgment that society needs to examine the whole concept of the aging process is long overdue. Studies demonstrating the effect of individual behavior and environmental conditioning on the aging process are exciting and challenging. Such research supports the contention that there is a strong interaction between individuals and their environment about health choices and responsibilities. There are a number of implications for professionals working with the elderly population. The first concern is individual professional responsibility. Because ageism can be quite subtle, service providers need to continually examine their own attitudes toward aging and elderly people. Health care professionals need to move away from using the term "age" as an explanatory variable and the assumption that after enough time certain "things" will happen to people. As Bodily (1991) pointed out, this assumption moves away from actual causes to the view that time is a sufficient cause and places the profession squarely in the biomedicalization model of aging. Instead, social workers and other health professionals need to focus on the causes of functional impairments, even the impairments that occur more frequently among older adults.

Professionals can also combat ageism through the types of programs offered and the way these programs are developed. Service providers need to actively involve elderly people in identifying what programs are needed and in designing, implementing, and managing the programs. Examples of such programs are Peer Counseling and Mentor Programs, where older people "buddy up" with high school students who are at high risk of dropping out. Programs could also be designed to target misconceptions about aging more directly in elderly people themselves. These programs would encourage them to examine how aging myths may be affecting their behavior and to experiment with acting differently. Such programs could have three main components: (1) direct challenge of aging myths, (2) skill-developing practice, and (3) a supportive environment for testing the new behavior. The advantage of this approach is that not only do participants learn new ways of responding, they also become more attuned to the manifestations of aging myths in society and the subtle effect they may be having on their own responses to aging and sense of well-being.

The second concern is professional training. Exposure to elderly people and to aging issues has been shown to reduce ageism (Gatz, Popkin, Pino, & VandenBos, 1984). Educational institutions in the health care and social sciences need to establish departments with subspecialties in gerontology, particularly at the graduate level (Storandt, 1983). These same educational institutions need to include aging issues in their continuing education programs, thus allowing working professionals to keep up to date on the gerontological literature and new trends in the field. Schaie (1988) criticized researchers and professionals working in gerontology for having a lack of awareness of relevant work in the existing aging literature.

The third area of concern is research. More research needs to be conducted on issues such as work and aging, individual differences in age-related change in behavior and performance, the magnitude of age changes and age differences, how to enhance health behaviors, and how to optimize the functioning of very old people. Research also needs to be aimed at identifying aging stereotypes and their effect on individuals and society, factors that contribute to their development and maintenance, and ways they can most effectively be changed. Researchers need to be educated about the biases that may be influencing their own research. As Schaie (1988) pointed out, much of the current aging literature can be dismissed because of these biases.

Finally, professionals working with the elderly population have an obligation to make a concerted effort to confront ageism in society as a whole. Older people's failure to make health changes may often be the result of the barriers society creates to block successful change. The stereotypes of aging discussed in this article may prevent elderly people from initiating change or may defeat them before they start. Much can be learned from other groups, such as the women's movement, about how to raise awareness of stereotyping and unfair practices, including concerted lobbying efforts to change government policy at all levels. And service providers must actively target stereotypical beliefs in themselves, their professional organizations, and their communities to bring about lasting change.

▰ REFERENCES

Adler, T. (1993). Experts in aging outline research, funding focus. *APA Monitor, 4*(10), 18.

Avorn, J., & Langer, E. (1982). Induced disability in nursing home patients: A controlled trial. *Journal of the American Geriatrics Society, 20,* 297–300.

Baltes, M., & Barton, E. (1979). Behavioral analysis of aging: A review of the operant model and research. *International Journal of Behavioral Development, 2,* 297–320.

Baltes, P. B. (1990, October). *A psychological model of successful aging.* Paper presented at the 19th Annual Scientific and Educational Meeting of the Canadian Association on Gerontology, Victoria, British Columbia.

Bandura, A. (1977). Self-efficacy: Toward a unifying theory of behavioral change. *Psychological Review, 84,* 191–215.

Bandura, A. (1982). Self-efficacy mechanism in human agency. *American Psychologist, 37,* 122–147.

Beck, A. T. (1991). Cognitive therapy: A 30-year perspective. *American Psychologist, 46,* 268–375.

Bodily, C. L. (1991). "I have no opinions. I'm 73 years old." Rethinking ageism. *Journal of Aging Studies, 5,* 245–264.

Botwinck, J. (1984). *Aging and behavior* (3rd ed.). New York: Springer.

Butler, R. N. (1987). Ageism. In G. L. Maddox & R. C. Atchley (Eds.), *The encyclopedia of aging* (pp. 22–23). New York: Springer.

Clarfield, A. M. (1989, November). *The geriatric imperative.* Paper presented at the 75th Annual General Meeting of the Pharmaceutical Manufacturers Association of Canada, Ottawa.

Clark, B. (1989, November). *The aging of North America: The shape of things to come.* Paper presented at the 75th Annual General Meeting of the Pharmaceutical Manufacturers Association of Canada, Ottawa.

Clark, P. G. (1988). Autonomy, personal empowerment, and quality of life in long term care. *Journal of Applied Gerontology, 2,* 279–297.

Doty, L. (1987). *Communication and assertion skills for older persons.* New York: Hemisphere.

Fordyce, W. E. (1976). *Behavioral and methods for chronic pain and illness.* St. Louis: Mosby.

Gatz, M., & Pearson, C. G. (1988). Ageism revised and the provision of psychological services. *American Psychologist, 11,* 184–188.

Gatz, M., Popkin, S. J., Pino, C. D., & VandenBos, G. R. (1984). Psychological interventions with older adults. In J. E. Birren & K. W. Shaie (Eds.), *Handbook of the psychology of aging* (2nd ed., pp. 755–787). New York: Reinhold.

George, L. (1987). Self-esteem in later life. In G. L. Maddox & R. C. Atchley (Eds.), *The encyclopedia of aging* (p. 593). New York: Springer.

Health and Welfare Canada. (1986). *Achieving health for all: A framework for health promotion* (Catalog No. H39-102/1986E). Ottawa: Ministry of Supply and Services.

Health and Welfare Canada. (1989). *The active health report on seniors* (Catalog No. H-39-124/ 1988E). Ottawa: Minister of Supply and Services.

Hillerbrand, E. T., & Shaw, D. (1990). Age bias in a general hospital: Is there ageism in psychiatric consultation? *Clinical Gerontologist, 2*(2), 3–13.

Katz, I. R., Curlick, S., & Nemetz, P. (1988). Functional psychiatric disorders in the elderly. In L. W. Lazarus (Ed.), *Essentials of geriatric psychiatry* (pp. 113–137). New York: Springer.

Katzman, P., & Carasu, T. (1975). Differential diagnosis of dementia. In W. S. Fields (Ed.), *Neurological and sensory disorders in the elderly* (pp. 103–104). Miami: Symposium Specialist Medical Books.

Kimmel, D. C. (1988). Ageism, psychology, and public policy. *American Psychologist, 11,* 175–178.

Langer, E., & Rodin, J. (1976). The effects of choice and enhanced personal responsibility for the aged: A field experiment in an institutional setting. *Journal of Personality and Social Psychology, 34,* 191–198.

Lazarus, R. S., & Folkman, S. (1984). *Stress, appraisal and coping.* New York: Springer.

Moody, H. R. (1988). *The abundance of life: Human development policies for an aging society.* New York: Columbia University Press.

National Advisory Council on Aging. (1989a). *1989 and beyond: Challenges of an aging Canadian society* (Catalog No. H37-3/10-1989). Ottawa: Ministry of Supply and Services.

National Advisory Council on Aging. (1989b). *Understanding seniors' independence Report No. 1: The barriers and suggestions for action* (Catalog No. H37-3/11-1-1989E). Ottawa: Ministry of Supply and Services.

Palmore, E. B. (1986). Attitudes toward aging shown by humor: A review. In L. Nahemow, K. McCluskey-Fawcett, & P. McGhee (Eds.), *Humor and aging* (pp. 101–119). New York: Academic Press.

Parnham, I. (1987). Perceived control. In G. L. Maddox & R. C Atchley (Eds.), *The encyclopedia of aging* (pp. 454–455). New York: Springer.

Persons, J. B. (1989). *Cognitive therapy in practice: A case formulation approach.* New York: W. W. Norton.

Reker, G. T., Peacock, E. J., & Wong, T. P. (1987). Meaning, purpose in life and well-being: A life span perspective. *Journal of Gerontology, 11*(1), 44–49.

Rodin, J. (1986). Aging and health: Effects of the sense of control. *Science, 233,* 1271–1276.

Rodin, J., & Langer, E. (1980). Aging labels: The decline of control and the fall of self-esteem. *Journal of Social Issues, 36*(12), 12–29.

Rowe, J. W., & Kahn, R. N. (1987). Human aging: Usual and successful aging. *Science, 237,* 143–149.

Roybal, E. R. (1988). Mental health and aging. *American Psychologist, 43,* 189–194.

Santos, J. F., & VandenBox, G. R. (1982). *Psychology and the older adult: Challenges for training in the 1980s.* Washington DC: American Psychological Association.

Schaie, K. W. (1988). Ageism in psychological research. *American Psychologist, 43,* 179–183.

Snyder, C. J., & Barrett, G. V. (1988). The Age Discrimination in Employment Act: A review of court decisions. *Experimental Aging Research, 14*(1), 3–47.

Storandt, M. (1983). Psychology's response to graying in America. *American Psychologist, 38,* 323–326.

Svanborg, A. (1990, October). *Aging, health and vitality: Results from the Gothberg longitudinal study.* Paper presented at the 19th Annual Scientific and Educational Meeting of the Canadian Association of Gerontology, Victoria, British Columbia.

Troll, L. (1989). *Continuations: Adult development and aging.* College Park: University of Maryland, International University Consortium.

Whitbourne, S. K., & Hulicka, I. M. (1990). Ageism in undergraduate psychology texts. *American Psychologist, 11,* 1127–1136.

World Health Organization. (1947). The constitution of the World Health Organization. *WHO Chronicles, 1,* 16.

Zautra, A. J., Maxwell, B. M., & Reich, J. W. (1989). Relationship among physical impairment, distress, and well-being in older adults. *Journal of Behavioral Medicine, 12,* 543–557.

Chapter 7

Advance Directives: Most Patients Don't Have One, Do Yours?

MARGARET W. BERRIO   MAUREEN E. LEVESQUE

The Patient Self-Determination Act states that patients in health care settings that receive Medicare or Medicaid funds must be given information about planning for health care decisions in advance of an incapacitating illness or injury. Despite the fact that patient notification must now be given regarding advance directives, many health care facilities find that only a handful of their patients have completed a living will or durable power of attorney for health care. Whose responsibility is it to broach this often difficult subject with patients? This chapter outlines staff education approaches used by one health care institution to facilitate greater compliance with this important patient education opportunity.

A nurse responding to Bill Powell's call light at 5 AM one Friday found him severely short of breath, with a pulse of 110. Mr. Powell had cancer. His color was dusky, he was flailing, and the pulse oximetry monitor showed his oxygen saturation was 82%. The physician was called, but by the time he arrived Mr. Powell wasn't breathing effectively. He was placed on 100% oxygen and a discussion ensued about what to do if he should go into respiratory arrest.

His physician planned to call a code. The nurse who admitted Mr. Powell was sure he'd mentioned that he didn't want to be intubated, but nothing to that effect was in his chart. There was no advance directive on record and now he was too ill to communicate.

Fortunately, Mr. Powell recovered from his respiratory crisis. He told his nurse afterward that he was worried about who would make decisions for him if he became incompetent. He knew that his time was limited. Some of his relatives lived nearby, but he wasn't on the best of terms with them. His girlfriend had taken care of him for years, and he wanted to make sure that she'd be "calling the shots" when the time came.

Because he got a warning that many patients don't, Mr. Powell was motivated to prepare an advance directive. As we'll see, his case was more the exception than the rule.

From *American Journal of Nursing* 96(8):25–28. Reprinted with permission.

TABLE 7-1 Essentials of the PSDA

To encourage patients to complete advance directives, Congress enacted the Patient Self-Determination Act (PSDA) in October 1990. The law, which went into effect in December 1991, requires hospitals, nursing homes, and hospices to:

- advise patients on admission of their right to accept or refuse medical care;
- advise patients of their right to execute an advance directive;
- document whether a patient has an advance directive;
- implement advance directive policies;
- educate their staffs and communities about advance directives; and
- in the case of managed care organizations and home health care agencies, provide the same information to each of their members on enrollment.

▰ LAW RAISED EXPECTATIONS

The Patient Self-Determination Act (PSDA) passes in December 1991 attempted to ensure that patients would be aware of their right to make health care decisions and to refuse treatment, even after they're unable to communicate (see *Essentials of the PSDA*; Table 7-1). This is accomplished primarily by informing patients about how to create an advance directive for health care (see *Designing an Advance Directive*; Table 7-2). It requires that a process of patient education be implemented by all institutions getting reimbursement from Medicare and Medicaid. The provisions for patient notification and documentation are also incorporated into current Joint Commission on Accreditation of Healthcare Organizations standards.

The patients we treat on our pulmonary medicine unit give us ample cause for concern about this issue. We see them over the continuum of their disease process: at first ambulatory and relatively self-sufficient, then gradually deteriorating, needing more medications to control the pain, and requiring supportive therapies to breathe.

TABLE 7-2 Designing an Advance Directive

Each state has specific laws that designate which types of advance directives are binding. Some allow treatment preferences to be binding; others may be more restrictive. When you're helping a patient design an advance directive, be certain that your recommendations take account of local laws.

- The *living will* is a document stating what medical treatment a person may choose to omit or refuse in the event that the person is unable to make those decisions himself and is terminally ill.
- The *health care proxy*, or *durable power of attorney for health care*, is a document that appoints a proxy agent, usually a relative or trusted friend, to make medical decisions on the patient's behalf if he can no longer decide for himself. This type of document is preferable to a living will because it has broader applicability and can include treatment preferences (both requests for and refusals of treatments).

Along the way, we get to know our patients' personalities and social support systems as well as their views on the changes in their physical status. At the end, when we see them struggling for air, we wonder if they truly want to be intubated and dependent on a ventilator for every breath for the rest of their lives. So we've tried to promote advance directives as a means of providing our patients some level of control over end-of-life decision-making and the circumstances of their death.

The PSDA was received with great relief by many health care professionals who believed they would finally have a guide to patients' wishes about heroic life-sustaining measures in advance of needing them. As we began to implement the law's mandates, it was expected that giving patients this information would dramatically increase the number of patients who completed advance directives.

Unfortunately, as demonstrated by numerous clinical examples, these expectations haven't been met.

▀ UNFULFILLED PROMISE

The procedures we devised to satisfy the PSDA are straightforward: the admitting clerk gives the patient a booklet explaining advance directives, the physician informs him about his health status and the implications for treatment, and nurses ensure that the patient understands and has been given the written information. The social worker for the unit is responsible for actual completion of the advance directive document with the patient (if he doesn't already have one) and filing it in his chart.

When the law was passed, a series of conferences were held to inform nurses, physicians, and social workers about their roles. At that time, most of us simply assumed that patients would follow through and create the documents once they were informed. But we found, to our dismay, that the issues surrounding advance directives, especially the low completion rate, aren't so easily disposed of (see *Barriers to Completion of Advance Directives*; Table 7-3).

TABLE 7-3   Barriers to Completion of Advance Directive

The following have been identified in the literature and in our experience as barriers to patients completing advance directives:

- procrastination, or waiting to do it later
- dependence on family for decision-making
- lack of knowledge about advance directives
- difficult topic to talk about
- waiting for the physician to initiate a discussion
- the physician waiting for the patient to initiate discussion
- believing they need a lawyer to fill out the forms
- fatalism, or acceptance of the "will of God"
- fear of "signing my life away"
- fear of not being treated

About three years after this policy had been established, we reviewed patients' medical records over two months on the pulmonary medicine unit. These patients often had poor prognoses and ought to have been good candidates to complete their advance directives. But the results showed that only nine out of 51 (17%) had done so.

That finding falls within the range of results of other studies, which show that although patients may express interest in advance directives, not many actually complete a formal document. In one of the more recent reports, researchers at Johns Hopkins Hospital found that only eight of 26 patients (31%) had completed an advance directive. Most of these patients (19) were in critical care, cardiac, or AIDS units. Seven were admitted to acute medical units. Other studies have shown completion rates as low as 4%.

▰WERE POLICY AND PROCEDURES TO BLAME?

Our first effort to pinpoint why there were so few advance directives on record was to review our policy. We believed that the way to improve our results was to reinforce the policy. If we gathered all the evidence about what part of the process needed to be fixed and systematically approached the corrective actions, we thought that a clear picture of the problem, and thus a simple solution, would emerge.

We conducted a chart review over a three-month period, using the nursing assessment form as our source of information. We noted how many patients had an advance directive on admission, how many wanted more information about advance directives, and whether the physician or social worker had been notified. We looked for an advance directive in the chart if the patient told us that he'd completed one.

The results showed a number of areas that could be improved:

- We had no mechanism for alerting staff to the presence of an advance directive document in a medical record.
- When a patient told us that he had an advance directive from a previous admission, we noticed that there were sometimes delays in obtaining the document from the medical records department for the current chart.
- We found that as many as 48% of patients didn't receive the pamphlet that describes advance directives on admission. There were a variety of reasons for this, including admissions through the emergency department, patients already having one, and some refusing the pamphlet. In a few instances the pamphlets had run out.
- Five patients were admitted to the unit wanting more information — even when they had completed an advance directive.
- There was no standardized procedure for noting when a patient wanted to speak to a social worker or physician about advance directives, except on the admission nursing history. Communicating patients' desires for more information wasn't formalized either.
- There was no mechanism to ensure that the physician or social worker had spoken to the patient once the request for contact had been made.

▬ NOBODY "OWNED" THE PROBLEM

To accomplish effective change, we knew that members of every discipline of the health care team needed to be included in discussing solutions to these problems. A brainstorming session was called to share the results of the initial survey. The physician chief of service, chief of unit administration, head nurse, a number of staff nurses, unit coordinators, chaplains, respiratory therapists, and dietitian attended.

In presenting data from the chart review to the team, it was important to stress that we were looking for solutions to a difficult problem — and didn't expect that any one approach would be definitive. Neither did we believe that any one discipline "owned" the problem; all disciplines participated in the process and shared in the problems.

The response from the team was mixed. Some questioned why we needed to concern ourselves with this issue, when we knew from the literature that there was little chance of increasing our percentage of completed advance directives.

We were surprised to realize that we needed to repeatedly return to the goal of the PSDA: to provide the patient with the knowledge and tools necessary to create an advance care document if he so desired. By the end of the meeting, everyone agreed to support a process to achieve the spirit of the law and meet regulatory standards.

▬ WORKING TOWARD A SOLUTION

Our first inclination was to plan for the more obvious changes that would result in concrete improvements. A notification routine to indicate that a patient had an advance directive could be created in the hospital computer system, thus communicating this information to all involved with one quick entry. This was done by the unit coordinator. We now see a notice that states that the patient has an advance directive each time a computer entry is made for a patient who has one.

Making sure that a document created during a previous admission was placed on the chart was more difficult, since it must come from the record room as part of the old chart, or from another facility as part of the transfer documentation. In response to this problem, we've established a system for duplicating the advance directives of patients who we believe are likely to return to our unit.

As we continued to discuss our findings, we noticed that despite all our efforts we weren't achieving the goal of getting our most fragile patients to create the document in the first place. There was much discussion about the purpose of the law as opposed to the letter of the law. This helped us to realize that the staff still needed to be educated about advance directives in order to create an open atmosphere, in which patients felt confident that any member of the health care team could answer their questions on the subject.

▬EDUCATION IS ONGOING

We faced an enormous education effort, and not only with our patients. All staff members needed to project a respectful yet healthy attitude about forming end-of-life decisions. We determined that our approach would be an inclusive, continuous, and open effort to educate all of our staff and all patients who were interested.

We asked the members of the initial brainstorming group to participate in a different approach to patient education. We wanted to offer patients information they needed when they wanted it in the form of an interactive presentation on the unit. We first developed a set of slides that any team member could use as a guide throughout the presentation for staff, patients, and their families. The slides helped to standardize the information presented and ensure that nothing essential was left out.

Members of the health care team — physicians, social workers, and chaplain's staff — were invited to review and comment on the presentation during the two to three weeks before full implementation. As new staff came to the unit, they were shown this presentation as part of their orientation.

We planned for everyone to participate in the patient education sessions by asking the physicians to introduce the topic generally, the nurses to give the details of the law and patients' rights, the social worker to present information about how to complete an advance directive, and the chaplains to discuss the religious and spiritual aspects of contemplating end-of-life issues.

▬BOTH STAFF AND PATIENTS BENEFIT

A posttest was created to determine the effectiveness of the education for patients. Initially, we wanted to use the rate of completed advance directives as a measure of effectiveness. But we've come to understand that the low completion rates at our hospital and elsewhere indicate more than simply a lack of education about the letter of the law, the advantages of having an advance directive, or patients' rights. Our completion rate didn't improve as a result of these sessions, but the posttest results show that our patients gain a better understanding of their right to determine the kind of care they will receive and learn where to go for more information when they're ready.

We've continued the on-unit patient information sessions for six months, and have received many positive comments from patients, family members, and staff. We've refined the participant posttests and developed an attitudinal survey about the program for our staff members to complete.

The survey results indicate that our staff members are pleased with the program. They feel more comfortable speaking with patients about advance directives, and they're willing to present the program to patients as part of their weekly routine. In short, they believe in the program and support the philosophy behind the PSDA.

And what happened to Mr. Powell? He decided to create an advance directive after much discussion with his nurse and the rest of the health care team. His girlfriend was designated to carry out his wishes via a durable power of attorney. About three weeks later, he died peacefully with his girlfriend and daughter in attendance at the hospital.

It takes work to create a climate that's both supportive and accepting of the patient's right to make decisions about health care measures before they're needed. But we believe that our efforts have made a positive difference, and we'll strive to maintain a climate that can help our patients work through this difficult self-directed process.

■ REFERENCES

ANA position statement on nursing and the Patient Self-Determination Act. *Prairie Rose* 61(2):10a, 13a, June–Aug. 1992.

Edinger, W., and Smucker, D. R. Outpatient's attitudes regarding advanced directives. *J. Fam. Pract.* 35:650–653, Dec. 1992.

Emanuel, L. L., et al. Advance directives for medical care — A case for greater use. *N. Engl. J. Med.* 324:889–895, Mar. 28, 1991.

Gamble, E. R., et al. Knowledge, attitudes, and behavior of elderly persons regarding living wills. *Arch. Intern. Med.* 151:277–280, Feb. 1991.

La Puma, J., et al. Advance directives on admission: Clinical implications and analysis of the Patient Self-Determination Act of 1990. *JAMA* 266:402–405, July 17, 1991.

Schneiderman, L. J., et al. Relationship of general advance directive instructions to specific life-sustaining treatment preferences in patients with serious illness. *Arch. Intern. Med.* 152:2114–2122, Oct. 1992.

Stelter, K. L., et al. Living will completion in older adults. *Arch. Intern. Med.* 152:954–959, May 1992.

SELECTED BIBLIOGRAPHY

Adams, P. & Dominick, G. L. (1995, Fall). The old, the young, and the welfare state. *Generations* 38–42.

Bandman, E. L. (1994). Tough calls: Making ethical decisions in the care of older patients. *Geriatrics 49*(12):46–51.

Bishop, S. M. (1989). Children and the elderly: Pitting generational concerns in the social policy arena. *Journal of Child and Adolescent Psychiatric and Mental Health Nursing* 2(3):85–86.

Callahan, D. (1996). Controlling the costs of health care for the elderly: Fair means and foul. *The New England Journal of Medicine 335*(10):744–746.

Fox, P. D. & Fama, T. (1996, Summer). Managed care and the elderly: Performance and potential. *Generations* 31–36.

Holstein, M. (1995, Fall). The normative case: Chronological age and public policy. *Generations* 11–14.

Jecker, N. S. & Schneiderman, L. J. (1994). Is dying young worse than dying old? *The Gerontologist 34*(1):66–72.

Johns, J. L. (1996). Advance directives and opportunities for nurses. *Image: Journal of Nursing Scholarship* 28(2):149–153.

Kingson, E. & Quadagno, J. (1995, Fall). Social security: Marketing radical reform. *Generations* 43–49.

Koitz, D. (1995). *Social Security: Brief Facts and Statistics.* Washington, DC: Congressional Research Service, Library of Congress.

Mezey, M., Bottrell, M. M., Ramsey, G., & the N.I.C.H.E. faculty (1996). Advance directives protocol: Nurses helping to protect patient's rights. *Geriatric Nursing 17*(5):204–210.

Rathbone-McCuan, E. (1985). Health needs and social policy: The health care of elderly women. *Women & Health 10*(2/3):17–27.

Sansome, P. & Phillips, M. (1995). Advance directives for elderly people: worthwhile cause or wasted effort? *Social Work 40*(3):397–401.

Yenerall, J. D. (1995). College socialization and attitudes of college students toward the elderly. *Gerontology & Geriatrics Education 15*(3):37–48.

Zimmerman, J. (1994). Good life, good death, and the right to die: Ethical considerations for decisions at the end of life. *Journal of Professional Nursing 19*(1):22–37.

Unit 2
Promoting Quality of Life and Longevity

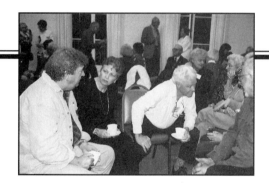

A mericans are living 25 years longer now than they did at the turn of the 20th century. We are experiencing this increase in life expectancy because of the impact of public health practices such as a safe water and milk supply, prenatal care, and immunizations against childhood diseases, flu, and pneumonia; advances in medical technology where diseases and injuries can be cured and/or treated; and the national abundance and variety of nutritional food.

For many Americans this addition to life expectancy will exceed all expectations; living to age 100 will be common, and increasing numbers of people will reach age 110. How healthy one will be and the quality of one's life during these additional years is of concern to us all, especially health care providers who work with older adults. It is within the capabilities of most people to conduct their lives in a way that will compress the years of dependence and infirmity while extending the years of health and wellness. However, people will need the help of knowledgeable caregivers to achieve a higher level of wellness and quality of life within the gift of these additional years. More years of life are not a gift if they cannot be lived well.

This unit focuses on chapters that consider the concepts of wellness, quality of life, and longevity. The unit begins with an overview of issues impacting the health of older adults developed by a group of nursing experts in the field of aging. It looks at national strategies for improving health and wellness. The following chapters focus on appropriate use of humor to assist with education, decrease stress, and relieve the depersonalization many elders feel; the Great Depression of the 1930s as an age-related relevant life experience as a factor for self-care behaviors; promoting the sexual health of elders, which is often not addressed with elders; empowering clients and their level of wellness through their perceptions of being strong; and finally, promoting health in the last third of a woman's life using menopause as an important marker.

Nurses and other health care professionals who work with older adults have similar goals for their clients. They want them to experience the healthiest life possible for as long as possible. When older adults are asked, this is also their goal. In order to achieve these mutual goals the nurse must have the information and related skills necessary to help elders improve the quality of their lives and to participate in activities that will enhance longevity. With the selection of chapters in this unit the nurse has the beginnings of information needed to enrich their understanding of what improves the quality of lives that will be longer.

Chapter 8

Wellness and Health Promotion of the Elderly

DOLORES M. ALFORD   MAY FUTRELL

This chapter represents the cutting edge work of two geriatric nurses in response to the American Academy of Nursing's Expert Panel on Older Adults. The panel asked for interested members to formulate a policy paper on wellness and health promotion of the elderly. The policy paper was published in *Nursing Outlook* and readers were invited to review and comment on the policy recommendations that were formulated. The reader will find recommendations for changes in curriculum, self-care, social policy, research, accessibility of care, and health/wellness care delivery to older adults within nursing models. The chapter concludes with additional recommendations, which include such changes as improving the health of practicing nurses to promote successful aging, restructuring the workplace to accommodate older workers in a proposed future of nonretirement, and making grants available for designing "think-tank" institutes of gerontologic nursing.

Promoting a healthy life-style is big business in the United States for younger people. Promoting healthy life-style behaviors for older persons, however, has been deemed unnecessary and undesirable. After all (as the prevalent attitude expounds), older people are ill, cannot be cured, and must use the Medicare services available to them. This myth of older people being ill or unhealthy must change if all citizens are to be helped to enjoy a high quality of life for as long as they live.

Undeniably the number of older persons (i.e., those over 65 years of age) is increasing in our society. The United States Census Bureau reports that a 40% increase in the number of older persons will have occurred between 1980 and 2000. The 35 million older Americans will represent a 10 million increase in just 20 years.[1] At present, approximately 10% of the population is 65 years or older. This number is expected to increase to 20% by the year 2000, with an 86-year life expectancy for men and 91 years for women in the year 2040.[2,3] The minority portion of the elderly is expected to be 17% in 2030.

From *Nursing Outlook* 40(5):221–226, 1992. Reprinted with permission.

Longevity and threats to longevity are changing. People are indeed living longer, not only because of their own life-style changes, but because of the technologic advances in every area of society.

For older persons, the concept of "health" must be restructured. Filner and Williams[4] suggest health might be defined as "the ability to live and function effectively in society and to exercise self-reliance and autonomy to the maximum extent feasible, but not necessarily as total freedom from disease." Disease, then, should not characterize old age. For the elderly of the next century, healthy independence will relate to the functional ability of older individuals and their needs for health promotion/protection, housing, and social services. No longer can health care itself be construed as the traditional concept of medicine, nursing, and various therapies. A comprehensive view of health — including social/environmental health in a holistic framework for the elderly — will be the model of health and wellness care in the 21st century.

Race and ethnicity also determine the beliefs in and use of health promotion/protection services. During the past decade, however, there has been a substantial growth in health-promotion activities for older adults of all ethnic backgrounds. Life-style changes being encouraged include engaging in exercise, eating a nutritious diet, and quitting smoking. Particular attention needs to be directed to ways to reduce the poor health status of many older persons, mainly in the black and Hispanic populations.

At present, the elderly over the age of 80 (old, old) require a greater proportion of health services than do the young old (55 to 65 years of age), but all older adults benefit from primary health care:

People over age 65 need regular primary health care services to help them maintain their health and prevent disabling and life-threatening diseases and conditions. Clinical preventive services include the control of high blood pressure, screening for cancers, immunization against pneumonia and influenza, counseling to promote healthy behaviors, and therapies to help manage chronic conditions such as arthritis, osteoporosis, and incontinence. For example, skin cancer screening can detect the majority of malignant melanomas and basal cell carcinomas.[5]

Successful aging for most people means coping and adapting. Atchley[6] states, "If older people are satisfied with their present and past lives, they have adapted to aging." Havighurst et al.[7] identified five components of life satisfaction: zest, resolution and fortitude, completion, self-esteem, and having hope. These components, of course, are as valid today, as older persons seek high life satisfaction, as they were in 1963.

Today's elderly are disadvantaged by attitudes of ageism, by sociopolitical policies that deny access to health care and demand illness before care is rendered, by a lack of adequate housing, transportation, and congregate/comprehensive services. Communities with high crime and abuse of citizens also affect the well-being of today's elderly.

Because there are more elderly people who are living longer, we are faced with many questions: the complex ethical decision making about the use of high technology for life support, the use of biotechnology for organ transplantation, and the use of new pharmacologic technology for treatment of disease with uncertain outcomes. Should the elderly be encouraged to die when the costs of maintaining their ravaged bodies becomes too high?

Added to these issues is one of having enough willing, competent, compassionate health care workers to care for older adults along the continuum of wellness/illness. The changing family structure also has a profound effect on today's elderly, as it will in the future. Health care workers will have to learn to be "family" for the elderly, and use the concepts of case management to meet the multiplicity of needs of the growing older population.

THE ELDERLY IN THE 21ST CENTURY

For their own protection, the elderly of tomorrow will have to learn to stay well and to become a powerful political force. To age well, one will have to practice a healthy life-style over the life course.

As they become politically active, older adults must demand their rights as citizens. Work in this direction is beginning with the adoption (by acclamation) of a set of Principles for Older Persons, proposed by the United Nations' Social Development Commission.[8] What is important about this document is that not only are rights of the elderly outlined, but the responsibilities of older adults are enumerated.

No one can force the elderly to promote and protect their health. As citizens, however, the elderly have an obligation to exercise that citizenship to the fullest by staying active in society, especially in the formulation of policy that affects their well-being. Older persons must stay active in business, in education, in the arts, and in social organizations, whether they are owners, employees, or volunteers. Older persons must continue to learn and to pursue opportunities that help them reach their fullest potential. They must not be afraid to be.

Some of the needs older persons will have in their quest for wellness and longevity are for housing that is affordable, safe, and convenient to services. Transportation services, tailored to older persons' needs, must be designed and implemented, perhaps by the elderly themselves. Social and health promotion/protection services must be in service centers, where the elderly can make use of many services in one location. Health services, mainly under the aegis of clinical nurse specialists expert in aging and wellness, will need to be designed for and offered to each older person in designated areas.

Older persons will have to plan for their health care and dying. They will have to develop their own caring families, if their biologic families are uninterested or unavailable. They will have to learn the developmental tasks dealing with change and loss; their adaptation techniques will be models for the young to follow.

NURSING'S PROJECTED ROLE

Philosophically, nurses have yet to define their "wellness" role, even though "health" has long been one of nursing's goals. For nurses to accept an advocacy role to help persons to age and die "well," nurses will have to learn these skills themselves.

If nurses are to accept the leadership role for promoting health and wellness in older persons, they must believe and practice what they are trying to promote. Therefore nurses themselves must be the picture of wellness, and their own behaviors must promote and protect health.

The same life-style behaviors and practices being taught to the elderly must be evident in nurses (i.e., weight control, no smoking, prudent eating of healthy food, control of alcohol intake, periodic exercising, wearing seat belts in vehicles, and control of stress).

Nurses must understand the aging process, know how to adapt health-promoting and health-protecting techniques to cope with age-related factors, and must actively provide the care and support of older persons as they seek wellness.

▬MODELS OF WELLNESS AND HEALTH PROMOTION

Ways of promoting health and encouraging wellness in the elderly are already being demonstrated. Some of the models include the Healthy Lifestyles for Seniors, sponsored by the Santa Monica Senior Nutrition and Recreation Program, the New Mexico Health Promotion with Elders project, sponsored by the state agency on aging, and the Wallingford Wellness Project, sponsored by a grant from the Administration on Aging.[9] The latest initiative is that which is being undertaken by the American Association of Retired Persons to carry out the recommendations of Healthy People 2000.

Many senior centers have planned periodic exercise programs, as well as talks on health-promoting topics. The various components of the media also promote healthy life-styles across the life span. Restaurants are beginning to add healthy foods to their menus. Airlines and many restaurants, churches, and businesses prohibit smoking on their premises.

What is being learned today will certainly be evident in the next few decades, as the present population ages. The habits of healthy living will be a way of life in the next century.

▬EDUCATION FOR A HEALTHY LIFE-STYLE

In nursing education today there is a lack of emphasis on the aging process and concepts of wellness in all levels of the curriculum. There seems to be a "gerontophobia" among nurse educators, who are handicapped with the same stereotypical myths concerning older persons and aging held by most other health professionals and the general public.

It is not enough to demand that gerontologic and wellness nursing be added to the curriculum. That is easy, for words may be written into curriculum plans. What is needed is for the words to be taken out of the plans and translated into teaching strategies and learning techniques. The content must be taught, understood, and practiced.

If we are to make such curriculum changes, we must prepare faculty to have a positive attitude about aging, health, and wellness. There are, at present, few faculty who are formally prepared in either gerontologic or wellness nursing.

The baccalaureate curriculum must include the aging process, as well as wellness- and health-promotion concepts. Students must have the opportunity in clinical settings to test these concepts. They must have the opportunity to work with well elderly, who are active and well integrated into society. This is a big change for colleges of nursing, for the curriculum emphasis has been illness, with the more complex illnesses being the most popular. Students need to see older persons continuing to fully function in business, government, teaching, recreation, socialization, and parenting. The sites we choose for our students to interact with the elderly will therefore have to change. Students need experiences with the elderly in senior centers/clubs, worksites, churches — wherever older adults are found. Students should have the opportunity to conduct health and life-style appraisals, provide short programs on healthy life-styles, assist individuals to work toward identified health/wellness goals, and provide the support necessary to maintain the desired goal. Students must also have the opportunity to see older persons die "well."

Even when students enter clinical experiences that are illness focused, they should have the opportunity to carry out wellness and health promoting techniques. For example, if a student is caring for an older man with a stroke, efforts should be made to encourage appropriate protection of his senses (e.g., checking his ears to ensure they are free of excess cerumen; determining if hearing aids would provide an adjunct to age-related hearing deficits; determining if vision could be enhanced with cataract extraction or change of glasses). Dental and foot health could be taught with specific recommendations for health maintenance. In this way, students would begin to see their patients/clients as more than a fascinating illness process — as human beings with potential. During health teaching on a daily basis and for discharge, students could remind the older patient to keep immunizations up-to-date, to have periodic health screenings, to control weight through prudent eating, to take care with the use of any type of medication, to maintain flexibility of all joints, and to promote their mental health. Students can provide resources for health promotion and continuity of care.

Graduate students at the master's level, should have the opportunity to followup specific groups of elderly to validate current gerontologic and health-promoting theories. This could be achieved at senior centers, geriatric clinics, and retirement housing.

Master's students should have opportunities in practice sites to validate studies in aging as they affect nursing. These students should have opportunity to question public policy concerning aging and the aged and to participate in advocacy groups. Classes in research theory and design should include not only how to conduct research on older subjects, but ways of conducting wellness research in older population samples. Master's-level students should have beginning opportunities to conduct original research studies under the aegis of a qualified gerontologic nursing researcher. Practice experiences should include producing and conducting wellness-

and health-promotion programs for older persons in group settings, as well as working with individual older persons and their families.

Doctoral-level students, under the mentorship of faculty who are experts in aging and wellness, should have the opportunity to conduct original research on wellness and aging, to critique available studies, and to forecast future research needs in wellness and aging. Research studies should be conducted in multisettings on elderly in complex situations (e.g., an older abused person in a dysfunction setting needing extensive health and social services). The learning climate should foster the establishment of new nursing theories of aging and wellness in a complex, high-tech society, the updating/revision of current nursing theories of aging and wellness, and the participation with other disciplines in their quest to develop new theories or update current ones.

Because we live in a global village, doctoral students should also have the opportunity to develop a world view of aging and health, including the political, social, and economic policies that shape these world views and that have an impact on the well-being of older persons.

There is a desperate need for longitudinal studies of all facets of wellness and health promotion of people as they age. For example, we do not know what effects our health-promotion efforts for younger persons will have on these people in 20, 30, or 40 years. Doctoral faculties must begin to do these longitudinal studies, using newer cohort compression techniques,[10] to obtain these vital data. Doctoral students must also be involved with their mentors in this type of research.

Continuing nursing education will remain one of the most important and effective ways to change attitudes and behaviors of nurses, as well as to give them current knowledge about wellness and health promotion in older persons.

Efforts must begin now with promoting health and wellness in nurses themselves. Then instruction in aging and health can be presented. Under the aegis of the nurse experts in aging and health, a cadre of instructors can be prepared to provide such continuing education. Input, approval, and cosponsorship from the Council on Gerontological Nursing of the American Nurses Association, as well as from the American Holistic Nurses Association, would help ensure that the content and style of the program offerings are designed to meet stated objectives.

■ NURSING'S PUBLIC POLICY ROLE

If the wishes of our profession concerning wellness and health promotion for the elderly are to come true, nurses will have to change social policy. To do so, nurses must be conversant about the social policies regarding older persons, as well as the diverse positions taken on these policies.

First, nurses should change their image so they are noted for their wellness- and health-promoting care, as well as for their illness care of older persons. Only then will nurses have the credibility to effect such changes.

Gerontologic nurses must be activists to shape public policy regarding wellness and health promotion in older adults. Nurses must speak before civic groups, senior citizen clubs and centers, political party functions, and other special-interest groups that are instrumental in helping to change social policy. Nurses must be unafraid to testify before legislative bodies as advocates of the elderly.

Recognizing that policymakers rely heavily on information given them, nurses will also have to have hard data to demonstrate that being healthy in old age is socially and politically appropriate. Nurses will have to learn the fine art of compromise as they testify and negotiate for changes from illness to wellness. Nurses will have to be creative in identifying options for the extremely politically and economically powerful "illness" industries to produce products and services for wellness. For example, hospitals are beginning to recognize the trend toward wellness in aging. Many hospitals have "Over 50" clubs and programs with a wellness focus, but with options to use the hospital's illness services if needed.

Older people must be viewed as healthy despite their having chronic diseases and conditions. Therefore health insurance plans must be designed to cover health-promoting and health-maintaining activities. This insurance would reduce the illness care emphasis so prevalent today. The present health maintenance organization model could be expanded to include social health maintenance organizations to provide comprehensive health services to older persons. This is not to say Medicare would not be needed; the program would still be needed for unavoidable illnesses. But the structure of Medicare would be different. The premium one pays for wellness/illness insurance would be based on an individual's degree of positive health habits practiced consistently. Individuals with illness/conditions resulting from negative health behaviors/practices would have higher insurance premiums to pay. Efforts would have to be made to bring later cohorts of elderly under this full plan, for at least two present generational cohorts will have to be excluded partially or fully from the penalties. (For example, in our present 30 to 60 year olds, damage to blood vessels, lungs, and skin are already producing costly acute and chronic illnesses that must be treated and managed.)

To effect such changes, nursing, along with other health disciplines, will have to conduct projects to demonstrate how effective these changes will be on the well-being of older individuals, the cost implementation and cost effectiveness of such programs, and the effects it will have on the politics of aging.

Political and social policy guiding services to older adults seeking wellness must address the role of nurses as primary caregivers/care managers on a parity with, or even above, physicians. Gerontologic nurses with a wellness focus should be able to manage their own case load of older adults in specifically identified areas.

Older persons with illnesses best treated by physicians should be referred to specific medical consultants. These medical consultants would have to understand the gerontologic nurses' role so the elderly patients are returned to their nurse's care for continuing management and surveillance.

▬RECOMMENDATIONS

This article is a set of recommendations for changes in curriculum, self-care, social policy, research, accessibility of care, and health/wellness care delivery to older persons in nursing models.

The following are some additional recommendations:

1. The American Nurses Association and The American Academy of Nursing should convene an expert panel on health/wellness in aging. These experts should be prepared to provide consultation to social policy-makers, to advocate for healthy aging in all types of media, to testify before governmental bodies, to provide consultation to colleges of nursing for curriculum development, to help develop creative ways for public and private sectors of society to work together to solve aging issues, and to help write the profession of nursing's position statements on aging and health.

2. The American Nurses Association, with the aid of the specialty organizations, should be responsible for helping practicing nurses to live healthier lives and to learn how to age successfully. An intense, creative campaign for such aid should use all types of learning strategies.

3. A media campaign should be mounted that portrays gerontologic nurses as models of health and as advocates for healthy, successful aging.

4. A massive campaign should be undertaken by the public and private sectors — through television, radio, newspapers, and community programs — to teach all citizens how to be responsible for their own health. Reinforcement of these responsibilities would continue as people age.

5. A public policy of nonretirement should be established.

6. The workplace should be restructured to accomodate older workers (e.g., brighter lights with less glare; adjusting heights of tables, chairs, and fixtures; easier grip tools; a slower work pace). Gerontologic nurse specialists should be on premises of the workplace if there are 50 or more older workers.

7. Lifelong learning for health and wellness should be promoted. Positive health behaviors must be reinforced as people age. Colleges of nursing should have some educational/consultative input into local schools and colleges, as well as into the workplace.

8. Public policy should be directed toward consolidating services for older persons (e.g., neighborhood services centers), services that could be housed in existing facilities such as senior centers and retirement housing or in shopping malls. Services provided would include nurse-managed wellness centers, Medicare/Medicaid office, Social Security office, social worker, transportation and housing coordinators, nutritionist, podiatrist, dentist, optometrist, and therapists. Demonstration projects should be undertaken to determine the feasibility of such centers and to demonstrate how the various disciplines would coordinate their services for older persons. Cost benefits of such centers should be included in the projects.

9. Grants should be available for the designing of institutes of gerontologic nursing in university programs offering doctoral preparation in nursing. The institutes should focus on being resource centers to nurses, other health professionals, and the community on the role and function of gerontologic nurses. The institutes would conduct ongoing research, especially longitudinal studies on aging well and on the well elderly.

   The institutes would have think tanks to forecast trends in aging, longevity, health/wellness, and ways nursing can address these trends, findings, and issues.

   Educational offerings on aging well for all levels of nurses, as well as for the elderly themselves, would be provided through such institutes. Curriculum development and consultation in aging and wellness would also be provided. The institutes would provide nurse mentors to students.

   Once such institutes were underway, they would bid to be the specialists in certain aspects of aging and wellness. (There is a crucial need for nurses to develop expertise in (1) the psychoneuroimmunoendocrinology of aging, as it applies to nursing, (2) gait, station, and mobility preservation through the adult life span, (3) nursing case management for families as they age, (4) psychogerontologic nursing, (5) health of older women, and (6) skin care and aging.)

   The institutes would develop and control their own practice settings in which to validate and update all nursing procedures used for eldercare; develop and test new nursing techniques and procedures, including the creation of new equipment and supplies; generate new theories of aging, wellness, and health promotion; and provide learning environments for students to validate the knowledge they are learning.

   Funding for such institutes of gerontologic nursing would come from public and private sources. Federal demonstration grants would provide the funds for start-up. Facilities — buildings, clinics, nursing homes, hospitals — available as government-owned properties could be purchased from the government and renovated to meet needs. Consortia of nursing schools and health-related businesses could be developed to underwrite field studies. Organizations concerned with aging issues, such as the AARP, could also provide monetary support for such institutes. Donations from individual private donors and foundations should be sought. If nursing had the "right" image and vision, the money would be available.

10. Social policy should be directed toward helping older persons to understand they have a responsibility to assist in forecasting health trends, validating or disproving theories of aging, and influencing public policy on their behalf. The elderly must be partners with nurses. The elderly should not expect nurses or anyone else to "do for them" when they can mobilize their own resources to help themselves. The elderly themselves should use the media to the fullest to promote positive values of wellness and aging. The elderly themselves must make war on the stereotypes of aging.

■ REFERENCES

1. Chellis R, Grayson P. Life care: a long-term solution? Lexington, Massachusetts: Lexington Books, 1990:XXI.
2. Dychtwald K. Age wave. Los Angeles: Jeremy P. Torcher, 1989.
3. Hess B. America's aged: who, what, when, where? In: Hess S, ed. Growing old in America. New Brunswick, New Jersey: Transaction Books, 1976.
4. Filner B, Williams T. Health promotion for the elderly: reducing functional dependency. In: Healthy people 2000. Washington: US Government Printing Office, 1979:365–87.
5. US Department of Health and Human Services. Health people 2000. Washington: US Government Printing Office, 1979.
6. Atchley R. Social forces and aging. 5th ed. Belmont, California: Wadsworth, 1988:250.
7. Havighurst R, Havinghurst R, Neugarten B, Tobin S. Disengagement, personality and life satisfaction. In: Hansen PF, ed. Age with a future. Copenhagen: Munksgaard, 1963.
8. Nusberg C. UN takes action on principles for older persons. Ageing Intl 1991;18(1):3–6.
9. Fallcreek S, Warner-Reitz A, Mettler M. Designing health promotion programs for elders. In: Dychtwald K, ed. Wellness and health promotion for the elderly. Rockville, Maryland: Aspen, 1986:219–33.
10. Fiske M, Chiriboga D. Change and continuity in adult life. San Francisco: Jossey-Bass, 1990.

Chapter 9

Humor: A Nursing Intervention for the Elderly

JANET R. HULSE

> Humor is not new to nurses; we have always used it as a method of coping with the stressors we experience in our discipline. Humor enhances all aspects of life and is being seriously studied by health care professionals. The use of humor with clients has been incorporated into their caregiving, formally in careplans and as institutional policy and perhaps more frequently, informally. Janet Hulse suggests using humor as a communication strategy, to enhance education, reduce stress, and relieve the depersonalization many older adults feel. Throughout the chapter ideas are shared on how to appropriately incorporate humor when interacting with clients, families, and caregivers, in their homes as well as in health care institutions, and the benefits one might expect from humor.

Although laughter and humor are a part of everyday life, the positive benefits of humor on health are often underestimated. Patients, families, and nurses can all benefit from humor. Humor can be used as a nursing intervention in treating the elderly because it creates a relaxed atmosphere that enables patients to be more receptive to learning and more willing to participate in their own care. Humor can be used to aid families through the difficult stressors of caregiving, and humor can lower the stress level of nurses' own daily routine.

Humor has been defined as both an emotional and a cognitive process that is unique to an individual and appeals to the comic sense.[1] It is considered spontaneous. It is interesting, but not surprising, that nursing practice has not focused attention on humor. Humor has not been considered a significant component of the daily role of the nurse. This is ironic, especially since humor is a major defense mechanism that allows one to cope with extremely difficult situations.[2] Nursing curriculum has fostered the scientifically based role of the nurse and the rational, serious nature of the profession.[3]

The concept of humor dates back to Plato and is even described in the

From *Geriatric Nursing* 15(2):88–90, 1994. Reprinted with permission.

Bible. Sociologists, psychologists, and philosophers have studied humor for centuries, but only recently have health care professionals devoted research to the implications of incorporating humor into practice.[4] One of the first, Norman Cousins, in 1977 described his experience with a life-threatening illness. In his book, Cousins explained how the use of humor and laughter cured him of collagen disease.[5] Cousins' therapy included 10 minutes of hearty laughter each day, which enabled him to sleep without pain. He attributed the cure of his illness to the use of humor and laughter.

■FUNCTIONS OF HUMOR

There are many theories and beliefs concerning the values and types of humor. Cognitive theorists study the social mechanisms of humor, and the psychologic and the physiologic effects of humor and laughter.[1] One universal assumption is that laughter and humor make one feel good.[5]

Socially, humor is used as a communication strategy and stimulus to facilitate social interactions and promote group cohesiveness.[7] Humor may be used as an "ice breaker" to establish rapport with patients and families. Communicating with humor conveys a message of caring and humanness.[8] Humor unites people, acknowledges acceptance of them, creates a common bond.[4] Humor has been used to enhance the learning process. An environment conducive to increased retention and to enhanced learning is established by incorporating humor and laughter into the experience.[9]

Self-perception may become negative as an individual's health declines.[10] Humor promotes a more positive attitude. Humor encompasses the realms of body, mind, and spirit.

Physiologically and psychologically aspects of humor may provide the patient with relief from anxiety, stress, and pain. The ability to laugh and use humor may be an indicator of a person's degree of mental maturity and health and may even demonstrate coping capacity.[11] The incorporation of humor in the workplace aids in relieving the feeling of burnout for the nursing professional. Smith Lee[4] suggested using these strategies to enhance the work environment: posting work-related cartoons on the bulletin board, placing pamphlets and books of humor in the staff lounge, and holding a monthly staff break dedicated to a humorous situation.

■PHYSIOLOGIC BENEFITS OF LAUGHTER

Humor that produces laughter provides physiologic benefits through improving oxygenation and energy levels. Laughter stimulates the skeletal, facial, abdominal, and thoracic muscles. When a person laughs, oxygenation is increased, the heart rate increases, and the thoracic and abdominal muscles contract. The body temperature rises a half a degree, and the pulse and blood pressure also rise above baseline values. Once the laughter subsides, the blood pressure and pulse return to normal. The increase in oxygenation and the use of the abdominal and thoracic muscles improve a person's energy level.[4,7,10,11]

Cousins thought laughter caused the release of endorphins.[5] Since that time, research has shown this to be a likely assumption. The combination of the release of endorphins and increased oxygenation causes a feeling of well-being. This is the same effect that exercise or aerobics has on an individual. For example, when a person uses a rowing machine for 10 minutes each day or laughs 100 times each day the effect on the person's feelings are the same.[12] The total physiologic effect of laughter creates a feeling of well-being in a person. After a period of laughter, there is a relaxation period and a heightened ability to deal with stressful situations.[7,13] Recent studies of psychoimmunology indicate that humor actually may enhance immune function through the release of endorphins.[3]

▬ HUMOR AND THE NURSE-PATIENT RELATIONSHIP

Humor can aid in developing a healing relationship between the nurse and the patient. Laughter and humor establish communication and allow the patient to establish an egalitarian position, enhancing understanding of self and situation.[2] This benefits the patient teaching process and allays fears and tensions surrounding unfamiliar experiences.

Enhanced nurse-patient communication allows patients to gain control over their own healing and wellness and explore new coping skills. Humor provides patients with a method of attaining knowledge of self from a different perspective.

Studies identifying the characteristics and needs of the elderly are abundant. Lower self-esteem and low morale are two issues frequently identified that can be addressed with humor. Humor may aid the elder in resolving conflicts and incongruities in difficult situations.[10]

▬ ASSESSING THE APPROPRIATENESS OF HUMOR

Sensitivity about the appropriate timing and use of humor as a therapeutic intervention is essential. The expert nurse must assess the patient to ascertain if humor should be used as a therapeutic intervention. It is important to discover what makes a person laugh and to realize that some individuals may not possess a sense of humor. A psychologic assessment will provide some clues regarding an individual's capacity to respond to humor. Previous methods of coping with stress must be examined, and the significance of humor in everyday life must be discovered.

If the patient feels threatened or vulnerable or does not understand the intent of the humor, it may build a barrier to communication. What is humorous to one patient may seem dull or even vulgar to another. If the humor exposes sensitive or embarrassing issues, it may be destructive rather than constructive. A patient may misuse humor (as wit or sarcasm) to deny a problem or illness. The patient's anxiety level or depression will affect the response to humor and may cause negative effects.[2,10]

For the elderly patient, family should be included to understand their views of humor and to provide input regarding the patient's level of humor. Interactions between the patient and family should be observed to identify if humor is a significant aspect of their communication. Leading questions may provide the nurse with an assessment of the practices and values of humor for the individual and family. Questions that may assist the nurse in assessing the level of humor include: What makes you laugh? When do you feel humor is a negative experience? Do you often look at the funny side of everyday life situations? If so, how?[1]

The nurse may use humor to avoid anxiety in a difficult patient situation. This misuse of humor may create negative consequences in the therapeutic alliance. Nurses should assess their own values and uses of humor and recognize when it signals anxiety in themselves or their patients. The questions that are asked of the patient are also relative to the nurse. When humor is used appropriately, it relieves the depersonalization and creates a caring atmosphere. Humor incorporated as a nursing therapy can relieve the stress and feelings of despair patients experience.

▰ NURSING INTERVENTIONS

Once the nurse has assessed the patient and identified that humor could be a useful component of daily activities, interventions should be incorporated into care. Humorous articles or books may be given to the patient to read or be read to the patient. Comic strips and joke books may also be given to patients to read. Interventions should be appropriate to identified deficits when physical or sensory impairments are present. Humorous stories of the past serve to stimulate families to recount stories of struggling with life and reminisce of times and treasures, and this may relieve stressful situations.[11]

A bulletin board placed in a central location on the unit can include humorous short stories and comics from the newspapers. Posters can be placed on the bulletin board. Such an example is currently in place at The Cornwall Hospital. A bulletin board is located in the unit activity room at a low level so that even the wheelchair-confined elderly patient can enjoy scanning the cartoons. The bulletin board is updated biweekly, and the old material is filed for future use. Often at mealtime, in the activity room, discussion revolved around the current postings on the bulletin board. Jokes with hidden meanings may also stimulate resident interest and curiosity.

A cartoon scrapbook can provide humor for patients confined to their rooms. This scrapbook can be augmented periodically to create an informal library of humor. A humor diary that the staff contribute to can also be entertaining. Staff can contribute short humorous stories or jokes for patients to read. It must be stressed that jokes and stories contributed are tasteful and nonthreatening to the patients.

A comedy shop can be developed to house audiotapes, silly games, videotapes, and joke books.[12] Volunteers can aid in activities. By organizing the materials, the volunteers will be able to have many different resources for humor available for their use.

Humorous videotapes can be incorporated on an informal or formal basis. Specific times can be designated for patients to view the videos. When the patients view the videos together it serves two purposes: Humor is

BOX 9-1 Suggestions for Audiovisual Aids for Humor in Geriatric Care

Videotapes
Abbott and Costello (numerous tapes available)
"The Bad News Bears"
"Biloxi Blues"
"Brighton Beach Memoirs"
"City Slickers"
"Father of the Bride"
"Home Alone"
"The Honeymooners" (Vol 1-7)
"The In-Laws"
"Its a Mad, Mad, Mad, Mad World"
"M.A.S.H."
Mel Brooks' "Life Stinks"
"Naked Gun"
"On The Road — Bing Crosby & Bob Hope" (numerous tapes)
"The Pink Panther"
"Planes, Trains, and Automobiles"
Red Skelton "Lost Episodes"
"The Revenge of The Pink Panther"
    "King of Laughter 1-2"
"Scrooged"
"Spaceballs"
The Best of Ernie Kovacs
The Three Stooges (numerous tapes available)
The Best of Laurel and Hardy (numerous tapes available)
"Three Amigos"
Tim Conway "Comedy Review"
"The Trail of The Pink Panther"
Victor Borge "On Stage"
    "Birthday Gala"

Audiotapes
Abbott and Costello (numerous tapes available)
Amos and Andy
The Bickersons (numerous tapes available)
Bill Cosby (numerous tapes available)
"Classics of Bob and Ray 1 and 2"
Jack Benny "Classics"
"Laughter from the Golden Age of Radio 1 and 2"

contagious, and conversation is stimulated through enjoyment of a common theme.

Videotapes of old movies such as those featuring Abbott and Costello or The Three Stooges can be shown. Movies featuring Danny Kaye or Jerry Lewis are enjoyable for some patients. A list of suggested videotapes and audiotapes has been developed to aid in choosing appropriate humor (Box 9-1). Residents should be surveyed regarding their preferences. This list should be added to periodically as new movies are discovered.

For these nursing interventions to be successful, the nursing unit members (staff and residents) must utilize the programs and periodically contribute to the humor library. One member of the health care team must be responsible for critiquing and updating all material and filing the used material.

A live comedian or a puppet show may also entertain the patients. Tennant[10] studied formal humor as an intervention for elders and found that a formal humor program promoted group cohesiveness and stimulated social interactions and relationships among the participants of the study. Discussion of movies or presentations after the viewing will stimulate communication and will evaluate the merits of the presentation.

▬SUMMARY

Researchers should investigate humor's value and impact on quality of life of elders. Humorous interventions should be studied and compared in elders. The effects of endorphin release during laughter is another aspect of humor to be studied.

Certainly humor is not the answer to all the discomforts encountered by older adults, but the positive effects on some cannot be disputed. Humor as a noninvasive modality and an adjunct to patient care can be of benefit not only to the patient and family, but also to the professional nurse who encounters the discomforts of the patient on a daily basis. Humor can aid in viewing the pleasures and pains of the world with new perspectives.

▬REFERENCES

1. Bellert J. Humor: a therapeutic approach in oncology nursing. Cancer Nurs 1989;12:65–70.
2. Kaplan H, Saddock B. Classification of defense mechanisms. In: Kaplan H, Saddock B, eds. Synopsis of psychiatry, 6th ed. Baltimore: Williams and Wilkins, 1991:184.
3. Rosenberg L. A delicate dose of humor. Nurs Forum 1989;14(2):3–7.
4. Smith LB. "Humor relations" for nurse managers. Nurs Manage 1990;21(5):86–92.
5. Cousins N. The healing heart. New York: Bantam Books, 1977.
6. Groves F. "A merry heart doeth good like medicine. ..." Holistic Nurs Prac 1991;5(4):49–56.
7. Lapierre E, Padgett J. What is the impact of the use of humor as a coping strategy by nurses working in geropsychiatric settings? J Psychosoc Nurs 1991;29(7):41–3.
8. Sumners A. Professional nurses' attitudes toward humor. J Adv Nurs 1990;15:196–200.
9. Ferguson S, Campinka-Bacote J. Humor in nursing. J Psychosoc Nurs 1989;27(4):29–34.

10. Tennant K. Laugh it off: the effects of humor on the well-being of the older adult. J Gerontol Nurs 1990;16(12):11–17.
11. Pasquali E. Learning to laugh: humor as therapy. J Psychosoc Nurs 1990;28(3):31–5.
12. Carlisle D. Comic relief. Nursing Times 1990;86(3):50–1.
13. White L, Lewis D. Humor: a teaching strategy to promote learning. J Nurs Staff Dev 1990;2:60–4.

Chapter 10

Health Behaviors and the Great Depression

JACQUELINE S. NOWICKI

> Life experiences and events have profound effects on people. Those who remember the assassination of John Kennedy, the Vietnam War, or the Oklahoma City bombing, know how the extent of the event impacted their lives. Those of us younger than age 60 cannot fathom the age-related relevancy of the Great Depression, an event that lasted for over 10 years, from 1929 to 1939. To most younger people it is only an event in the history books. For older adults, growing up during that time, it is a lived experience that has significantly influenced health values, thrift, self-reliance, and compliance. These behaviors are described in one case study exemplifying how a person was influenced by the Great Depression. The chapter concludes with effective strategies for the health care professional to work successfully with older adults considering the impact of the Great Depression in their lives.

The present older adult population in this country was highly influenced by a very dramatic event — the Great Depression of 1929 to 1939. This was a time of widespread poverty. By understanding the implications of Depression-era beliefs and values on elders, with its effect on health behavior throughout the life span, health care professionals can assist these clients to change behaviors toward a more healthy lifestyle.

According to Matarazzo,[1] assessment of longitudinal development can assist the health care professional to understand the health behavior of a client. Wilson and Trost[2] state that coping techniques and styles do not seem to change with age and may persist for more than 70 years.

The Great Depression caused a great deal of mental and physical suffering, especially for those who were unemployed or lost their savings. For example, it was estimated at one point that 15 million people were out of work in the United States. The severe unemployment directly affected some 37.5 million men, women, and children. Millions more in service professions and occupations were also severely, although

---

From *Geriatric Nursing* 17(5):247–250, 1996. Reprinted with permission.

indirectly, affected. One family doctor stated that as many as half of his patients were charity cases. Dentists complained that much of their work consisted of pulling neglected teeth that could no longer be treated any other way.[3]

Evictions were frequent. Most landlords were willing to allow a few apartments to remain vacant rather than to appear soft-hearted and collect no rent at all. Foreclosures were also common. Tax sales in daily newspapers were as long as 24 pages.[3]

For those still employed, pay cuts were accepted without a murmur. Cuts of as much as 10% were common.[3]

Numerous settlements of tar paper huts, called "Hoovervilles," sprang up in cities like New York. Here families lived reluctantly like gypsies, cooking whatever they had over open fires. Former businessmen peddled apples along city streets. Charities worked with city, state, and local governments to find the resources to prevent hunger. Private charities and organizations were stretched to the limit. The unemployed waited for hours in breadlines for a meal.[3]

As the demands on public and private funds increased, relief was spread very thin. In Toledo, Ohio, the allowance was 2.14 cents per meal for each person. No relief money was available for medical or dental care. The meager relief money was generally spent on food for subsistence.[4]

Surprisingly, there is no evidence that the general health of society was compromised during this time. Life expectancy continued to increase from 57.1 years in 1929 to 63.7 years in 1939, and the death rate decreased from 11.9/1000 to 10.6/1000.[5]

There was a steep decline in food prices, and those who still had jobs could buy staple items at reduced prices. Calorie consumption for the unemployed ranged from 2600 to 2900 calories for an adult man. Although calorie intake was adequate, diets tended to be concentrated in grains and vegetables rather than more expensive milk, meat, and fresh fruits. However, with the monotony of everyday life, those with a little money looked forward to buying sweets or wine whenever possible.[5]

As the Depression continued, governments of several countries, including the United States, encouraged citizens to grow their own food. Land was frequently allocated on the edge of cities and towns for gardens.[5]

Miners in West Virginia's coal mines were hit especially hard. Families lived in mining camp shacks. They had coal for heat and walked miles to receive flour from the Red Cross when it was issued. Gardens were started from charity seed. To a large extent these people lived on wild blackberries.[4]

During the early 1930s there was no national system of unemployment benefits or welfare programs, although various programs were discussed. The federal government seemed unable to agree on some way to address the magnitude of the situation.[5] Volunteerism was encouraged, and community and charitable organizations assisted in the relief effort. With the extreme intensity of day-to-day survival, routine medical and dental care was neglected by the unemployed. Priorities were shifted to food, shelter, and safety.[5]

In summary, the culture of the Great Depression left its mark on those growing up in those years. Values of thrift, self-reliance, and prioritizing basic physiologic and safety needs became most important.

CASE STUDY

Mrs. M., at age 72, exemplifies a person influenced by the Great Depression. The following is a summary of her health status: she is 5'5" tall, weighs 165 pounds, and underwent heart angioplasty 3 years ago for moderate to severe angina. At present, she has few symptoms of angina. She has been advised by her physician to follow a cardiac diet, lose 20 pounds, and participate in mild aerobic exercise at least 3 times per week.

Mrs. M. considers losing weight to be the most important action to improve her health in terms of her chronic heart problems. She states that she tries to eat large amounts of vegetables and to decrease her intake of fats and sugars, but she is often unsuccessful in doing this. Although her doctor has given her written diets to follow, Mrs. M. says that she knows what to eat and has hardly looked at the diets. She has lost a total of 5 pounds since diagnosis and treatment 3 years ago. Mrs. M. enjoys gardening as a hobby and spends a considerable amount of time each summer and fall working in the garden and freezing and canning vegetables. She occasionally does volunteer work with her church helping to cook and serve at an inner city soup kitchen. Mrs. M. states that she gets exercise walking on her frequent shopping trips, but she does no planned aerobic exercise.

Mrs. M. was a latency-age schoolchild and adolescent/youth during the Great Depression, 1929–1939. Her lifestyle at that time became a basic conditioning factor and has had a major impact on Mrs. M.'s health attitudes. The Great Depression was occurring while Mrs. M. was learning strategies for engaging in the tasks of everyday living and developing a philosophy and mature set of values.[6] During this critical developmental stage, she was faced with developing coping strategies for food choices and values regarding food that would shape her self-care agency.[7] Mrs. M.'s health values and compliance to diet and exercise appear to have been significantly influenced by the Great Depression.

Compliance with diet can be further explained by certain theories of health behavior. One of these theories is the health belief model revised by Becker and Maiman.[8] One aspect of this theory is that the perceived severity of the possible illness is very low if the client has no symptoms. When the perceived severity is low, motivation to act is low.[9] Dean et al.[10] state the perceived seriousness of an illness is the most important step to a self-care response. The perceived threat of myocardial infarction for Mrs. M. does not seem as severe without the symptoms of frequent angina. In addition, Mrs. M.'s latency or formative years occurred during the Great Depression, when it was difficult to acquire even one of the most basic needs as listed in Maslow's hierarchy of needs — food.[11] The perceived threat of myocardial infarction probably does not seem as serious as the necessity of food. Kondo and Foreyt[12] state that scarcity at one time in one's life can make a "clean plate and full belly" an essential value.

Conflict theory can also explain health behavior. According to this theory, the coping pattern is determined by the presence or absence of three conditions. One of these conditions is the hope of finding a better alternative. If the hope of finding a better alternative is not met, defensive avoidance will be the primary coping pattern.[13] If Mrs. M.'s formative years were spent during the Great Depression, with little hope of finding a better alternative of changing food patterns, then avoidance of change would be the primary coping pattern. This pattern would perpetuate itself into her adult life. Mrs. M. would then follow some of the same basic food patterns acquired during the Depression.

Food itself can be looked on as a value or status symbol. During the Depression the wealthy and fortunate had a variety of foods to eat, leisure time for inactivity, and a car to drive rather than walk. Modern research has shown that these very habits that were valued during the Depression are now considered risk factors for heart disease.[14]

Mrs. M. says that she knows what kinds of food to eat to lose weight and avoid heart problems. She says that she eats fruits and vegetables and tries to avoid fats and sugars. However, according to Mrs. M., she does not lose weight because she eats too much sugar and fat. She also states that she cooks and eats more food than she needs. Mrs. M. grows her own vegetables and cans large quantities of food, a common practice during the Depression. She also keeps large quantities of sale items of food and other necessities stored in her home. She credits this storing of food to her experience with shortages during the Depression.

According to Mrs. M., she received a nickel from her grandmother once a week, which was used to go to the candy store. She states that it took a great deal of time to decide how to spend the money on the perfect treat. This valuing of sweets that was present during her formative years has persisted into her present value system concerning food.

The basic conditioning factor of the Depression as an age-related relevant life experience has been both a facilitating and a limiting factor for Mrs. M.'s self-care agency. Mrs. M. realizes the importance and value of good food. She is accustomed to cooking and eating vegetables and fruits that can be grown in gardens and orchards. Because she assumes the responsibility for her food choices, she also feels a responsibility to pay attention to what is said in the media concerning a healthy diet. She always has plenty of healthy food on hand because of her habit of storing items. She values the importance of proper nutrition. This is evident in the fact that she does volunteer work with an inner-city soup kitchen.

Mrs. M.'s experience during the Great Depression has resulted in some limiting effects to Mrs. M.'s self-care agency. Although she realizes the importance of healthy food intellectually, she also values sweets as a symbol of pleasure and joy, a common view during the Depression. The client says that she understands what good food is but eats too much of it. As was noted earlier, scarcity at one time in a person's life can lead to overeating. Because Mrs. M. is used to making her own food choices, she has rarely looked at the heart diet that her physician has given her.

■ STRATEGIES

This analysis of the Great Depression related to health values can lead health care professionals to a greater understanding of elders. It is easier to deal with problems of compliance when the causes are understood. Furthermore, several strategies can be used to deal with these attitudes. The positive aspects of Depression-era health attitudes can be emphasized with clients. Elderly clients can be praised for making food choices such as whole grains and vegetables, and for taking responsibility for their own diets, but *with* professional guidance. Consumption of healthy food choices that were scarce during the Depression and considered a luxury, such as citrus fruits and chicken, can be encouraged. Patients who have an interest in gardening can be encouraged to pursue this hobby for providing both fresh wholesome vegetables and for the opportunities for exercise that it offers. Reminiscence emphasizing the "good old healthier days" when everyone walked everywhere can be encouraged.

Social support of the patient is a useful tool in encouraging compliance. The support and participation of family and friends can be enlisted in encouraging the patient to lose weight. The family relationship needs to fit several criteria to have the potential for constructive involvement. Mrs. M. needs to have a generally supportive family where conflict is not excessive. Social support can help Mrs. M. adapt to better choices in diet.[12]

Social support can also be used in encouraging the client to exercise. Gillett,[14] in a study of an exercise program involving 38 overweight women, achieved a 94% adherence rate. The credit for this high rate of adherence was given to social support through group homogeneity, carpooling, and the social networks that developed.[15]

A "foot in the door" strategy to shape behavior can also be used. A minimal change in behavior should be requested of the client. This change must be enough to produce a minimal positive clear result.[16] The client should be praised for these positive results (such as Mrs. M.'s initial loss of 5 pounds) and encouraged to greater sequential steps toward the ultimate goal of permanent weight loss, proper diet, and regular exercise.

Health values and compliance are poorly understood. Traditional methods of teaching health values have been through modeling, limiting choices, persuading and imposing rules. Raths,[17] in 1966, proposed values clarification. According to this strategy, values can be arrived at by cognitively choosing, prizing, and acting. Choosing needs to be freely done by use of alternatives, with careful consideration of the consequence of the alternatives. The client must be pleased with or "prize" the choice and be willing to act on the choice repeatedly and form it into a life pattern.[18] These steps can be used by health care professionals in assisting elderly clients to plan a diet and exercise program. Perhaps if Mrs. M.'s diet had been planned with her rather than given to her, it might have been more successful.

Self-affirmation is another strategy that can be used. The client repeats a sentence 20 times a day dealing positively with what they want to do or become. This will help evoke emotions that could assist in changing selfcare patterns.[16]

Contracting is a strategy that has been used for assisting clients to take charge of their own health actions with the assistance of a health care professional. The client is perceived as a partner in the plan of care. The terms of the contract are mutually agreed on. The problem needs to be identified and responsibilities and activities clarified. Periodic evaluation and renegotiation are needed. Rewards on completion of the contract need to be planned. The most effective rewards are often self-administered.[16]

Six steps can be used to assist clients in their self-care. First, a client should be carefully assessed. Clients over age 60 probably possess health values influenced by the Great Depression. These values need to be reviewed with the client.

Second, health care problems and goals for treatment need to be evaluated with the client. Consideration must be given to the client's values and attitudes.

Third, plans for care must be established. These plans need to incorporate appropriate strategies by use of the most positive aspects of the client's health care values and build on these.

Fourth, appropriate time tables for achievement of steps toward the ultimate goal need to be established. Again, this is done with the client or by the client with the assistance of the health care professional.

Fifth, after an established period of time, progress needs to be evaluated with the client. Any adjustment in the overall plan should be made.

Finally, ultimate goal accomplishment needs to be acknowledged and rewarded. Plans for a lifelong program of health can be established *with* the client at this time.

It is apparent that clients meet their self-care needs on the basis of their cultural and cohort backgrounds.[7] The present elderly population's health values have been significantly shaped by the Great Depression. However, by emphasizing the positive aspects of Depression-era health attitudes and using planned strategies of change, health care professionals can successfully assist the older adult population in dealing with their self-care needs.

▬ REFERENCES

1. Matarazzo JD, Weiss SM, Herd JA, Miller NE, Weiss SM, eds. Behavioral health. New York: John Wiley & Sons, 1984.
2. Wilson NL, Trost R. A family perspective on aging and health. Health Values. 1987;2(2):52–7.
3. Bendiner R. Just around the corner. New York: Rinehart & Co., 1967.
4. Mitchell B. Depression decade. New York: Rinehart & Co., 1947.
5. Garraty JA. The great depression. San Diego: Harcourt Brace Jovanovich Publishers, 1986.
6. Murray, RB, Zenter JP. Nursing assessment & health promotion through the life span. 3rd ed. Englewood Cliffs, N.J.: Prentice-Hall, 1985.
7. Orem DE. Nursing: concepts of practice. 4th ed. St. Louis: Mosby–Year Book, 1991.
8. Becker MH, Maiman LA. Sociobehavioral determinants of compliance with health and medical recommendations. Medical care, 13, 12. Philadelphia: JB Lippincott, 1973.
9. Feuerstein M, Labbe EE, Kuczmierczyk AR. Health psychology. New York: Plenum Press; 1986.
10. Dean K, Hickey T, Holstein BE, eds. Self-care and health in old age. London: Croom Helm, 1986.
11. Beck CM, Rawlins RP, Williams SR. Mental health-psychiatric nursing. St. Louis: CV Mosby, 1984.
12. Kondo AT, Foreyt JP. A family perspective on weight loss and maintenance: health values. New York 1987;2(2):47–52.
13. Gentry WD. Handbook of behavioral medicine. New York: Guilford Press, 1984.
14. Harper A. The health of populations. New York: Springer Publishing, 1986.
15. Gillett PA. Self-reported factors influencing exercise adherence in overweight women. Nurs Res 1988;37(1):25–9.
16. Ryan P. Strategies for motivating life-style change. Cardiovasc Nurs 1987;1(4):54–66.
17. Raths LE, Harmin M, Simon SB. Values and teaching: working with values in the classroom. Columbus, Ohio: Chas E Merrill, 1966.
18. Whitman NI, Graham BA, Gleit CJ, Boyd MD. Teaching in nursing practice, a professional model. East Norwalk, Conn.: 1992.

Chapter 11

Promoting the Sexual Health of Geriatric Patients

MOLLY T. LAFLIN

Health care providers are adept at assessing elders for medication use, sleep and dietary patterns, activity and mobility, and the amount, color, and consistency of all types of bodily fluids. However, when it comes to a client's sexual health, nurses and others fall short of even discussing sexual issues. In this chapter Dr. Molly Laflin presents 10 concepts needing to be understood by health care providers in order to promote the quality of life issues related to the sexuality of their clients. What is shared here will perhaps encourage nurses to develop the skills needed to provide holistic care, which includes promoting a client's sexual health.

At times the accepted behaviors of healing professionals seem difficult to rationalize to an outsider. For example, it can be argued that it seems odd that in an attempt to improve the health and quality of life of their patients, health care professionals hesitate to ask even the most basic questions about sexual practices, yet they seem perfectly at ease probing for information about medications ingested; sleep patterns; food consumed (variety and quantity); range of motion; ambulation; and amount, color, and consistency of all excretions (urine, fecal material, or pus). Why is this?

Few topics evoke so much distress and pleasure, agony and longing, communication and silence as the erotic possibilities of our bodies. Dealing with the sexuality of others is no less troublesome. Most of us experience some discomfort talking with patients about sexual matters. When it comes to older patients, many ease this discomfort by denying the need for such discussions. After all, older patients who have need of rehabilitation services certainly have lost all sexual competence and interest. If not, surely they must be perverted or mentally ill. Geriatric patients are generally old enough to be our parents or grandparents. Thinking of these patients as individuals with sexual feelings comes too close to thinking about our parents as sexual beings.

From *Topics in Geriatric Rehabilitation* 11(4):43–54, 1996. Reprinted with permission.

Such prejudice against older people neuters and dehumanizes them and diminishes their quality of life. It also portends a dismal, self-fulfilling prophecy for one's own sexual future. For to be prejudiced against an older person is to be prejudiced against one's future self.

The role of a rehabilitation specialist is to help patients learn to function at their optimal level despite physical or emotional setbacks. Although the focus of the treatment plan is the presenting symptoms, it is the patient as a whole who must be treated. It has been said that "If sexual behavior is integral to a person's lifestyle, then part of rehabilitation is enabling the patient to adapt sexually."[1(p367)] For the purposes of this article, *sexuality* encompasses the psychologic, physical, and social qualities that contribute to the subjective sense of oneself as a sexual being. There are 10 concepts that geriatric rehabilitation specialists should understand in order to address quality of life issues related to the sexuality of their patients:

1. Change is constant: we are evolving and adapting at every age.
2. Demographics affect sexual opportunities and expression.
3. Societal attitudes toward sex and aging influence patient sexual behaviors, as do the attitudes of health care workers.
4. As one ages there are predictable, normal physiologic changes in sexual functioning.
5. Sexual fitness does not mean "use it or lose it."
6. Sexual enhancement is possible at any age.
7. Sexual adaptations can be made to accommodate illness or injury.
8. Nursing homes and retirement homes present special problems as well as opportunities.
9. Rehabilitation specialists should develop a comfortable environment in which patients can discuss sexual issues.
10. Resources are available.

Each of these concepts is discussed separately in the text that follows.

▰CHANGE

Human development is, in part, the product of the interaction between individual needs and abilities and societal expectations. Many older people have a need for a good sexual relationship even though they must adapt to gradual physical and mental changes. "Age brings changes at 70 just as it does at 17. But you never outgrow your need for intimate love and affection."[2(p8)]

Although most men accept that they are no longer as strong (or fast) athletically as they were at a younger age, it is difficult for them to accept this same difference in their sexual performance. Older men want the quick response that they experienced in their youth. The fact is that erection rigidity peaks in the late teens and then gradually declines throughout adult life. The changes for women are not related as much to limited sexual response as they are to limited available partners. Due to the imbalance between the numbers of available women and available men, heterosexual

women may cease sexual activity or find outlets other than sexual intercourse. Unfortunately, cultural taboos often mitigate against choices other
than sexual expression with a male partner.

■ DEMOGRAPHICS

How do you define such terms as middle age, mature, aging, old, retirement
age, and geriatric? When I was in first grade, mature and old seemed
identical to me, and they were epitomized by eighth graders. A 40-year-old
woman told me recently that she was incensed when she visited her physician
and he told her that her gallbladder problem was common among middle-
aged people. "Middle aged," she said. "I'm not middle aged!" Clearly, as
we ourselves age, our concepts of these milestones shift. Membership in
the American Association of Retired Persons (AARP) can begin at age 50.
Hostel for older persons is available to 55-year-olds. Full Social Security
retirement benefits currently start at age 65. Most people agree that there
is considerable variability in development from ages 1 to 50, yet few people
blink when ages 51 through 100 are put in the same category. Certainly,
when considering sexual behavior and aging, it is important to distinguish
that sex for a 55-year-old is generally quite different from sex for a 95-year-
old individual.

Just what is sex, then? Unfortunately there is no simple answer. Freud
defined *sexual* as "improper, that which must not be mentioned."[3(p247)]
Most dictionaries define sex as biologic maleness and femaleness or physical
activity involving the genitals.[4] Most people define sex as heterosexual sexual
intercourse. Defining sex as intercourse obviously limits one's capacity for
sexual pleasure. A broader definition is needed to incorporate a wide variety
of erotic behaviors. Regardless of one's definition, when it comes to sex,
as in other areas, most people want to know if they are normal.

Surveys cannot tell us what is normal or erotic, but, with certain limitations, they can tell us the frequency of various behaviors and what practices
people say they enjoy. Most surveys indicate that sexual intercourse is the
preferred form of sexual expression. Andrew Greeley analyzed two surveys
involving 5,738 people and found that 37% of married people over age 60
have sex once a week or more, and 16% have sex several times a week.[5]
He also found that "The happiest men and women in America are married
people who continue to have sex frequently after they are 60. They are
also the most likely to report that they are living exciting lives."[5(p2)]

Most studies have found that although sexual activity persists in later
life, it is generally less frequent than among young people today. Because
of the limitations of the research it is unclear whether this difference is
due to aging itself or to a cohort effect. The best predictor of sexual patterns
in old age appears to be one's pattern of sexual activity in earlier years.[6]

Reliable data on the sexual practices of older lesbian and homosexual
men are scarce. Estimates of the percentage of homosexuals in the population are currently quite controversial and range from Kinsey's 10% (10%
of white males aged 16 to 55 reported that they had had predominantly gay
contacts for at least 3 years; only 4% said they were lifelong homosexuals) to

Battelle's 2.3% (2.3% reported homosexual contacts in the last 10 years; just over 1% of the total said they were exclusively gay in that period).[7]

Not everyone has the opportunity to maintain a sexually active life with a partner despite an interest in doing so. There are now 3.5 unmarried women over the age of 65 for each unmarried man in the same age range.[8] If all the unmarried men over age 65 were paired with women over the age of 65, there would still be over 7.5 million women without a partner. The problem is further exacerbated by the fact that older men are more likely than older women to choose younger partners.

Some sexologists have speculated that homosexuality might be the answer for the vast majority of women who are without a partner. However, as Cross indicates, "Sexual orientation, although potentially fluid throughout a life-span, is more complicated than the suggestion implies. While some women discover lesbian sexuality at an older age, it is rarely the result of a decrease in the availability of male partners."[9(p8)] In their survey of sex and sexuality in the mature years, Starr and Weiner[10] found that although 64% of their respondents believed that homosexuality was all right for those who choose it, the vast majority were not interested in seeking homosexuality as a personal life style. This same study found that even masturbation was taboo for many of their female respondents.[10]

▬SOCIETAL ATTITUDES

Hudson and colleagues[11] and Keller and associates[12] found that today's older people have a higher degree of sexual guilt, more conservative sexual attitudes, and more restricted sexual behaviors than today's youth. These attitudes, coupled with social pressures associating sexual attractiveness with youthful bodies and sexual activity with marriage, make it difficult for many older people to feel comfortable expressing their sexuality. The popular view of older people as impotent, devoid of sexual interest, and sexually nonfunctional becomes a self-fulfilling prophecy for many older people. Because human sexual response is highly sensitive to emotional and other psychologic processes, the sexual behavior of older people is likely to suffer as much or more from exposure to prevailing social attitudes as from physiologic changes.

Society's admonition to older people to "act their age" is, in fact, a demand that they stop listening to their bodies' needs to be touched, stroked, cuddled, and caressed. It is unbecoming to feel sexual, appropriate to feel ill. Interestingly, it is not uncommon for an older person who has complained about numerous physical ailments for years to stop complaining when he or she starts dating, falls in love, moves in with a lover, or marries.

Grown children of divorced and widowed older Americans often discourage their parents from behaving as sexual beings. Their feelings may stem from a Freudian discomfort with parental sexuality, fear of loss of inheritance if the parent remarries, aversion to change, jealousy at having to share a parent's time or attention, fear of eventually having to care for a new family member, or a sense of religious or moral outrage.

Like other older Americans, homosexuals and lesbians face illness, reduced income, loss of friends and family, and increased isolation as they age. Their needs are the same as the rest of the older population, but they may be less likely to risk rejection by asking for help. The death of a long-term companion is similar to the death of a marital partner. The grief process, pain, and feelings of loss and abandonment are the same; however, society often does not validate the experience because the relationship was not validated. There may be serious financial consequences for the remaining partner as well. Gay people often are frustrated in trying to plan their estates. Their families may not be supportive of their life styles, and state inheritance laws may present a major obstacle. Health benefits, retirement funds, Social Security, and even wills do not provide for the needs of the remaining partner.

It is important for rehabilitation specialists to examine their own attitudes about sex and aging because their attitudes undoubtedly will influence their patients. Denial of an older person's sexuality not only colludes with the ageism of society, but also makes it difficult to recognize and understand some of the dilemmas inherent in providing personal care services to older persons. For example, the sexual potential of close physical contact when assisting with dressing or bathing must be addressed.[13]

▬PHYSIOLOGIC CHANGES

Age-related physiologic changes appear gradually and generally can be accommodated. Health care workers should be familiar with these changes and with techniques that facilitate adapting behaviors to enhance sexual pleasure.

As men age they do not expect to run or walk a mile in the same time they did at age 18. They can also anticipate that their erections will be less frequent; take more time and direct stimulation to achieve; and be less firm, large, or straight. Ejaculations may come with a shorter warning period (or none at all), require more time, be less forceful, involve fewer contractions, and contain less semen. In fact, many older men report a decreased need to ejaculate, perhaps ejaculating every third sexual episode. The refractory period (the length of time that must pass after ejaculation and before stimulation to another climax) may lengthen from just a few minutes at age 17 to as much as 48 hours or more by age 70. Some men deal with this elongated refractory period by learning to experience orgasms without ejaculating, thus bypassing the refractory period. Sexual satisfaction for an older person can be as high or higher as in early adulthood.

For emotional as well as physical reasons, some women find menopause to be distressing, others find it liberating. Changes in sexual functioning tend to develop during this time and are primarily the result of a decline in female hormones. Vaginal lubrication takes longer. The lining of the vagina thins, and the vaginal barrel is reduced in length and width. The vagina, bladder, and urethra become more susceptible to irritation. A reduction in the acidity of vaginal secretions increases the likelihood of vaginal infections. The amount of pubic hair decreases, the labia majora loses fullness, the clitoris decreases in size, and the clitoral hood atrophies, as does the fat pad over the mons. The orgasmic and resolution phases are shorter in duration. However, the capacity for multiple orgasms remains.

An understanding of normal sexual aging may help patients decrease their anxiety and enhance their sexual enjoyment. For example, if an aging male realizes that his lack of instant responsiveness to his partner or his sluggishness in reaching orgasm is normal, he is less likely to develop secondary impotence or blame himself or his partner. For women, decreased female lubrication should be expected and is not a signal that sexual behavior is no longer appropriate. Vaginal dryness can easily be rectified by using saliva, a water-based lubricant, or, after consultation with a physician, hormone replacement therapy (HRT). Many of the other age-related sexual changes (e.g., vaginal elasticity and integrity) can be rectified with HRT, and HRT also reduces bone loss (osteoporosis) and protects against heart disease and onset of Alzheimer's disease. For these reasons and more, some view estrogen, America's number one selling prescription drug, as an "elixir of youth." However, estrogen replacement therapy has recently been associated with various cancers, most notably, breast cancer.[14] Women must consult with their physicians and carefully weigh the benefits and risks when making the choice to use or not use HRT.

◼SEXUAL FITNESS

"Use it or lose it" is a catchy phrase, but in this context it can easily be misunderstood. While it is possible that age-related genital changes (e.g., decreased lubrication or thinning vaginal tissues) may tend to be less pronounced in those who are sexually active (masturbation or intercourse), a period of abstinence, however long and for whatever reason (e.g., lack of partner, illness, boredom), does not doom one to permanent celibacy. In addition, there is ample evidence that the old adage, "You can't teach an old dog new tricks" does not apply to sex and the older person. As with any form of fitness, however, a resumption of activity and achieving one's full sexual potential may require some practice.

◼SEXUAL ENHANCEMENT

It is important to recognize that not all people, young or old, wish to be sexually active. For some people the power of touch can be a healing antidote to frustration, the pain of physical or emotional losses, the threat of loneliness, and fears of reduced income or an unclear purpose in life. However, older people who never enjoyed sex in their youth will probably use aging as an excuse to stop engaging in sexual behavior. Boredom, overeating, marital problems, and heavy alcohol use are all associated with low levels of sexual activity.

Some older couples find renewed love, intimacy, and sexual vitality in their retirement years. They have better communication, more understanding and tolerance of each other, increased leisure time, relaxed roles, and less stress. In their study of sex in the mature years, Starr and Weiner[10] received overwhelmingly positive responses to questions about sexual enjoyment. Here are some of the responses:

Male, married, age 69: Sex is one of the pleasures of life. It is also one way in which men and women overcome loneliness and frustration. There's the added pleasure as we grow older, we can still enjoy sex.[10(p37)]

Female, married, age 65: It's a natural way to ease the loneliness inherent in being an individual. It feels good and now I learned it's good for arthritis.[10(p37)]

While sexual pleasure is enhanced with aging for some people, others face obstacles to sexual fulfillment. Lack of a partner probably accounts for discontinuance of sexual activity in many older people, but illness also steals the sex lives of many more. Forty percent of Americans aged 65 and older have activity limitation, and 24% have major activity limitation.[8] Losses and limitations must be acknowledged, but it is important to focus on what is possible. For many people the key to maintaining personal sexual fulfillment is the ability to adjust old patterns to meet ongoing changes. Attitudes and practices that increase sexual participation include:

- Understanding normal changes associated with aging.
- Increasing communication on nonsexual topics as well as improving communication of sexual feelings and preferences.
- Not hurrying. Enjoying each moment. Decreasing performance anxiety.
- Using sexual positions (such as side lying or sitting) that do not require support of the body on isometrically contracted arm muscles.
- Using sexual positions that do not put pressure on joints or areas prone to pain or muscle strain.
- Using Kegel exercises to improve muscle tone and to achieve more vigorous vaginal contractions during sexual activity. (Men can benefit from Kegel exercises because they improve bladder and rectal strength.) Kegel exercises should be performed several times a day by contracting the pubococcygeal muscle 20 to 30 times. Kegel exercises can best be described as pretending to hold back from urinating and defecating.
- Practicing oral–genital stimulation.
- Stimulating partner's genital area digitally.
- Using a vibrator alone or with a partner.
- Masturbating alone or as part of sexual activity with a partner.
- Consulting a physician concerning treatment for impotence. Treatment options include psychologic intervention; inflatable, flexible and semirigid prostheses; injection therapy; or a vacuum constriction device.
- Using a technique called "stuffing," in which the penis is stuffed into the vagina before a full erection is obtained. The penis will often become more erect as a result of the stimulation of being inside the vagina.
- Exploring the pleasures of touch and massage. Use of creams and massage oil can be fun. A deemphasis on intercourse can be pleasurable for both men and women and can decrease performance anxiety for men.
- Using a water-soluble lubricant during sexual intercourse or masturbation. Some women prefer vegetable oil because it lasts longer.

- Engaging in fantasizing, reminiscing, hugging, kissing, stroking, talking, and laughing.
- Living a healthy life style: get plenty of rest (and plan a time of day for sex when feeling rested and relaxed), exercise moderately, take precautions against sexually transmitted diseases, do not smoke, eat, or drink excessively (wait 3 to 4 hours after eating a large meal or drinking alcohol before having sex, have no more than one drink on days when having sex).
- Be imaginative and romantic (lighting, clothing, flowers, locations, music, travel, compliments). Purchase and use a book offering romantic tips (e.g., *A Husband's Little Black Book* by Robert J. Ackerman, *1001 Ways to Be Romantic* by J. P. Godek).
- Show respect by paying attention to personal hygiene and grooming (bathing, shaving, and so forth) and taking care to make one's partner feel attractive.[1]

SEXUAL ADAPTATIONS

Rose and Soares[13] have developed eight patterns of sexual adaptation to aging, ranging from accommodation (modifications in sexual behavior between partners to accommodate changes in health and functioning) to revitalization (increased sexual activity after years of sexual inactivity). The focus in this section will be on accommodation.

Sexual concerns for chronically ill patients can range from chronic fatigue and pain to fear of rejection. Men are likely to deny sexual desire when disease impairs erections. Women are most vulnerable to illnesses or surgeries that affect their appearance.[15] In this society where sexual desirability is based on physical attractiveness, a chronic illness can be devastating to self-confidence.

There are several excellent sources of information on sexual adaptations to specific illnesses or injuries. It is not within the purview of this article to cover this material in detail. However, the following list contains answers to the most common questions about sex and illness:

- A patient who can comfortably climb one or two flights of stairs or take a brisk walk around the block is ready to resume sexual activity — usually 4 to 5 weeks after a coronary attack.
- The likelihood of a heart attack during sex is very small. Deaths during coitus account for 0.6% of all sudden deaths; of these, 80% occurred during intercourse with an extramarital partner.[16]
- Although arthritis may limit some forms of sexual behavior, there is evidence that regular sexual activity decreases the effects of the arthritis and decreases stress as well.
- Timing sexual activity around a pain medication schedule so that pain is not a limiting factor can increase sexual participation.
- If nudity causes self-consciousness or discomfort for the cancer survivor, suggest avoiding positions in which the partner looks directly at a scar.
- Emphasize stimulation of areas that are still sensitive to touch.

▪ Most prostatectomy patients recover from surgery within a couple of months and are fully able to resume sexual activity.

▪ Approximately 25% of sexual problems in men are caused or complicated by medications.[17(p1737)] Tranquilizers, antidepressants, and some high blood pressure medications can cause impotence; other medications can lead to reduced sexual desire or impaired ejaculation.

▬NURSING HOMES AND RETIREMENT HOMES

Approximately 7 million people used some form of long-term care in 1990.[18] By the year 2040, the number of people requiring these services may increase to 18 million. Approximately one third of the people who require long-term care live in an institutional setting. Sex complicates things in an institutional setting, and a sex history is rarely taken as part of the activities of daily living (ADL) assessment or medical history.

Most nursing home procedures are designed to facilitate a smooth operation and to meet the needs and desires of staff and families rather than to please the patients. In most cases, staff discomfort, customs, rules, and lack of privacy severely inhibit sexual expression by residents. Occasionally patients act out sexually. Wiggling out of bed clothes, soiling oneself, or touching others may be a ploy by a lonely, touch-deprived patient to receive touch. However, the patient is often punished instead of nurtured, and becomes further depressed and lonely.[19]

Steffl[19] suggests that caregivers can redirect inappropriate sexual expression to more healthy outlets by

▪ providing more human touch;
▪ providing touching and feeling objects (yarn, prayer beads, stuffed animals) to handle;
▪ accepting and allowing masturbation;
▪ bringing live pets into the setting and allowing residents to handle them;
▪ providing more music;
▪ encouraging opportunities for opposite sexes to meet, mingle, and spend time together;
▪ providing double beds for married couples;
▪ counseling families about sexual needs of older people; and
▪ developing a bill of rights for sexual freedom in their facility.

Personnel in long-term care facilities need to examine their attitudes, values, and beliefs regarding aging and sexuality. To be effective in helping older people who seek counseling on sexual concerns, they need to be alert to their own nonverbal messages. Steffl[19] suggests that the professional should assess his or her skill level in initiating communication, observing verbal and nonverbal cues, and creating an atmosphere conducive to discussion of sexual concerns.

Staff should bear in mind that intimacy is an important component for most people's quality of life. Intimacy brings people together to give and receive affection. Close relationships with family and friends can provide rewarding opportunities for nonsexual intimacy. Although sexual intimacy is not the only form of physical intimacy, for many older people sexual intimacy remains an important part of expressing love.

ROLE OF REHABILITATION SPECIALISTS

Sexual health assessment should be included in the ADL assessment of all patients, married or unmarried. Unmarried or gay patients, fearing staff disapproval, may be even more hesitant to bring up sexual concerns than married clients.

It is important for health care workers to examine personal attitudes and beliefs about aging and sexuality. Professionals should ask themselves the following questions: Are you comfortable discussing the sexual concerns of your patients, particularly as they relate to the disability you are treating? Can you give necessary sexual information without being judgmental? Are you comfortable providing emotional support, procuring lubrication, scheduling a needed medical examination, or facilitating privacy for frail older persons who have opportunities and desires for sexual activity? Are you too embarrassed to inquire about the sexual concerns of your patients because you believe "old people do not like to talk about something they do not do any more"? Are you like the medical student at a lecture on sex and aging who asked, "How can I tell an older male patient to be excited about his wife when I think how unexciting it must be to think of and see flabby breasts, an unshapely body, and an old face? I wonder how it will be in 30 years when I feel that way about my wife, and how will she feel about me?"[10(p3)]

One way to approach the subject is to ask questions or include comments about sexual function in matter-of-fact discussions of overall health status, raising more specific concerns as necessary. Another approach is to ask the patient if he or she has any questions or would like to discuss sexual adjustments necessitated by the injury or illness. An example would be, "Do you have any sexual concerns related to your arthritis?"

Sometimes patients just need basic sexual information or "permission" to behave as sexual beings. Other patients may need a referral to a urologist, gynecologist, or a therapist certified by the American Association of Sex Educators, Counselors, and Therapists. Acknowledge whatever feelings the patient expresses (e.g., fear, embarrassment, loneliness, anger at sexual losses) and avoid patronizing statements about how wonderful they "should" feel about their condition. Such "pep talks" are usually delivered with the best of intentions, but can come across as insensitive and condescending.

RESOURCES

The appendix lists resources that can help build a strong base of information for dealing with the multitude of issues facing older persons. By understanding these issues, quality of life, including sexual health, will be easier to promote.

The role of a geriatric rehabilitation specialist is to help patients acquire the skills to function optimally despite physical setbacks. Although the focus of the treatment plan is the presenting symptoms, it is the patient as a whole person who must be treated. Geriatric rehabilitation specialists are in a unique position to enhance the quality of life of their patients by conveying a humanistic, pleasure-oriented view of sexual adjustment to aging and illness. Whether patients seek intimacy through companionship and non-sexual touching or through various forms of sexual activity, human touch is a powerful healer.

▬REFERENCES

1. Laflin MT. Sexuality and the elderly. In: Lewis CB, ed. *Aging: The Health Care Challenge.* Philadelphia, Pa: F.A. Davis; 1996.
2. Sexuality and aging: what it means to be sixty or seventy or eighty in the '90s. *Mayo Clin Health Let.* 1993;February:1–8.
3. Freud SA. The sexual life of man. In: Riviere J, trans. *Introductory lectures on psychoanalysis.* London: Heron Books; 1970:247.
4. Masters WH, Johnson VE, Kolodny RC. *Human Sexuality.* New York, NY: HarperCollins College Publishers; 1995.
5. Greeley A. *Sex After Sixty: A Report.* Chicago, Ill: National Opinion Research Center; 1992.
6. George LK, Weiler SJ. Sexuality in middle and late life. *Arch Gen Psychiatry.* 1981;38: 919–923.
7. Billy JOG, Tanfer K, Grady WR, Klepinger DH. The sexual behavior of men in the United States. *Fam Plan Perspect.* 1993;25:52–60.
8. US Department of Commerce, Bureau of the Census. *Marital Status and Living Arrangements: March 1993.* Washington, DC: Government Printing Office; 1994.
9. Cross RJ. What doctors and others need to know. *SIECUS Rep.* 1993;21(5):7–9.
10. Starr BD, Weiner MB. *The Starr-Weiner Report on Sex and Sexuality in the Mature Years.* New York, NY: McGraw-Hill; 1981.
11. Hudson WH, Murphy GJ, Nurius PS. A short-form scale to measure liberal vs conservative orientations toward sexual expression. *J Sex Res.* 1983;19:258–272.
12. Keller JF, Eakes E, Hinkle D, Hughston GA. Sexual behavior and guilt among women: a cross-generational comparison. *J Sex Marital Ther.* 1978;4:259–265.
13. Rose MK, Soares HH. Sexual adaptations of the frail elderly: a realistic approach. *J Gerontol Social Work.* 1993;19:167–178.
14. Colditz GA, Hankinson SE, Hunter DJ, et al. The use of estrogens and progestins and the risk of breast cancer in postmenopausal women. *N Engl J Med.* 1995;332:1589–1593.
15. Schover LR, Jenson SB. *Sexuality and Chronic Disease: A Comprehensive Approach.* New York, NY: Guilford; 1988.
16. Dagon EM. Sexuality and sexual dysfunction in the elderly. In: Lazarus LW, Jarvik LF, Foster JR, Lieff JD, Mershon SR, eds. *Essentials of Geriatric Psychiatry: A Guide for Health Professionals.* New York, NY: Springer; 1988.
17. Slag MF, Morley JE, Elson MK, et al. Impotence in medical clinic outpatients. *JAMA.* 1983;249(13):1736–1740.
18. Williams ME. *The American Geriatrics Society's Complete Guide to Aging and Health.* New York, NY: Crown Publishers; 1995.
19. Steffl BM. Sexuality and aging: implications for nurses and other helping professionals. In: Solnick RL, ed. *Sexuality and Aging.* Los Angeles, Calif: University of Southern California Press; 1978.

▬APPENDIX RESOURCES

Al-Anon Family Groups, PO Box 862, Midtown Station, New York, NY 10019. Telephone: (212) 302-7240. This national organization publishes information that is helpful to both alcoholics and their family members.

Alcoholics Anonymous (AA), General Services Board, 468 Park Avenue South, New York, NY 10016. Telephone: (212) 686-1100. AA publishes information that is helpful to both alcoholics and their family members.

Alzheimer's Association, 70 E Lake Street, Suite 600, Chicago, IL 60601. Telephone: (800) 572-6037.

American Association of Retired Persons (AARP), 601 E Street, NW, Washington, DC 20049. Telephone: (202) 434-2277. Single copies of the booklets *Divorce After 50: Challenges and Choices* and *On Being Alone* are available at no cost.

American Cancer Society. Telephone: (800) ACS-2345 to reach your state organization.

American Diabetes Association, 1660 Duke Street, Alexandria, VA 22314. Telephone: (800) ADA-DISC. Single copies of *Impotence* are available for a nominal fee.

American Heart Association, 7272 Greenville Avenue, Dallas, TX 75231. Telephone: (214) 373-6300. Single copies of *Sex and Heart Disease* are available at no cost.

American Urological Association, 1120 N Charles Street, Baltimore, MD 21201. Telephone: (410) 727-1100. This organization is committed to combating urologic disease and improving the standards and practice of urology for urologists and their patients.

Arthritis Foundation, PO Box 19000, Atlanta, GA 30326. Telephone: (800) 283-7800. Single copies of *Living and Loving: Information About Sex* are available at no cost.

American Association of Sex Educators, Counselors, and Therapists (AASECT), 435 N Michigan Avenue, Suite 1717, Chicago, IL 60611. Telephone: (312) 644-0828. This association will provide a registry of members by city and state and a copy of the Code of Ethics for Sex Therapists.

Impotence Foundation, PO Box 60260, Santa Barbara, CA 93160. Telephone: (800) 221-5517. The foundation is a national information service run by a maker of penile prostheses.

Impotence Information Center, Department USA, PO Box 9, Minneapolis, MN 55440. Telephone: (800) 843-4315. This center is run by a maker of penile prostheses.

National AIDS Hotline. Telephone: (800) 342-AIDS, (800) SIDA (Spanish language), (800) AIDS-TTY (hearing impaired).

National Cancer Institute, National Institutes of Health. Telephone: (800) 4-CANCER. The Cancer Information Service can answer many questions about prevention and treatment and will send you a copy of its helpful booklet. *Diet, Nutrition, and Cancer Prevention: A Guide to Food Choices.*

National Institute on Aging (NIA), Building 31, Room 5C35, Bethesda, MD 20205. The NIA has a list of free and low-cost publications that describe exercise programs, nutrition, and aging.

Senior Action in a Gay Environment (SAGE), 208 W 13th Street, New York, NY 10011. Telephone: (212) 741-2247. SAGE was established to advocate for high-quality, professional help for gay and lesbian seniors. SAGE is the prime resource for national and local print and broadcast media seeking information and background on issues affecting older gay Americans.

Widowed Persons Service, American Association of Retired Persons (AARP), 601 E Street, NW, Washington, DC 20049. Telephone: (202) 434-2277.

Chapter 12

A Heideggerian Hermeneutical Analysis of Older Women's Stories of Being Strong

MARGARET F. MOLONEY

Margaret Moloney explores the quality of older women's lived experiences in this study of women's stories recalling examples of being strong. Three patterns of strength emerged that can help female nurses better understand themselves and their female clients. The patterns of survival, finding strength, and gathering the memories . . . seeing the patterns, emerged from the analysis of the 12 participant's stories. The exercise of visualizing and verbalizing examples of one's strength is an empowering experience that can potentiate the health of older women and men. Using this story telling technique and analysis has potential for nurses to develop an appreciation of older adults. It assists nurses to look beyond stereotypical expectations and toward new visions of caregiving.

Historically, research specifically focused on women has tended to perpetuate the stereotypical view of women as sick and weak. Normal life events such as menopause have been treated as disease states (MacPherson, 1992). Studies of older women have often focused on those in nursing homes, ignoring the 95% of older women who lead active, independent lives (McElmurry & Librizzi, 1986). Research that does emphasize women's health has centered primarily on women's maternal roles, viewing women solely in terms of their reproduction (Duffy, 1985; Dunbar, Patterson, Burton, & Stuckert, 1981; Woods, 1982, 1988). Therefore, it is not surprising that nurses, physicians, and psychologists, among others, have used male-centered models to focus on women's illnesses and "weaknesses," rather than on women's strengths.

To state that women can be strong is a contradiction in terms, given the historical images of women (Cixous, 1980; de Beauvoir, 1974). However, feminists have begun to create alternative definitions of "woman." De Beauvoir (1974) described woman as "becoming," not as a static creature

From *Image* 27(2):104–109, 1995. Reprinted with permission.

but as one who changes and grows. Kristeva (1980) and Cixous (1980) asserted that a rigid model of a woman is impossible. Hooks (1984) reminded us that when we say woman, we must ask, "Which woman?" Daly (1978, 1987) urged women to celebrate such negative labels as "spinster" and "crone," and use these names to create new strong images of women. Other researchers have begun to uncover the stories of women who have created lives that defy the traditional images of womanhood (Bateson, 1989; Heilbrun, 1988, 1990; Luttrell, 1989; The Personal Narratives Group, 1989; Robinson, 1985). These stories have the potential to provide other women with positive models of life experience and effectiveness.

A fundamental assumption underlying this study was the belief that all women in our culture possess the potential for inner strength; that this quality of inner strength is developed through living in the world into which they are born; and that inner strength varies from woman to woman depending on her life experiences. The purpose of this study was to discover some of the possible meanings of inner strength in women's lives. The inquiry sought to elicit older women's stories about times in their lives that exemplified meanings of "being strong."

■ BACKGROUND

The term "women's inner strength" has been used in at least one study (Rose, 1990) and has its foundations in other work (Belenky, Clinchy, Goldberger, & Tarule, 1986; Gilligan, 1982; Miller, 1986). Miller (1986) stated that women begin to perceive forms of strength based on their life experiences. However, Heilbrun (1988, 1990) concluded that it is difficult for women to learn how to live rich independent lives if they do not have role models. Recent research focusing on women's lives and experiences may provide women with new models. Five studies of women's lives provide stories of women's inner strength. Rose (1990) analyzed the stories of nine mostly European-American, well-educated, relatively young women. This phenomenologic study focused on these women's perceptions of their inner strength, identifying such qualities as centering, introspecting, and embracing vulnerability. Connors (1986) conducted a fascinating exploration of the lives of six elderly Irish-American women who believed that their stories were not worth telling. *A Woman of the Land* is an ethnographic portrait of an elderly Australian woman (King, 1989) who made her life by relying on herself. The meaning of spiritual well-being in the lives of 13 European-American Appalachian women was explored by Barker (1989). Finally, Bateson (1989) used her life and the lives of four of her women friends to illustrate the ways in which "composing a life" is like using seemingly disconnected threads to create a tapestry.

■ METHOD

Heideggerian hermeneutic phenomenology was the research method used to gather and analyze the data. Heidegger (1962) believed that people are all situated in the world and that their understanding of the world comes from their experiences within the world. Heidegger's approach, which is well-suited to an examination of the meaning of women's lives, was used to identify some common patterns of meaning among the experiences of a group of older women.

Participants were sought who were 65 years or older. People who were physically or mentally infirm were excluded from the study (for example, women who were bedridden or who had a health condition that interfered with communication or the ability to reflect thoughtfully). A total of 12 women, 5 African-American and 7 European-American, was recruited and interviewed throughout 1993. Two of the participants were women I knew slightly; the other 10 were referred by friends, colleagues, and other research participants. Nine of the women were widowed and two were never married. One participant had been divorced earlier in her life, was married at the beginning of the study but became widowed during the study. The participants were 65 to 87 years of age. Education ranged from completion of the seventh grade to a doctoral degree, with the majority having completed 12 grades of high school.

Interviews were conducted in person with 11 of the participants. Because the twelfth lived in another state, interviews with her were conducted by telephone. This woman also sent me stories of her life which she had written earlier. I read these stories before we began the first phone interview. Followup interviews were conducted with 9 of the 12 participants.

A letter describing the research project and a copy of the consent form were sent to most of the participants following an initial phone contact, before the first interview. In several cases, there was not sufficient time between the phone contact and first interview to send these papers. In these cases, the project and consent form were described in detail on the phone and again in person. Most of the interviews took place in participants' homes. Many of the women made coffee; several offered coffee cake or cookies. I took something with me to one or the other of the interviews, usually flowers. During the initial visit, before we began the actual interview, the other woman and I spent some time getting to know each other. I then began the interview by saying, "Tell me a story, a time you'll never forget, about being strong." Some women had notes which they had prepared. Several had talked with their children about which stories to tell me. Often I was shown pictures, high school yearbooks, paintings, or framed awards. The interviews averaged about 1.5 hours, with very few pauses between stories. Each interview was transcribed, reviewed, and analyzed before the second interview took place; the transcript was also sent to the respective participant for her review before the second interview. During the second interview, the participant shared her corrections and editing with me, told new stories, and provided feedback on my initial analysis.

The data were analyzed using the circular hermeneutic process described by Heidegger (1959) and explicated by Diekelmann, Allen, and Tanner (1989). I read each new transcript, first trying to gain a sense of the overall meaning of the stories, and then wrote a short summary of the interview. Following this, I went line-by-line through the transcripts to identify the themes, gradually grouping these into larger themes. As this analysis proceeded, I also conducted first interviews with other women and transcribed those. During this time, I was also engaged in group analysis of the interview data with members of my research team, a group of qualitative nurse researchers whose assistance enhanced credibility, provided consensual validation, and helped in grouping the themes into larger constitutive patterns.

▬ FINDINGS

The constitutive patterns, and the themes that comprised the patterns, emerged for me from the participants' words. The three constitutive patterns that emerged were: "Surviving," "Finding strength," and "Gathering the memories . . . Seeing the patterns."

In most of the interviews, participants began by talking about times that were difficult and then went on to describe their perceptions of the origin of their strength to survive the hard times. Finally, they reflected on what telling the story actually meant and reviewed the meanings of their stories in the context of their whole lives.

Surviving

Four major themes reflected the women's stories of survival. These themes were "Living with loss," "Living through hard times," "Being different," and "Putting it behind you."

All the women told stories of having lost people they loved. They also talked about the loss of a home or sometimes the loss of a way of being. In addition, the stories reflected the losses these older women faced as they began to experience the necessity of learning to live with the limitations of aging: loss of bodily function, loss of family and friends, and the possible imminent loss of home.

Often the stories of loss were the first ones told in the interview, and usually involved the loss of a mate or family member. Ophelia told of how she felt when she heard that her mother had died. She said:

> *I almost fainted that night. I was standing and he caught me, 'cause I would have hit the porch. . . . As I said, the first time I'd ever had a death. And it just struck me, that's my mother.*

Many of the stories of survival involved living through hard times. All the women had memories of the Great Depression of the 1930s, as well as World War II in the 1940s, and in some cases, World War I. In addition to their all having memories of not having enough, there were frequent stories of coping with a government bureaucracy that made the experience even more difficult.

Jane, who is now 87, was a young adult during the years of the Depression. She talked about what it was like to live through that time. She and her husband had gone to work in Detroit. When all the automobile factories closed, they moved back to the Midwest to be near their families. She said:

> *We sold all our furniture in Detroit in order to have money to come back here. . . . We just got the bare necessities that we had to have, you know, to live*

in this little place. It was a nice little place, and lo and behold, we couldn't make any payments, so what did the furniture company do but come and took everything out of our house . . . except one company left the washing machine because they knew that we had a child, you know . . . well, it just happened at that time when [our daughter] died, so they left that . . . even took the linoleum off the floor. . . .

The women who were European-American had a difficult time surviving the economic shortages of the Great Depression. Going to college was difficult or impossible for women then because of the lack of resources and because women were frequently not admitted to universities. But for African-American women facing the added oppression of racism, the struggle was even more difficult.

All the women told stories that demonstrated how being female, or being African-American, or, in some cases, being Southern created constraints in their lives that limited their choices or actually created hardships. For the African-American women, the difficulty they faced because they were female was compounded by racial oppression.

Merrell reminisced about her memories of growing up as the stepdaughter of an African-American sharecropper. She remembered:

They weren't making anything. He worked on this farm so hard, and then in the fall when the harvest time come around, you really hadn't made anything . . . because you were sharecropping. . . . By the time the White man would take out for the expenses for your farm, and then he had to take your part out of that. And that left you hardly with anything. And you just only had a little money to go shopping once a year for clothes, or things like that. And so it were hard.

She went on to say:

For my father, if he had been a White man, he would have been making more, and maybe I wouldn't have had to drop out of school to help support the family. . . . Well, now the true part of it . . . it's always harder for Black women. It's harder for Blacks. . . . I had wanted to attend school longer, but I did not, because I had to start work, to help my stepfather.

Woven through the stories of grief, loss, hardship, and oppression were the women's philosophies of survival. All the women talked about putting difficulties behind, looking forward, and moving on. Jane talked about what it was like to move into her own apartment at the age of 70, away from her daughter. Throughout her stories, one could see how she moved forward, having the courage to make changes, and not looking backward: "So I just said, 'Well, this is it, a change, but I think it's going to be for the better.'"

Finding Strength

The women in this study clearly described their inner strength as a quality that developed out of the experiences of their lives. The hard times and losses were times in which they had to be strong, but it was the everyday events of living in the world that strengthened them. Throughout the stories, there were common themes about the process of finding strength:

"Being close to others," "Drawing strength from others," "Being at home," and "Feeling good about myself."

A meaningful part of the lives of all these women was their relationships with other people. The women reminisced about relationships with parents, siblings, husbands, and friends. They told stories of raising children, caring for others, and getting along with family members. They also gave examples of others who had helped them to be strong. Frequently these stories were about learning by example from elders. Many of the stories were about mothers and grandmothers. Marjorie told me about her granddaughter, who is caring for her congenitally ill infant:

> *I know [my granddaughter] asked her Dad recently, 'Where do I get the strength to go through this?' And he says, 'You've got a grandmother and great-grandmother that you are following.'*

Lugene told me about an older woman she knew, whose words helped her when her husband died and she was planning the funeral.

> *One thing stuck in my mind, I just love to sit around old people and hear them talk. You get a lot of wisdom from them. . . . When [Aunt Sue's husband] died, when somebody would come in the door, she would say, 'Oooh. . . .' and she would break down, and then she'd push open that door and she said, 'Li'l Jean, you cry with one eye open and the other shut because you got to watch everything when your husband dies.' That never left me. . . . But what she was doing, she was keeping her eye on everything. . . . I remember when we stayed in the country, people would come and that's when they would steal and take things from you. . . .*

Many of the women described having found strength through their faith in God. Many grew up in households that were religious, where prayer was a way of life. Endy said, "I came from a very religious family . . . and it seems my mother was always on her knees."

People experience the world as a home and the making of a home is a distinctively human way of being (Heidegger, 1971). Although a house may be a home, there are times when one is not at home in her own house, and times when one is most at home with other people. The women talked of being at home with others and of losing their homes when their family and friends were gone.

There were stories of leaving home, of losing one's home, of staying home, and of coming home. Throughout all these stories was woven the desire to create a safe, comfortable place in which to dwell. The theme of creating a home was a thread that ran throughout the narratives. Often the women talked about how their mothers and grandmothers had kept the home together, providing for children and instilling responsibility and values. Many of the women described making homes for their mothers or grandmothers or of having taken others into their homes. Ophelia told a story of "tricking" her mother so as to get her to move into Ophelia's house and Endy remembered her sister buying a larger house to accommodate her dead sister's children.

Throughout the narratives, there were stories that reflected the women's pride in their accomplishments, in their lives outside the home, and in the care they had given to their children and other family members. Edith told stories of what it had been like to be a nurse educator when it was thought that nurses did not need college education. She talked about continuing to fight uphill battles for this and of how she thought the work she did was a part of God's plan.

Others described the pride they felt in their current appearance, their independence, and their ability to take care of themselves. Following Julia's hospitalization, she was moved to a nursing home. She said:

> *Then they sent me for 2 weeks to [a nursing home]. And my doctor said, 'Oh, she'll never go back up to [her apartment building].' Both times now, he said that! So when I went to see him, I said, 'I fooled ya, didn't I!' [laughs]. . . . They thought I wasn't gonna be able to do anything when I got back.*

Several of the women told stories of how they had had to be the strong one in their families. In this story, Ophelia was telling about what happened after the death of her mother.

> *And my baby sister was here but she depended on me. She said, 'Ophelia, what we gonna do about so and so, what we gonna do about so and so?' WE meant ME! What was I gonna do. So I said, 'I'm gonna wait;' I said, 'Now I don't believe in calling the undertaker too quick and I'm gonna wait. . . .'*

This constitutive pattern, "Finding strength," is composed of all the strands of everyday life that gave these women strength. The connectedness with others that is embodied in the theme "Being close to others," the strength drawn from other people or from religious faith, the strength found in being at home in the world, and the pride of feeling good about one's self, are all characteristics that enabled these women to find strength in themselves.

Gathering the Memories. . . . Seeing the Patterns

The process of telling the stories was a pattern in itself. As the women told stories of their lives, they reflected on what it all meant, and frequently made it clear that they were able to see the meaning only now, in looking back. For many of the women, telling these stories enabled them to reflect on their lives but it was also a way of passing on their stories. A number of the women shared transcripts and tapes with their children. One participant edited the transcript to give to her daughter. The themes that emerged included: "Telling my story," "Having regrets," "Living today," "Knowing my strength," and "Looking back over."

Although in many cases, the stories were about experiences that had occurred more than 20 years earlier, the details were clear and complete. The richness of these details reflected what Heidegger called "the nearness of the far," the experience we have of being taken in our memories or imagination to a place which may be far away in time or space. The details of the stories are also part of what makes the narrative a story. They give form and substance to the memory, so that, in the sharing of the story, the listener is also transported.

The narratives were characterized by poetry, colorful detail, and humor. In this story of Eleanor's, she talked about life with her grandparents.

Grandma dressed us as she probably did her own children. I wore a Ferris waist with buttons sewed all around the waistline. On this were buttoned long knit drawers, a flannel petticoat and an embroidered white petticoat. Our hygiene consisted of a 'hot wash' from a basin of water warmed in a tank on the kitchen stove, set up on a chair. We were ensured privacy for this function and always admonished to 'Wash behind our ears.'

Finally, the storytellers expressed their feelings and thoughts about the meaning of having told the stories. Merrell, who edited her transcript before our second interview, wanted to have a copy for her daughter because, "I never told my daughter, really, about all these things." For Mabel, as well as some of the other women, telling these stories was an emotional outlet.

The storytelling was also a way to examine life. One of the outcomes of this examination for the women was being able to express regret. This regret was an expression of the understanding that life, and the decisions made in life, had not been perfect. In spite of their regrets, the women all expressed a philosophic attitude that, "What's done is done." Mabel said: "There are some things I would do differently if I had to go back over and do it again. But, basically, I didn't do too badly. I've had a long life and a good life."

As the women reflected on their lives, they invariably began to make comparisons between the way things should be, and the way things actually are. Most of the women were eager to convey their perceptions of changes that they thought should be made in society. This critique usually accompanied details about their present lives, including where and how they now live, their relationships with others, and how they stay involved with the rest of the world. Loneliness was often a theme, the result of the losses of aging.

Throughout the narratives, the women talked about being strong, the meaning of strength, whether they actually possessed strength, what it is like not to have strength, and how their own strength developed. Almost all the women clearly stated they were strong. Merrell, in the opening statement of the narrative she prepared beforehand, said it this way: "I want to talk to you about some of the things I have experienced in my life that have made me strong." When I asked Mary, a very traditional woman who was a housewife all her life, if she considered herself a strong woman, she answered: "I think I consider myself strong. If I want to do something, I do it. . . . Whenever I do something, I know before I do it that I can do it."

Julia and Eleanor both told me initially that they were not strong. However, later, in the midst of telling me a story about how she had had to be strong, Eleanor said, "But I was just normal." I said, "So being strong is normal?" She replied, "Yes. You do what you have to do, and that's all there is to it. There's no way you can back out once you put your shoulder to the wheel."

I asked several of the women if they thought that there was a difference between women's strength and men's strength. Virginia described women's strength as having to do with "the intuitive part of living." Marjorie concurred.

It's a different type of strength. More a silent strength. Not a macho one. Men's is usually more on the macho side . . . although there are some amazing men in their strength, what they do. . . . Men usually broadcast it a little bit more.

Toward the end of the interviews, most of the women engaged in a summing-up and took a clear look at the present. Several of the women expressed their feelings about dying or about losing their independence. There was usually an expression of having come to peace, of accepting the way things had been in the past and feeling comfortable about the future. Virginia expressed her impressions of her life as a whole, saying, "The high moments and the low moments blend together into a fabric of your life. . . ."

For most of the women, there was a sense that events in their lives had been ordered for a reason, even if it was a reason they could not understand. Edith concluded.

But when you look back on it and you see what happened, and you know what you accomplished wasn't your doings, it had to be in the patterns of things to happen and to come. . . . When you look back on it . . . you see the pattern was there all the time. . . .

▬ DISCUSSION

To understand strength from a woman's perspective can change the ways nurses view themselves and their female clients. Understanding the possibility that an older woman perceives herself as strong, instead of assuming that she sees herself as weak, changes the ways in which nurses assist others. Helping women verbalize their strength may help them visualize themselves as strong in a way that potentiates health.

The stories in this study illustrate the empowering nature of narrative (Diekelmann, 1991; Hartman, 1991; Heilbrun, 1988; Hutchinson, 1994; Sandelowski, 1991). There was often a catharsis at having told the stories. In telling their stories, many of which had not been voiced before, the women also found a way to reflect on the meaning of their lives. There was a sense, through the storytelling, of coming to peace with one's life, as well as a recognition that the wisdom one possessed could be of value to others. Storytelling can be thought of as a way of caring: caring for the individual who is telling the story by providing her with a vehicle for looking over her life, and caring for the listener who gains from the wisdom of the storyteller's experiences. For a nurse to encourage the telling of life stories can be as enriching for herself as for the storyteller.

In addition, for nurses as women to voice their own strengths, and their pride in their work, is an empowering act. For nurses, it can also be empowering to realize that their own stories can give other women "plots" on which to build their life stories (Bateson, 1989; Hartman, 1991; Heilbrun, 1988, 1990).

For the nurse who cares for women of a different race, class, or age than her own, the understanding of how their experiences compare to hers can enable her to help women find and use their strength. Understanding the connections and contrasts of life experiences can also begin to create a better appreciation of others' experience (Lugones & Spelman, 1990). As the number of aged persons in our society increases, seeing beyond stereotypes of the aged and appreciating and honoring the strengths of older women and men are crucial to helping older people.

This study illustrates the value of exploring "life in the margins" (Bateson, 1989; Daly, 1992). The lives of older women are not usually considered worthy of attention; most older women are not important or powerful. The power of these stories and the insights of these women have important implications for the lives of others.

Nurses might also be considered to be in the margins, since most are women and their work is often directed by others. For example, the work of advanced practice nurses is especially marginal, close to the boundaries of mainstream nursing practice and infringing on the boundaries of medical practice. According to Bateson (1989), it is in these margins "where new visions may be born." It is in these margins that nursing research must continue to explore new visions of practice and new visions of health care.

Research methods such as the one used in this study, Heideggerian hermeneutics, encourage the voicing of women's experiences and emphasize understanding the meaning of experience from the individual's perspective. Narrative, in this study, can be seen as a powerful mode for communicating strength, as well as for sharing strength. The use of narrative, as well as the use of poetry and other creative art forms, may have potential for demonstrating women's strengths and the importance of women's experiences. The power of these stories and the insights of these women suggest that the creativeness that lurks close to the boundaries of society has important implications for the lives of everyone. Researchers must save these stories, because as Edith said, "When an old person dies, it's like a library burning down."

■ REFERENCES

Barker, E. (1989). Being whole: Spiritual well-being in Appalachian women, a phenomenological study. Unpublished doctoral dissertation. University of Texas, Austin.

Bateson, M. C. (1989). Composing a life. New York: Plume.

Belenky, M., Clinchy, B., Goldberger, N., & Tarule, J. (1986). Women's ways of knowing. New York: Basic Books.

Cixous, H. (1980). Sorties. In E. Marks & I. de Courtivron (Eds.), New French feminisms (90–98). New York: Schocken Books.

Connors, D. (1986). I've always had everything I've wanted — but I never wanted very much: An experiential analysis of Irish-American working class women in their nineties. Unpublished doctoral dissertation, Brandeis University.

Daly, M. (1978). Gyn/ecology. Boston: Beacon Press.

Daly, M. (1987). Websters' first new intergalactic wickedary of the English language. Boston: Beacon Press.

Daly, M. (1992). Outercourse. San Francisco: Harper Collins.

de Beauvoir, S. (1974). The second sex. New York: Vintage Books.

Diekelmann, N. (1991). The emancipatory power of the narrative. In Curriculum revolution: Community building and activism (41–62). New York: The National League for Nursing.

Diekelmann, N., Allen, D., & Tanner, C. (1989). The NLN criteria for appraisal of baccalaureate programs: A critical hermeneutic analysis. New York: National League for Nursing.

Duffy, M. (1985). A critique of research: A feminist perspective. Health Care for Women International, 6, 341–352.

Dunbar, S., Patterson, E., Burton, C., & Stuckert, G. (1981). Women's health and nursing research. Advances in Nursing Science, 2(2), 1–10.

Gilligan, C. (1982). In a different voice. Cambridge: Harvard University Press.

Hartman, E. (1991). Telling stories: The construction of women's agency. In E. Hartman & E. Messer-Davidow (Eds.), Engendering knowledge (11–34). Knoxville: The University of Tennesee Press.

Heidegger, M. (1959). An introduction to metaphysics (R. Manheim, Trans.). New Haven: Yale University Press.

Heidegger, M. (1962). Being and time. New York: Harper & Row. (original work published in 1927)

Heidegger, M. (1971). Poetry, language, thought (A. Hofstadter, Trans.). New York: Harper & Row.

Heilbrun, C. (1988). Writing a woman's life. New York: Ballantine Books.

Heilbrun, C. (1990). Hamlet's mother and other women. New York: Ballantine Books.

Hooks, B. (1984). Feminist theory: From margin to center. Boston: South End Press.

Hutchinson, S. A. (1994). Benefits of participating in research interviews. Image: Journal of Nursing Scholarship, 26, 161–164.

King, P. (1989). A woman of the land. Image: Journal of Nursing Scholarship, 21, 19–22.

Kristeva, J. (1980). Woman can never be defined. In E. Marks & I. de Courtivron (Eds.), New French feminisms (137–141). New York: Schocken Books.

Lugones, M. C., & Spelman, E. V. (1990). Have we got a theory for you! Feminist theory, cultural imperialism and the demand for "the women's voice". In A. Al-Hibri (Ed.), Hypatia reborn (18–33). Bloomington, IN: Indiana University Press.

Luttrell, W. (1989). Working-class women's ways of knowing: Effects of gender, race, and class. Sociology of Education, 62, 33–46.

MacPherson, K. I. (1992). Cardiovascular disease in women and noncontraceptive use of hormones: A feminist analysis. Advances in Nursing Science, 14(4), 34–49.

McElmurry, B., & Librizzi, S. (1986). The health of older women. Nursing Clinics of North America, 21(1), 161–171.

Miller, J. (1986). Toward a new psychology of women (2nd ed.). Boston: Beacon Press. (original work published 1976)

The Personal Narratives Group. (Eds.) (1989). Interpreting women's lives. Bloomington, IN: Indiana University Press.

Robinson, C. (1985). Black women: A tradition of self-reliant strength. In J. Robbins & R. Siegel (Eds.), Women changing therapy (135–144). New York: Harrington Park Press.

Rose, J. (1990). Psychologic health of women: A phenomenologic study of women's inner strength. Advances in Nursing Science, 12(2), 56–70.

Sandelowski, M. (1991). Telling stories: Narrative approaches in qualitative research. Image: Journal of Nursing Scholarship, 23, 161–166.

Woods, N. (1982). Women's health: Perspectives for nursing research. Nursing Clinics of North America, 17(1), 113–119.

Woods, N. (1988). Women's health. Annual Review of Nursing Research, 6, 209–236.

Chapter 13

Menopause: A Holistic Look at an Important Transition to the Last and Best Third of Life

SUSAN E. D. DOUGHTY

A woman's life can be divided into three ages. Birth to about age 25 focuses on physical growth and learning. From the mid-20s until about age 60 women raise families and devote time to a career. The third age is a new period nonexistent in previous centuries. With women living into their 80s and 90s this third age is developing into a long third that can be a healthy part of life. Menopause transitions women into this last third of life and is an often overlooked physiological and psychological phenomenon experienced by women. In this chapter Susan Doughty explores the impact of menopause on the health of women, including osteoporosis and the pros and cons of hormone replacement therapy. Nurses who have a richer understanding of menopause and the health of women in the last third of life will be better prepared to assist women in making healthful choices.

The average age when a woman in the United States has her last menstrual period is 51.5 years. In 1900, fewer than 5 million American women were older than 50, since the life span of women at that time peaked at approximately 50 years. In the years 2000 to 2010, it is projected that more than 21 million women will reach the age of 50,[1] joining the 35 million women already 50 years or older. This group will constitute more than one third of the total female population of the United States. With current life expectancy ranging from 80 to 92 years of age, American women can expect to live more than one third of their lifetime after menopause. In order to ensure quality of life throughout the entire life span, women need to understand what is happening to their bodies.

Menopause is the process of the female ovaries ceasing egg production, estrogen levels dropping considerably, and the ending of reproductive capacity. Until recently, most women suffered in silence as they experienced

---

From *Topics in Geriatric Rehabilitation* 11(4):7–15, 1996. Reprinted with permission.

the signs of menopause: night sweats with insomnia, hot flashes, inability to focus thinking, and vaginal dryness. In addition, many women experienced heavy periods causing anemia, and were relieved to have their uterus and ovaries removed — a surgical menopause — because they "wouldn't need them anymore."

Some women became profoundly depressed, suicidal, or exhibited atypical behavior. But, because they could not talk about what was happening, many were afraid. Physicians did not know how to help, so many women felt isolated and abandoned at worst, and patronized at best. Of course, there were a few women who simply stopped having menstrual periods without any of the difficulties mentioned, and felt relieved not to have such difficulties. To this day, health care providers do not know why one woman will suffer in the extreme, while another will progress easily through the transition. What is known currently is that all women experience menopause, and more women are talking about it. Many questions still remain because research is inadequate and conflicting.

This article, written from a holistic health perspective, discusses what is known about the physiology of menopause and presents related health concerns including osteoporosis, cardiovascular disease, sexuality, and the pros and cons of hormone therapy. Particular emphasis is accorded to natural alternatives to hormones and to the role of the body as teacher of women as they move into the last and best third of their life span.

■PERIMENOPAUSE

The perimenopausal period of time may extend from 2 to 15 years prior to the last menstrual period or the onset of menopause. This transitional time can be more uncomfortable than actual menopause, and, because no accurate method exists to predict when the final menstrual period will come, most women over age 45 are considered to be perimenopausal. Two factors are known. First, the age when the individual's mother experienced her last menstrual period seems to be the most accurate predictor. Second, smoking brings on menopause 2 to 5 years earlier.

Menopause is the cessation of all ovarian activity and occurs one year after the last menstrual period. A woman needs to use birth control to prevent conception until that time. Perimenopause is the time period just before menopause, and postmenopause occurs 2 to 6 years after the final menstrual period when the physical signs of low estrogen, such as hot flashes, cease. Vaginal dryness is the only sign of menopause that does not disappear in postmenopause unless hormones are taken.

■MANAGING PERIMENOPAUSE

Prior to perimenopause, the menstrual cycle starts with the onset of bleeding with a period. The uterine lining sloughs off producing a bloody discharge, but estrogen is being secreted by the ovaries causing its level to rise in the circulating blood. This rising estrogen signals the period to stop and the uterine lining to thicken once again to receive a fertilized egg.

The ovary, with hundreds of thousands of eggs present since before birth, allows many eggs to compete for ovulation but just one egg is ripened to maturity. Approximately 14 days from the onset of that last period the egg is evacuated from the egg sac to travel down the fallopian tube to the uterus. If the egg is not fertilized, it is expelled through the vaginal opening. The egg sac remains, however, and secretes progesterone into the bloodstream, the hormone that signals the lining of the uterus to organize itself for a possible implanted, fertilized egg. If no egg remains, the organization of the tissue in the lining allows it to slough off neatly and efficiently with the next period. After 14 days of progesterone secretion along with estrogen secretion, if no fertilized egg exists, secretion of both hormones drops quickly, which signals the lining once again to slough off, starting the next menstrual cycle.

Women in their 40s do not ovulate every cycle because their egg supply is low. When they do not ovulate, they do not secrete progesterone. Estrogen is circulating, however, and stimulates a thick spongy lining without the organizing effect of progesterone. Thus, some women spot at mid cycle or bleed quite heavily with their periods. If the estrogen level has started to fall, follicle stimulating hormone (FSH) from the pituitary gland will rise to stimulate ovarian activity. But without estrogen stimulation a woman may skip a period and many even have some hot flashes, signaling the onset of the transition into perimenopause.

As the changes begin to occur, a woman may see a health care provider. If she becomes anemic from too much blood loss with her periods, progesterone is usually prescribed the last half of her cycle to offset the effect of lack of progesterone from lack of ovulation. Unfortunately synthetic progestins may cause side effects such as depression, pelvic cramping, bloating, headache, or elevated blood pressure and cholesterol. Natural progesterone, however, compounded from the root of the giant Mexican yam or the soybean, can be ordered from a compounding pharmacy as an alternative. Natural progesterone has very few side effects, specifically, sleepiness in high doses. Most women prefer natural progesterone to synthetic progestins for this reason, but may have difficulty convincing their provider to prescribe it, because most research in this area has not been published. However, the postmenopausal estrogen/progestins intervention (PEPI) trial, published in January 1995, showed natural progesterone to be as effective as synthetic progestins in organizing the uterine lining.[2] This finding is very important because prolonged disorganization of the lining from low progesterone levels could possibly lead to endometrial cancer, especially in obese women who tend to secrete more estrogen from body fat. This status is referred to as unopposed estrogen, and sometimes it causes profound premenstrual syndrome–like symptoms of mood swings, sore breasts, sugar/carbohydrate cravings, and bloating. Often, natural progesterone will help ameliorate these signs in perimenopause and can sometimes be found in the form of a wild yam cream in a health food store. Because no prescription is needed for the cream, many women get great relief by applying one quarter teaspoon to the soft areas of the skin such as inner thighs, buttocks, abdomen, or triceps areas, twice daily on days 14 to 28 of their menstrual cycle. It is best to rotate the sites of application to prevent saturating the area. One cannot get an overdose of the cream, because any extra is excreted, and there are no common side effects.

Sometimes women will see a health care provider with hot flashes and night sweats. A blood test will be done measuring FSH and thyroid stimulating hormone (TSH), because hypothyroidism can cause a similar response. If the TSH is normal and the FSH is below 12 pg/dL, the FSH will often fluctuate and periods will be irregular. In this instance, it would be premature to start exogenous estrogen. Vitamin E (400 IU two times daily) and bioflavonoids with vitamin C (500 mg two to four times daily), along with natural progesterone cream (one quarter teaspoon two times daily) usually will ameliorate the night sweats and hot flashes. It also helps to avoid stimuli that trigger hot flashes, such as certain foods (citrus, chocolate, spicy foods); hot drinks, especially with caffeine; alcoholic drinks; hot, humid weather; synthetic fiber clothing; warm bed covers; and anxiety or stress.

Some providers may suggest low-dose oral contraceptives designed for women in perimenopause, especially if birth control is an issue. Contraceptives will help even out low estrogen and progesterone levels and eliminate the signs of menopause quite efficiently, especially heavy bleeding. If a woman does not have a history of liver or gallbladder disease or blood clots, and she is known not to have breast, ovarian, or uterine cancer, low-dose oral contraceptives can be an option. If a woman smokes or has high blood pressure or high cholesterol, an alternative is usually sought because oral contraceptives can aggravate heart disease or stroke in these women. Oral contraceptives are similar to hormone therapy but are administered in slightly higher doses to prevent conception. Hormone therapy alone will not prevent conception if a woman is still intermittently ovulating. Some women continue oral contraceptives into their 50s and then switch to hormone therapy when their blood levels of estrogen indicate the menopausal state.

During the perimenopausal period, it is important for a woman to prepare for menopause. Many women find it helpful to talk with other women about what eradicates discomfort. Menopause groups are being formed all over the country, providing a medium for women to confide in each other and assist each other along the way. Occasionally family-of-origin issues arise and counseling is indicated; some women need antidepressant therapy as well. If physical exercise has not been a part of their routine, aerobic exercise 30 to 45 minutes three to six times per week has shown to eradicate discomfort. Exercise also helps to keep high-density lipoprotein (HDL) cholesterol elevated to protect against arteriosclerotic plaque formation. Rehabilitation professionals are aware that exercise plays a major role in reducing the negative effects of osteoporosis on quality of life. High-intensity strength training exercises have been shown to preserve bone density while improving muscle mass, improving strength and balance even in postmenopausal women.[3] Many controlled empiric studies reveal the importance of both strength training and regular aerobic exercise to improve the quality of life and prevent many negative effects of the typical aging process.

▬ OSTEOPOROSIS

A woman needs 1,000 mg of calcium daily prior to menopause and 1,500 mg per day after menopause to help prevent osteoporosis.[4] Research is being done on calcium uptake at the moment, but most agree that the best source of calcium is food. Dark green leafy vegetables with vinegar or lemon juice to free the calcium, rhubarb, seaweed, soy products such as soy milk or tofu, molasses, crushed sesame seeds, or low-fat dairy products are foods rich in calcium. Calcium supplements with magnesium are best taken before bed. Vitamin D (400 IU daily) is necessary for adequate calcium absorption in those geographic areas where sunlight is not tropical.

Perimenopause is a very special time in a woman's life as she prepares for the rite of passage of menopause. If she has not concluded child-bearing, it is important to work with an endocrinologist to conceive safely and carry to term. For those women who are ready to stop child-bearing, a period of grieving the loss of reproductive ability may be very important. As her body changes, it is important for a woman to focus on herself in a self-enhancing manner that brings about balance and stress reduction. Yoga, regular massage, and acupuncture all can help in the transition and create health. Regardless of what a woman experiences physically in perimenopause, if she is able to listen to her body to receive its wisdom and work with a health care provider, her spiritual and emotional growth can be quite profound.

▬ MENOPAUSE

As a woman's level of estrogen drops significantly, the uterine lining gets thinner, periods are skipped, and finally monthly bleeding ceases. One year after the final menstrual period the time of menopause begins. However, some women do restart their monthly periods even after several years without a period, especially if they have experienced menopause before age 50 or engage in a new intimate relationship (or both).

Osteoporosis and heart disease are considered the two major risk factors for menopausal women, manifesting 10 to 15 years after their final period, long after the acute signs of menopause have lifted.[1,5] Current research supports the use of low-dose estrogen/progesterone therapy to offset the effects of low estrogen and progesterone that exist after menopause to prevent osteoporosis and early death from heart attack. Much controversy surrounds hormone therapy, and many health care providers are not current with the research or they take a stand for or against hormones and then impose that decision on their clients. Each woman needs to become informed about the controversy and make the decision herself. Unfortunately, much of the information that comes from the media is biased when it is financed by pharmaceutical research. To arrive at a sound decision about hormones, both the provider and the client must talk out the pros and cons in terms of that client's individual risk.

Risk for heart disease includes obesity, hypertension, high low-density lipoproteins (LDL) and triglyceride cholesterols, low HDL cholesterol, history of heart attacks before age 50 in the family, diabetes, and smoking. Risk for osteoporosis includes family history of osteoporosis; small bones; light skin; early hysterectomy before age 45; chronic thyroid or steroid medications; anorexia; bulimia; lack of menstrual periods from exercise, low body fat, or chronic stress; smoking; sedentary life style; excess caffeine and alcohol intake; and lower than normal bone density.

▄HORMONE THERAPY — PROS AND CONS

The biggest concern about hormone therapy is its relationship to the rising incidence of breast cancer. Since 1975, many studies have examined that relationship, but the results have never been consistent. Estrogen as a hormone is known to play a fundamental role in the origin of breast cancer, but a causal relationship between hormone therapy and breast cancer has not been clearly and consistently proven. Available evidence[6] suggests that use of hormones in menopause for less than 5 years is not associated with increased risk of breast cancer. Use of estrogen more than or equal to 10 years may be associated with a 30% to 80% risk increase. Addition of progestins has not been shown to affect risk.

Once a woman's risk is evaluated, including her risk for breast cancer, it is helpful to read about the pros and cons of hormone therapy. Many books are being published about this topic, and a library can provide an idea about a book before a woman purchases it to use as a guide. At the conclusion of this article the author lists several books in the suggested reading that are good resources.

Overall advantages to taking hormones include:

- elimination of hot flashes, night sweats, anxiety attacks, insomnia, and unfocused thinking;
- elimination of vaginal soreness and dryness;
- reduced risk of calcium depletion from bones;
- reduced risk of atherosclerotic plaque formation;
- possible reduced risk of Alzheimer's dementia; and
- other personal advantages.

Overall disadvantages of taking hormones include:

- possible increased risk of breast cancer after age 55;
- possible increased risk of liver or gallbladder disease;
- possible growth of uterine fibroids;
- possible exacerbation of endometriosis;
- possible continued periods or irregular bleeding;
- more expense through cost of hormones and more frequent visits to health care provider; and
- other personal disadvantages.

As a woman is weighing personal values along with her risk in making this decision, questions about sexuality may arise. For many women, the fear of drying up and almost disappearing, especially sexually, is a huge concern as they approach menopause. Others experience even better sexual pleasure. The variation in response is in large part due to the psychologic nature of sex, once the physical constraints of vaginal soreness or decreased sex drive (libido) are managed. Self-stimulation once to twice weekly has been shown to keep vaginal tissue more moist and responsive. Lubricants can be found in the drug store, Astroglide being the most like human mucous, or in the kitchen, such as almond or sesame oil. The holistic approach to health care emphasizes that the spiritual grounding that often comes in the 40s helps a woman stay centered on her inner beauty, which then radiates regardless of age. Women's groups help a woman find her voice to ask for what she needs from her sexual partner, and good nutrition and exercise help unblock energy that adds to sensuality and well-being. Women who choose hormone therapy may find no alteration in sexual response or possibly an increased libido once the fear of conceiving is gone. Some women choose celibacy and remain quite content in that choice. Whatever the choice, it is important for a woman to communicate thoroughly with her partner so that her needs are met.

■ INDIVIDUALIZING THE THERAPEUTIC PROGRAM

Once a woman has weighed the pros and cons of hormone therapy with her personal risks, one more step can be helpful. Many times a decision such as this one is best arrived at by inner wisdom or intuition, regardless of what logic or intellect would suggest. If a woman cannot imagine herself taking a pill or pills daily or applying cream or a patch on a regular basis without feeling she is ill or something is wrong with her, it is hard to imagine she will persist with hormones once her initial discomfort is gone. Indeed, studies[7,8] indicate poor adherence to hormone therapy when prescribed.

Some women do not realize it is not necessary to continue monthly periods on hormones especially when their provider insists that it is necessary. This area becomes a real quality of life issue. Many studies now support low-dose progesterone along with estrogen on a daily basis for a woman with an intact uterus, eliminating monthly periods. Other women resist hormones for years, only to find themselves less vibrant or "folding in on themselves." Then, they choose to try hormones to determine if, in fact, their bodies respond favorably and the quality of their life improves.

When a woman takes estrogen and progesterone, nuisance side effects such as breakthrough bleeding, breast tenderness, or fluid retention can be managed by manipulating dose, type, and route of administration. Some women choose natural rather than synthetic hormones, compounded from plants and taken in pill, patch, or cream form. If a woman chooses hormones, it is very important to work with an informed provider to tailor her regimen for her safety and comfort. Unexplained vaginal bleeding must always be assessed in menopause, with or without hormones, to decrease undetected endometrial (uterine) cancer. Pelvic examinations every 6 months to every year with an annual Pap smear, as well as monthly self-breast examination and an annual breast examination are also essential to create health in menopause.

Data indicate the onset of risk for heart disease and osteoporosis starts when one stops hormone therapy,[9] so many women choose to continue hormones. Others gradually wean off hormones after hot flashes and rapid calcium depletion stop, about 5 years after the onset of skipped or absent periods. Many women live well into their 90s without taking hormones. Others take hormones into their 80s without any breast cancer.

Two factors not often discussed in the literature have the potential to make a big difference in the quality of a woman's life in menopause by decreasing risk. First is the prevention of osteoporosis. In addition to adequate calcium and regular weight-bearing exercise, if a woman receives support from her loved ones and visualizes her bones as supporting her, then she lives a constantly changing energy system, positively affecting her body. It has been proven that each cell of the body believes what the individual thinks is true, regardless of the "truth" of the idea.[10] In other words, women can influence their bodies to respond in a desired way through visualization.

The second factor deals with heart disease prevention. A well-known study[11] at Ohio State University revealed that all rabbits fed high-cholesterol, high-fat diets developed plugged coronary arteries and heart attacks, except those rabbits held and cuddled at feeding time. Their coronary arteries showed little evidence of obstruction. Heart disease is more than the outcome of lack of exercise and poor nutrition. Risk for coronary artery disease can be influenced by an ongoing relationship in which one loves and feels loved, as well as by reducing stress and managing hostility around time urgency. Northrup[12] suggests that the best way to protect the heart in menopause is to live with passion and joy so that the heart energy is available throughout the body. Women can be encouraged to identify their needs and get them met.

As baby boomers move into their 50s, a new era of evolution is occurring referred to as "the third age."[13] The first age, from birth to about 25 years, centers on biologic development, learning, and survival. The second age, from about ages 26 to 60, concerns raising the family and productive work. The third age is evolving as individuals live healthier lives over longer periods of time. The third age allows the individual reflective time to further the development of the intellect, memory, imagination, emotional maturity, and spiritual identity. It is also a period of giving back to society lessons, experiences, and resources collected over the years and becoming a living bridge between yesterday and tomorrow, a critical role that no other age can perform. By 2025, Americans over age 65 will outnumber teenagers by more than two to one. The American culture has the perfect opportunity to uproot ageism and gerontophobia, expelling the archetype of the old woman alone in the woods found in many fairy tales. Letting go of the notion that chronologic age defines an individual makes room for embracing the cycles of human existence and the contributions that older adults have made.

Menopause is a rich time for growth and coming into one's own power. Gone are the days when a woman feels useless or no longer attractive when her reproductive capacity is gone. The opportunity to learn how to create health through menopause into the third age is a gift that inevitably will enhance quality of life and benefit the culture as a whole. Growing beyond traditional youth-oriented values to discover a positive, expanded vision of who one is capable of becoming is critical for quality of life. This opportunity is made uniquely possible in therapeutic relationships with a holistic perspective. Health care providers are in a unique position to assist women to realize this opportunity.

▆ REFERENCES

1. Gibbons J. *The Menopause, Hormone Therapy, and Women's Health.* Washington, DC: Government Printing Office; 1992. US Congress, Office of Technology Assessment, OTA-BP-BA-88.
2. Miller V, La Rosa J, Barnabei V, et al. Effects of estrogen/progesterone regimens on heart disease risk factors in postmenopausal women. *JAMA.* 1995;273:199–208.
3. Nelson M, Fatarone M, Morganti C, et al. Effects of high-intensity strength training on multiple risk factors for osteoporotic fractures. *JAMA.* 1994;272:1909–1914.
4. Reid I, Ames R, Evans M, et al. Effect of calcium supplementation on bone loss in postmenopausal women. *N Engl J Med.* 1993;328:460–464.
5. Berg G, Hammar M, eds. *The Modern Management of Menopause.* New York: Parthenon Publishing Group; 1994.
6. Ewertz M. Hormonal replacement therapy and incidence of breast cancer. In: Berg G, Hammar M, eds. *The Modern Management of the Menopause.* New York, NY: Partheon Publishing Group; 1994.
7. McKinlay S. *Massachusetts Women's Health Survey.* Boston, Mass.: Cambridge Research Center Report; 1986.
8. Ravinkar V. Compliance with hormone therapy. *Am J Obstet Gynecol.* 1987;156:1332–1334.
9. Daly E, Vessey MP, Barlow D, et al. Hormone replacement therapy in a risk-benefit perspective. In: Berg C, Hammand M, eds. *The Modern Management of the Menopause.* New York: Parthenon Publishing Group; 1994.
10. Levine B. *Your Body Believes Every Word You Say.* Lower Lake, Calif: Aslin; 1991.
11. Nerem R, Levesque M, Cornhill J. Social environment as a factor in diet-induced atherosclerosis. *Science.* 1980;208(4451):1475–1476.
12. Northrup C. *Women's Bodies, Women's Wisdom: Creating Physical and Emotional Health and Healing.* New York, NY: Bantam; 1994.
13. Dychtwald K, Flower J. The third age. *New Age J.* 1989;6(1):50–59.

▆ SUGGESTED READINGS

Burton J. *Drawing from the Women's Well: Reflection on the Life Passage of Menopause.* San Diego, Calif: Lura Media; 1992.

Cone F. *Making Sense of Menopause.* New York, NY: Simon & Schuster; 1993.

Greenwood S. *Menopause Naturally.* San Francisco, Calif: Volcano Press; 1984.

Lark S. *The Menopause Self-Help Book.* Berkeley, Calif: Celestial Arts; 1990.

Lark S. *The Estrogen Decision.* Berkeley, Calif: Celestial Arts; 1990.

McCain M. *Transformation Through Menopause.* New York, NY: Bergin and Garvey; 1991.

Taylor D, Sumerall E, eds. *Women of the Fourteenth Moon: Writings and Menopause.* Freedom, NH: Crossing Press; 1991.

SELECTED BIBLIOGRAPHY

Baltes, M. M. & Carstensen, L. L. (1996). The process of successful ageing. *Ageing and Society* 16: 397–422.

Dellasege, C., Clark, D., McCreary D., Helmuth, A., & Schan, P. (1994). Nursing process: Teaching elderly clients. *Journal of Gerontological Nursing* 20(1): 31–38.

Duffy, M. E. (1993). Determinants of health-promoting lifestyles in older persons. *Image: Journal of Nursing Scholarship* 25(1): 23–28.

Evans, W. J. (1995). Exercise, nutrition, and aging. *Clinics in Geriatric Medicine* 11(4): 725–734.

Kaye, R. A. (1993). Sexuality in the later years. *Aging and Society* 13: 415–426.

Kick, E. (1989). Patient teaching for elders. *Nursing Clinics of North America.* 24(3): 681–686.

Perls, T. T. (January 1995). The oldest old. *Scientific American* 272: 70–75.

Roberts, B., Dunkle, R., & Haug, M. (1994). Physical, psychological, and social resources as moderators of the relationship of stress to mental health of the very old. *Journal of Gerontology: Social Sciences.* 49(1): S35–S43.

Running, A. F. (1996). "The Measure of My Days" Critiques by the oldest old. *Image: Journal of Nursing Scholarship* 28(1): 71–74.

Schulz, R. & Heckhausen, J. (1996). A life span model of successful aging. *American Psychologist* 51(7): 702–714.

Siu, A. L., Hays, R. D., Ouslander, J. G., Osterwell, D., Burciaga Valdex, R., Krynski, M., & Gross, A. (1993). Measuring functioning and health in the very old. *Journal of Gerontology: Medical Sciences* 48(1): M10–M14.

Trice, L. B. (1990). Meaningful life experience to the elderly. *Image: Journal of Nursing Scholarship* 22(4): 248–251.

Wagnild, G., & Young, H. M. (1990). Resilience among older women. *Image: Journal of Nursing Scholarship* 22(4): 252–255.

Wiley, D. & Bortz, W. M. II (1996). Sexuality and aging — usual and successful. *Journal of Gerontology: Medical Sciences* 51A(3): M142–146.

Unit 3

Age Segregation, Grandparenting, and Ethnicity: Sociocultural Issues in an Aging America

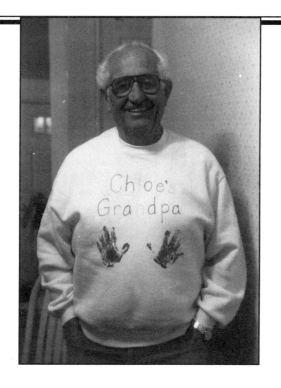

O ur lives are shaped by many social and cultural influences. At any age, the influence of our social structures and environments can be felt. Many roles that we assume in our lives have attendant expectations grounded in our immediate family or cultural group, as well as the larger society. It is not surprising that the roles of elders in our society have changed in response to these sociocultural forces.

135

As we live longer, we are spending a greater percentage of our lives in retirement. Yet, productive work can be an incentive for older adults to remain active and involved. Many elderly are seeking opportunities for part-time employment or volunteer activities in order to sustain their level of functioning and to feel challenged. Another way to stay engaged and sharp is to return to school. College attendance for those 65 and over is increasing, and many colleges are actively recruiting older students.

Older people now serve as caregivers to their disabled spouses or their own oldest-old parents as a result of our increased longevity. The changing face of families has led to important changes in the roles grandparents play in the lives of their grandchildren. Today, many grandparents are primary caretakers because the parents are unable or unwilling to care for their children. And in cases of divorce, the rights of grandparents in child custody cases are beginning to be considered.

Not only our families are changing, but the cultural and racial mix of our country is shifting. The population of ethnically diverse elders is growing at a rapid rate, with all groups expected to increase in proportion to White elders by the year 2030. Of these ethnic "minority" groups, elders of Hispanic origin are projected to show the largest rate of population growth. Rates of poverty in the elderly are also increasing, despite social programs that were instituted to protect older adults.

In order to be more effective practitioners, we must have a greater understanding of our clients' social environments and expected roles. Much of the information we need to synthesize will depend on the population groups with whom we work. This unit looks at some larger societal influences as well as more group-specific factors. Ethnicity, along with other sociocultural issues such as evolving grandparenting roles and the segregation of students, workers, and retirees by age, comprise the focus of this unit. The chapters that follow discuss the need for greater age integration in our society as well as the role and influence of grandparents, including ethnically diverse grandparents. There are also chapters delineating how ethnicity and cultural values and beliefs can affect older adults' health behaviors, specifically addressing health behaviors of Mexican American and Chinese American elders. The final chapter covers survey research that illustrates poverty as a barrier for access to health care in a group of older adults.

It is important to take social and cultural factors into consideration when planning care for elderly clients, and readers may find the selected bibliography at the end of this unit helpful in locating further resources.

Chapter 14

Age Integration and the Lives of Older People

MATILDA WHITE RILEY   JOHN W. RILEY, JR.

Dr. Matilda White Riley, a Senior Social Scientist for the National Institute on Aging, and her husband, Dr. John Riley, posit that our age-differentiated society will evolve into a more age-integrated one where age will no longer constrain the entry, exit, and performance within education, work, and retirement. As people's longevity and quality of life have been markedly improved, our social structures have not kept pace. Should healthy, capable elders be relegated to lives without work or education? The authors of this chapter suggest that it would be better for middle-aged workers to be able to intersperse periods of leisure and education throughout their careers, and for elders to no longer be simply "retirees."

Over the next several decades, the familiar social structures of work, retirement, and education will be virtually transformed. *Age* will have lost its current power to determine when people should enter or leave these basic social structures; nor will age any longer constrain expectations as to how people should perform. This structural revolution can mean a greater *age integration* of society. Beginning with older people, it can enhance the lives of people of every age.

We present this theme as a challenge toward current planning for future research, public policy, and professional practice. While the prediction may be visionary, our argument is not without scientific guidance. It rests on a basic proposition from the sociology of age: that, in all known societies, human aging and changing social structures are distinct but interdependent dynamisms. Each influences the other (Riley, Johnson, & Foner, 1972). In modern societies, however, a perplexing problem has been developing for many decades: the dynamism of aging has been outrunning the dynamism of structural change. This is the problem we call "structural lag" (Riley, 1988). Essentially, there is an imbalance between the mounting numbers of long-lived people (the unprecedented transformation of aging) and the lack of productive and meaningful role opportunities — or places in the

From *The Gerontologist* 34(1):110–115, 1994. Reprinted with permission.

social structure — that can recognize, foster, and reward these capacities. We draw attention now to the need for age integration, before the 21st century inundation of "baby boom" cohorts can exacerbate the structural lag and overwhelm the societal order.

▬ STRUCTURAL LAG

The 20th century has experienced a revolution in people's lives, now well-known and documented. With increases in longevity at birth, nearly three decades have been added to the average length of life, more than was previously added in all of human history. These added years have been accompanied by dramatic alterations in the ways people grow up and grow old. For older people, nearly one-third of adult life is now spent in what has become "modern" retirement (cf. Torrey, 1982). Yet ironically, only a minority of older people are so frail or disabled as to need support *from* society; instead, the majority are comparatively "robust" (to use Richard Suzman's term) and capable of making contributions *to* society. Figure 14-1 gives graphic evidence of the overwhelming numbers of older people today who are robust (neither fully disabled nor institutionalized) — and of the greatly enlarged numbers who will be robust in the 21st century (cf. Suzman, Harris, Hadley, Kovar, & Weindruch, 1992). The projections do not include

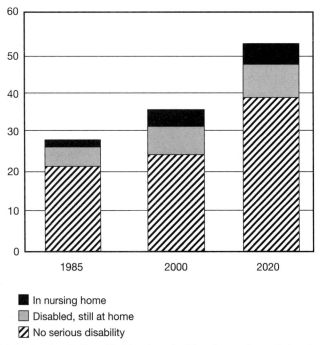

■ In nursing home
▨ Disabled, still at home
▨ No serious disability

FIGURE 14-1   Frail vs "robust" older people 65 and over (population in millions). (Source: Manton, Stallard, and Singer, 1992)

the most recent indications that, on the average, age-specific functioning may be improving.

In contrast to the revolution in people's lives, however, there has been no comparable revolution in the age structures of society. To be sure, many changes have been made in ways of caring for the frail and disabled, but meaningful and institutionalized role opportunities for the robust and capable have lagged behind. Thus, a structural revolution now awaits the 21st century. Increasing numbers of capable, motivated, and potentially productive older people cannot long coexist with empty role structures. Something has to give.

There is a message here: imminent changes (to use Sorokin's term) are underway that can help to offset the structural lag. These changes—though latent—are intrinsic to the continuing societal interplay between changing lives and changing social structures. In this article, we first examine such revolutionary changes by counterposing two ideal types of age structures: a familiar or "age-differentiated" type which is characterized by the lag, and a new or "age-integrated" type which theoretically has the potential to reduce it. We then note a few evidences of age integration in the structures of modern societies, and propose that further scientific professional, and policy attention be paid to these evidences and their implications.

■ "IDEAL TYPES" OF AGE STRUCTURES

These "ideal types" of age structure, as schematized in Figure 14-2, are but heuristic devices to aid understanding. In Max Weber's sense, they are artificially simplistic. They may never exist in reality, but are idealized

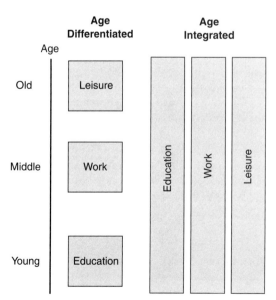

FIGURE 14-2 Ideal types of social structures.

selections from it. Yet they prompt us to think of key elements of one type as reflective of the reality of the recent past, and key elements of the other as potentially prophetic of real directions for the future. Let us be more specific.

Age-Differentiated Structures

At one extreme (at the left of Figure 14-2), age-differentiated structures divide societal roles into three parts: retirement or leisure for older people, work roles for the middle-aged, and educational roles for the young. This type of structure is commonplace today. It so closely approximates the actual experiences of the 20th century as to allow detailed scientific analysis (e.g., Henrichs, Roche, & Sirianni, 1991; Mayer & Schoepflin, 1989). Today, however, we believe that these age-based structures and norms can often be seen as vestigial remains of an earlier era when most people had died before their work was finished or their last child had left home. For example, age 65, established as the criterion for insurance eligibility in 19th century Germany, is still widely used under utterly changed contemporary conditions.

Despite its failure to accommodate people's changing lives, this conventional age differentiation is continually reinforced. It has been appropriate for societies where paid work is the predominant role, and achievement (or material "success") the predominant value. In particular, this age-differentiated type is bolstered by "ageism," the mistaken but stubborn belief in universal and inevitable decline because of aging: e.g., older workers, even those in their 50s, are erroneously believed to have inevitably lost their efficiency. Moreover, the familiar age-based divisions among education, work, and retirement offer many advantages: they provide orderliness as they have become "institutionalized" in people's lives; they are a societal convenience; and they are typically accepted without question. Examples of their persistence are easy to find. Thus, as the baby boom cohorts in the United States flooded entry-level jobs in the workforce, there were heavy social pressures and corporate inducements for older people — well before age 60 — to make room for them through "early retirement." Paradoxically, while the age of exit from work has been declining, the age of exit from education and entry into work has been rising. Martin Kohli (1988), writing about the "tripartite" division of the life course, states the absurd extreme this way:

If we extrapolate the trend of the last two decades, we shall, somewhere in the second half of the twenty-first century, reach the point where at the age of about 38, people move from the university directly into retirement.

Yet, history is not unidirectional and trends in one direction cannot persist indefinitely. Lives are changing, but structures lag behind.

Age-Integrated Structures

Age-integrated structures, at the right of Figure 14-2, stand in sharp contrast to the ideal type of age-differentiated structures. Here (within the limits set by biology) the age barriers are removed. Role opportunities in *all* structures — education, work, and leisure — are open to people of *every* age. This means that throughout society people of all ages are brought together — they are "integrated." Neither teenagers nor retirees are excluded from worksites because of age. There are nursery schools for the very young, and universities are open to adults of all ages, including the old. Extended opportunities for leisure and freedom from work are available even to those in the typically overburdened middle years, rather than being reserved almost exclusively for the "roleless role" of older people, to use Ernest Burgess' well-known expression.

Ideally, such age-integrated structures would have revolutionary consequences. They would open to older people the full range of role choices. And, in changing the opportunities for older people, new opportunities would be unlocked for everyone. For the middle-aged, there would be reductions in the strains imposed by multiple roles — when work is combined with family, homemaking, and health care, as well as with leadership in politics, religion, and community service. Ideally, too, such age-integrated structures would lead to the often proposed "reconstruction of the life course," providing options for people over their entire lives to intersperse periods of work with periods of education and of leisure. And for the society, these structures would broaden the economic base for support of that minority of older people who are frail and needy.

In reality, as ideal types confront real-world exigencies, we have little first-hand experience for specifying the nature of age integration under modern conditions. For example, how might an age-integrated society cope with the widely shifting economic balance between demand and supply for labor (e.g., Sheppard, 1989)? Can mechanisms be designed for spreading more evenly across the range of ages those jobs that are actually available at particular times? Or if age criteria were no longer to control access to work roles, or to other roles in education, family, and health care institutions, what new criteria — of achievement or of need — could be fashioned to replace them (cf. Riley & Schrank, 1972)? Such issues have not gone unnoticed in the gerontological literature: witness, for example, the earlier discussion of an "age irrelevant" society by Bernice Neugarten (Neugarten & Hagestad, 1976); or Barbara Silverstone's (1992) call for a "new view of aging" that would raise to 75 the age of eligibility for Social Security in the United States.

Fuller analytical understanding of how these ideal types might correspond to reality is needed — and urgently. Already the increases in numbers of capable retired people are far outstripping the numbers of younger people who are actively contributing to the economy (cf. Binstock, 1992). And already the metamorphoses in longevity and technology, and the long-range shift toward "contingent" rather than lifetime careers, are pressing toward the flexible boundaries that would characterize age-integrated structures. Paradoxically, while the typical life course becomes *longer*, the half-life of most occupations becomes *shorter*. Medical doctors and nurses, after many years of training, find themselves out-of-date after only a few years of practice. As workers over their lifetime change jobs (and sometimes occupations) as many as eight times, engineers, insurance salespersons, taxi drivers, bankers, computer operators, practicing gerontologists — indeed everyone — is required to relearn and to seek ways of interspersing periods of work with periods of learning and retraining. Thus, strong pressures are already operating to alter societal structures in the age-integrated direction.

▬TOWARD AGE-INTEGRATED STRUCTURES

Where does this typology leave us? It alerts us, we believe, to real tendencies toward age integration which are already emerging, and which hold far-flung implications and issues for both individuals and society.

Alterability

Parallel to the fallacious belief that the aging process is fixed and immutable is another belief — also fallacious — that social structures, because they ordinarily persist beyond the lifetimes of the individuals passing through, are impervious to alteration. Yet institutions and roles continually change and can often *be* changed, as history has demonstrated. Familiar evidence of structural alterability are the changing ages for marrying, bearing children, leaving school, or leaving the labor force. Somewhat less familiar is the variability in the United States in the age of entry into school. Historians (cf. Angus, Mirel, & Vinovskis, 1988) tell of 19th century "infant schools" where 3-year-olds were taught to read and precocity was encouraged. This was followed, however, by a drastic raising of the age of "reading readiness" as a fear of early learning, even leading to insanity, developed. Only recently has this age criterion for school entry relaxed again, with the current development of nursery schools and infant day care. Even less well-known are the historical changes in age criteria for serving in the military: during the American Civil War, soldiers were reported to range in age from 11 to 61 (Vinovskis, 1989), a far cry from the age requirements in the military today. Such evidences of alterability in the past make clear the future possibilities for age flexibility in social structures.

Evidences of Change

Today, in many countries and in diverse domains, research is beginning to disclose numerous evidences that structures are indeed changing, that the familiar age barriers are weakening, and that deliberate interventions to offset structural lag are feasible. Various aspects of the ideal type of an age-integrated society may not after all be purely visionary. Here are a few examples:

In education, roles are no longer confined largely to the young. Opportunities are being made for older people to engage in teaching (e.g., teaching adults who cannot read, or immigrants who cannot speak the language). Other opportunities are being made for older people to go back to school. For example, according to some U.S. reports, nearly 1,000 colleges now make plans for students over age 65. And, as such structural interventions are focused on older people, they tend to integrate people of all ages.

Thus, in a college classroom, making room for older adults brings them together with traditional students who are younger, and with teachers who too are often younger.

Similarly, at work, roles are less exclusively confined to the middle years. Given the ups and downs in the economy, and the recent reorganization of firms to increase productivity per worker, the age patterning of work has become more variable (Henretta, 1992). In the late 1980s in the U.S., various reports showed that 44% of all employers had programs for part-time work, 14% sponsored sabbatical leaves, 40% made "flextime" available (Dychtwald, 1989). Some companies have model programs for "unretirement," rehiring retired employees, providing part-time employment, retraining older adults or preparing them for new occupations. There are opportunities for some older people to become entrepreneurs, and for others to "moonlight" in work that is not officially reported. There are growing demands for older people in the role of care*giver* (rather than care*receiver*). There are increasingly varied and significant opportunities for many kinds of volunteer jobs.

At the other end of the age range, many teenagers work part-time, often alongside middle-aged and older workers who may serve as mentors. Despite its rigidity as a "tracking" system, the German model of combining schooling of the young with on-the-job apprenticeship to the mature is having an impact on educational systems elsewhere. The rising numbers of working mothers often mean that even very young children have assigned tasks along with their elders in the home; and educators are discovering the reciprocal advantages of children teaching children.

Particularly important for the emergence of age integration are public policies and their latent consequences. As one example, Anne Marie Guillemard (1990) has analyzed reports from several European countries that show how the pathways leading from work to retirement are being rerouted because of the transformation of the welfare system. Public pension plans, which once sustained *age-differentiated* structures, are breaking down with the rise of insurance programs for disability and for unemployment — which operate irrespective of age. As Prof. Guillemard puts it, age criteria for leaving work are giving way to functional criteria, and "old age, retirement, and withdrawal from the labor force no longer coincide."

All such structural interventions are tending to produce new and more flexible roles; and this means wider options for people of every age, and in particular for the competent elderly. If given such options, some old people will opt to remain in the economic mainstream of society. (One U.S. study shows that substantial minorities of early retirees would prefer to work if opportunity afforded, see Harris, 1990.) Other older people will choose education. Others will opt for leisure activities, often combined with householding. Still others will undertake volunteer roles. Today, older people are widely heterogeneous (cf. Nelson & Dannefer, 1992); ideally, they require a wide diversity of roles. But one thing is clear: the wish of *all* older people is *not* for roles in which they are disregarded, denigrated, or dependent.

Unintended Consequences

Many such considerations, then, are providing the fuel for the imminent changes which are operating below the surface of our conventional age-differentiated society. These changes show that the difficulty of reducing the structural lag lies, not in any inevitable inflexibility of age structures, but rather in understanding how the changes occur and how particular *interventions* can operate to benefit, rather than damage, both individuals and society (Riley & Riley, 1989). Unguided interventions to reinforce the inherent tendencies toward age integration can sometimes have unintended, even undesired, consequences. For example, if flexibility of age criteria were pushed too far, the well-known dangers of exploiting the labor of children or older people could rear their ugly heads. Or, entitlements to leisure and relaxation in retirement — as these might be distributed more fairly than at present — could be threatened. Clearly, a broad vision of the future and a sound knowledge base are essential here for guiding interventions — as interventions, explicit or implicit, are continually being undertaken through public or private policies, professional practice, or people's everyday lives.

▄OTHER SOCIETAL CHANGES IMPLICATED

Social science theories point immediately to other revolutionary aspects of this broad vision. Among them, we conclude this article by noting forms of societal integration and change that are implicated in the potentially emerging ideal type of an age-integrated society, and that raise future issues of gerontological concern.

Most immediately, age integration emphasizes that older people cannot be viewed in isolation. Changes affecting older people tend to ramify throughout the society to affect those of every age and, in turn, to have further consequences for older people themselves (cf. Foner, 1982; Riley, 1978). Lessons learned from aging research disclose many primordial truths about humanity.

Moreover, age integration evokes new forms of *institutional integration*. As roles in work, education, or leisure intersect with roles in other social institutions, old structures give way to new hybrids. For example, corporations become integrated with schools as they provide worker education, and also with families as they provide daycare for employees' children and frail parents, or as technological advances allow jobs to be performed in the home.

Gender integration is already being produced by the extraordinary increases in women's participation in the labor force which bring men and women together at work as well as in the family. Yet the changes in women's roles have primarily affected the years of adulthood prior to retirement. Thus the dual burdens of work inside and outside the home are heavily concentrated among the middle-aged. And the structural lag is exacerbated.

In addition, age integration raises critical issues of *values*, as the norms to which today's middle-aged people have been socialized encounter the exigencies of old age in an utterly changed future society. What changes in achievement values and consumption aspirations would be needed in an age-integrated society if many older individuals, rather than retiring, were to undertake new assignments that bring rewards and benefits lower than their former levels of pay or prestige? What added increments of social involvement would justify the economic decrements? Already in the U.S., some companies have been experimenting with programs to convince middle-aged employees, even business school graduates, that they can find rewards and satisfaction by moving laterally, rather than upward, on occupational ladders. For the future, is it likely that nonmonetary rewards of "success" and "consumerism" will be modulated by renewed emphases on other rewards, such as new types of recognition in the world of work, affection and response from family and friends, recognition for cultural pursuits, or pleasure in new adventure? Is it likely that the current principle of "rights" for older people will be counterbalanced by the principle of "responsibilities" for those capable older people who are competent and motivated to be active participants in society? Resistance to such change is illustrated by the abortive efforts by the International Federation on Aging, in preparing for the 1992 World Assembly on Aging, to include "responsibilities" along with "rights" in its declaration.

▬FUTURE ISSUES

In this brief research-based essay, we have outlined possible revolutionary changes from a social structure that is primarily age-differentiated toward one that may encompass major elements of age integration. We have suggested that changes toward age integration will implicate broader changes as well: institutional integration, gender integration, changes in values. We have noted latent tendencies that, if they in fact coalesce toward a new societal integration, will reduce structural lag. These inherent tendencies will mean that many people in their later years will be productive assets, rather than burdens, on the economy. And in turn, these inherent tendencies will also unlock future potentials for people's lives: providing wider options for shaping the entire life course; reducing middle-age burdens of piled up responsibilities of work and family; protecting against ageism and discrimination for those elders still wanting to work; enhancing the health and well-being which comes (as massive gerontological research has shown) from all types of sustained active participation.

Like other structural changes sweeping through the world today, such tendencies toward structural integration raise new issues demanding new attention. These tendencies will reach their potential only through innovative, even radical, policies and practices that emanate from laborious and often unglamorous scientific research, and from evolving understandings. In our time, few efforts have been made to reach such understandings (but see Riley, 1978; Riley & Riley, 1991). While much has been learned about aging processes and the dynamic aspects of human lives (cf. Riley & Abeles, 1990; Riley & Riley, 1992), relatively little has been learned about the roles, institutions, and cultural norms that shape these lives and, in turn, are shaped *by* them. One current effort in search of deeper understandings is the Program on Age and Structural Change (PASC) at the National Institute on Aging. Involving a network of scholars, PASC focuses on this neglected area: it aims toward understanding *structural* opportunities and constraints (in Robert Merton's sense) that affect the quality of aging from birth to death.

We salute this objective, and we seek suggestions, criticisms, and help from interested members of the gerontological community.

■ REFERENCES

Angus, D. L., Mirel, J. E., & Vinovskis, M. A. (1988). Historical development of age stratification in schooling. Columbia University, *Teachers College Record, 90,* 211–236.

Binstock, R. H. (1992). The oldest old and "intergenerational equity." In R. M. Suzman, D. P. Willis, & K. G. Manton (Eds.), *The oldest old* (pp. 394–417). New York: Oxford University Press.

Dychtwald, K. (1989). *Age wave: The challenges and opportunities of an aging America.* Los Angeles: Jeremy P. Tarcher.

Foner, A. (1982). Perspectives on changing age systems. In M. W. Riley, R. P. Abeles, & M. S. Teitelbaum (Eds.), *Aging from birth to death: Vol. II, Sociotemporal perspectives.* (pp. 217–228). AAAS Selected Symposium 79, Boulder, CO: Westview.

Guillemard, A.-M. (1990). Reorganizing the transition from work to retirement: Is chronological age still the major criterion determining definitive exit from work? Paper presented at the XII World Congress of Sociology, Madrid, July 9–13.

Harris, L., & Associates (1990). *Aging in the eighties: America in transition.* Washington, DC: National Council on the Aging.

Henretta, J. C. (1992). Uniformity and diversity: Life course institutionalization and late-life work exit. *The Sociological Quarterly, 33,* 265–279.

Henrichs, C., Roche, W., & Sirianni, C. (1991). *Working time in transition.* Philadelphia: Temple University Press.

Kohli, M. (1988). *New patterns of transition to retirement in West Germany.* Tampa, FL: International Exchange Center on Gerontology, University of South Florida.

Mayer, K. U., & Schoepflin, U. (1989). The state and the life course. *Annual Review of Sociology, 15,* 187–209.

Manton, K. G., Stallard, E., & Singer, B. H. (1992). Projecting the future size and health status of the U.S. elderly population. *International Journal of Forecasting, 8,* 433–458.

Nelson, E. A., & Dannefer, D. (1992). Aged heterogeneity: Fact or fiction? *The Gerontologist, 22,* 17–23.

Neugarten, B. L., & Hagestad, G. O. (1976). Age and the life course. In R. H. Binstock & E. Shanas (Eds.), *Handbook of Aging and the Social Sciences* (pp. 35–55). New York: Van Nostrand Reinhold Company.

Riley, M. W. (1978). Aging, social change, and the power of ideas. *Daedalus, 107,* 39–52.

Riley, M. W. (1988). The aging society: Problems and prospects. *Proceedings of the American Philosophical Society, 132,* 148–153.

Riley, M. W., & Abeles, R. P. (1990). *The behavioral and social research program at the National Institute on Aging: History of a decade.* Working Document. Bethesda, MD: Behavioral and Social Research, National Institutes of Health.

Riley, M. W., & Bond, K. (1983). Beyond ageism: Postponing the onset of disability. In M. W. Riley, B. B. Hess, & K. Bond (Eds.), *Aging in society: Selected reviews of recent research* (pp. 243–252). Hillsdale, NJ: Lawrence Erlbaum.

Riley, M. W., Johnson, M., & Foner, A. (1972). *Aging and society, Vol. III: A sociology of age stratification.* New York: Russell Sage Foundation.

Riley, M. W., & Riley, J. W., Jr. (1989). The lives of older people and changing social roles. In M. W. Riley & J. W. Riley Jr. (Eds.), *The quality of aging: Strategies for interventions,* special issue of *The Annals* of the American Academy of Political and Social Science (pp. 14–28). Newbury Park, CA: Sage.

Riley, M. W., & Riley, J. W., Jr. (1991). Vieillesse et changement des roles sociaux. [The lives of older people and changing social roles]. *Gerontologie et Societe, 56,* 6–14.

Riley, M. W., & Riley, J. W., Jr. (1992). Die individuellen und gesellschaftslichen potentials. In P. Baltes (Ed.), *Das Alter and und die Zukunft der Gesellschaft.* [Individual and social potentials]. Berlin: Walter de Gruyter.

Riley, M. W., & Schrank, H. (1972). The work force. In M. W. Riley, M. Johnson, & A. Foner (Eds.), *Aging and society, Vol. III: A sociology of age stratification* (pp. 160–197). New York: Russell Sage Foundation.

Sheppard, H. L. (Ed.) (1989). *The future of older workers.* Tampa, FL: International Exchange Center on Gerontology, University of South Florida.

Silverstone, B. (1992). A gerontological perspective on the 1992 presidential election and beyond. Beattie Award Lecture, conference of the State Society on Aging of New York, Albany.

Suzman, R. M., Harris T., Hadley, E. C., Kovar, M. G., & Weindruch, R. (1992). The robust oldest old: Optimistic perspectives. In R. M. Suzman, D. P. Willis, & K. G. Manton (Eds.), *The oldest old* (pp. 341–348). New York: Oxford University Press.

Torrey, B. B. (1982). The lengthening of retirement. In M. W. Riley, R. P. Abeles, & M. S. Teitelbaum (Eds.), *Aging from birth to death: Vol. II: Sociotemporal perspectives.* Boulder, CO: Westview Press.

Vinovskis, M. A. (1989). Have historians lost the Civil War? Some preliminary demographic speculations. *Journal of American History, 76,* 34–58.

Chapter 15

Grandparenting at the Dawn of a New Century

As this collection of thoughts from six authors bring to life, grandparents play an important role in our society, passing along sociocultural expectations to their children and grandchildren, and acting as the link between past and future generations. The importance of this role is even more evident in nondominant ethnic groups. However, changing cultural norms and family structures can lead to role strain. Increasingly, grandparents are raising their grandchildren due to the inability of their own children to parent — frequently owing to problems with drugs and alcohol. Divorce and remarriage muddy the waters, and some older adults may have difficulty defining their grandparenting roles and functions.

Keepers of Community in a Changing World

AMANDA SMITH BARUSCH   PETER STEEN

Elders traditionally serve as witnesses to history, preserving the memories and transmitting the values of a culture. Grandparents can serve as conduits of cultural identity, transmitting the meaning and importance of distinct traditions to succeeding generations. Although critical to maintenance of a culture, this role is vulnerable to disruption in times of social dislocation.

Considerable theoretical work has focused on ethnic identity and its relationship to the role of elders. A good example is a recent book on aging and group identity, *The Cultural Context of Aging: Worldwide Perspectives* (Sokolvksy, 1990). The focus of the book's chapters is on how the social milieu determines the social construction, character, and importance of the elder. Under this view, culture defines the elder role, and "groups differentiated by ethnicity or subcultural heritage have contrasting orientations toward age and aging" (Bengtson, 1979:10). While the role of elders is to a great extent determined by culture, the elders themselves can have

From *Generations* 49–52, 1996, Spring. Reprinted with permission.

substantial influence on that culture. A second main focus concerning the relationship between elders and culture is on grandparents as maintaining culture, serving as "keepers of community." Bengtson and Robertson (1985), for example, suggested that one of the central functions of grandparents within a family context was as "participant in the construction of family history," responsible for interpreting and transmitting an understanding of key events and actors.

When asked, grandparents themselves often identify the role as an opportunity to link the past and the future. Kornhaber and Woodward (1981) interviewed numerous grandparents and grandchildren and summarized the social functions of grandparents. Several of these functions involve transmission of cultural identity: acting as mentors, role models, connections with the past, and connections with the future. Helen Kivnick's (1982) book, *The Meaning of Grandparenthood,* also described the elder as a unifying element between the past and future. In this and other work, Kivnick defines this connecting function as providing "symbolic meaning," which involves grandparenthood in "historical connectedness and symbolic immortality" (1982:11). Kivnick also emphasizes the value society ascribes to the wisdom of the elder. These features of the elder role enable grandparents to become keepers of community. In this view, the culture values the elder as a wise person, and the elder maintains the culture by passing it on to young members.

This interactive view of the relationship between a culture and its elders has intuitive appeal. But, as historians have noted, social and technological changes force the redefinition of generational roles (see Haber, 1983; Achenbaum, 1978; and Fischer, 1977), as can be seen, for example, in a look at two discrete cultures, the Chamorro people of Guam and Navajo living in the four-corners area of the Southwest.

Like people of many cultures, the Chamorro and Navajo face significant external challenges to their distinctive identities. U.S. educational policies, outmigration of young adults, and technological changes have brought the beliefs, practices, and values of the majority culture into their lives, dramatically changing the role of grandparents as keepers of community.

▬ GRANDPARENTING ON GUAM

Guam is a U.S. territory located in Micronesia. Colonization of the island began with the arrival of Ferdinand Magellan in 1521. Guam was a Spanish territory until 1898, when it was ceded to the United States. Apart from a three-year Japanese occupation during World War II, the island has remained a U.S. possession.

Although not the first to colonize Guam, the United States exerted the most control over the island and had the greatest effect on its culture and people — primarily through social and economic assistance. A primary means of establishing an American presence was the institution of an American-style educational system that sought to create a base of common language and American values among the native populations. This process supported U.S. efforts to secure the land necessary for Western Pacific military bases and to exert economic and military influence in the region (Colletta, 1976).

During the centuries prior to the influx of American education, Guamanians acquired knowledge, beliefs, and language informally through the extended family network. This smooth, informal transmission of culture from one generation to another was disrupted by Americanization. In addition to learning English, Guamanians were indoctrinated with American ideas and exposed to the American lifestyle. As the push toward greater U.S. involvement in Micronesian affairs was felt in the early 1960s, students in Guam (as well as the rest of Micronesia) began, like their counterparts in the United States, to see education as the key to success in the new way of life. Henny (1968) noted that the process of "credentialling" became increasingly important, with heavy reliance on standard achievement tests that "actually measure[d] proficiency in the English language rather than general achievement . . ." (p. 404). The result of the growing importance of acculturation and English proficiency is a generation of young people who share American ideals and aspire to an American lifestyle.

No previous generations of Guamanians have experienced this kind of pressure to put aside their language and culture and adapt to new and foreign ways. Because it is only within the last twenty to forty years that English has become the language of commerce on Guam, those who went through adolescence prior to 1944 are generally not proficient in English. Those who were born and raised on Guam after World War II, and especially those born since 1960, are proficient in English. Indeed, many members of these younger generations are fluent in English only and are unable to communicate in the language of their elders.

Grandparents on Guam were raised with very different expectations from those of members of the same age cohort on the U.S. mainland, growing up as they did prior to the post–World War II expansion of American involvement on Guam. During their adolescence and young adulthood, family life on Guam was embedded in a system of reciprocal obligations; with Americanization came great change. Their response was documented by our 1989 study.

In this study of 60 grandparents on Guam, 65 percent reported that their grandchildren spoke only English and were unable to communicate with the elders in their preferred language. For these grandparents, the results of Americanization were reduced family contact and intergenerational assistance and a modest decline in life satisfaction. Our results were consistent with those of other studies (Forsyth, Roberts, and Robin, 1992; Kivnick, 1981) that have reported a relationship with grandchildren as a strong predictor of satisfaction among grandparents and a decline in satisfaction if the relationship diminishes.

In addition, many of the younger generation emigrated to the United States, placing great geographic distances between the elderly who remained behind and their grandchildren. According to the 1990 Census, 49,935 of Guam's residents were native Chamorros. The same year, almost the same number — 48,000 Chamorros (identified in the Census as "Guamanians") — lived on the U.S. mainland.

Once separated from their community of origin, Chamorro children often experience pressure to assimilate into the majority culture. Elders typically remain on Guam. So they become, not daily forces in their grandchildren's lives, but holiday friends and pen pals. So outmigration reduces the opportunities for grandparents to transmit cultural identity.

■ GRANDPARENTING ON THE NAVAJO RESERVATION

The Navajo Reservation occupies an area about the same size as West Virginia, encompassing the northeast section of Arizona as well as strips of bordering land in New Mexico and Utah. Much of the change on the reservation since the childhood of the current Navajo elders has involved the inrush of social and technological features of the wider American society. Two major technological changes have appeared. First, there has been some expansion of the physical infrastructure of roads to include more reservation areas in the circulatory system of the wider American economy (American Indian Policy Review Commission, 1976; Young, 1955). Even so, the physical infrastructure of towns bordering the reservation is still more complete than that found in most areas of the reservation (Natwig, 1986). (We will return to the impact of this uneven development.) The second major technological change is the wider availability of electricity. With electricity comes television, which has brought a mass of non-Navajo values derived from the wider American consumer market (Downs, 1972). These changes affect both the ethnic identity of the Navajo and the role of the elders in preserving this identity (Stavenhagen, 1987).

The literature on the Navajo is replete with studies completed in the mid to early part of this century that draw a static picture of Navajo society. The elder was placed at a central location in this static conception of traditional society and was seen as a wise one, as a source of important and useful information. Through the elders, the past was brought to the present and given to the children to transmit to the future. This practice provides an excellent example of Kornhaber and Woodard's findings, which posit a role for grandparents establishing a connection with the past for their grandchildren. In the traditional Navajo society, the elder was a central conduit of identity between generations, supported by a broader social network that highly valued transmission of Navajo identity to young people.

In the past, the elder's stories served at least a double purpose. First, the stories related practical experience from the lives of the older people, which contained valuable information for how the young person might lead a materially successful life. Second, these stories conveyed identity. By acting as family historian, the elder delivered the meaning of being a member of a particular family unit. The family was part of a tightly sewn quilt of smaller immediate families coming together into matrilineal clans and then into a whole called the Dine (Navajo).

These days, Navajo society is increasingly penetrated by American lifestyle and values. One measure of this is the prevalence of the English language. Presently, the Navajo Nation is moving to ensure that its young will be able to communicate in the language of their ancestors. But many generations have been cut off from each other by the past policy of English-only instruction in schools (Dodge, 1946). An elder who is cut off from grandchildren because of language is cut off from the wealth of roles assigned to grandparents.

Many living on the reservation have witnessed the impact of transportation and television on the role and importance of the Navajo elder. Television affects the relationship between the elders and young people in several ways. First, its content is alien to the traditional values of the Navajo. Television is replete with visions of materialistic success that put forward a vision of *good* that is implicitly or explicitly demeaning to the standards of accomplishment that might have governed the norms and values of the elders.

In the face of this onslaught by mainstream American messages, the elder is pushed to the periphery. Elder life experiences become colorful tales of the past rather than practical lessons for the young. The successes of the past become less meaningful amid all the messages of material gain. The images and norms brought by television weaken both the role and the importance of the elder as the vision of norms and values delivered by modern technology floods the families, clans, and whole of the native people. The elder is no longer supported by a total societal framework that works to bring young people together with ancestors; instead, the young are drawn away from the elders and their messages of community.

On another level, the transportation revolution and its attendant spatial organization of living and work affects the relationship elders have with the young. In the past, the people lived in family-centered arrangements that ensured the geographical proximity of elders to young people. With modern transportation, people move *to* jobs. The physical infrastructure of the "border towns" is more complete than that found on much of the reservation and siphons off much economic activity from within the reservation and draws people to the towns (Natwig, 1986). The Navajo who move to the border towns to work and live are drawn out of the reservation and the family-centered form of spatial organization. Many Native Americans have left reservations in search of jobs (Navajo Nation, 1993). But even within the reservation, people move to jobs, and the elders are often left behind.

Like their counterparts in mainstream America, more Navajo grandparents have assumed the role of parent. This role can be incompatible with the role Weibel-Orlando (1990) described as that of "cultural conservators." The key here is intention. Grandparents who assume custodial responsibilities *because* they want to pass on cultural beliefs and values redefine the "parenting" role to include these aspects of grandparenthood.

■GRANDPARENTING IN MODERN AMERICA

Weibel-Orlando (1990) argues that the role of "cultural custodian" has relevance only for ethnic minorities struggling to maintain a distinct tradition in the midst of a dominant culture.

The Chamorro and Navajo have both experienced social and economic dislocation brought by an inrushing sea of mainstream American culture. In this context, heroic efforts are required by grandparents who want to convey a unique ethnic identity to their grandchildren.

But drawing from the work of Kivnick as well as Kornhaber and Woodward, we can argue that grandparents in mainstream America also play an important role in the definition and maintenance of identity. Like the Chamorro and the Navajo, residents of mainstream America have experienced profound social and technological change during the past four decades. Transportation and communication technologies have expanded the geographic opportunities for individuals even as they have brought public events and ideas into homes.

Even as geographic distance, technological advances, and changing values may mitigate against grandparents as "keepers of community," other trends serve to support that role. For example, the U.S. Bureau of the Census (1991) estimated that 3.2 million children under the age of 18 live with their grandparents. Although this number has been variously attributed to such negative factors as rising divorce rates, drug addiction, and adolescent pregnancy (Minkler and Roe, 1993), simple physical proximity of the generations does represent a significant opportunity. One key to successful coresidence may be grandparents who regard the experience as an opportunity to pass knowledge, values, and beliefs to the next generation. A continuing challenge for gerontology practitioners will be to foster and support grandparents in their essential role as "keepers of community."

■ References

Achenbaum, W. A. 1978. *Old Age in the New Land: The American Experience Since 1790.* Baltimore, Md.: Johns Hopkins University Press.

American Indian Policy Review Commission. 1976. *Report on Reservation and Resource Development and Protection. Task Force Seven: Reservation and Resource Development and Protection. Final Report to the American Indian Policy Review Commission.* Washington, D.C.: Government Printing Office.

Barusch, A. S., and Spaulding, M. L. 1989. "The Impact of Americanization on Intergenerational Relations: An Exploratory Study on the U.S. Territory of Guam." *Journal of Sociology and Social Welfare* 16(3): 61–79.

Bengtson, V. L. 1979. "Ethnicity and Aging: Problems and Issues in Current Social Science Inquiry." In D. E. Gelfand and A. J. Kutzik, eds., *Ethnicity and Aging: Theory, Research, and Policy.* New York: Springer.

Bengtson, V. L., and Robertson, J. F., eds. 1985. *Grandparenthood.* Beverly Hills, Calif.: Sage.

Colletta, N. J. 1976. "Cross-cultural Transactions in Ponapean Elementary Classrooms." *Journal of Research and Development in Education* 9: 113–23.

Dodge, C. 1946. Statement. In U.S. Senate, 79th Congress, 2d Session. *Navajo Indian Education* (pp. 4–6). Washington, D.C.: Government Printing Office.

Downs, J. F. 1972. *The Navajo.* New York: Holt, Rinehart and Winston.

Fischer, D. H. 1977. *Growing Old in America.* New York: Oxford University Press.

Forsyth, C. J., Roberts, S. B., and Robin, C. A. 1992. "Variables Influencing Life Satisfaction Among Grandparents." *International Journal of Sociology of the Family* 22(2):51–60.

Haber, C. 1983. *Beyond Sixty-Five: The Dilemma of Old Age in America's Past.* Cambridge: Cambridge University Press.

Henny, L. M. 1968. "Education and the Americanization of Micronesia." *Sociologische Gids* 15: 402–7.

Kivnick, H. Q. 1981. "Grandparenthood and the Mental Health of Grandparents." *Ageing and Society* 1(3), 365–91.

Kivnick, H. Q. 1982. *The Meaning of Grandparenthood.* Ann Arbor, Mich.: UMI Research Press.

Kornhaber, A., and Woodward, K. L. 1981. *Grandparents/Grandchildren: The Vital Connection.* Garden City, N.Y.: Anchor Press.

Minkler, M., and Roe, K. M. 1993. *Grandmothers as Caregivers: Raising Children of the Crack Cocaine Epidemic.* Beverly Hills, Calif.: Sage.

Natwig, E. 1986. "Institutional Barriers to Financing Development Projects in Indian Country." In U.S. Senate, 99th Congress, 2d Session. *An American Indian Development Finance Institution: A Compendium of Paper. Select Committee on Indian Affairs* (pp. 59–82). Washington, D.C.: Government Printing Office.

Navajo Nation. 1993. *1990 Census: Population and Housing Characteristics of the Navajo Nation.* Window Rock, Ariz.: Division of Community Development, The Navajo Nation.

Peterson, G. 1979/80. "Breadfruit or Rice? The Political Economics of a Vote in Micronesia." *Science and Sociology* 43: 472–85.

Sokolvsky, J., ed. 1990. *The Cultural Context of Aging.* New York: Bergin & Garvey.

Stavenhagen, R. 1987. "Ethnocide or Ethnodevelopment: The New Challenge." *Development: Seeds of Change* 1: 74–8.

U.S. Bureau of the Census. 1991. *Current Population Reports: Marital Status and Living Arrangements: March 1990.* Washington, D.C.: Government Printing Office.

Weibel-Orlando, J. 1990. "Grandparenting Styles: Native American Perspectives." In J. Sokolovsky, ed., *The Cultural Context of Aging.* New York: Bergin & Garvey.

Young, R. W. 1955. *The Navajo Yearbook of Planning in Action.* Window Rock, Ariz.: Navajo Agency.

No Place Without a Home: Southeast Asian Grandparents in Refugee Families

DANIEL F. DETZNER

There are few better examples of multigenerational families in a long-term "crisis" than those who are in transit as refugees, immigrants, and displaced persons. In 1995, the number of world refugees exceeded 20 million persons, the largest forced relocation in human history. An estimated 25 million more persons are internally displaced in their own countries as a consequence of war, famine, or ethnic conflicts. Countless others are also on the move in search of food, economic opportunity, or escape from natural disasters. Refugees and immigrants who relocate in other countries must reorganize their daily lives and family interaction patterns, thereby creating intergenerational tensions that often continue for several generations (Detzner, 1993).

Since 1975, more than 1.2 million refugees from Southeast Asia have fled to the United States seeking safety. Although elders are key sources of information concerning the family's development as well as important contributors to family well-being, most previous studies of Southeast Asian elders have focused on their individual problems — for example, subsistence incomes, absence of language proficiency and job skills, cultural isolation, physical health problems, and post-traumatic stress (Lee and Lu, 1989; Kinzie, 1989).

Although little is known specifically about the families who migrate under duress (Liu and Fernandez, 1988), we do know quite a bit about Southeast Asian families in general. Asian-Pacific Islanders are the fastest growing and poorest ethnic group in the United States (Rottman and Merideth, 1982). Southeast Asians value strong families, they believe current situations are influenced by past events, they prefer to avoid conflict, and they emphasize self-discipline and respect for authority (Boyer, 1991; Gozdziak, 1989; Henkin and Nguyen, 1981).

We also know that filial piety is central to their beliefs, with all family members, both living and deceased, arranged hierarchically by generation and gender into a network of obligation and authority (Seabloom, 1991). Threads of continuity connect the family to ancestral generations and determine the patterns of family relationships. In Southeast Asian cultures, a loss of place in the web of family, culture, and history means a forfeiture of identity (Boenlien, 1987). Within the structure of filial piety, a tension between generations is inherent; however, it is often suppressed by the elders' expectations of respect and devotion. Nevertheless, families are the arena in which these tensions often emerge because filial piety emphasizes reverence for the past, for traditional Asian practices, and for the elders'

From *Generations* 45–48, 1996, Spring. Reprinted with permission.

generation at a time when the younger generation's attention is focused on the future, adaptation to Western culture, and youth.

Although there are of course distinct differences in history, language, culture, and beliefs among Southeast Asians, collectively elderly refugees from this part of the world share many similar experiences. They have survived the horrors of war, dangerous escape attempts, crowded refugee camps, resettlement in a Western country, and the multiple pressures of adjustment (Nicassio, 1985). Their families have been forever disrupted at a stage in life when they expected to become respected elders, moral leaders, and sages. This study is based on forty life-history accounts of Vietnamese, Cambodian, Laotian, and Hmong elders that were gathered to elicit a pattern of feelings, motives, and life experiences that could be grouped around a particular locus of concern or dominant theme (Hess and Handel, 1959). These themes express a recurring fundamental view of reality from the perspective of the oldest member of a multigenerational family. For the purposes of this study, the dominant themes are conceptualized as family types and used as a framework through which intergenerational relationships and grandparenting are analyzed.[1]

▬ GRANDPARENTS IN CONTEXT

Although there is usually a clearly discernable dominant theme in the life-history narratives, most cases actually include several themes that are intertwined. Dominant themes were discerned through a process that revealed problems, dilemmas, or issues recurring frequently or with intensity across the life course. In this way, the contemporary concerns of elders are located within the context of their individual lives and family histories.

Separated Families

The eight elders whose families were classified as separated have experienced fragmentation of their family systems over the course of many years. Families were separated when the men left to fight as soldiers, when they were incarcerated after defeat or capture, during the process of escape and refugee camp internment, and during the resettlement process. Two cases illustrate the difficulties elders have fulfilling grandparenting roles in separated families.

A 76-year-old Cambodian man explains how separations occurred in a dramatic escape story as he and approximately 20 members of his extended family moved around the countryside seeking to avoid the Khmer Rouge forces and the Vietnamese invaders. "We just moved away again and again until we are in Battambong. There I made a house, day and night so that we could live happily" (CM2:1283–1288).[2] He had just finished the house when fighting erupted nearby and the family was forced to flee again. "Everyone left. Whoever stayed, they killed them all. We just went and stayed wherever we wanted . . . Afterwards, when they went around and saw that you lived there, they told you to move somewhere else" (1351–1374).

During the course of these movements, his family was disconnected, his wife died, and several family members were moved into different Thai refugee camps. Today, he lives with a second wife and his youngest daughter in the United States. A son and his family with six grandchildren live nearby, and a daughter lives in California with eight grandchildren. Three adult children and nine grandchildren remain in Cambodia. Three children and nine grandchildren were in Thai camps at the time of the interview, and two adult children were missing and presumed dead.

A 69-year-old Laotian woman's family separations began at the age of seven when her father died. Later, her husband was killed in an accident, leaving her with ten children to raise alone. One of her sons was then killed by the Communists, and, since both she and her husband had worked for the Laotian army, she felt unsafe when the Communists took control of the government. At age 57, she left eight adult children and eleven grandchildren in Laos to escape through the jungle with a daughter and nephew. After three years in a Thai refugee camp, she came to the United States to live with a granddaughter who had escaped earlier. Although she has many grandchildren in Laos, there are few relatives in the United States. Most of the time she is alone, and her thoughts often return to the past ". . . when my family was together like my children and my husband, how happy we were. Now I live alone and it's sad" (LFI:568–576).

She says she would like to visit relatives in other states, but transportation costs are prohibitive with her minimum Supplemental Security Income. She spends her time cleaning the house and talking to her granddaughter: "Mostly I tell her to do well in school and don't go out too much. I teach her about Laos culture. I tell her to be respectful" (1098–1103).

Conflicted Families

The four elders whose narratives are filled with conflict are an unusual group, since overt conflict is typically avoided in Southeast Asian families (Detzner, 1992). Conflict that does occur often involves disagreements about who in the family is supposed to be fulfilling what role(s). In many cases, conflict involves the elder's belief that the young should perform traditional filial piety practices involving respect, deference, and absolute obedience. Although the younger generations continue to show respect, the absence of many traditional rituals of deference is a recurring source of conflict. Despite their reluctance to discuss family conflict directly, there is evidence of it in almost every life-history case, across cultural groups, in both genders, throughout the life course.

A 51-year-old Vietnamese woman, the oldest child in a family with 13 children, illustrates how expectations for traditional practices of filial piety create intergenerational and social conflict. She believes that in the United States, "children have too much freedom. For example, parents aren't allowed to punish their kids with sticks. In Vietnam, children respect their elders, but not in the U.S. I knew a friend who had a teenage daughter. His daughter didn't study hard, she went out with her boyfriend every day. So her father punished his daughter by hitting her with a stick. His daughter went to tell her counselor at school that her father abused her. So finally, the agency moved the daughter from the father and put her into a foster home. Her father is very depressed now" (VF2:1210–1234).

Conflictual interactions between elders, adult children, and grandchildren, seldom experienced in Southeast Asia, are more likely in the United States. Elders report disobedience, confrontations with schools, a loss of humility on the part of youth, and other generational conflicts. Most grandparents are in the middle of the conflict, since they continue to play important roles within the family, especially in caring for grandchildren. In some conflicted families, however, when there is a divorce, geographic separation, or a history of conflict, elders are cut off from grandchildren. A 72-year-old Laotian woman reports that her granddaughter no longer listens to her advice: "She can listen or not, but as long as she doesn't talk back. In my head I love her very much. That's why I discipline her. I don't want her to be a bad person. I want her to be like a Laos lady" (LF2:1513–1524).

Lost Families

Eight of the elder's families are classified as lost because their narratives are filled with multiple losses extending across the life course. All refugees experience multiple losses (Mollica, Wyshak, and Lavelle, 1987); however, the families of elders in this category are coping with an overwhelming number of nonnormative losses. Perhaps most difficult is the loss of the honored position within families. Though elders continue many functional roles in families, they no longer have important status roles as economic provider, sage, family head, and moral leader because their experience is perceived by the young as not relevant in the American context (Detzner et al., 1989).

This loss of an important place within the family is especially difficult because elders have distinct memories of their own grandparents as revered storytellers, teachers, role models, and keepers of the past. A 60-year-old Cambodian woman who survived the holocaust in her country expressed fear about her adult children and grandchildren in the United States: "The feeling of insecurity is always in me. I'm afraid that they might not be what I want them to be because in this country the children are very unpredictable" (CF2:1367–1372). "I just pray that my children will study hard and be good. I no longer have the authority to tell them what to do ... If they do something wrong I just give them advice. If they listen then it is good. ... I don't like to talk too much, because the more you talk the less respect they have toward you" (1399–1407).

Intergenerational conflicts that arise in lost families are often related to the forfeiture of family headship and economic provider roles. The dilemma is best expressed by a 65-year-old widowed Hmong man, the father of twelve children and five grandchildren: "We Hmong never had a history of dependency on welfare or other people. Now ... most of the older people are dependent on welfare, because we didn't have any education and can't go to work. However, most of the younger people who had little education, they [are] already working and don't depend on welfare" (HM2:2088–2100). Normative developmental roles are reversed in the new environment as youth assimilate faster than elders, finding work roles and a place in the new society, while elders must accept dependency and the loss of esteem.

Resilient Families

The twenty elders whose families are classified as resilient compose the largest group in the study. Although many have experienced separation, loss, and conflict during their difficult lives, the dominant theme that emerges from their life histories is flexibility, hardiness, and tenacity in the face of major obstacles.

A 58-year-old Cambodian woman who lost her family explains the importance of her only living relative to her purpose in life: "I want to stay alive because I want to see my son finish school and get a good job, so I can live with him. My son can take care of me. I don't have to depend on strangers anymore. For now, I know my son is going to take good care of me, but in the future when he has his own family, he might change" (CFI:26–30). The importance of staying together through life's difficulties was the lesson learned when seven adult children and all her grandchildren were killed by the Khmer Rouge. When her twenty-three-year-old son returns home to visit from college "I can't sleep," the woman says. "I just sit there watching his face while he is asleep. When I see his face I think about my other [deceased] children. I keep myself alive because of my son. I don't want him to be alone. We've been through a lot of hardship together. You're happy here only if you have family with you" (CFI:10–15).

A 69-year-old Vietnamese man with nine adult children and five grandchildren living in the United States expressed the challenges confronting his grandchildren: "In my family, the [grand]children must be respectful to the elders and polite to the guests. They must bow their heads, greet the elders, and they must serve tea to the guests in the proper way. The children must speak Vietnamese at home. When they are at home they are Vietnamese, and when they leave home, they are Americans" (VM5:1970–1977). The emphasis on bicultural adaptability is an important characteristic of most resilient families.

In some resilient families, traditional expectations held by elders often create generational differences. An older Hmong man expressed concern about the ongoing tensions: "In the U.S., there are a lot of problems of understanding between the younger and the older. The younger saw and followed what American kids did, but the elders want their children to do it their way. So it creates a big problem between the younger and the older" (HM3:1346–1356). This man's solution to the dilemma is customary: "The oldest child must listen to their parent. The younger should listen to the older brother or sister so they can be a brother and sister and live very close together. So they will get along with other people around them" (1478–1485).

■ DISCUSSION

The impact of modernization and loss of continuity with the past is a significant issue in the intergenerational relations of Southeast Asian families. Efforts to reestablish traditional family practices in the United States are a functional adaptation strategy for elders seeking to maintain some element of coherence; however, these efforts often create problems between generations with very different developmental agendas. Vestiges of traditional family practice continue to be a part of everyday life, but the status of elders, especially the male patriarchs, is diminished by their efforts to hold on too strongly to the past. For grandchildren born in the United States, filial piety is difficult to practice in the nostalgically remembered ways that the elders believe to be proper.

Tensions between grandparents and grandchildren can be interpreted as a clash between modern and traditional values and between continuity and change (Weinstein-Shr and Henkin, 1991). The young are reported by their elders to be eagerly embracing individualism and materialism, while the elders consistently emphasize retention of culture and the importance of family. Many traditional practices of deference, obedience, and self-denial are in opposition to the modern values of self-expression, freedom, and individuality. It should not be surprising that intergenerational conflict would erupt in families that have been repeatedly separated, buffeted by multiple losses, and cast into a cultural value system so different from their own. With each generation having such different experiences and developmental agendas, what is surprising is the resilience evident in so many narratives.

Perhaps the most important lesson of a long life lived in the context of war and international strife is the importance of accommodation. This lesson is central to understanding intergenerational relations in these refugee families. On one hand is the centrality of family structure, hierarchy, and filial piety taught by Confucian philosophy. On the other hand is the acceptance of fate and the values of bending with the winds of change and survival taught through Buddhist religious beliefs. Although in some ways these two philosophies may appear contradictory, they might also be seen as fostering a continuing and useful dialectical process between generations in which they can address fundamental values in the dramatically altered contexts of their lives.

▬ NOTES

1. The life-history narratives are examined using a grounded theory (Strauss and Corbin, 1990), comparative cast study approach. The processes for analyzing cases follow Yin's (1984) model for multiple case comparisons and Abramson's (1992) model for the treatment of a case study within life-course and ecosystemic contexts (Bubolz and Sontag, 1992). The process of analysis is inductive, comparative, and grounded in the words, actions, and constructed accounts of elders.

2. Quotations are referenced by the culture, gender, and identifying number of the person interviewed (CM2 = Cambodian male, no. 2; LFI = Laotian female, no. 1; VFI = Vietnamese female, no. 1) and by numbered lines in an Ethnograph software text file located in the Refugee Studies Center at the University of Minnesota.

■REFERENCES

Abramson, P. 1992. *A Case for Case Studies: An Immigrant's Journal.* Newbury Park, Calif.: Sage.

Boenlien, J. K. 1987. "Clinical Relevance of Grief and Mourning Among Cambodian Refugees." *Social Science Medicine* 25: 765–72.

Bubolz, M. M., and Sontag, M. S. 1992. "Human Ecology Theory." In P. G. Boss et al., eds., *Sourcebook of Family Theories and Methods: A Contextual Approach.* New York: Plenum.

Detzner, D. F. 1993. "Transnational Families: Immigrants and Refugees." IN K. Altergott, ed., *One World, Many Families.* Minneapolis, Minn.: National Council on Family Relations.

Detzner, D. F. 1992. "Conflict in Southeast Asian Refugee Families: A Life History Approach." In J. Gilgun, K. Daly, and G. Handel., eds., *Qualitative Methods in Family Research.* Newbury Park, Calif.: Sage.

Detzner, D. F., et al. 1989. "Continuity and Change in Vietnamese and Cambodian Refugee Families: Elder Roles, Family Values, and Filial Piety." Paper presented at the 51st Annual Scientific Meeting of National Council on Family Relations, New Orleans, La.

Godziak, E. 1989. "New Branches . . . Distant Roots: Older Refugees in the United States." *Aging* 359: 2–7.

Henkin, A. B., and Nguyen, L. T. 1981. *Between Two Cultures: The Vietnamese in America.* Saratoga, Calif.: Century Twenty One.

Hess, R., and Handel, G. 1959. *Family Worlds: A Psychosocial Approach to Family Life.* Chicago: University of Chicago Press.

Kinzie, J. D. 1989. "Therapeutic Approaches to Traumatized Cambodian Refugees." *Journal of Traumatic Stress* 2(1): 75–91.

Lee, E., and Lu, F. 1989. "Assessment and Treatment of Asian-American Survivors of Mass Violence." *Journal of Traumatic Stress* 2(1): 93–121.

Liu, W., and Fernandz, M. 1988. "Asian Immigrant Households and Strategies for Family reunification." In W. Liu, ed., *The Pacific/Asian Mental Health Research Center: A Decade Review.* Chicago: Pacific/Asian American Mental Health Research Center.

Mollica, R., Wyshak, G., and Lavelle, J. 1987. "The Psycho-Social Impact of War Trauma and Torture on Southeast Asian Refugees." *American Journal of Psychiatry* 44(12): 1567–72.

Nicassio, P. 1985. "The Psycho-Social Adjustment of the Southeast Asian Refugee: An Overview of Empirical Findings and Theoretical Models." *Journal of Cross Cultural Psychology* 16(2): 153–73.

Rottman, L., and Merideth, W. 1982. "Indochinese Families: Their Strengths and Needs." In L. Stinnet et al., eds., *Family Strengths: Positive Support Systems.* Lincoln: University of Nebraska Press.

Seabloom, M. 1991. "Filial Piety Beliefs in the Life Histories of Ten Vietnamese Elders." Master's thesis. St. Paul: Family Social Science Department, University of Minnesota.

Strauss, A., and Corbin, J. 1990. *Basics of Qualitative Research: Grounded Theory Procedures and Techniques.* Newbury Park, Calif.: Sage.

Weinstein-Shr, G., and Henkin, N. 1991. "Continuity and Change: Intergenerational Relations in Southeast Asian Refugee Families." *Marriage and Family Review* 16: 351–67.

Yin, R. 1984. *Case Study Research.* Beverly Hills, Calif.: Sage.

Grandparents Remembered: Granny

ROBERT C. ATCHLEY

My earliest memories are of life in a close-knit, three-person, three-generation "broken home." Within a year after my birth in the Fall of 1939, my
father had left for parts unknown, and my mother's mother, Laura Louella
Maddux — my Granny — had made the long trip from Tennessee to Texas,
to live with Momma and me. It was a good arrangement, I think. Granny
was 71 in 1940. She had a tiny pension from Social Security, not enough
to live independently. My mother, Roberta Atchley, was 35 at the time, and
she worked a lot of twelve-hour days at a succession of challenging and
demanding jobs managing stores, supervising regional operations, and
troubleshooting ailing businesses for national ladieswear chains, and she
needed someone to take care of me. We seldom lived anywhere very long,
usually less than six months. We each had a small trunk for our clothes
and personal belongings, and we had one big trunk for our radio, dishes
and kitchen utensils, towels, linens, and so on. For us, household simplicity
was a practical necessity. Granny lived with us full-time until I was six and
off and on until her death at age 80, just before my tenth birthday. Mom
and I used to joke about our being so much alike because we had the same
mother, and in many important ways, we did.

Granny was from the hills of middle Tennessee. She had little formal
schooling, but she could read well and enjoyed it. She was a tiny woman.
When she came to live with us, I'm told she suffered from arthritis, osteoporosis, and a heart condition. But I don't remember her ever being sick
until I was about eight. What I remember most is her absolute personal
integrity, her strong will, her work ethic, her soothing deep alto voice, and
her gentle touch.

For my fifth birthday (1944), Granny gave me *The Golden Book of Bible
Stories,* a large, thick book with deep blue binding, big print, and beautiful
color prints depicting biblical scenes. We were living in a small city in the
North Carolina mountains then, and the weather was chilly and dreary a
lot that Fall. We had a wide cast-iron grate in the living-room fireplace,
where we burned huge chunks of coal to warm the small brick house.
Granny and I got in the habit of sitting close together on the overstuffed
horsehair couch, and in the flickering light she would read aloud those
exciting and inspiring stories. We did this just about every day, and by my
sixth birthday I could read them to her. I feel fortunate to have first learned
these great biblical legends as simple stories designed to be spoken and
understood by children.

There was a terrible housing shortage during World War II, and being
on the move a lot meant that we got stuck in some pretty rough accommoda-

---

From *Generations* 71–72, 1996, Spring. Reprinted with permission.

tions. Granny and I shared a bed much of that time. Granny invariably dressed in drab print dresses and "grandma shoes," and she always wore her hair in a severe bun. But at bedtime a metamorphosis occurred. She wore colorful flannel nightgowns, and she let down and brushed her long silky-fine white hair. She would often give me just a hint of a smile and say, "Last one in bed is a rotten egg!"

In 1947, when I was 8 and Granny was 78, we were living in Bristol, Virginia, in an airy second-floor apartment with lots of windows and a big four-poster bed in the large bedroom Granny and I shared. For some reason, I remember this time quite vividly. We'd put out the lights, I'd lie on my stomach and while Granny patiently and gently scratched my back — a luxurious sensation that I always looked forward to — she told stories about her life, my mother's life, and our family's history.

There were plenty of funny stories, especially about me and all the mischief I got into when I was younger. The good humor with which Granny relished these stories communicated her complete forgiveness of whatever "wrongs" I might have done. But, a lot of Granny's stories were neither pretty nor uplifting. Laura Louella Maddux had given birth to eleven children, and by 1947 all but three of them were dead. Hard-scrabble farm life, dangerous factory work, tuberculosis, smallpox, and alcoholism had taken her children, often leaving her to care for her grandchildren. I was the last grandchild of many she had taken care of.

I remember the details of these nighttime stories only haphazardly. I mostly remember how warm and safe I felt snuggled up to Granny, how thoroughly included I felt. I also felt tied through this gritty, emaciated old woman to a family that had so far managed to prevail against enormous odds. It was a head-held-high, working-class family history, one that my mother was desperately trying to leave behind back then, but Mom came to appreciate it again toward the end of her life, when she, as Granny Atchley, began to tell the family stories to my children.

Grandparents Remembered: Grandfather Chin

JENNIE CHIN HANSEN

My paternal grandfather, Grandfather Chin, was the only grandparent I ever met, since my mother's parents died before I was born, and my other grandmother never left Hong Kong. *Ah Yeah*, which translates into "father of my father" (there would be a different title for my mother's father, as there is a specific title for one's particular role in the Chinese family) was the kindly and humorous old gentleman I remember.

When I was between six and eight, my grandfather ended up being my surrogate parent because of the long hours my parents worked at their restaurant in New Jersey. I recall that he was of slight build and rather hunched, making his short height even more marked. It wasn't until years later, upon seeing his photo, that I realized that he had blue eyes — quite remarkable given the Asiatic genetic trait of brown eyes! I somehow later pieced together that there was some definite mixing somewhere along the generations.

Grandfather didn't live with us, but he did stay for extended periods. It's funny to think back to his stays; we lived in such a small flat that I have no idea where he even slept!

He painted murals and silk hangings, which were of landscapes and flowers. His work covered the walls of my parents' Chinese restaurant (a great pro bono interior designer!). Since we didn't at the time have a Chinese peer group, I didn't go to Chinese school, as many others did in the larger cities, but ended up copying the calligraphy of the Chinese newspaper that we would occasionally have access to. I recall that Grandfather was tickled to see my efforts and took particular interest in seeing that I would have "good penmanship."

During this period of my life, I had constant tonsillitis, which affected my eating ability (certainly hard to even imagine this problem now!). My grandfather would have "contests" with me to see if I could finish my food before he would. Needless to say, I pretty well knew what he was trying to do, but I would try to humor him as well. It's interesting to realize that children tune in well to the games that we adults play and often play along with us.

One other memory I have of him includes our going shopping for a particular Easter dress, one that I vividly remember to this very day. Somehow I didn't consider it at all unusual that I was going to pick out this pretty blue dress with him, despite how old and frail he already was at that time. I guess we were an "odd couple," yet I certainly never felt it, since I never looked at it through another's eyes at that time.

From *Generations* 75–76, 1996, Spring. Reprinted with permission.

These have been disparate thoughts and remembrances, but I guess they have imprinted on me the significance of that brief relationship (he died not long after these remembered events occurred). I recall the feel of holding his hand as we walked down the street, watching his intense mischievous eyes, and his walking me home from the restaurant at nights when my parents were still hard at work. There is a special trust and comfort that I had with him and a sense that he was old, yet not really. He was a part of my young life that became memorable, and perhaps that is in some measure why I have been so committed to intergenerational activity (as we have at On Lok) — to assure that continuity of caring and value from one generation to the next.

Grandparents Remembered: Andrea Arrendondo Raya

FERNANDO M. TORRES-GIL

My earliest childhood recollection of my grandmother was of her helping me with my physical therapy. She was a self-taught masseuse who would patiently work with me to help me walk. I was one of her first grandsons, and she took special pride and concern about my welfare. As I went through the early stages of polio — trips to the hospitals, recuperation, therapy — she was there, along with my mother, to provide love, support, and comfort. She was a strong figure, teaching me my prayers and my Spanish. Through the years, I came to realize that she was much more than just my support. She was the anchor that kept our extended family together — she represented the history of our family's emigration from Mexico, and she was the source of and inspiration for the values we hold today. For me, she remains one of the fundamental influences in my life.

Andrea Arredondo Raya was born in 1890 in Valle de Santiago, a small farming community in the rural areas of the state of Guanajuato. She grew up just prior to the turmoil of the Mexican Revolution, a time of haciendas and great disparities of wealth and poverty. Her early childhood was comfortable — her family was relatively well-off. But her mother died when Andrea was 13 years old, and she was raised and educated by her aunts. Her life took a dramatic turn during the Mexican Revolution. Her family lost their property and possessions and, like millions of others at the time, faced great uncertainty and insecurity. At a young age, she married my grandfather, Antonio Raya. Antonio was a humble and poor man from a village outside of Valle de Santiago, a widower with one son. He would often travel to the United States for extended periods to find work.

It was during one of his travels to the United States in the early 1920s that my grandmother, along with her husband's brother and the brother's wife, decided to immigrate to the United States. By then my grandmother had another child and was pregnant with my mother, Maria. They set out on the arduous trek not knowing where they would go and what they would do. In fact, they did not know where my grandfather was — he had disappeared. According to family folklore, on one of his trips to California he was shanghaied and taken to Alaska to work in the fish canneries. My grandmother and her relatives traveled by way of Texas to Los Angeles (where her husband had last been seen), with Andrea in the back of a pickup on a makeshift sling to protect her unborn child from the rough roads. Eventually, while in Los Angeles, and through a great stroke of luck, our grandfather found his family.

Once reunited, part of the family decided to stay in Southern California seeking work as gardeners, while my grandfather decided to try his fortune

From *Generations* 73–74, 1996, Spring. Reprinted with permission.

as a farm worker. Thus began their migrant sojourn throughout California. Being from a traditional Mexican family, Andrea would follow her husband wherever he deemed necessary. And so they wound up traveling throughout the San Joaquin Valley and the California coast, working in whatever crops would give them work, living in tents, barns, and whatever shelter they could obtain. Their life was hard. Andrea had the full responsibility of raising a rapidly expanding family (ten children) and handling the frequent moves, while her husband (and their kids) worked in the crops. Antonio eventually became a labor contractor. By 1931, they found themselves in Moss Landing and then in Castroville, where Andrea, having saved her precious dollars, had the good fortune and foresight to purchase property. Our family to this day has a family home in Castroville.

Andrea Arredondo Raya was the spiritual and emotional strength for her family. Through the worst of times — and there were times when they were not sure what they would eat or where they would sleep — she kept her family together. It was she who instilled the love of learning in her children as well as her strong faith in God and her belief in discipline. My aunts and uncles and their growing families looked to her as the thread that bound them all together. On her death in 1980, the family resolved to keep close ties, even though the extended family was spread throughout California. And today, annual family reunions are held, alternating between Northern and Southern California, with the memory of Andrea's strength and love sustaining the emotional and historical bonds of her legacy.

As I grew up and spent time with her, on her visits to Salinas where we lived in housing projects, or on our summer visits to the town of Tracy, where our grandfather had established a large ranch, I remember vividly how she would gather our growing clan of cousins together to teach us (whether we wanted it or not) the Bible, prayers, Spanish, and discipline. And woe to any of us who disobeyed her. She was a firm disciplinarian, but she was bright, vivacious, and deeply committed to her grandchildren.

This spirit of learning certainly had an impact on my mother and our siblings. Although my mother never went beyond the sixth grade, she followed her mother's example and kept books and musical instruments (my grandmother loved music and poetry) around our house and pushed us all to excel academically. When her nine children were older, my mother became a volunteer translator in the county welfare office and eventually retired from the Monterey County Department of Social Services, where she worked in the general assistance program.

Andrea, in her later years, never stopped trying to make life better for her family and others. She loved the United States and was deeply grateful to this country for the opportunities provided to her family, however difficult their experiences might have been. She was patriotic and was proud that many of her children and grandchildren served in the U.S. armed forces. Two of her sons served in World War II. She would use maps to chart their travels throughout the European and Pacific theaters of operations. Her life-long dream was to become a citizen. She attended Salinas High Adult School for six months to learn American history and English. And in her early 60s, she proudly became a U.S. citizen.

Andrea's husband died in the 1950s, and she lived until 1980. But until her very last days, without fail, she would attend church regularly, helping out with parish activities. And she would be the core of our family gatherings. One of my most rewarding moments, just prior to her death, was to bring her younger brother to Tracy on her birthday and to see them both dancing together. Andrea had raised her siblings, after the death of her mother, and here they were, both in their 70s and 80s, dancing like school kids, relishing a cherished moment, and bringing to all of us present a connection to our early history.

What Andrea represents is now solidly entrenched in her children — my aunts and uncles — and her grandchildren and great grandchildren, my cousins. She exemplifies the essence of dignity, integrity, and perseverance. She has shown that however tough life might be, believing in oneself and keeping faith with God, family, and duty is the mark of a successful and good life.

To this day, I attribute my own sense of civic duty, family, and love of country to my grandmother and my mother. Whenever I worry that perhaps what is occurring today with politics and society is a harbinger of bad times, I think of my grandmother's constant faith and optimism, and I recall how difficult her life was, yet how much she enjoyed the simple things in life, and how she never lost hope that faith and charity would overcome all obstacles.

Chapter 16

The Role of Ethnicity in Elder Care

VERONICA F. REMPUSHESKI

> Our ethnic identity provides us with a sense of origin, a set of rituals surrounding birth, death, health and illness, and a distinctive value and belief system. Similarities and differences exist across, and within, all cultural and ethnic groups. It is especially important to consider ethnicity in the care of our older clients, as they have had a very long time to incorporate cultural beliefs into their daily habits and behaviors. It is also good to note that the health care system has its own cultural milieu that may be very foreign to our clients. This chapter addresses methods of assessment and strategies for interpretation, as well as perceived biases and expectations on the part of the elder and the nurse.

The word "ethnicity" may evoke an image of an elder patient speaking a language you do not understand, performing a ritual that is strange to you, displaying icons that are unknown to you, or eating foods that have names unfamiliar to you. What part do these observable differences play in nursing care? What beliefs and meaning underlie these observable differences? How is an elder's ethnic identity reflected in perceptions of expected and received care? How does a nurse incorporate an elder's ethnic beliefs into daily practice?

The purposes of the following discussion are to examine (1) the concept of ethnicity within the context of elder care, (2) issues in the assessment of ethnicity, and (3) ways to incorporate ethnicity data into an elder's plan of care. The underlying assumptions of this discussion are that everyone has some kind of ethnic identity, that elders have had a lifetime to incorporate the beliefs of their heritage into what to them is everyday behavior, and that a health care setting represents a foreign land wherein professionals speak a foreign language, use strange signs and symbols, and, as strangers, probe intimate areas of one's body and mind.

■ CONCEPT OF ETHNICITY

What is ethnicity? Ethnic identity involves origins, rules, and contrasts[5] and answers three questions. The first question is, "Where are we from?" This question refers not only to a country of origin of ancestors, but also to

From *Nursing Clinics of North America* 24(3):717–724, 1989. Reprinted with permission.

geographic and historical dimensions of that country as well as to regional/intraregional differences. For example, not all people emigrating from one country, such as Poland, are the same. They will vary according to whether they lived in a rural or urban setting, in the mountains of southern Poland, along the sea coast of northern Poland, in a river valley, or in the plains. They will vary according to bordering countries and the relationship that exists between the bordering countries, now and in the past (for example, today Poland borders the Soviet Union to the west, Germany to the east, Czechoslovakia to the south, and the Baltic Sea to the north). They will vary according to their social standing in the country, their religious beliefs, and intraregional differences that result from the interplay between historical and ecological factors. During the period of greatest influx of Poles into the United States (1870 to 1913) for example, Poland did not exist as a country; it was partitioned into Austria, Prussia, and Russia. Immigration records for 'country of origin' reflected the immigrant's perception of his country, not the name of the geographical partition at the time of his entry into the United States. A similar situation can occur today; when the borders of Poland were redefined after World War II, some Poles found themselves living in Russia or Germany. An elder emigrating from Russia or Germany today therefore may declare himself as a Pole rather than a German or a Russian, reflective of his perception of his country of origin and ethnic identity and not of the country that now occupies those borders.[17,18]

Ethnicity is symbolized in ritual practice, which in itself dramatizes continuity with the past. A ritual is a ceremony or sequence of actions based on a belief and involving one or more persons. It is important to examine those rituals that mark transitions in the life cycle — for example, rites of passage — that yield the most valuable information regarding their association with aging.[15] What are the rites of passage in old age? Are physical signs and symptoms of disease ignored because they are thought to be a necessary part, a "rite of passage," to "getting old?" How do these rites of passage differ? They not only differ by ethnic identification but also according to the degree to which the elder has incorporated modern health care beliefs into his ethnic beliefs about health.

The second question is, "What must we do?" Ethnicity is part of a gradual and continual definition of self. It is a moral commitment. The answer to this second question includes what the elder must do to promote his own health, to give care to self in time of illness, and to give care to others in time of health or illness. In that same regard, it includes expectations that are held for receiving care from others.

The third question is, "How are we different?" A person's behavior tells him who he is and to what group he belongs. Others who behave differently are not part of this group. Therefore, we know who we are by knowing who we are not. A health care professional may be part of the group if certain traits are revealed, for example, ethnicity symbolized in a family name, language, or appearance.

The historical focus of question one integrates roles and differences (addressed in questions two and three); however, the thrust is on following the way our ancestors did things. The combined answers to these three questions constitute an individual's ethnic identity or ethnicity.

"Ethnicity generally expresses the fact that certain people are defined socially as belonging together by virtue of common descent."[7] Ethnicity may be portrayed superficially, without incorporation of beliefs into everyday behavior. This kind of ethnicity has been labeled "symbolic ethnicity" or a "nostalgic allegiance to the culture of the immigrant generation."[8] An individual therefore may find it convenient to express his ethnicity in association with a festive or popular event, not because of belief in the meaning of the rituals or the event, but because he is looking for new ways to establish differences from others. Greeley[10] asks: Under what sets of circumstances do which people express what sort of identification? When is ethnicity relevant and for whom? Is it when there is actual or potential political or economic power in the group? When it is a member of a highly visible group or a sophisticated (sought after) group?

Ethnicity in Elder Care

All of the questions just mentioned have implications for elder care, regardless of the setting in which care is delivered. Whether behaviors expressed by elders are manifestations of symbolic ethnicity or strongly held beliefs, incorporation of these behaviors into care is essential. Ethnicity is an issue in elder care because of its integrating character. An elder's "meaning of caring is symbolized in ritual practice, moral commitment, and behaviors unique to an ethnic group. Roles for caring actions and exchanges, unique to each ethnic group, determine the kind of caregiving–care receiving relationship developed between elder client and nurse."[17]

A bridging of the ethnicity and age concepts is apparent in an anthropological community study approach. The community case study approach has had a strong influence on the anthropological study of old age and certainly has implications for nursing care. A critical issue in community studies is defining the territory/geographical area, limits, or boundaries. Three themes of community assist in the defining process: (1) the idea of territory or place as a "geographical experience"; (2) the idea of group membership or a "we feeling," a shared ethnic identity; and (3) the idea of social organization or structure, defined by an insider or outsider.[6]

The ethnic community gerontological studies conducted by Guttmann (with Euro-American ethnic communities in Washington, DC, and Maryland) and Cuellar (with minority ethnic groups in San Diego) are combined[11] to reflect the potential barriers to health care. The barriers that predominate are lack of English language and communication skills and the discrepancy found between services extended to the elderly by health care providers and the expressed needs specific to an ethnic group. These authors emphasize the need for ethnic group input into the US health care system.

An overlap exists in discussing community studies specific to gerontology and ethnicity, and studies that focus on health beliefs and practices of ethnic or culture groups. Some of these studies also take a community approach; they are not all specific to elders, however.

Ethnicity studies in the United States that relate to health care in some way (for example, care, health beliefs, practices, access to health care) have focused mainly on minority groups, such as Asians, blacks, Mexican Americans, Native Americans, and Puerto Ricans, and very little attention has been given to study the health care of specific white ethnic groups. All white ethnics are aggregated together, assuming they believe and act similarly, despite differential cultural backgrounds.

Clinton[1] supports the notion that white American are heterogeneous in terms of their ethnic identity and patterns of health. Her research data demonstrate that ethnicity plays an important part in what some Euro-Americans believe and do about health. Clinton therefore cautions practitioners against assuming that ethnic differences among European descendants disappear after the first generation.

A major problem revealed by one study[4] of white ethnic groups is that many professionally staffed programs or services tend not to be successful in serving elderly ethnic clients. In this study, the norms of professional caregivers were in conflict with the norms of Irish, Italian, and Polish American elders.

Although socioeconomic factors play an important role in health care, practice issues based on cultural beliefs and perceptions about health care have emerged from the research literature.[2,3] If immigrants believe in folk illnesses, for example, they will not use a Western scientific health care system; they will use both a Western scientific health care system and a folk care system; they will perceive health care professionals as lacking an understanding of folk illnesses, and this lack of understanding affects the professional's behavior when the immigrant seeks care.

■ ASSESSMENT OF ETHNICITY

Biases — for example, likes, dislikes, and stereotypes — may be grounded in ethnicity and revealed partially in behaviors. Biases also are revealed in expectations of self and others. Strong moral commitments to a belief may underlie a behavior. A multifaceted assessment of ethnicity includes eliciting an elder's perceptions of biases and expectations of care. The nurse also must examine his or her own biases and expectations of giving and receiving care.

Nature of the Assessment

A Catch-22 situation exists in assessing ethnic identity. On the one hand, there are questions that can elicit the necessary information. On the other hand, some of these questions may be perceived as sensitive by the elder and thus set up a defensive reaction. One key to a successful assessment interview is sensitivity to behavioral cues of the elder, prior to and during the interview, and sensitivity to your own reactions and feelings. Cues can help guide the interview toward specific topics if the nurse is alert and responds to cues with an inquiry related to the elder's care — for example, comfort level, needs.

Although some ethnic identity assessment tools exist that potentially are useful in a variety of clinical settings,[13,18] a functional assessment tool eliciting information regarding usual care activities, such as personal hygiene, eating, elimination, sleeping, comfort level, and so on, can be used. Most important is not to assume that your own perspective on a kind of ritual, for example, the bathing ritual, is the norm for all elder patients. Table 16-1 lists assessment categories and suggested areas to explore with the elder when eliciting rituals, beliefs, and symbols of care activities. Three care activities — sleep, personal hygiene, and eating — are used as examples.

TABLE 16-1   Assessment Categories with which to Elicit Rituals, Beliefs, and Symbols of Care Activities

---

Sleep

Condition of room/environment: occupancy of room and bed/sleeping surface, kind of bed/sleeping surface and other furniture, condition of room (temperature, lights, doors and windows open or closed, other artifacts/symbols in room).

Kinds of covering, comforting materials: pillow/head support (height/number of supports used, type, positioning); covering (blanket type, sheet type, other).

Sleepwear: covering on head, body, legs, feet (type and variation by season or event).

Care of bed linen: kind of cleaning, frequency, how, by whom.

Bedtime ritual: time, tasks, others involved, food or liquid consumed, sensory stimulation, symbols/icons used.

Rules for sleeping: when, with whom, how, in what positions, where, beliefs related to rules.

Rules for awakening: by whom/what, how, mechanisms used.

Awakening rituals: time, tasks, others involved, food or liquid consumed, sensory stimulation, symbols/icons used.

Personal Hygiene

Tending one's body: rituals for mouth care (tools and substances used, time, who can assist); rituals for body and hair care (how, when, where, how often, substances used, taboos, gender rules, symbols, beliefs associated with aspects of ritual).

Associations with health/illness: care associated with body fluids/excretions, symbolism, body temperature, activities of tending one's body, substances used in rituals, seasonal/climate taboos, kinds of activities, time of day/year, gender rules, beliefs.

Eating

Kinds of foods: preferences, dislikes, specific to an event, ritual, specific to time of day/week/month/year, seasonal, rules or taboos for hot foods, cold foods, rules for amount, type, composition, beliefs, and symbolism associated with specific foods.

Schedule of foods: rules for when/when not to eat; amount related to time of day; healthy/ill status; associated with certain rituals, beliefs, symbols; before/after meal rituals, symbols/icons used/present.

Environment for eating: place, people, position, taboos/rules, symbols/icons used/present.

Implements/utensils: kind, number, rules for use of each, taboos, utensils as symbols.

Perceived Biases and Expectations: Elder's Perspective

An elder may choose a kind of food because, he says, "I like butter. It is better for you than margarine; it doesn't have all those additives." Butter may be an ethnic symbol and an elder has incorporated this belief into a behavior that is socially acceptable, expressed as a "like." In the Rempusheski study,[18] one Polish American elderly woman talked about when she was ill at home with the flu and her neighbors brought her chicken soup. She says:

> When I was sick that one time, I had German chicken soup, Italian chicken soup, Irish chicken soup, Jewish chicken soup, and (my husband made) Polish chicken soup. They were all chicken soup, and I ate them. I didn't care how they made them. I was tickled pink they brought it. And there was a difference. We finally ended up saying Polish chicken soup is better. (Quoted from Janina, p. 90.)[18]

Janina's expectation of care was that her husband make chicken soup even though she certainly was being "cared for" by many others with their chicken soup. She is not ungrateful for what others had done for her but she expressed her bias (like) for the soup that is symbolic of her ethnic identity.

The biases of an elder may be revealed in his choice of a nurse, perhaps believing a nurse with the same or similar ethnic beliefs will "understand" the behavior revealed. Understanding is more than the words and symbols that are communicated. Understanding or meaning is derived from the ideas, beliefs, and knowledge of a group. There may exist a unique dimension of understanding, therefore, between an elder and a nurse who hold the same or similar ethnic beliefs. Calling on the assistance of a nurse colleague who speaks the same language as an elder you are to assess is extremely helpful in eliciting biases and expectations. The nurse and elder may not have the same biases and expectations, but the elder may be more comfortable revealing them to a nurse whom he believes understands the underlying ethnic beliefs. This is revealed in the following clinical example:

Mr and Mrs H. One of the nurse specialists in the hospital where I am employed called to tell me about an elderly woman with Alzheimer's disease who was admitted from a nursing home to one of the medical units. Her husband accompanied her and was present in the hospital most of each day. I was told this story because Mr. and Mrs. H. and I share an ethnic identity and the nurse specialist observed care behavior that was supported by strong ethnic beliefs.

Mr. and Mrs. H. emigrated from the Soviet Union in 1981 to reunite with family and spend their retirement years in the United States. The medical unit staff considered this couple Russian and sought out the assistance of a Russian interpreter to communicate with Mrs. H. when her husband was not present. Staff were unable to perform a mental status examination on Mrs. H. to determine her orientation because the words she spoke were not English. The nurse specialist's assessment of Mr. H. revealed that they were Polish and both held officer positions in the Polish army during World War II. The land where they lived became Russian territory in 1945. Their first language was Polish; they also spoke Russian, German, and English, however.

Mr. H. was eager to share his heritage with me, asking where my Polish grandparents were born, and responding to my comments with his recollections of Poland. He also busied himself caring for his wife, frequently repositioning her in bed and checking her decubitus dressing after the primary nurse had just done the same. He was the primary caregiver for Mrs. H. at home for 7 years before she was placed in a nursing home within the past year. She had been diagnosed with Alzheimer's disease soon after their arrival in the United States. Both are frail elders. He talked to me as he took care of his wife and explained that there were certain things he knew she liked and other aspects of care, for example, reinforcement of decubitus dressing, were done because of certain "beliefs." Mr. H. was not dissatisfied with the care his wife was receiving. He praised the nurses for taking such "good care" of her.

The nurses revealed their frustration at returning to Mrs. H's room to find her dressings changed or reinforced, her position in bed changed, and other aspects of her care done her husband's way. My discussions with the primary nurse for this elderly couple revealed a different set of biases and expectations.

Perceived Biases and Expectations: Nurse's Perspective

Who are you? What beliefs ground your practice? There are Western scientific beliefs, an individual's ethnic and religious beliefs, and ethical beliefs underlying the profession of nursing. These beliefs are exhibited in care behavior, in choice of patients to whom we give care, in choices of care strategies, attitudes about self-care, shared care, colleagial contacts, and a host of other daily activities. The language we choose to speak is a combination of health care/nursing jargon, English, and other languages. The nurse's ethnic identity may be revealed to patients in his or her language. Or a person may reveal an ethic identity without a language component and be highly criticized for lacking such language skills. The elderly Jewish informants in Myerhoff's study of a senior center in Venice, California, asked how she could claim to be Jewish if she did not speak Yiddish.[14]

A nurse's ethnic biases and stereotypes are grounded in beliefs. These may be revealed in how a patient and family are perceived or cared for by a nurse. The health care providers in the Phillips and Rempusheski study[14] revealed ethnic stereotypes in assessing elders and caregivers in the home. For example, one of their subjects stated, "He is a man from Greece. I can see why maybe somebody would get upset with him because he's from a different culture and his reactions to things are different." The rationale given by the health care provider was based on a stereotypic view of persons from a "different culture."

In the aforementioned clinical example of Mr. and Mrs. H., the staff caring for them also viewed them stereotypically, as coming from a "different culture." The language barrier with Mrs. H. deterred their usual assessment strategies for determining cognitive function and the care provided by Mr. H. was perceived as an "interference" rather than a complimentary component of care. How might the care provided by Mr. H. (and other aspects of their ethnic beliefs) have been incorporated into a plan of care?

■ INCORPORATION OF ASSESSMENT INTO ELDER CARE PLAN

Beliefs, Rituals, and Symbols

Language, food, family name, and form of dress may be symbols of an ethnic identity, some of which may be incorporated into health care activity rituals and most of which are associated with the beliefs of an ethnic identity. The following are examples of incorporating symbols into an elder's care plan.

LANGUAGE AS A SYMBOL.   When assessment reveals an elder's primary language is not English and observations of the elder's behavior reveal use of his primary language with significant others or family members, the nurse could elicit the assistance of the elder to learn a greeting or other words in his language. Specific words in an elder's language may be reserved for certain health care rituals and he may wish to share these with a nurse in an attempt to increase understanding of a ritual and underlying beliefs.

FOOD AS A SYMBOL.   Certain kinds of foods may be symbolic of ethnic beliefs or unique to one's ethnic identity. Ethnic foods may be reminiscent of ethnic events involving family and friends and thus evoke a positive feeling in an elder. This was the situation in a southeastern US nursing home where a frail French woman was placed when her husband died. She had no other family in the United States. In an attempt to incorporate some of the elder's food preferences into the traditional "Southern" menu, a team composed of the nursing home administrator, nursing director, and dietitian explored possible interventions and decided to purchase "French pastry" for special treats once a week for this elder. The result was the emergence of an elder who displayed her ethnicity with great pride and shared her heritage with other residents and staff.

Specific kinds of foods may be identified with certain ethnic-affiliated institutions (or in the previous example, identity by regional preferences) and create bias in staff if so perceived. Gould-Stuart[9] describes one way to bring about an awareness about ethnic foods and remove the bias and complaints they had toward what they believed to be "Jewish food." Although this New York nursing home was Jewish affiliated, the chef was not Jewish and he prepared such "international" foods as *arroz con pollo* (chicken with rice) and *empanadas* (fried dumplings stuffed with beef). After a series of group sessions examining various cultures, their beliefs, and traditions, staff expressed a willingness to accept residents' unique ethnic behaviors and incorporate ethnic symbols into their care. Food was one of the highly charged topics and each staff member expressed personal "ethnic" food preferences. What was revealed by these group sessions was how a symbol, behavior, or preference may be *mis*interpreted by a nurse or, more accurately stated, that there may exist two or more different interpretations of the same behavior, preference, or symbol — for example, a nurse's interpretation and an elder's interpretation.

Nurse's Interpretation versus Elder's Interpretation

One aspect of care that is open to the nurse — elder dichotomous interpretation is following a treatment regimen. The regimen may involve dressings, applications of substances, ingestion of liquids or pills, and many other possibilities. An elder's interpretation of what a nurse taught may be quite different from what the nurse actually said. The elder's interpretation may include incorporation of folk practices or beliefs; the resultant behavior may be viewed as noncompliance from the nurse's perspective. Hess[12] illustrates this phenomenon in her study of Chinese elders' use of over the counter (OTC) drugs, wherein folk practices were transferred to perceptions of Western science/health OTC drugs. Preparations sought out by the Chinese elders in her sample were in liquid form. She suggests that the Chinese preference for teas and topical preparations for symptom relief may be explained by the use of single-dose liquid preparations in Chinese folk practices. This was in conflict with the Western medical practice of multiple dosage, in tablet or capsule form.

The previous suggestions are not inclusive of all the possibilities for incorporating ethnic assessment data into an elder's plan of care. Rather, they are examples of some of the ways others have attempted to acknowledge the uniqueness we all bring to a situation from our ethnic identity perspectives.

■SUMMARY

This article has attempted to illustrate (1) how the concept of ethnicity is related to elder care, whether that care is given at home, in a hospital, or in a nursing home; (2) some of the issues inherent in the assessment of ethnicity; and (3) some of the ways to incorporate the symbols of ethnic identity into an elder's plan of care. Essential to the assessment process are examination of perceived biases and expectations of care from both an elder's and a nurse's perspective. Incorporation of assessed ethnicity involves interpretation of an elder's behavior, rituals, and symbols — for example, preferred foods and language — and mutual planning of care that meets the priorities of the elder's ethnic beliefs.

■REFERENCES

1. Clinton J: Ethnicity: The development of an empirical construct for cross-cultural health research. West J Nurs Res 4:281–300, 1982
2. Chavez LR: Doctors, curranderos, and brujas: Health care delivery and Mexican immigrants in San Diego. Med Anthro Q 15:31–37, 1984
3. Clark M: Health in the Mexican-American Culture. New Brunswick, New Jersey, Rutgers University, 1959
4. Cohler BJ, Lieberman MA: Personality changes across the second half of life: Findings from a study of Irish, Italian, and Polish-American women. *In* Gelfand DE, Kutzik AJ (eds): Ethnicity and Aging. New York, Springer, 1979, pp 227–245

5. DeVos G, Romanucci-Ross L: Ethnicity: Vessel of meaning and emblem of contrast. *In* Devos G, Romanucci-Ross L (eds): Ethnic Identity: Cultural Continuities and Change. Palo Alto, California, Mayfield, 1975, pp 363–390
6. Eckert JK: Anthropological 'community' studies in aging research. Res Aging 5:455–472, 1983
7. Francis EK: Interethnic Relations: An Essay in Sociological Theory. New York, Elsevier, 1976, p 6
8. Gans HJ: Symbolic ethnicity: The future of ethnic groups in America. Racial Studies 2:1–20, 1979
9. Gould-Stuart J: Bridging the culture gap between residents and staff. Geriatr Nurs 7:319–321, 1986
10. Greeley AM: Why Can't They Be Like Us? Facts and Fallacies About Ethnic Differences and Group Conflicts in America. New York, Institute of Human Relations Press, 1969
11. Guttman D, Cuellar JB: Barriers to equitable service: Generations. Q J West Geront Soc 6:31–33, 1982
12. Hess P: Chinese and Hispanic elders and OTC drugs. Geriatr Nurs 7:314–318, 1986
13. Martinelli PC: Ethnicity in the Sunbelt: Italian American Migrants in Scottsdale, Arizona (Doctoral Dissertation, Arizona State University, 1984). Dissertation Abstracts International 45:2664A, 1984
14. Myerhoff B: Number Our Days. New York, EP Dutton, 1978
15. Myerhoff B: Rites and signs of ripening: The intertwining of ritual, time, and growing older. *In* Kertzer DI, Keith J (eds): Age and Anthropological Theory. Ithaca, New York, Cornell University, 1984, pp 305–330
16. Phillips LR, Rempusheski VF: A decision-making model for diagnosing and intervening in elder abuse and neglect. Nurs Res 34:137, 1985
17. Rempusheski VF: Caring for self and others: Second generation Polish American elders in an ethnic club. J Cross-Cultural Geront 3:223–271, 1988
18. Rempusheski VF: Exploration and Description of Caring for Self and Others with Second Generation Polish American Elders (Doctoral Dissertation, University of Arizona, 1985). Dissertation Abstracts International 46:3785B, 1986

Chapter 17

Aging and Health Behaviors in Mexican Americans

KYRIAKOS S. MARKIDES   SANDRA A. BLACK

In this chapter, the selected health behaviors of smoking, alcohol consumption, obesity and physical activity, and cancer-screening are examined in the elderly Mexican American population. Sociocultural factors such as socioeconomic status, language barriers, and level of acculturation may significantly influence these health behaviors. In order to design more culturally specific and appropriate interventions for this group of elders, gerontological nurses must have a clear knowledge of the prevalent health risks and intervening barriers to health promotion.

During the past two decades there has been a growing interest in the health status and health care behavior of the Hispanic population of the United States, the nation's second largest minority population, estimated at 22.4 million in 1990.[1] Most of this interest has been directed toward Mexican Americans, who constitute approximately 60% of Hispanics and live principally in the five southwestern states of Texas, New Mexico, Colorado, Arizona, and California.

A recurring conclusion about the health of Mexican Americans since the mid-1980s is that their relatively favorable profile is much closer to the Anglo population than to the African American population, to whom they are more similar socioeconomically.[2,3] Mexican Americans enjoy low mortality rates from diseases of the heart and cancer, at least among men.[2,4] This generally favorable mortality profile has been attributed to selective immigration, since immigrants appear to be healthier than native-born people,[5] and to possible protective cultural factors.[2]

Recent analyses of data from the National Longitudinal Study found lower death rates for middle-aged and older Mexican Americans of both genders than for "other white."[6] Thus, it appears that even elderly Mexican Americans may enjoy a morality advantage despite their rather poor socioeconomic conditions. However, the extent to which low mortality translates into better health is not clear. Data on functional limitations, for example,

From *Family & Community Health* 19(2):11–18, 1996. Reprinted with permission.

suggest that elderly Mexican Americans fare slightly worse than other white people but better than African Americans.[7,8] The same appears to be true with respect to self-ratings of health.[9]

Mexican Americans have high rates of diabetes (a risk factor for heart disease), high rates of obesity, and low rates of physical activity.[4] It does not appear that Mexican Americans, including the elderly, have lower rates of hypertension[4,7] than earlier thought.[10] In addition, smoking rates and alcohol consumption have been relatively high among Mexican American men.

This article provides a brief overview of recent knowledge on selected health behaviors of Mexican Americans, with particular attention to the elderly. Even though the Mexican American population is still relatively young, it is growing rapidly but remains socioeconomically disadvantaged relative to the general population. Understanding important health behaviors and practices will help in planning health promotion programs and delivering health care to this expanding segment of the population.

■ SELECTED HEALTH BEHAVIORS
Smoking

A reason traditionally given for Mexican Americans' low cancer and heart disease morality has been the population's low smoking rates.[4,11,12] However, it has been women's lower rates of smoking that have accounted for the population's overall lower rate, with Mexican American men smoking at rates equal to or higher than those of the general population.[13-15] Data from the Hispanic Health and Nutrition Examination Survey (Hispanic HANES), for example, showed high rates of smoking among Mexican American men of all ages, including the elderly, during 1982 to 1984.[16] Approximately 41% of Mexican American men aged 65 to 74 were current smokers in the Hispanic HANES, a considerably higher percentage than among elderly men in the general population.[17] Smoking rates for older Mexican American women were considerably lower than those for other women, and both Mexican American men and women smoked significantly fewer cigarettes. Level of acculturation was positively associated with the probability of being a smoker among both older men and women.[16]

The high rates of smoking by older Mexican American men during the early 1980s have received little attention in the literature. A recent analysis of data from a probability sample of Mexican American elderly people residing in the southwestern states (the Hispanic Established Populations for Epidemiologic Studies of the Elderly, or Hispanic EPESE) found significant declines in smoking rates of both men and women aged 65 to 74 from 1982 to 1984, when the Hispanic HANES was conducted, to 1993 to 1994 (Markides KS, Miller TQ, Ray LA. 1995. Unpublished data). Rates for men dropped from 41.2% to 19.6%, and rates for women fell from 19.2% to 9.8%. This encouraging trend was interpreted to mean that the broader public health message causing the general population to quit smoking is reaching elderly Mexican Americans so that they now smoke at rates similar to the general population of elderly people.[17] Nevertheless, room for further reductions exists.

Alcohol Consumption

Over the past few years alcohol consumption among Hispanics, especially Mexican Americans, has received increasing attention. This literature has shown relatively low rates of consumption among women and older people.[18-21] Mexican American men have been found to be relatively infrequent drinkers but appear to have a disproportionate number of heavy drinkers,[20-22] a pattern also observed among men in Mexico.[23] Moreover, alcohol consumption appears to be highest among the least acculturated men[24] but increases with acculturation among Mexican American women, especially younger ones.[19,25,26]

Another interesting pattern among Mexican Americans is that rates of heavy drinking remain high until late middle age[20,21,27] and then decline drastically in old age, probably because of health problems[27] and financial problems. One study found that the strongest correlate of alcohol consumption among older Mexican American men was income.[20]

Lower rates of alcohol consumption among older Mexican American men are consistent with the literature on elderly people in the general population.[28-30] One analysis of data from the 1982 to 1984 Hispanic HANES[27] found that the drop in consumption among Mexican American men in old age was considerably higher than among Cuban Americans, who exhibited consumption patterns similar to those of the general population. Further examination revealed that much of this decline is related to health problems among previously heavy drinking Mexican American men.[27]

A recent study using national data found significantly lower alcohol consumption rates in 1990 than in 1984 among white people. However, no declines were observed among Hispanics.[29] Unfortunately, no data on trends were available for elderly Hispanics. However, it is possible to examine trends using data from the Hispanic HANES (1982 to 1984)[21] and data from the Hispanic EPESE (1993 to 1994), both of which have representative samples from the southwestern states. Among Mexican American men aged 65 to 74, 32.8% reported consuming alcohol during the month prior to the interview in 1993 to 1994, down from 46.8% in 1982 to 1984. A similar decline was observed among women aged 65 to 74, down to 6.8% in 1993 to 1994 from 14.2% in 1982 to 1984. No significant trends were observed with respect to frequency and volume of consumption.

It appears that alcohol consumption is a problem among Mexican American men until well into late middle age, when health problems force them to abstain or reduce their levels of consumption significantly. In addition, it is not clear how many do not survive to old age because of alcohol-related mortality; mortality from cirrhosis of the liver is considerably higher among Mexican American men than among other white men.[2,3]

Obesity and Physical Activity

It has long been established that rates of obesity are higher among Mexican Americans than among the general population and that obesity is implicated in the population's high rates of diabetes.[2-4] It has also been found that Mexican Americans are less physically active, at least with respect to nonwork or leisure-time activity such as exercise.[4,31,32] However, knowledge about obesity and physical activity has generally been limited to middle-aged and younger subjects. Although obesity rates appear to continue to be high in the older years,[2] it is not clear what happens with physical activity. Since physical activity in old age is mostly limited to nonwork or leisure-time activity, it is probable that exercise rates are low among elderly Mexican Americans. Yet one study of Medicaid recipients in California found higher levels of exercise among elderly Mexican Americans than among non-Hispanic white people.[33] Another study of Latino adults in California found that vigorous physical activity was positively associated with self-efficacy, support from friends, eating a heart-healthy diet, and physical activity in childhood.[34] Clearly, much more remains to be learned about both obesity and physical activity in elderly Mexican Americans and how they relate to health and quality of life.

Cancer Screening

Limited literature suggests that cancer screening rates are much lower among Mexican Americans than among other groups. Data from the 1987 National Health Interview Survey (NHIS), for example, indicate that Mexican Americans use cancer screening tests less frequently than African Americans and non-Hispanic white Americans.[35] These data also suggest that lower screening results from lack of knowledge and that ethnic differentials disappear when Mexican Americans are aware of such tests.

Two areas that have received attention among Mexican Americans are screening for breast and cervical cancer. Kaplan and colleagues,[36] for example, demonstrated that the rates of cervical cancer screening are much lower among Mexican American women than among non-Hispanic white women. Data from the NIHS revealed that Hispanic women were over three times as likely not to have ever had a Pap smear.[37] At particularly high risk were Hispanic women over 65 who lived below the poverty level. Suarez[38] found that rates of cervical cancer screening decreased dramatically with age, from almost 62% among Mexican American women aged 40 to 49 to about 28% of women aged 70 and older. An important ethnic difference is that non-English-speaking women are much less likely to know what a Pap smear is.[39]

Mexican American women also are less likely to participate in breast cancer screening.[37,38,40-43] For example, Calle and colleagues[37] found that Hispanic women, particularly those over 65, had lower rates of ever having had a mammogram or having had a mammogram in the past year. Although one study found that the low rates of breast cancer screening in Mexican American women varied little with age,[38] another study found the rates of mammography to be markedly lower among Hispanic women over the age of 75.[40]

Lower mammographic screening rates are attributed to lack of access to regular medical care, cost, and lower educational attainment. One study found that the prevalence of breast cancer screening was lower in Hispanic women in Texas than in black women, raising the question of whether language and cultural barriers negatively influence mammographic screening, as well as rates of clinical breast examination and breast self-examination, in Hispanic women.[43] Hispanic women were less likely than Anglo women to report a physician referral for mammography. This finding is consistent with the observation that primary care physicians caring for predominantly Hispanic patients are less likely to recommend mammography than are physicians of predominantly Anglo patients.[44] It has also been found that greater insurance inadequacies, poorer quality of life, and greater concern about breast cancer among Hispanics interfere with the maintenance of screening behavior.[45]

The importance of language barriers was recently highlighted in a study of screening behavior of older Hispanic women in Los Angeles.[42] This study found that language acculturation (greater understanding and use of English) was associated with greater exposure to media-based health information. Media exposure, in turn, was associated with higher rates of cancer screening and knowledge of cancer symptoms, controlling for acculturation, age, education, and health insurance coverage.

■IMPLICATIONS FOR HEALTH PROMOTION

Although recent evidence suggests a relatively favorable health profile for Mexican Americans, especially with respect to mortality indicators, it does not appear that this favorable health profile is present among elderly Mexican Americans. However, data on the health of elderly Mexican Americans have been scarce. The Hispanic EPESE, a large-scale epidemiologic study of the health of elderly Mexican Americans currently under way, promises to generate much-needed information.

Examinations of how important health behaviors influence the health of Mexican Americans have not yielded definitive conclusions. However, it is probable that negative health behaviors in early life influence the health status of elderly people. Smoking and alcohol consumption rates have been found to be high among Mexican American men in the middle and younger years. What this means for the health of older Mexican Americans has not been well documented. A hopeful sign is recent declines in both smoking and drinking among elderly Mexican Americans in the Southwest, particularly men.

Another important area is obesity and physical activity. Rates of obesity are high among Mexican Americans, including the elderly, despite relatively favorable diets.[46] The evidence on levels of physical activity is inconclusive, although it appears that Mexican Americans engage in less leisure-time activity such as exercise, which is particularly relevant among older people, the vast majority of whom do not benefit from work-related physical activity. In addition, clear disadvantages are observed in health screening among Mexican Americans, particularly for cancer screening such as Pap smears and mammograms.

Many disadvantages in health behaviors are related to socioeconomic and possibly cultural factors. Clearly, Mexican Americans are socioeconomically and educationally disadvantaged relative to the general population. In addition, they have low health insurance coverage,[47] which likely influences health status in the later years. Insurance coverage is less of a problem among elderly Mexican Americans, of whom an estimated 87% are covered by Medicare.[7] Although this percentage has increased significantly in recent years, it remains considerably below the figure for the general elderly population.[48] Moreover, few Mexican Americans have supplemental private insurance[7] to cover gaps in Medicare coverage, and attempts by Congress to reduce Medicare spending are likely to disproportionately affect Mexican Americans and other minority elderly people.

Another critical barrier for Mexican American elders is language. English language ability is highly associated with exposure to media-based information regarding health and health screening practices. Low screening rates are clearly related to educational and language barriers rather than to any inherent cultural factors.

Interventions to improve the health status of Mexican Americans, including the elderly, are much needed. Interventions to reduce smoking and alcohol consumption, especially among younger and middle-aged men, are necessary in the family, school, community, and worksite to counteract advertising campaigns by cigarette and alcohol companies directed at Hispanic communities.[3] Similar interventions to promote physical activity and reduce obesity are needed at every age, including among elderly people. Spanish-language, media-based interventions are especially important to increase health screening rates, especially among elderly Mexican American women, as are interventions aimed at physicians caring for elderly Mexican Americans. The success of any intervention is likely to depend on the extent to which cultural factors related to family, church, and other community supports are incorporated.

We are only now beginning to understand the special health and health care needs of elderly Mexican Americans. Even though they constitute a small proportion of the Mexican American population, this proportion is rising rapidly. Better understanding of how health behaviors and related socioeconomic, cultural, and genetic factors earlier in life influence health in the older years is much needed, as are interventions aimed at improving the health of the Mexican American population in general.

■ REFERENCES

1. U.S. Bureau of the Census. *Race and Hispanic Origin.* Washington, DC: U.S. Bureau of the Census; 1991. 1990 Census Profile, no. 2 (June).
2. Markides KS, Coreil J. The health of Southwestern Hispanics: an epidemiologic paradox. *Public Health Rep.* 1986;101:253–265.
3. Vega WA, Amaro H. Latino outlook: good health, uncertain prognosis. *Annu Rev Public Health.* 1994;15:39–67.
4. Mitchell BD, Stern MP, Hazuda HP, Patterson JK. Risk factors for cardiovascular mortality in Mexican Americans and Hispanic whites. *Am J Epidemiol.* 1990;131:423–433.
5. Stephen EH, Foote K, Hendershot GE, Schoenborn CA. *Health of the Foreign-Born Population: United States, 1989–90.* Hyattsville, Md: National Center for Health Statistics; 1994. Advance Data from Vital and Health Statistics, no. 241.
6. Sorlie PD, Backlund MS, Johnson NJ, Rogat F. Mortality by Hispanic status in the United States. *JAMA.* 1993;270:2646–2648.

7. Markides KS, Rudkin L, Angel RJ, Espino DV. Health status of Hispanic Elderly in the United States. In: Martin LJ, Soldo B, Foote K, eds. *Racial and Ethnic Differences in Late Life Health in the United States.* Washington, DC: National Academy Press. In press.

8. Wallace SP, Levy-Storms L, Ferguson LR. Paid help for disabled elderly: do Latinos differ from non-Latino whites? *Am J Public Health.* 1995;85:970–975.

9. Angel JL, Angel RJ. Age at migration, social connections, and well-being among elderly Hispanics. *J Aging Health.* 1992;4:480–499.

10. Pappas G, Gergen PJ, Carroll M. Hypertension prevalence and the status of awareness, treatment, and control in the Hispanic Health and Nutrition Examination Survey (HHANES), 1982–1984. *Am J Public Health.* 1990;80:1431–1436.

11. Lee ES, Roberts RE, Labarthe DR. Excess and deficit lung cancer mortality in three ethnic groups in Texas. *Cancer.* 1976;38:2551–2556.

12. Menck H, Henderson B, Pike M, et al. Cancer incidence in the Mexican American. *J Natl Cancer Inst.* 1975;55:531–536.

13. Haynes SG, Harvey C, Montes H, Cohen BH. Patterns of smoking among Hispanics in the United States: results from the HHANES 1982–84. *Am J Public Health.* 1990;80(suppl):47–53.

14. Marcus AC, Crane LA. Smoking behavior among US Latinos: an emerging challenge for public health. *Am J Public Health.* 1985;75:169–170.

15. Markides KS, Coreil J, Ray LA. Smoking among Mexican Americans: a three-generation study. *Am J Public Health.*1987;77:708–711.

16. Coreil J, Ray LA, Markides KS. Predictors of smoking among Mexican Americans: findings from the Hispanic HANES. *Prev Med.* 1991;20:508–517.

17. Centers for Disease Control and Prevention. Cigarette smoking among adults — United States, 1993. *Morbidity Mortality Weekly Rep.* 1994;43:925–930.

18. Caetano R. Drinking patterns and alcohol problems among Hispanics in the US: a review. *Drug Alcohol Depend.* 1983;12:37–57.

19. Caetano R. Acculturation and drinking patterns among US Hispanics. *Br J Addict.* 1987;82:789–799.

20. Markides KS, Krause N, Mendes de Leon CF. Acculturation and alcohol consumption among Mexican Americans. *Am J Public Health.* 1988;78:1178–1181.

Chapter 18

Conformity With Nature: A Theory of Chinese American Elders' Health Promotion and Illness Prevention Processes

YEOU-LAN DUH CHEN

Chinese immigrants are a rapidly expanding group, and their health care practices and beliefs are sometimes difficult for non-Asian health professionals to understand. In order to give culturally competent nursing care, we must have a better grasp of the similarities and differences between the underlying belief systems of the mainstream culture and this important ethnic group. Common beliefs and behaviors of health promotion among Chinese American elders, garnered through the use of qualitative research methods, are described in this chapter.

The Chinese, one of the largest groups of Asian immigrants in the United Stats, are increasing more rapidly than any other immigrant group.[1,2] According to Weeks,[3] 98% of Chinese elders in the United States were foreign born. Language barriers, unfamiliarity with services offered in the health care system, and misunderstanding and misinterpretation on the part of American health care providers with regard to Chinese health beliefs and health-related behaviors have been identified as barriers to care for Chinese elders.[4,5] Concepts of health and illness and health-related attitudes and behaviors are influenced by the Chinese cultural heritage. To provide culturally relevant nursing care, nurses must take these influences into account.[6-9]

The research described in this article sought to generate a substantive theory that explains the worldview of health and illness and the beliefs and behaviors with respect to health promotion and illness prevention among Chinese elders. The following research question guided this study: What are the health and illness beliefs and social processes of health-related behaviors among Chinese elders in the United States?

From *Advances in Nursing Science* 19(2):17–26, 1996. Reprinted with permission.

▰ BACKGROUND

Confucianism, Taoism, and Buddhism are three philosophies or religions that strongly influence the Chinese way of living and thinking, including beliefs and behaviors about health and illness.[10-13] The teachings of Confucius, which are principles for social interaction, have had the greatest influence on Chinese behavior. "Jen" (benevolence), "Yi" (righteous), "Chung" (loyalty), "Hsia" (filial piety), and "Te" (virtue) are five characters that represent important concepts of Confucianism.[10,14]

"Tao," or Way, is the major concept of Taoism: "Man models himself on earth, earth on heaven, heaven on the way, and the way on that which is naturally so."[15(p82)] Taoism teaches that human beings should be in harmony with nature, that is, Tao.[16,17]

The theory of "Yin" and "Yang," which was expanded by Taoism, dominates concepts of health and illness in traditional Chinese thought.[18,19] In Chinese medicine, health is viewed as harmony between the forces of Yin and Yang within and between the body and the environment. Illness, in contrast, is viewed as an imbalance or disequilibrium of these forces.[20,21] The forces of Yin and Yang formulate the Qi (or Chi), which is classified into human, heaven, and earth Qi.[22] Qi is called "vital energy" in the West[23]; "Qi is the source of life" and is defined as "the energy circulating in the human body."[22(p10)] The study of human Qi relates to health and longevity. The traditional Chinese physician focused on the interruption or blockage of Qi, the driving force (or energy) of the cosmos and of human life. This system formed the basis for the diagnosis and treatment of illness, as well as for promoting health and preventing illness.[24,25]

Mercy, thriftiness, and humility are the three treasures of Buddhism. "Inn" and "Ko" (cause and effect) is the principle that encourages people to do "good" and "right" and to receive "good" in return.[17,25]

For this study, symbolic interactionism[26,27] provided the underlying theoretical foundation. Symbolic interactionism helps in understanding an individual's behaviors related to health and the meaning of those behaviors based on interaction with others.

▰ METHODOLOGY

The grounded theory method, an approach to understanding how people define reality through social interactions, was used to conduct this study.[28] The grounded theory method captures and describes the process of health promotion and illness prevention.[29-33]

Participants

Theoretical and convenience sampling were used to select the participants. The four selection criteria were (1) age of 60 and older; (2) immigration from Taiwan, Republic of China; (3) minimum of 6 months' United States residency; and (4) noninstitutionalization. Informed verbal consent from the participants was obtained and their confidentiality assured. Initial participants were recruited from a Chinese Christian church. Later, these elders introduced their friends to the study. The completed study included 21

Chinese elders aged 60 to 90 years living in Salt Lake City, Utah. Eleven were women, and 12 had post-high school education. All had been married, but nine were widowers or widows. Seventeen of the Chinese elders had lived in the United States from 5 to 15 years.

Data Collection and Analysis

Data were collected through two interviews 2 weeks apart, observations during interviews, personal health diaries of one week's duration, and the researcher's memos and journal. The key questions asked at the first interview were, "What are your beliefs and behaviors in promoting health and preventing illness?" "Why do you believe this?" and "What do you do to stay healthy?" The second interview validated and clarified data from the first and gave each participant a chance to elaborate on his or her initial responses. Interviews were conducted in Mandarin Chinese and were tape-recorded in each Chinese elder's home. The diaries and taped interviews were translated into English by the researcher. A second nurse, also fluent in Mandarin Chinese, listened to the tapes to validate the translation.

Observations were used to provide information that might have been overlooked by the interviewing method alone. For example, one elder did not mention taking herbs to promote his health. However, on the table the researcher noted Tu-Chun tea, ginseng tea, and ginseng root. The elder even urged the researcher to drink some ginseng tea saying, "It is good for your health." Observational notes were written immediately after each interview. The diaries documented the participant's health activities. The interviews, observations, and diaries served as triangulation to enhance the credibility of the study. The researcher's personal memos and journal provided another source of data. All data were analyzed by constant comparative analysis.

Data analysis and collection were concurrent. Coding and categorizing formulated a tentative framework. Key words used by the elders were coded as substantive codes. For example, a woman stated, "Respect from other people can provide happiness and promote an elder's health." Respect and happiness were coded as substantive codes. As the data were coded and compared, clusters and patterns of categories emerged. A detailed decision trail was formulated to enhance transferability.

Reduction of categories, selective sampling of the literature to support the data, and emergence of the core variable were used to expand the emerging conceptual framework. Literature explaining the Yin and Yang theory was selected to support the idea of health and illness discussed by the Chinese elders. An American researcher served as peer debriefer. Study participants were asked to validate their statements during the second interview and at the time of the final draft. An audit trail provided detailed information and evidence of the research process. This audit trail and all of the data, including written documentation, were kept to ensure the dependability and confirmability of the study. Rigor was examined and trustworthiness enhanced through credibility, transferability, dependability, and confirmability, as described by Lincoln and Guba.[34]

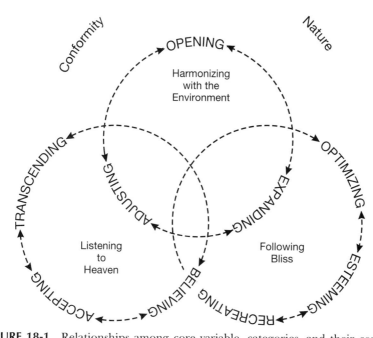

FIGURE 18-1 Relationships among core variable, categories, and their complementary properties.

▰FINDINGS

Conformity with nature, the substantive theory that was generated from this study, is the process of knowing nature and trying to modify oneself to best fit nature's flow. Through this process, a person achieves health and wellness. *Nature* is defined by this study's data as all things and events that surround one, such as air, mountains, plants, animals, people, society, and even Supreme Nature. Nature forms rhythms or patterns such as cultural dynamics, changes in seasons, and the series of changes from birth to death. Three categories — harmonizing with the environment, following bliss, and listening to heaven — interrelate to form the core variable, conformity with nature. The theory is depicted in Figure 18-1.

Harmonizing with the Environment

Harmonizing with the environment is a process of discovering and attempting to be in balance with nature through opening, adjusting, and expanding, three complementary properties.

Opening is the process of allowing oneself to gain access to, experience, interact with, and be aware of nature. Accessing and accepting nature, obtaining information about nature, and using natural resources were ways the Chinese elders reached opening.

The Chinese elders were likely to walk or exercise outdoors. They believed that the natural scene gives them peace of mind and that fresh air promotes their health. Being open in the aging process means being aware, seeking valid information, and accepting this change. A Chinese proverb quoted by several elders, "Follow the culture wherein you live," made it easier for the elders to be open and adjust to the American social environment. One elder stated, "Even though we elderly have language and transportation difficulties, I still believe we should attend activities which are offered in American society. It can give us a chance to know the society and culture. However, it is hard to do it."

Adjusting is the process of modifying oneself to harmonize with nature. The elders believed that nature provides the elements necessary for one to live. Therefore, to achieve health, an individual must modify the self to fit natural rhythms. Most of the Chinese elders used the theory of Yin and Yang to guide and make adjustments to their body's constitution and environment. Summer is a Yang season, and winter is a Yin season. The elders believed that living differently in each season was important. Particular herbs and foods were used to adjust one's Yin and Yang. One elder stated, "during winter we need to eat more Yang type foods, and during summer we should eat more Yin type foods." Another observed, "Chinese herbs work as either 'Boo' or 'Shu.' Herbs either add to or remove excess Yin and Yang from our bodies. . . . When we use herbs, we need to be aware of the seasons, the body's constitution, and the herbs' characteristics."

Regarding adjustment to biological changes associated with aging, the Chinese elders believed that it is important to do things based on actual abilities. Overdoing and underdoing were not considered good for health. In exercising, the elders began with gentle types of traditional Chinese movements rather than the vigorous exercises that were possible when they were young.

Expanding is the process of generating an expansive lifestyle by adjusting to one's dynamic environment and events. The study participants believed that Chinese values do not need to be completely replaced with American values: The Chinese values they believed were good were kept, but some were abandoned if inappropriate to the American environment. Through this a healthy, happy, and expansive lifestyle could be generated and practiced.

All elders agreed that aging is a natural process. Therefore, they wanted to accept and adjust to it and not be afraid. They wanted to realize and use their abilities to live fulfilling lives. One elder explained, "Though physically we cannot contribute much to society, we can contribute our wisdom and experience to the community." Another noted, "I teach an American friend Tai-Chi movement every morning. That is the way I see myself contributing to American society."

Following Bliss

Following bliss is sensing or seeing a goal that "fits" with one's idea of happiness in life and living to achieve that goal. All elders stated that following bliss means doing things that make them happy while not

threatening others' happiness, especially that of family members. All participants agreed that "All goes well in a harmonious home." Optimizing,
esteeming, and re-creating are the three properties of following bliss.
A person who reaches the level of recreating is considered to be highly
blissful.

Optimizing is the process of dealing with daily events positively and openly.
All elders believed that optimizing based on open-mindedness is the most
effective way to achieve bliss: Problems appear less serious, and solutions
are more apparent. Religion is one way the elders encouraged positive and
hopeful attitudes. Several elders expressed the following thoughts: "In our
lives, eight out of ten events do not happen as we wish. We should deal
with these things with an open and positive attitude. Otherwise, we would
easily give up this tough life."

Optimizing and open-mindedness can be learned from Chinese philosophies such as Confucianism and Taoism. Many Chinese proverbs encourage
perceiving events in an open and optimizing manner. Two examples
were frequently stated by elders: "When it comes to the bridge, the boat
will straighten," and "Heaven never leaves a person absolutely no way
out."

Esteeming is the process of cultivating self-worth. Esteeming includes self-
respect and respect from others. All elders stated that being respected by
their children was very important to their happiness and health. If they
wanted respect from others, they must first consider whether they deserve
it. To obtain self-respect from others, they must practice upright behavior
(eg, being honest, dependable, socially acceptable, and trustworthy), take
care of themselves, keep their knowledge current, respect and love their
adult children, and help their adult children with housework. Helping with
housework can also increase satisfaction with life and happiness. A 90-
year-old woman stated, "Doing housework as a form of exercise not only
improves your physical health but can also increase your self-worth and
make you happy."

Re-creating is the process of making a new life and reviewing daily activities
to make life more blissful. The Chinese elders stated that a busy, but not
hurried, daily schedule and being active are important for life satisfaction
and health promotion. A man commented, "Retirement means one retires
from one's job but not from one's activities."

Having a routine or regular lifestyle that follows natural rhythms and
includes exercising, eating balanced food (more vegetables and bean
products), enjoying hobbies, staying active, and believing in God is the
way to re-creating a healthy and meaningful lifestyle for these elders.
A Chinese proverb quoted by several elders, "Diseases enter the mouth,"
guided their dietary activities. Food should be fresh and light, and one
should consume "eight out of ten" (80% of satiety). The elders walked,
gardened, or practiced traditional Chinese movements such as Tai-
Chi, Y-Tan-Kun, Swai-so, and Pa-Dun-Gin for exercise. These Chinese
movements also serve as therapy. After performing 1,000 Swai-so movements twice daily for a year, a woman reported that she recovered
markedly from right hemiparesis that followed a cerebrovascular accident.

Listening to Heaven

Listening to heaven is knowing and accepting the divine purpose in life and living in the knowledge of that purpose. It focuses on "the things not seen" — that is, the spiritual dimension of existence. Three properties of this category are believing, accepting, and transcending.

Believing is the process of crediting God or a supreme being with providing meaning to life events. All participants believed first that there is at least one supreme being who is powerful and controls all events. Second, they believed that everything that happens in one's life (including health status) occurs for a reason. Third, they saw being healthy as a blessing from God, while illness may be either a warning, a punishment, or a blessing. A belief in God is an effective way to promote health. The elders explained:

> *Fate, Inn, and Ko are the main factors that determine health. Fate is just like a net that is made up of many different threads. Each thread is connected to another, and all are attached. Each thread affects all others. Therefore, always doing good to others and being a good person are very important.*
>
> *When you believe in God, you will be more aware of your behaviors and will be encouraged to be good. Then you will have no guilt and feel more peaceful, which can promote your mental health.*
>
> *Believing in God can change an individual's view of the meaning of events, which then makes life less threatening and stress producing.*

Accepting is the process of trusting God's will. Practicing acceptance gives more peace than believing in God alone. Accepting provides confidence in the midst of uncertainty, a means for coping with difficulties, protection from danger, consolation from sin or mistakes, comfort from pain, and care of self and others. A Christian man stated, "Our bodies are God's dwelling. Therefore, we should take good care of ourselves. Also, we should love and care for other people because that is God's will." A Buddhist woman observed, "Caring and helping people can accumulate goodness. In the concept of Inn and Ko, the good causes will become good effects. Therefore, caring for people is not only a benefit to others but also a benefit to ourselves."

All elders expressed that the highest acceptance of God is to "Listen to heaven and follow fate." That is, when things happen, the individual should try his or her best, be positive, and leave the outcome to God. Meanwhile, they should let God lead the way.

Transcending is the process of achieving ultimate well-being. The ultimate level of believing in God is worshipping God totally and placing oneself entirely into God's hands. A man explained, "When people reach this stage, they can forget their pain and convert the pain into helping others." Helping others produces real happiness and peace of mind — the highest goal of ultimate well-being.

Believing, accepting, and transcending are complements. When one reaches the level of transcending, one is considered to have achieved ultimate well-being.

■DISCUSSION

Conformity with nature, the substantive theory for Chinese elders, promotes health and prevents illness by enabling the elders to adjust to and conform with nature to achieve harmony, center on family and society to follow bliss, and accept the will of heaven to achieve ultimate well-being. Conformity with nature is viewed not as being passive but as doing one's best and going with the flow. Once the effort is made, the outcome is accepted peacefully.

This theory reflects a holistic view of the individual and world that is strongly influenced by Chinese culture. It reflects the teachings and thoughts of Confucianism, Taoism, and Buddhism. Harmony with all others and a lack of self-centeredness, respect for parents, and loyalty to family are the main teachings of Confucianism.[12] Harmony with nature, simplicity, and selflessness are the major tenets of Taoism.[16] Love, faith, and compassion for the living are emphasized in Buddhism.[17] Even though several participants in this study were Christian, the influence of Buddhism, so central to Chinese culture, was still expressed. All of the elders valued Chinese medicine, and most used Chinese herbs to promote health and prevent illness.

This study demonstrates that Chinese elders believe in and seek a satisfying social life, happiness, and peace to promote health and prevent illness. A satisfying social life means harmony with the social environment. Language barriers and transportation difficulties limit social interactions, and the tendency to socialize primarily with the Chinese community is a common phenomenon among Chinese immigrants.[5,13] Happiness is reached through respect from others, especially adult children, and being open-minded. A peaceful mind is gained through devotion to a religion or to God.

The goals of promoting health and preventing illness are similarly valued by Chinese and American elders.[35,36] However, the methods to approach the goals and the meaning behind the methods are different. For example, in the Chinese diet, "foods are considered for their flavor, energies, movement, and common or organic actions"; in the Western diet, "foods are considered for their protein, calories, and carbohydrates."[37(p3)] The Chinese believe that elders should eat more vegetables and bean products such as tofu for a healthy, long life.[38] In this study, elders not only chose foods to achieve the above purposes, but also added herbs to enhance the functions.

For the Chinese, exercises that involve movement are designed to guide ("Daogi") and activate ("Xingi") the Qi.[39-41] The movements are known as "preventive against old age and sickness, but also serve to cure certain diseases, chronic and acute."[39(p225)] The types of movement this group of elders chose depended on their physical condition and their purpose. For example, a woman chose Y-Dan-Kun to treat her high blood pressure. In Western culture, exercise places more emphasis on cardiovascular fitness. For happiness, the Chinese elders emphasized the harmony of family; an individual would sacrifice a personal interest if it would not benefit the family as a whole.[11] In America, the focus is more on individual happiness.

The response from family members or society is crucial to Chinese elders' self-worth and happiness, but it receives less emphasis in Western society.

■IMPLICATIONS FOR NURSING
The theory of conformity with nature provides nurses a subjective and philosophical basis for understanding Chinese elders' worldview, beliefs, and practices regarding health promotion and illness prevention. This theory can be used to design nursing care strategies and to target areas of risk. Nurses need to be aware of several points when they assess Chinese elders and plan their care: To achieve harmony with the environment, the elders prefer to obtain and use natural resources. For example, they prefer opening a window to using an air conditioner, eating fresh foods to eating canned foods, and taking Chinese herbs or natural products for promoting health and preventing illness. To maintain harmony with the social environment, Chinese elders usually do not argue with health care providers, even when they disagree. Chinese elders value consideration of other people and will withdraw their ideas if they believe they would inconvenience others. Nurses need to be patient and to encourage elders to express their thoughts, to respect what the elders say, and to follow up by checking with family members. Because home harmony is highly valued, nurses need to consider family opinions and ideas when making plans for elders. Health education must be delivered to the family as a unit.

Multiple research methods are needed to test, validate, and refine this theory. Studies of this theory's applicability to other ethnic and age groups are warranted.

■REFERENCES
1. Gardner RW, Robey B, Smith PC. Asian Americans: growth, change, and diversity. *Popul Bull.* 1985;40:1–44.
2. U.S. Bureau of the Census. *Statistical Abstract of the U.S. 1993.* Washington, DC: U.S. Dept. of Commerce; 1993.
3. Weeks JP. *Aging: Concepts and Social Issues.* Belmont, Calif: Wadsworth: 1984.
4. Carp FM, Kataoka E. Health care problems of the elderly of San Francisco's Chinatown. *Gerontologist.* 1976;16(1):30–38.
5. Chang K. Chinese Americans. In: Giger JN, Davidhizar RE, eds. *Transcultural Nursing.* St. Louis, Mo: Mosby; 1991.
6. Andrews MM, Boyle JS. *Transcultural Concepts in Nursing Care.* Philadelphia, Pa: Lippincott, 1995.
7. Chae M. Older Asians. *J Gerontol Nurs.* 1987;13(11):11–16.
8. Leininger MM. The theory of culture care diversity and universality. In: Leininger MM, ed. *Cultural Care and Diversity and Universality: A Theory of Nursing.* New York, NY: National League for Nursing; 1991.
9. O'Hara EM, Zhan L. Cultural and pharmacologic considerations when caring for Chinese elders. *J Gerontol Nurs.* 1994;20(10):11–16.
10. Allinson RE. *Understanding the Chinese Mind: The Philosophical Root.* Hong Kong: Oxford University Press; 1989.
11. Chen-Louie T. Nursing care of Chinese-American patients. In: Orque MS, Blouch B, Monrroy L, eds. *Ethics in Nursing Care: A Multicultural Approach.* St. Louis, Mo: Mosby; 1983.
12. Hansen C. *A Daoist Theory of Chinese Thought.* New York, NY: Oxford University Press; 1992.

13. Spector RE. *Cultural Diversity in Health and Illness.* Norwalk, Conn: Appleton & Lange; 1991.
14. Graham AC. *Studies in Chinese Philosophy and Philosophical Literature.* Albany, NY: State University of New York Press; 1990.
15. Lau DC. *Lao Tzu: Tao Te Ching.* London, England: Penguin; 1963.
16. Lao-Tze. *The Canon of Reason and Virtue.* La Sulle, Ill: Open Court; 1991.
17. Ching J. *Chinese Religions.* Maryknoll, NY: Orbis; 1993.
18. Hoizey D. *A History of Chinese Medicine.* Vancouver, BC, Canada: University of British Columbia Press; 1993.
19. Owson M. *Chinese Medicine.* New York, NY: William Morrow; 1988.
20. Beinfield H, Korngold E. *Between Heaven and Earth: A Guide to Chinese Medicine.* New York, NY: Ballanine; 1991.
21. Porkert M, Ullmann C. *Chinese Medicine.* New York, NY: Holt; 1990.
22. Yang J. *Chinese Qigong Massage.* Jamaica Plain, Mass: Yang's Martial Arts Association; 1994.
23. Moffet HH. Acupuncture and oriental medicine update. *Alternative Complementary Ther.* 1994;1(1):46–47.
24. Beinfield H, Korngold E. Chinese traditional medicine: an introductory overview. *Alternative Therapies.* 1995;1(1):44–52.
25. Capra FM *The Tao of Physics.* New York, NY: Bantam New Age Books; 1991.
26. Blumer H. *Symbolic Interactionism: Perspective and Method.* Englewood Cliffs, NJ: Prentice-Hall; 1969.
27. Mead GH. *Mind, Self and Society.* Chicago, Ill: University of Chicago Press; 1955.
28. Glaser BG, Strauss AL. *The Discovery of Grounded Theory: Strategies for Qualitative Research.* Chicago, Ill: Aldine; 1967.
29. Chenitz WC, Swanson JM. Qualitative research using grounded theory. In: Chenitz WC, Swanson JM, eds. *From Practice to Grounded Theory: Qualitative Research in Nursing.* Menlo Park, Calif: Addison-Wesley; 1986.
30. Hutchinson S. Grounded theory: the method. In: Munhall PL, Oiler CJ, eds. *Nursing Research: A Qualitative Perspective.* Norwalk, Conn: Appleton-Century-Crofts; 1986.
31. Stern PN, Allen LM, Moxley PA. Qualitative research: the nurse as grounded theorist. *Health Care Women Int.* 1984;5:371–385.
32. Stern PN, Pyles SH. Methodology to study women's culturally based decisions about health. *Health Care Women Int.* 1985;6:1–23.
33. Wilson HS. Usual hospital treatment in the United States community mental health system: a dispatching process. In: Chenitz WC, Swanson JM, eds. *From Practice to Grounded Theory: Qualitative Research in Nursing.* Menlo Park, Calif: Addison-Wesley; 1986.
34. Lincoln YS, Guba EG. *Naturalistic Inquiry.* Beverly Hills, Calif: Sage; 1985.
35. Cox LC, Spiro M, Sullivan JA. Social risk factors: impact on elders' perceived health status. *J Community Health Nurs.* 1988;5:59–73.
36. Fletchen KR. Health promotion. In: Hogstel MO, ed. *Nursing Care of the Older Adult.* Fort Worth, Tex: Delmar; 1994.
37. Liu HC. *Chinese System of Food Cures: Prevention and Remedies.* New York, NY: Sterling; 1991.
38. Lin A, Flaws B. *The Tao of Increasing Longevity and Conserving One's Life.* Boulder, Colo: Blue Poppy Press; 1991.
39. Despeux C. Gymnastics: the ancient tradition. In Kohn L, ed. *Taoist Meditation and Longevity Techniques.* Ann Arbor, Mich: University of Michigan; 1989.
40. Miura M. The revival of Qi: Qigong in contemporary China. In: Kohn L, ed. *Taoist Meditation and Longevity Techniques.* Ann Arbor, Mich: University of Michigan; 1989.
41. Ding L. *Acupuncture, Meridian Theory, and Acupuncture Points.* San Francisco, Calif: China Books & Periodicals; 1992.

Chapter 19

Health Care Access of Poverty-Level Older Adults in Subsidized Public Housing

JUDITH A. MALMGREN   MONA L. MARTIN   RAY M. NICOLA

Does poverty impede access to health care for older adults? And, if so, how? Because elders have a greater proportion of health problems and many also have limited resources, it is imperative that nurses working with them address barriers to appropriate health care and social services. Needs assessments are one method that can be used. Questionnaires or interviews that assess an elderly client's knowledge and utilization of available services can help the nurse pinpoint specific barriers and plan for necessary outreach programs or special services. This interview survey of elderly housing authority residents revealed, among other things, that visiting nurse services were remarkably effective.

Low-income and poverty-level older adults are one of the most invisible and difficult to reach groups in our society. They have limited financial resources to draw on in paying the out-of-pocket expenses associated with Medicare[1] — partly because they spend a greater proportion of their total income on health care relative to other expenses than those under the age of 65.[2] In addition, health problems (such as restricted activity days, bed days, and chronic conditions requiring ongoing care) are more frequent in low socioeconomic groups, creating more demand on their incomes to pay for health services.[3] Despite these prevailing conditions, a thorough review of the literature did not reveal any current reports on the unmet health care needs of poverty-level older adults.

We conducted a community survey to gather descriptive information on the health behaviors, health status, barriers to health care access, and unmet needs of adults 62 and older living in Seattle Housing Authority (SHA) facilities. In 1990, 1,872 elderly (ages 62 and older) persons resided in dwellings provided by SHA. The median age was 76 years, 92% lived alone, and 69% were female. The 1990 median income for high-rise community

From *Public Health Reports* 111:260–263, 1996. Reprinted with permission.

residents where the majority of the elderly live, was $5655.[4] All SHA residents were below the 1990 federal poverty-level income eligibility requirements of $6652 per year for an individual.

In 1983, Visiting Nurse Services of the Northwest began conducting monthly Wellness Clinics in space provided by the SHA with funding from the United Way. The clinic staff provides health screening and education, foot care, and flu immunizations. They also provide assessment and monitoring of chronic health problems and referrals to other health care providers when appropriate. Clinic nurses maintain contact with home care staff and resident managers to promote continuity of care. In turn, resident managers can alert clinic nursing staff to residents in need of medical care.

We used quote sampling to survey residents ages 62 and older in 28 SHA facilities distributed throughout the Seattle area. Each site was sampled until the number of men and women surveyed matched the 1990 reported sex and age distribution of the total SHA elderly population. Potential subjects were contacted by building managers and if they agreed to be interviewed were then contacted by our survey project staff for an appointment. Appointments were scheduled for 148 interviews, and 125 were completed. The 23 scheduled but not completed were due to people refusing interviews ($N = 4$), time conflicts or scheduling problems ($N = 13$), illness ($N = 2$), or an inability to understand the interview process ($N = 4$).

To develop the interview survey, we held resident focus groups to identify appropriate and relevant topics within our *a priori* identified areas of interest and to elicit the residents' own needs and concerns for inclusion as topics in the survey. The survey instrument included mental and physical health, functional state, and demographics. It also included measures to assess residents' ability to access health care, factors affecting health care utilization, and personal living situation. Questions addressing the Healthy People 2000 national objectives for older adults[5] and the *Guide to Clinical Preventive Services* periodic health examination schedule for persons ages 65 and older[6] were included. The 112-question survey was interviewer administered in an average of 60 minutes and included open-ended as well as standardized response questions. We used the Institute of Medicine's *Access to Health Care in America* framework to identify and define barriers to access.[7] We classified the responses to the question "Which of the following have ever made it hard to get care?" into three categories: financial, personal, and structural. T-test mean and chi-square test mean and chi-square test comparisons were done between those encountering and not encountering barriers to care.[8] Multivariate analysis was done using logistic regression to compute adjusted comparison statistics.[9]

■ RESULTS

In all, we surveyed 125 SHA residents. Their mean age was 77 (range: 62 to 98), 71% were women, and they were predominately white (77%) (See Table 19-1). A large proportion (41%) had not graduated from high school. Forty-two percent described their health as fair or poor; the rest said their health was excellent, very good, or good. Forty percent of those we surveyed

TABLE 19-1 Demographic Characteristics of 125 Older Adults Living in Subsidized Public Housing, Seattle, WA, 1990

VARIABLE	NUMBER	PERCENT
Age (years)		
62–74	58	46
75–98	67	54
Gender		
Female	89	71
Male	36	29
Ethnicity		
White	71	77
African American/Asian American/Native American/ Hispanic/Other	29	23
Education		
College graduate/some college	50	40
High school graduate	23	18
Less than high school	52	42
Ran out of money before month's end	41	33
Self-Reported Health		
Excellent/very good/good	47	58
Fair/poor	53	42
Stayed in Bed Due to Illness at Least Once During Previous Year	50	40
Needs More Help With Transportation Than Currently Available	36	29

reported that they had stayed in bed due to illness or injury at least once in the past 12 months. Running out of money before the end of the month and needing more help with transportation than currently available were commonly encountered living problems.

In response to the question "Do you know a place to go if you needed the following?" over 90% of the total survey population said they knew where to get physical exams; eye exams; and illness, injury, and emergency care. However, 46% of these poverty-level older adults reported having had problems obtaining health care (Table 19-2). A total of 36 people (29% of the total surveyed) reported having encountered one or more financial barriers. Lack of money or private health insurance was the most frequently encountered barrier to accessing health care. Nine percent of the residents reported encountering doctors who wouldn't accept Medicaid/Medicare payment. Eleven percent could not afford to fill prescriptions. Transportation problems comprised the majority of structural barriers encountered including having no transportation to get to the doctor and the distance being too far. Personal barriers were reported less often but included having been treated badly when trying to make an appointment and being too embarrassed or scared to go.

TABLE 19-2 **Barriers to Obtaining Medical Care, Counseling, or Dental Care Reported by 125 Older Adults Living in Subsidized Public Housing, Seattle, WA, 1990**

REASON	NUMBER (N = 57)	PERCENT
Financial Barriers (n = 36)		
No money or no private health insurance	27	22
Physician wouldn't take Medicare/Medicaid	11	9
Couldn't afford to fill prescription................................	14	11
Personal Barriers (n = 11)		
Too embarrassed or scared to go.................................	12	10
Was treated badly when tried to make appointment	4	3
Structural Barriers (n = 30)		
Had to wait too long for an appointment	16	13
Didn't know where to go to get care............................	12	10
No transportation	13	10
Too far...	12	10
Other	17	14
None of these	70	54

NOTE: Respondents gave all reasons that applied; therefore, the sample does not add to 100%.

The 20 people responding in the affirmative to the question "Have you ever tried to get health care for yourself but were denied or turned away?" were asked more in-depth questions. In response to "Who denied you care?" these people mentioned private doctors, clinics, and hospitals. In response to "What kind of care were you seeking when you were denied care?" they reported routine physicals, injury, illness, dental, or hospital care. In response to "Why were you denied or turned away?" they reported inability to pay, clinic scheduling problems, and refusal of the clinic or doctor to accept Medicaid or Medicare payment.

In a forced fit logistic regression model including age, ethnicity, education, and self-reported health, two factors — insufficient income to meet personal needs and needing more help with transportation — were significantly associated with encountering financial and structural barriers. Staying in bed due to illness or injury in the past 12 months was significantly associated with financial barriers, and being a woman with structural barriers.

Table 19-3 shows a comparison between the frequency of exams and procedures in the group we surveyed and the Year 2000 recommendations.[5] SHA residents have a high level of exam frequency, with the exception of dental care, pap smears, and mammograms. The pap smear and mammogram data do not exactly coincide with the recommended exam schedule, as our questions only addressed the year prior to the interview.

TABLE 19-3   **Frequency of Exams among 125 Older Residents of Seattle Housing Authority Facilities in Relation to Year 2000 Objectives**

EXAM OR PROCEDURE	PROPORTION OF RESPONDENTS WHO HAD EXAM OR PROCEDURE IN PAST 12 MONTHS	YEAR 2000 OBJECTIVES
Men and Women (N = 125)		
Flu shot............................	58%[a]	60–80% yearly
Fecal blood test.................	46%	50% every 1–2 years
Blood pressure check........	97%*	40% yearly
General physical...............	71%	40% yearly
Eye exam	65%	40% yearly
Dental exam	38%	60% yearly
Women (n = 89)		
Pap smear........................	33%	70% every 1–3 years
MD breast exam	67%	60% every 1–2 years
Mammogram past year	39%	60% every 1–2 years

[a] Service provided on site by Visiting Nurse Services of the Northwest.

▬ DISCUSSION

The Seattle Housing Authority population has lower education levels, worse health, and lower income than most of their elderly counterparts in the United States.[2,10] More than 90% of residents knew where to obtain care, and their exam frequency compared very favorably with Year 2000 objectives, yet 46% reported encountering financial, personal, and structural barriers. The primary barrier to care encountered by our study population was lack of money or private health insurance (22%) and an additional 9% said that they had been refused care due to their Medicare or Medicaid status. Low Medicare reimbursement schedules are seen by some experts as the source of reduced physician interest in treating elderly patients.[11]

A number of studies have found a larger burden of health care expense and a reduced ability to access care among the elderly with poor health and few financial resources.[12,13,14] Among the people we surveyed, those who encountered barriers to care did not have enough money to meet their monthly expenses, had significantly more bed days, and more transportation problems than those not encountering barriers.

In six out of nine categories of nationally recommended exams and procedures, SHA resident exam schedules for the previous twelve-month period met or exceeded the stated target levels.[5] The high level of exam frequency reported in our survey indicates the success of the outreach and advocacy program provided by Visiting Nurse Services. Examples of other programs aimed at improving care access for low-income elderly include the Tulsa County Medical Society Very Important Person (VIP) program — which enables physicians to identify elderly persons with limited resources who need special assistance in accessing care[15] — and Project Safety Net, started by the UCLA School of Medicine, which provides comprehensive geriatric assessment in community-based outreach programs operating from senior service centers, meal delivery sites, churches, and low-income housing units.[16]

We identified areas of unmet need for potential intervention, specifically, provision of better transportation options and identification of doctors willing to take Medicare/Medicaid patients. Gaps between needed services and Medicare coverage could be addressed by legislative action to correct entitlement schedules and reduce out-of-pocket expenses. The primary strength of our study is the detailed nature of the in-person interviews, in which open-ended questions about health and general living concerns were included. The cross-sectional design of our study limits our findings to noncausal associations between factors of interest. Future research evaluating care delivery programs such as the Visiting Nurse Services of the Northwest's Wellness Clinics could provide effective model guidelines for improving the health of our poverty-level urban elderly population. Needs assessments of similar populations that do not have access to the services provided by such clinics would likely reveal greater levels of need and barriers to care than those found among SHA residents. Reducing the burden of health care expense and increasing access to care are clearly identified areas needing improvement.

▰REFERENCES

1. Rowland D. Fewer resources, greater burdens: medical care coverage for low income elderly people. US Bipartisan Commission on Comprehensive Health Care (The Pepper Commission). Washington, DC 1990.

2. Aging America: trends and projections. Washington, DC: Department of Health and Human Services, 1991. DHHS pub. no. (FCoA) 91-28001.

3. Kaplan GA, Haan MN, Syme SL, Minkler M, Winkleby M. Socioeconomic status and health. In: Amler RW, Dull HB, editors. Closing the gap: the burden of unnecessary illness. New York: Oxford University Press, 1987:125–129.

4. Seattle Housing Authority. Annual population report. Research report series no. 45. Seattle, WA: Housing Authority of the City of Seattle, 1990.

5. Public Health Service [US]. Healthy people 2000: national health promotion and disease prevention objectives. Washington, DC: Government Printing Office, 1990. DHHS pub. no. (PHS) 91-50212.

6. U.S. Preventive Services Task Force guide to clinical preventive services: an assessment of the effectiveness of 169 interventions. Report of the U.S. Preventive Services Task Force. Baltimore, MD: Williams and Wilkins, 1989.

7. Millman M, editor. Access to health care in America. Committee on Monitoring Access to Personal Health Care Services, Institute of Medicine. Washington, DC: National Academy Press, 1993.

8. Norusis MJ. SPSS for Windows Base System User's Guide, Release 6.0. Chicago, IL: SPSS Inc., 1993.

9. EGRET. Seattle, WA: Statistics and Epidemiology Research Corporation, 1991.

10. Adams PF, Benson V. Current estimates from the National Health Interview Survey. National Center for Health Statistics. Vital Health Statistics 1991;10(181):112.

11. Butler RN, Brame JB, Kahn C, McConnell S, Myers RJ, Pollack R, Rowland D. Health care for all: a crises of cost and access. A roundtable discussion: part 1. Geriatrics 1993;47:34–36.

12. Thomas C, Kelman HR. Unreimbursed expenses for medical care among urban elderly people. J Community Health 1990;15:137–149.

13. Berk ML, Wilensky GR. Health care of the poor elderly: supplementing Medicare. Gerontologist 1983;25:311–314.
14. Kiefe CI, McKay SV, Halevy A, Brody BA. Is cost a barrier to screening mammography for low-income women receiving Medicare benefits?: a randomized trial. Arch Intern Med 1994;154:1217–1224.
15. Campbell JG, Rhode RE. Preserving access with dignity for the elderly: Tulsa's VIP Program. Arch Otolaryngol Head Neck Surg 1991;117:488–489.
16. Reuben DB, Hirsch SH, Chernoff JC, Cheska Y, Drezner M, Engelman B, et al. Project Safety Net: a health screening outreach and assessment program. Gerontologist 1993;33:557–560.

SELECTED BIBLIOGRAPHY

Ailinger, R. L. (1989). Self-assessed health of Hispanic elderly persons. *Journal of Community Health Nursing* 6(2): 113–118.

Allen, V. R. & Miller, M. D. (1986). A model for assessing health needs of the rural elderly: Methodology and results. *Journal of Allied Health* 15(3): 213–224.

Angel, J., Angel, R., McClellan, J., & Markides, K. (1996). Nativity, declining health, and preferences in living arrangements among elderly Mexican Americans: Implications for long-term care. *The Gerontologist* 36(4): 464–473.

Attico, N. B. (1996). Wellness and the elderly. *The Indian Health Service Primary Care Provider* 21(5): 55–62.

Cox, C., Spiro, M. & Sullivan, J. (1988). Social risk factors: Impact on elders' perceived health status. *Journal of Community Health Nursing* 5(1): 59–73.

Evans, C. A. & Cunningham, B. A. (1996). Caring for the ethnic elder. *Geriatric Nursing* 17(3): 105–110.

Jones, D. C. & van Amelsvoort Jones, G. (1986). Communication patterns between nursing staff and the ethnic elderly in a long-term care facility. *Journal of Advanced Nursing* 11(3): 265–272.

Karp, N. (1996, Spring). Legal problems of grandparents and other kinship caregivers. *Generations* 57–60.

Mellor, M. J. (1996). Special populations among older persons. *Journal of Gerontological Social Work* 25(1/2): 1–10.

Moon, A. & Williams, O. (1993). Perceptions of elder abuse and help-seeking patterns among African-American, Caucasian American, and Korean-American elderly women. *The Gerontologist* 33(3): 386–395.

Mullen, F. (1996, Spring). Public benefits: Grandparents, grandchildren, and welfare reform. *Generations* 61–64.

Nolan, K. (1992). Addressing cultural diversity through transcultural nursing. *Caring* 11(10): 20–26.

Pruchno, R. A. & Johnson, K. W. (1996, Spring). Research on grandparenting: Review of current studies and future needs. *Generations* 65–70.

Riley, M. W. (1994). Aging and society: Past, present, and future. *The Gerontologist* 34(4): 436–446.

Schostak, Z. (1994). Jewish ethical guidelines for resuscitation and artificial nutrition and hydration of the dying elderly. *Journal of Medical Ethics* 29(2): 93–100.

Unit 4

Innovative Programs in Gerontological Nursing

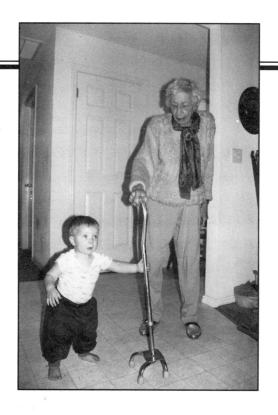

People approach aging in unique ways. Some go into old age feeling no different than they did in their 30s or 40s. They feel well, maintain a busy schedule of activities, have a rich network of interests and support systems, and if they
have any chronic illnesses they are adequately managed and do not interfere with
activities of daily living. Other people, for a variety of reasons, do not feel or act

well, have not built the broad spectrum of resources needed, have limited periods of good health, and are not managing old age well.

It is through an interrelated mesh of supportive services and promotion of self-care abilities that people are nourished and able to promote their quality of life throughout old age. In Unit IV we explore selected programs that have a positive effect on the lives of elders. The chapters focus on innovative health care delivery models and services for well elders and those who are attempting to successfully manage chronic illnesses at home or in alternative settings.

About half of the population over the age of 85 needs assistance to maintain activities of daily living. With increasing years people have more aspects of daily living that they cannot manage independently. Driving may become difficult or impossible at night, limiting independence. Preparing meals, light housekeeping, and self-care begins to take the bulk of the day and may become too challenging. They may become so frail or suffer some form of dementia or Alzheimer's disease, that they need the services provided in an assisted living center or skilled nursing facility. For 20% of our population, long-term care settings eventually become home; a home where supportive nursing care and other professional and social services are provided.

Since the over-85-year-old population is the fastest growing group in the United States, the last two chapters in this unit focus on programs that improve the quality of care and the quality of life for those who reside in long-term care settings. It is impossible to adequately cover the bevy of innovative programs that exist in the country in one section of a book. Every community has services for elders that are unique to the geographic area or the needs of the population. Nurses interested in the well being of older adults need to familiarize themselves with the services provided locally for older adults, identify the gaps, and become involved in the grassroots efforts to initiate the development of needed services. This unit serves as an introduction to the possibilities that exist.

Chapter 20

Preventive Nursing Care: A Keystone in Health Care for the Well Senior

RUBY M. VAN CROFT

This innovative program is a community-based case management program provided by the Visiting Nurse Association (VNA) in Washington, D.C. A multitude of health, social, and preventive services are provided to residents of senior housing units. Staff who provide the services form an interprofessional team of senior housing managers, registered nurses (who are seniors themselves), and student nurses. The resources from voluntary community agencies are identified and used along with medical specialists who donate their time, such as podiatrists. The nurses on the team function as advocates, coordinators, and clinicians with the goal of keeping seniors at a functional level and at home.

Since 1972 the Visiting Nurse Association of Washington, DC (VNA), has been providing preventive health service within senior citizen buildings. The agency participates with the senior citizens, community agencies, and housing authorities in a preventive health maintenance program that actively facilitates the individual's participation in positive self-care measures and in early and appropriate use of health, social, and medical resources in the community. The District of Columbia Office on Aging has provided financial support since 1982, the United Way since 1975. The objectives of the Senior Health Program are as follows:

- to counsel citizens residing in senior citizen buildings in preventive health care on a continuous basis;
- to provide updated information on community resources to senior citizens and other agencies on request;
- to maintain senior citizens within the community at the highest possible level of functioning;
- to provide senior citizens with the support that encourages self-reliance, continuation of good health habits, and adherence to medically advised treatment; and

From *CARING Magazine* 32–34, 1994. Reprinted with permission.

- to participate in the planning and implementation of a health screening program designed to prevent and detect health problems.

Over the years agency nurses have given care in six senior citizen buildings, two geriatric day care centers, and a low-income housing development. In 1974 the VNA served a total of 1,340 seniors, making more than 7,000 encounters through the service given to seniors. During fiscal year 1994 the senior health nurses saw a total of 1,805 seniors in six senior buildings in Washington, DC, with an average of 190 encounters each month. The profile of a senior receiving this service is usually female, age 70 years or older, widowed, and living alone. Many are active in the various programs planned by the management of the senior buildings. These can include shopping trips, pleasure trips locally and out of town, congregate meals, and the prevention program.

▄ DEVELOPING THE PROGRAM

As the VNA developed the concept for this program, the following process allowed the agency access to the seniors in the senior buildings.

- Develop program purpose and objectives.
- Set up meetings with the manager in each building to explain the program and how it could benefit the residents.
- With input from the managers and Senior Councils in some buildings, modify the program to meet their particular needs.
- Share information between buildings to help in problem solving, i.e., how to involve families as residents became unable to care for themselves.
- Share the list of community resources that would be particularly helpful in assisting in meeting seniors' needs.

Staffing the Sites

The VNA used several different methods to staff the senior building sites. At first the agency used staff from the area office in which the senior building was located. The nurses enjoyed working with this population, and it gave them an opportunity to work within a preventive framework from the beginning of their contact with the senior citizens.

However, referrals to a home care agency are usually for acute care, so prevention is an adjunct to the primary diagnosis. The use of regular staff continued until the pressure of increasing referrals began to erode the time allotted to the senior program. The agency then hired separate staff for the program and had as many as six part-time staff within the program, with a senior health nurse supervisor responsible for coordinating all senior services. The staff were usually the younger nurses who had families or who were working on their degrees. The current staff consist of two retired nurses who are seniors themselves. Budget cuts eliminated the senior health nurse supervisor position. The director of community affairs assumed those duties, delegating some responsibilities, particularly those of coordinating community resources, to the senior health nurses.

Responsibilities of Senior Health Nurses

The senior health nurses are responsible for planning, implementing, and coordinating the various activities at each senior building. They also must look at the special needs for each site. The activities related to the above responsibilities include the following:

- assessing the residents' health status emphasizing health/wellness behaviors such as nutrition; balance of rest and activities; drug, alcohol, and tobacco use/abuse; socialization/recreation; and self-esteem;
- monitoring residents' existing health problems and screening for new problems;
- helping to plan and conducting group meetings on common health, social, and financial problems;
- coordinating the use of other professional and supportive disciplines needed by the residents;
- keeping the residents informed about community resources and assisting them in obtaining the services when needed;
- functioning as the residents' advocate by teaching seniors how to make their needs known, speaking out in behalf of the seniors, and integrating them into the mainstream of care; and
- maintaining appropriate records of each senior on his or her health, social, and financial conditions.

▬ USING COMMUNITY RESOURCES

By using community resources, the senior nurses broaden their base of expert care for the seniors. The development of a solid working relationship with these resources has enhanced the nurses' ability to keep the focus on prevention. On a continuing basis, the senior health nurses have been preventing health crises through activities such as blood pressure screening, review of medications, diet instructions, exercise programs, limited bereavement counseling, and working directly with seniors' physicians to resolve health and other problems.

These services have been enhanced by the ongoing support and guidance the VNA has received from the American Heart Association, American Cancer Association, American Diabetic Association, Nutrition Council, and Arthritis Foundation; as well as sight, dental, and cholesterol screening through the District of Columbia Health Department; speech and hearing screening through the Washington Hearing and Speech Society; and the use of a podiatrist who donates his or her time — to name a few. These community resources have readily supplied their services at no cost to the seniors. In 1993 and 1994 the VNA has been one of the agencies coordinating the "Fight the Flu" program to protect the seniors from the most deadly strains of these viruses. This service has been provided in several of the senior buildings when the senior health nurse was present.

Student Nurses

Another resource the senior health nurses have been able to tap is student nurses from some of the area's schools of nursing. The VNA nurses have been able to act as preceptors as the students use their new skills to develop prevention programs for sessions with the seniors. Other volunteers have been some of the seniors themselves. In one instance, an experienced diabetic senior set up a program of instruction under the supervision of the senior health nurse, to teach new diabetics urine testing, blood sticks, use of the glucometer, care of the feet, and administration of insulin.

Building Managers

The senior health nurses are in the senior buildings usually on a weekly basis for two to four hours, averaging 50 hours each month. The senior health nurses work out these scheduled visits with each senior building. The managers in each building cooperate by providing space for the senior health nurse to have some privacy with each senior to discuss their concerns. Notices are posted to remind the seniors of the senior health nurse's visit for that week. During these site visits, the senior health nurse sees anywhere from 25 to 35 residents. Included in this service are seniors living in the community around the building, as well as the staff working in the buildings.

▬PROACTIVE PREVENTION

Although the VNA has received funding support from the District of Columbia Office on Aging and the United Way, funds are becoming more scarce. Therefore, the VNA knows it must try to be proactive through:

- increasing use of volunteers
- encouraging seniors to make small contributions for the service
- looking to other funding sources such as churches, businesses, etc.

Responses from the seniors, building managers, and seniors' physicians indicate that this is a worthwhile program that has been an important factor in helping to maintain the "well" senior at a functional level within the community.

Chapter 21

Perceptions of Senior Residents About a Community-Based Nursing Center

CECELIA B. SCOTT   LINDA MONEYHAM

This chapter describes a phenomenological study conducted on senior residents who had access to a community-based nursing center. Unlike the first chapter in this unit, this chapter focuses on the client's perception of such services. This view is important when such a service is being considered. Residents participated in four focus-group sessions and their perceptions were elicited using open-ended questions. The findings of the study offer an understanding of the value of community-based nursing centers to elders and provide strong support for case management provided by nurses.

In the movement toward health-care reform, it has been suggested that community based nursing centers have significant potential as an alternative model of health care delivery that can provide cost-effective services to high-risk populations (Mikulencak, 1993; National League for Nursing, 1993). The elderly frequently make up a significant portion of the clients of such centers. Of the estimated 250 nursing centers in the United States, 21% provide services solely for the elderly (National League for Nursing, 1993). However, there is little research to support assumptions frequently set forth about nursing centers. Little is known about the meaning of nursing center services to consumers or the influence that nursing services have on their health. The purpose of this study was to examine the perceptions of nursing services provided in a community-based nursing center for community-dwelling older adults and the meaning the nursing center held for these people.

▬ BACKGROUND

The literature on nursing centers has focused primarily on description of the development and implementation of the nursing center concept (Barger, 1986a; Barger, 1986b; Barger, 1986c; Barger, 1991; Glanovsky &

From *Image* 27(3):181–186, 1995. Reprinted with permission.

Provost, 1984; Hawkins, Igou, Johnson, & Utley, 1984; McEvoy & Vezina, 1986; Sharp, 1992). The earliest studies focused on identifying and locating nursing centers (Barger, 1986b; Boettcher, 1986). More recently, a small number of studies have focused on describing the characteristics of nursing centers, such as the populations served and type of services offered (Barger & Bridges, 1990; Barger, Nugent, & Bridges, 1993; Higgs, 1989; National League for Nursing, 1993). Nursing centers for older adults have been described in the nursing literature (Foster & Moses, 1987; Grimes & Stamps, 1980; Hawkins, Igou, Johnson, & Utley, 1984; Hazard & Kemp, 1983; Newman, Sloss, & Andersen, 1984). However, data about such centers have primarily been limited to reports of the number of client visits, the most common presenting problems, and client demographics.

Although it has been suggested that nursing centers are an alternative model of health care delivery that could play a major role in health-care reform, research is needed to influence health policy and make a strong argument for reimbursement of nursing care (Riesch, 1992a). Existing data about nursing centers is limited by a number of conceptual and methodologic deficiencies and by numerous questions about nursing centers that have not been addressed (Riesch, 1992b). Conspicuously absent in the literature are qualitative studies of the lived experience of nursing center clients (Riesch, 1992b). An important question is, "What meaning do consumers attach to nursing services delivered through community based nursing centers?" The perspective of the recipient of nursing care is a virtually untapped resource for identifying how nursing affects the health and well-being of the consumers of nursing care. Our study attempted to examine such a perspective.

▬METHOD
A phenomenological research design was used to explore the experiences of older adults using nursing center services. A focus-group approach was the primary data collection method. Focus groups are a widely used qualitative data collection method (Keller, Sliepcevich, Vitello, Lacey, & Wright, 1987; Krueger, 1988; Morgan, 1988; Morgan, 1993). In phenomenological research, the focus-group approach is used to elicit the shared meaning of every-day experiences from particular sub-groups (Calder, 1977; Gray-Vickrey, 1993). It is generally recommended that groups be limited to 10 to 12 participants to allow for maximum participation (Krueger, 1988; Morgan, 1988). The advantage of the focus-group approach is the synergy created among the group members. This group synergy: (a) fosters the production of information that is difficult to obtain in individual interviews (Kingry, Tiedje, & Friedman, 1990); (b) emphasizes participants' interactions and points of views (Morgan, 1988); (c) provides opportunities for participants to validate information shared by others (Gray-Vickery, 1993); and (d) clarifies arguments and reveals diversity in perspectives (Morgan, 1993).

Sample and Setting
The study was implemented during a 2-month period beginning in February 1993. The population of interest was community-dwelling older adults. A systematic random sample was selected from the 650 residents of an apart-

ment community designed for older adults in a large city in the southeastern United States. The community is unique in that an academic nursing center that provides a variety of nursing services is located there. The nursing center is cosponsored by a school of nursing and the apartment owners. Services provided include a nursing clinic, home visits, educational programs, screening programs, and care management. At the time of the study, the center was staffed by one full-time gerontologic nurse clinician and one part-time registered nurse.

Focus-group participants were randomly selected from four major subgroups in the community population: (a) Group 1 was community residents who served in the nursing center auxiliary group and volunteered at the nursing center on a regular basis; (b) Group 2 was community residents who had never used the services of the nursing center; (c) Group 3 was community residents who had used the services of the nursing center on a regular basis during the past 6 months; and (d) Group 4 was community residents who had used the services of the nursing center in the past, but who had not done so in the previous 6 months. Criteria were developed to recruit people with varying perceptions of needs and services who would most likely represent various subgroups in the community. Criteria for exclusion included mental or physical impairments that precluded participation in a group discussion. To obtain groups that allowed for maximum participation, the names of 12 people were randomly selected from lists of residents who met the criteria for each of the four subgroups.

Twenty-seven of the 48 individuals recruited agreed to participate. The characteristics of participants are shown in Table 21-1. The auxiliary volunteers (Group 1) made up the largest group with 11 participants; Group 2, consisting of those who had never used the services of the nursing center, was the smallest group with two participants.

PROCEDURES

In addition to the investigators, the research team consisted of an intermediary who conducted selection and recruitment of participants, a group moderator who led all four focus-groups, and research assistants who served as non-participant observers during group sessions. Members of the research team were selected and trained by the investigators and were not associated with services offered by the nursing center.

Recruitment and selection of participants was conducted by an intermediary to ensure confidentiality and avoid any sense of coercion. Recruitment letters were sent to potential participants inviting them to take part in the study and a follow-up letter was sent. Each person who agreed to participate was called 2 days before the meeting as a reminder and demographic information was collected at that time.

Interviews were audiotaped and transcribed, omitting any identifying information. Following preliminary review of the transcripts, the groups were again interviewed within 4 weeks to clarify previous comments and to confirm the investigators' interpretations of the data. After each session, observation notes were recorded by the group moderator and the non-participant observers, who then met with the investigators to discuss activities during the meeting. The study was approved by an institutional review

TABLE 21-1 Focus Group Participants

	GROUP 1 n = 11	GROUP 2 n = 2	GROUP 3 n = 6	GROUP 4 n = 8	TOTAL n = 27
Gender					
Male			4	3	7
Female	11	2	2	5	20
Age					
Range	56–82	78–79	64–84	60–86	56–86
Mean	70	78.5	77.3	73	74
SD	7.0	0.5	6.9	7.2	7.5
Marital Status					
Single		1		1	2
Married	5	1	3		9
Divorced				2	2
Widowed	6		3	3	14
Education					
Less than high school				1	1
High school graduate	3	1	1	1	6
Training after high school	6	1	3	2	11
College graduate	1		1	2	4
Post-graduate education	1		1	2	4
Living Arrangement					
Alone	5	1	3	3	12
With spouse	6		3	5	14
With sibling		1			1

board and informed consent was obtained for each participant. In addition, participants were asked to sign a confidentiality statement agreeing to keep confidential the identity of all other group participants.

Data Analysis

Verbatim transcripts from the audiotapes, observation notes, and demographic data provided the data base for the study. Analysis was completed using a phenomenological methodology developed by Colaizzi (1978) and adapted by Scott (1990, 1993) whereby themes are organized based on common phenomena from group sessions. Data were analyzed by both investigators who met regularly to review all tapes and transcripts. The essence of the group sessions and the development of themes across all four groups were reviewed by the research team for credibility.

▬ FINDINGS

Context

To more fully understand the participants' perceptions of the nursing center, consideration was given to the context — that is, to the conditions and circumstances that affected perceptions. Several contextual factors emerged in the data, including participants' views on aging, concerns for the future, and views on health care.

A contextual factor that emerged during discussion in all four groups was the commonly accepted belief that a loss of health and function are an inevitable part of growing older. Comments such as "There's nothing wrong with me except my age which you can't do anything about" were frequently expressed and suggested that a negative view of aging was present and influencing actions in everyday life.

This loss-oriented view of aging was evident in participants' descriptions of their concerns about the future. These concerns were expressed reticently as leading to increased dependency on others and included concerns about safety, transportation, and finances. For example, one participant described her fear of kitchen fires, "My mother lived in a retirement community. She almost burned the place down. Her eyesight became so bad she could not see to adjust the flame on the stove . . . I realized that that's going to be my problem someday."

Another finding, which contributed to a more in-depth understanding of the data, was related to participants' views on health care. The following comments from a 78 year old provided insights:

> *The majority of residents eligible to use the services of [nursing center] were born between 1902 and 1933 . . . and know very little about health care except as they were told by their doctors. Most of the residents have Medicare or other insurance which will pay a doctor [not a nurse] or for a clinic visit which is supervised by a doctor . . . [most residents] have the impression that health care is for one identified ailment and not for inclusive 'health' services.*

The participants' views of health care, as this participant suggested, were based on what was most familiar, a medical model of care. The care provided in this model, as they know it, is problem-oriented and delivered by physicians. This problem-orientation to "health" care was clearly evident in each of the groups. One participant stated, "Most of us came here [senior community] because we knew there was a nursing service here, those of us who had health problems."

The problem-oriented perspective of health care was most evident in Group 2 participants who had never used the services of the nursing center. Lacking experience of the nursing center model, they were unable to describe how nursing services could be useful to them unless they were to develop health problems. This was in stark contrast to participants from the remaining groups who had used the services of the nursing center and were able to describe various ways in which nursing center services, and interaction in which the nurses of the center, were of value.

The ageist perspective that a loss of health and function are an inevitable part of growing old seemed to create a sense of insecurity, valuelessness, and concern — particularly in relation to health care and the resulting costs. Further, the concerns or problems experienced by these older adults were not always viewed as topics that physicians should or would be willing to address. The nursing center personnel were viewed as an approachable and trusted source of care as reflected in the three major themes of feeling valued and respected, opening doors to self-care, and decreasing self-care costs.

Feeling Valued and Respected

A fundamental human need is to feel valued and respected. One aspect of the nursing center that was particularly meaningful to participants was the way in which the design of the services and the actions of the nurses supported this need for respect.

The nursing center was designed to provide prevention and health promotion services with the ultimate aim of assisting older adults to care for themselves. The nursing center model is conceptually different from the medical model that encourages dependence on medical authorities for care. Although the predominant use of the nursing services was for illness prevention and health-promotion, self-care was continuously addressed by the RNs. Direct client contacts and written materials conveyed messages that signified the strengths, capabilities, and self-worth of older adults.

Participation in the nursing center auxiliary, which provides full-time clerical coverage for the center, seemed to buttress self-esteem. One participant without previous secretarial experience said, "I had never done any kind of office work at all . . . But it did prove to me that I could do something."

An element central to the theme of feeling valued and respected was the positive relationship participants had with nurses. Participants viewed the RNs as trustworthy, caring, competent caregivers who valued and respected them as people. Being valued and respected for individual differences seemed to build the necessary confidence required for self-care. Evident in participants' descriptions of their experiences with the nursing center was a shift in responsibility for care from others to self. For instance — one older adult said, "They [doctors] don't want you to know too much. This is exactly the opposite of what I got here [nursing center]. It is great you should take some control over your own health."

The sense of being valued and respected also seemed to influence people's decisions about when to seek assistance. One participant stated:

Even though we all have our doctors, there's times that we have questions that we don't want to bother our doctor, because we're afraid our doctor will laugh at us for asking a dumb question. And we can come to the nurse or we can come here and ask the question and we're given respect, and any stress we might have had is gone . . . without seeing our doctor.

The data also indicated that the nurses' approachability and trustworthiness provided access to what participants saw as valuable assistance. The need to have someone listen attentively during a time of concern was prominent throughout the interviews, "No matter how busy the nurse is, she never appears too busy when you talk to her. She is all yours. Not like a doctor who is always in a hurry to get to the next person." Feelings of being valued and respected were expressed throughout all of the interviews and were strongly reflected in the other two major themes.

Opening Doors to Self-Care

Government authorities assert that older adults, more than any other age group, seek health information and are willing to make changes to maintain their health and independence (Office of Disease Prevention and Health Information, 1990). The data from this study support this assertion. Reflected in participants' comments was the perception of having increased access to the health care resources needed for self-care and made possible by the nursing center. Older adults spoke of a number of ways in which access was increased and in which their concerns related to maintaining independence were addressed.

Participants viewed RNs as sources of needed information and knowledge. Information related to illness prevention and health maintenance was noted as important. One stated, "I had a physical on the 17th of December and . . . my cholesterol was way up, so I came in and talked to the nurse one day and she made some suggestions and I followed them." Another commented, "I am mildly diabetic and since I have gotten into the exercise program and come to the clinic regularly, my blood sugar has dropped from 277 to 119." It is important to note that these residents were aware of their health condition, but the information from the nursing center RNs expanded their understanding. One said, "You don't usually get the information that you get from the nurses in the clinic. I think it is a very special thing, really I do." Another noted, "Here they don't want to contradict what the doctor said, but they try to ease it so you will understand, so it is not so unusable."

The nurses' knowledge of other community health resources was also viewed as helpful to self-care. For instance, residents were informed of two community exercise and walking programs designed for health promotion purposes. While participation in both of these programs was initiated by the nursing center, after the first year participation was coordinated totally by residents, including three levels of exercise programs offered to the senior community on a daily basis. Participants also saw the nursing center RNs as knowledgeable of other health care providers. For example, one said, "The nurse knows the doctors in the area that are at a convenient location . . . so the referral counsel is helpful." Convenience was a key factor, as many were concerned with the inability to drive in the future and related costs of transportation services.

The nursing center services and staff were viewed as a way to gain access to services that were otherwise inaccessible, for a variety of reasons. Many of the services offered by the nursing center did not exist in the locality, and hence, were not purchasable. A few of the available nursing center services that were discussed within the groups included the volunteer transportation system, medication review and counsel, and free evening and weekend consultation. Another valued service was hospital visitation as a part of the care management program. One resident said, "When my husband was up there in intensive care on a respirator and a feeding tube . . . and a center nurse went right up there. You know it's kind of like somebody's intervening for you and they can kind of tell you what's gong on." Although not without its limitations, the nursing center provided access to services aimed more toward prevention and health maintenance. For example, one participant with labile hypertension needed daily blood pressure monitoring during medication regulation and she explained it this way, "Not only did it [blood pressure] go down to where it stays the same all the time, he [doctor] said it [stability via medication] was because it could be taken at the same time everyday . . . so I have always thought that the clinic was very valuable for a lot of reasons."

Participants also viewed the nursing center RNs as instrumental in facilitating communication with physicians and other providers. In times of difficulty, the RN was seen as someone with authority who could initiate and negotiate access to their physicians. One participant shared how the nurse assisted her during an episode of acute illness:

> *I had called my doctor repeatedly and 2 hours had gone by and no return call. . . . The nurse called his office and finally I heard her say 'I know he has a beeper and I want him to return my call in 10 minutes.' She finally did get a prescription called in for me to get some suppositories to stop the vomiting and to change the medicine.*

Education, demonstration, and confidence in the older adults' abilities were key components in building a foundation for self-care. In the process of moving toward self-care, participants expressed increased assurance that their concerns about aging would be addressed.

Decreased Self-Care Costs

In all four groups, concerns about actual and potential loss were discussed. Finances, increasing dependency, changing health status, and safety were among the concerns producing stress and anxiety. Participants provided numerous examples of how utilization of the nursing center diminished their worries and hence, decreased factors impinging on self-care. Decreased doctor visits, assistance with decision-making, regular screening services, and collaboration with the health-care community and the apartment managers, were noted.

Participants related that obtaining services through the nursing center helped decrease the number of visits to their primary physicians. One stated, "The RN gave me vitamin B12 and iron shots once a month, and it kept me from having to go to the doctor's office. Things like that really help." Reducing the number of doctor visits not only reduced the financial costs, but it also lessened the tension associated with getting to the doctor's office. For some, the reduced number of doctor visits translated into not having to arrange transportation or depend on others, thereby lessening their feelings of dependency.

Regular screening services coordinated through the nursing center and RN collaboration with the health care community were also identified as major factors influencing self-care costs. For example, one participant discussed the usefulness of a prevention program for his wife:

> *My wife comes here to the nursing center more than I do. She has a number of pills and so forth. So the nurse went through all the medications she took, and*

they, in connection with my wife's private doctor, were able to eliminate some of them.

Programs obtained through the nursing center such as medication review served to reduce the number of doctor visits and the costs of more intensive services which might be needed if early intervention were not available.

Many participants admitted, albeit hesitantly, that they were often uncertain about when to seek medical care and this created a source of tension. A nurse, from the nursing center or from community agencies negotiated by the nursing center, was identified as someone who assisted with decision-making in this regard. The following example illustrates how the services offered through the nursing center allayed worries and provided a sense of security, "As long as the clinic is here, I feel somewhat secure to know that I can get down here and if I really feel the need to do so, that I'm going to be seen and be told whether I should get an ambulance, go to the hospital, or go home." Using the services of the nursing center to assist with decision-making served to facilitate more appropriate use of the health care system. Without this assistance, medical services are apt to be used when unnecessary or not used when necessary.

The nursing center provided support and security to residents. For some, these feelings came from receiving the center's regular services. For others, the sense of support and reassurance came from the services provided during emergencies. The comment, "It is a good thought to know the nursing center is here if we need it" was voiced by a number of participants, reflecting their comfort even if they did not use the center.

It is important to note that being from middle and upper income groups and having comprehensive insurance coverage, the participants in this study were a privileged class of health-care consumers. Despite having the resources needed to access services, these resources in themselves did not always contribute to improved self-care because services which promote and support self-care have not traditionally been available or purchasable. As reflected in the three major themes, the data suggest the services provided by the nursing center are needed, valued, and contribute positively to participants' health.

■SUMMARY AND IMPLICATIONS

The outcomes and cost-effectiveness of health care are traditionally assessed using data gathered after care is delivered. Disease-specific variables such as disability, morbidity, and mortality are frequently used as measures of effectiveness. While these variables are important, they offer only a partial perspective on the quality of older people's lives and provide little information about nurses' contribution to health. From a nursing perspective, health is considered a process which is influenced by multiple factors and as more than the absence of disease. Health can be experienced even when chronic illness is present. Data generated from this phenomenological study offer a broader perspective into the process of health and support the assertion that nursing centers can have a positive affect on health and the cost-effectiveness of care (Mikulencak, 1993; National League for Nursing, 1993).

The three major themes found in this study evolved from the context of the everyday lives of older adults. Participants seemed to operate from a belief system which: (a) stripped hope for a healthy future; (b) asserted that "appropriate" use of the existing health-care system was for problems only; and (c) undermined individual abilities, created an unwarranted dependency, and influenced the way in which health care was utilized. Personal stories shared by participants demonstrated that access to the nursing center created an alternative on which to base actions. The data strongly indicated that feeling valued and respected, one of the major themes, was pivotal to the way in which older adults viewed health and their participation in health care.

Feeling valued and respected seems to instill older adults with a sense of confidence, competence, and hope. The interrelation of feeling valued and the process of health is deceptively simple due to its universal acceptance. However, the data suggested that the conveyance of this message, through non-hierarchical relationships with nurse providers, influenced participants' health care transactions in several ways.

Viewing RNs as trusted sources of care, participants demonstrated a willingness to use the nursing center services. This action is significant in that it reflects a broadened perspective of the nurse's role in health care. Moreover, participants repeatedly shared stories of how they used center services for primary prevention and health promotion, or how their interactions at the nursing center led to secondary prevention and health maintenance. These experiences denoted a changing view of health possibilities and a more informed perspective on healthy behaviors.

Participants' descriptions lend strong support for care management provided by nurses. Access to services provided by the center RNs helped to increase the older adults' knowledge of healthy behaviors, prevented potential problems, and maintained or improved current level of health. Many of the experiences related by participants indicated that without the nursing center services, their health needs and concerns would have gone unaddressed, potentially leading to illness or disability, or would have required more frequent use of more costly physician services. The type of services offered through the nursing center, as well as how the services were delivered, were key factors shaping the process of health and the cost-effectiveness of health care for these older adults.

The future of nursing centers rests on nurses' ability to demonstrate the effectiveness of the care delivered in such centers. The findings from this study offer a beginning understanding of the value of community-based nursing centers to older adults. However there are several limitations. The study used a sample drawn from a relatively homogeneous population of older, middle class adults who were willing to share their perceptions in a group. Further research is needed to determine if the needs and perceptions identified in this study are shared by older adults from a more diverse background.

■ REFERENCES

Barger, S. E. (1986a) Academic nursing centers: A demographic profile. Journal of Professional Nursing, 2, 246–251.

Barger, S. E. (1986b). Nursing center: From concept to reality. Journal of Community Health Nursing, 3, 175–182.

Barger, S. E. (1986c). Academic nurse-managed centers: Issues of implementation. Family and Community Health, 9, 12–22.

Barger, S. E. (1991). The nursing center: A model for rural nursing practice. Nursing and Health Care, 12, 290–294.

Barger, S. E., & Bridges, W. C. (1990). An assessment of academic nursing centers. Nurse Educator, 15(2), 31–36.

Barger, S. E., Nugent, K. E., & Bridges, W. C. (1993). Schools with nursing centers: A 5-year follow-up study. Journal of Professional Nursing, 9, 7–13.

Boettcher, J. M. H. (1986). A national overview of nurse-managed centers. Paper presented at the Third Biennial Conference on Nurse Managed Centers, Scottsdale, AZ.

Calder, J. (1977). Focus groups and the nature of qualitative marketing. Journal of Marketing Research, 14, 353–364.

Colaizzi, P. F. (1978). Psychological research as the phenomenologist views it. In R. Vaile & M. King (Eds.), Existential phenomenological alternatives for psychology (48–71). New York: Oxford University Press.

Foster, B. E., & Moses, R. K. (1987). Satellite clinics for elder health care. Geriatric Nursing, 8, 188–189.

Glanovsky, A. R., & Provost, M. B. (1984). The ELMS College Nursing Center: An independent setting for translating theory into practice. Journal of Nursing Education, 209–211.

Gray-Vickrey, P. (1993). Gerontological research: Use and application of focus groups. Journal of Gerontological Nursing, 19(5), 21–27.

Grimes, D., & Stamps, C. (1980). Meeting the health care needs of older adults through a community nursing center. Nursing Administration Quarterly, 4(3), 31–40.

Hawkins, J. W., Igou, J. F., Johnson, E. E., & Utley, Q. E. (1984). A nursing center for ambulatory, well older adults. Nursing and Health Care, 5, 208–212.

Hazard, M. P., & Kemp, R. E. (1983). Keeping the well-elderly well. American Journal of Nursing, 83, 567–569.

Higgs, Z. R. (1989). Models of academic nurse-managed centers. In Nursing centers: Meeting the demand for quality health care (103–108). New York: National League for Nursing.

Keller, K. L., Sliepcevich, E. M., Vitello, E. M., Lacey, E. P., & Wright, W. R. (1987). Assessing beliefs about and needs of senior citizens using the focus group interview: A qualitative approach. Health Education, 18(1), 44–49.

Kingry, M. J., Tiedje, L. B., & Friedman, L. L. (1990). Focus groups: A research technique for nursing. Nursing Research, 39, 124–125.

Krueger, R. A. (1988). Focus groups: A practical guide. Newbury Park, CA: Sage.

McEvoy, M. D., & Vezina, M. (1986). The development of a nursing center on a college campus: Implications for the curriculum. Journal of Advanced Nursing, 11, 295–301.

Mikulencak, M. (1993). The "graying of America"—Changing what nurses need to know. American Nurse, 25(7), 1, 12.

Morgan, D. L. (1988). Focus groups as qualitative research. Qualitative Research Methods Series, Vol. 16. Newbury Park, CA: Sage Publications.

Morgan, D. L. (1993). Successful focus groups: Advancing the state of the art. Newbury Park, CA: Sage Publications.

National League for Nursing. (1993). A promising trend in the American health care scene: Findings from the Metropolitan Life Study of Nursing Centers. Prism: The NLN Research and Policy Quarterly, 1, 3–5.

Newman, J., Sloss, G. S., & Andersen, S. (1984). Evaluation of a health program. Geriatric Nursing, 5, 234–238.

Office of Disease Prevention and Health Promotion. (1990). Healthy older people: The report of a national health promotion program. Washington, DC: U.S. Department of Health and Human Services.

Riesch, S. K. (1992a). Nursing centers: An analysis of the anecdotal literature. Journal of Professional Nursing, 8, 16–25.

Riesch, S. K. (1992b). Nursing centers. Annual Review of Nursing Research, 10, 145–162.

Scott, C. B. (1990). The meaning of adult day care within the context of the caregiving relationship: Perspectives of older adults and their female caregivers. Unpublished dissertation. Georgia State University, Atlanta, GA.

Scott, C. B. (1993). Circular victimization in the caregiving relationship. Western Journal of Nursing Research, 15, 230–245.

Sharp, N. (1992). Community nursing centers coming of age. Nursing Management, 23(8), 18–20.

Chapter 22

Cluster Care: An Alternative to Traditional Care

YVONNE LANE GRAY   NELLIE C. BAILEY

The authors of this chapter, Gray and Bailey, state that Cluster Care is going to be the wave of the 21st century. Because of this, nurses need to be knowledgeable and creative so that this new model will be acceptable to its recipients. This model (also referred to as the shared aide model) is task-oriented rather than time-oriented and includes a group care plan in addition to individual plans, along with registered nurse supervision as in traditional care models. Clients in close proximity to each other get services based on tasks needed during different times of the day rather than a specific number of hours of service. For instance an aide can shop for three clients, prepare lunch for one, clean for another, and return to the first for late afternoon bathing assistance. This makes the model cost-effective while still providing the services needed. A vignette is provided to illustrate the model and clients' reactions to Cluster Care.

In this time of fiscal constraint and the need to contain healthcare costs, the Human Resources Administration (HRA), under the auspice of the Department of Social Services, has the objective of providing a home care service that is as cost effective and efficient as it is caring.[1] Presently, the elderly represent 12% of the population in the United States.[2] Those now older than 65 years old, which number some 32 million, constitute the fastest growing population today in the United States and are the majority recipients of home care service. Consequently, this population will command at least 50% of the total healthcare expenditures nationwide.[3]

Longevity predisposes the elderly to chronic health conditions as well as diminished physical activity, which increases their dependency on others and on the healthcare system. Some 40% of those older than 65 years old require assistance with activities of daily living such as feeding, dressing, and toileting.

From *Home Healthcare Nurse* 13(2):11–44, 1995. Reprinted with permission.

▄HOME CARE PROGRAMS IN NEW YORK CITY

Since the early 1980s, home care in New York City has become one of the fastest growing sectors within the human service system. Three of the four major home care programs in New York City include (1) HRA Home Care Services (Home Attendant, Housekeeper, and Homemaker programs); (2) Certified Home Health Agencies (CHHAs); and (3) Long Term Home Health Care Program (LTHHCP), also called the Nursing Home Without Walls Program.[4] The services provided by HRA are under the auspices of "social organizations"; CHHA and LTHHCP workers are employed by "health providers."[5]

In the past, home healthcare programs established a means of providing skilled service and nonskilled service for clients. According to Medicare regulations, skilled services are defined as those required by an individual that are reasonable and necessary for treatment of an illness or injury. Factors used to evaluate and determine the degree of skilled services included (1) complexity of service and condition of client; (2) performance or supervision of performance by a registered nurse or a registered physical therapist; (3) teaching of service by skilled professional; and (4) whether the service can be accomplished by a nonmedical person. Nonskilled services are those that do not fit the Medicare definition of skilled service.[2]

Certified Home Health Agencies

Certified Home Health Agencies provide skilled nursing care on an intermittent basis, or physical therapy, speech therapy, occupational therapy, or a home health aide. For CHHAs, the client must meet the coverage criteria for any skilled nursing and/or healthcare services for which Medicare provides coverage.

To be eligible for any home care coverage, a Medicare beneficiary must demonstrate that he or she is confined to the home and is in need of skilled nursing care on an intermittent basis or in need of one of the qualifying therapy services.[6]

The home health aide is directly supervised by the home care nurse or physical therapist. The role of the home health aide is to help clients reach their level of independence by temporarily assisting with personal hygiene. The home health aide implements the plan of care established by the nurse or other health professionals to reinforce teaching. Unlike the home attendant, the home health aide services are discontinued at the discharge of the client by the nurse or the physical therapist.

Long Term Home Health Care Program

The LTHHCP provides a range of professional and supportive services at home to clients needing care for an extended period. Individuals of this program must have Medicaid, be Medicaid-eligible, or elect to pay privately for services. Services offered may include professional nursing, physical therapy, occupational therapy, speech and audiology services, medical social work, nutritional counseling, respiratory therapy, personal care worker, home health aide, homemaker, and housekeeper.[7]

▬MODELS OF CARE

Traditional Care Model

Generally clients receive nonskilled service through a Traditional Care (time-oriented) model. This means one paraprofessional worker (also referred to as personal care worker, home health aide, or, in some agencies, a home attendant) is assigned to one client for a certain number of hours per day or week.[5] With this time-oriented model, the worker is in the home for a period of time, a minimum of 4 hours. Needless to say, this model facilitates a considerable amount of "empty time" in which the worker at times may sit and talk to the client, or read or watch television between tasks; or if the worker has completed the necessary tasks for that day, he or she watches the clock to fulfill the required hours.[8] Although this model helps to foster the development of a companionship between client and worker, it has resulted in the expenditure of more than $1 billion of Medicaid dollars annually in New York City alone.[9] This factor, along with the continued increase cost of healthcare particularly for the elderly home care clients, has brought the need for a new service delivery model that is cost effective.[9] Cluster Care is an alternative to the Traditional Care service delivery model presently existing.

Cluster Care Model

The increased cost of home healthcare for eligible Medicaid clients has led to New York City's HRA's decision to implement an alternative means of providing service to clients without a reduction in efficiency of care. Cluster Care has become the new cost effective alternative means of providing services to clients in their home environment if institutionalization is not required. Presently, the Cluster Care and Traditional Care models are used to provide activity of daily living assistance to clients who are Medicaid eligible and are in need of nonskilled services such as personal care and household chores. Cluster Care is designed to provide services to a group of clients residing in a designated geographic area, while providing quality care.[10] In this model, a paraprofessional worker might make multiple visits to one client during the same day, or might perform functions and tasks, such as shopping or doing laundry, for multiple clients simultaneously.[10] Unlike Traditional Care, Cluster Care is task oriented rather than time oriented and includes a group care plan in addition to an individual care plan.

Cluster Care, also referred to as the shared aide model, is a task-oriented method for which a Social Services district authorizes a paraprofessional to provide one or more nutritional and environmental support functions, personal care functions, or health-related tasks for one or more clients who reside with other clients in a designated geographic area or in close proximity (such as in the same apartment building).[11] The Cluster Care concept consists of two variations: (1) One paraprofessional worker services the client two to three times during the same day to perform one or more tasks specified in a client's care plan; and (2) two to three different workers provide service to one client at different times during the same day to perform one or more tasks. In each instance, the worker does not remain with the client for a predetermined period.

The intent of Cluster Care is to provide an entire team, not just a single worker, and higher-quality care.[12] Although Cluster Care may provide fewer hours, it is not necessarily intended to provide less service. For example, the paraprofessional worker might perform a shopping task for Client A in the morning, visit Client B to prepare a meal, and return to Client A in the afternoon to prepare a meal.

The Cluster Care team is composed of a case manager, two registered nurses, a site coordinator, a special group of personal care workers, and a community resource liaison who work together to provide the clients with the particular services needed.[12] The concept of working with a team is expected to increase productivity and the feelings of being professional.

Effects on the Elderly

Because Cluster Care is a new concept recently implemented in New York, the clients who are receiving Cluster Care currently, for the most part, were at one time a client of the Traditional Care (one-on-one) model. For many clients, this change is difficult. In addition, this change creates a disruption in the client's previous lifestyle of having a worker remain in the home for an extended period. It is especially difficult for the elderly because they generally experience difficulty adjusting to change.

An essential requirement for participation in the Cluster Care program is that the clients have to be available to admit and discharge the worker at least two to three times a day, depending on the number of workers they have. This activity often interferes with the clients' usual schedule, such as taking naps, resting, watching television programs, or participating in social activities outside the apartment. This scheduling also may create anxiety and affect the client physically when the worker is delayed at the previous client's home. Clients most suitable for the Cluster Care program include those who are alert, fully oriented, psychologically stable, ambulatory, without limited range of motion of upper extremities, and able to manage safely alone when the worker is not present.

Clients who are not appropriate for Cluster Care include those who have psychological problems, such as dementia or severe organic brain syndrome; need continuous safety supervision; are unable to provide access to the home, such as clients who are totally disabled or bedbound; have a history of paranoid episodes, such as chronic schizophrenics. Additional clients who are not appropriate for Cluster Care are those who need one-to-one extended care; dying clients, because of their emotional and physical needs; or clients who are receiving chemotherapy and might need to be out of the home for extended periods during the day, or who might not be physically able to cope with the added stress of providing access to the worker after chemotherapy treatment.

The following vignettes illustrate some clients' reactions to Cluster Care.

Mrs Porter is 92 years old and has had coronary heart disease for 20 years; noninsulin dependent diabetes mellitus for 50 years; and arthritis for 30 years, which she says has become worse during the past 5 years. She has been receiving Cluster Care for 9 months. Two to three workers visit at various times during the day to assist her with tasks. For example, one worker might visit at 7 AM to assist with bathing, dressing, and preparing her for breakfast, and leave at 9 AM to go to another client's home to perform scheduled household chores. Another worker will return to Mrs Porter's home at 12 PM to prepare lunch and do necessary shopping or errands, then leave to visit another client. At 5 PM, the third worker visits Mrs Porter to prepare dinner and assist with bed preparation.

Mrs Blake is 78 years old and has one worker that does tasks twice a day. The worker comes in the morning to assist with household chores for 2 hours, and then leaves to assist another client within the same building. She returns to Mrs Blake at 1 PM to perform errands or shopping.

Mrs Smalls is 75 years old and lives with her spouse who is 81 years old. She has one worker who visits her twice a day, and also sees other clients in between visits. Because of Mr Smalls' age and medical conditions, he is not able to care for his wife or perform household tasks. Mrs Smalls is totally dependent in all activities of daily living, is verbally unresponsive, and has a history of Parkinson's disease, diabetes mellitus, peripheral vascular disease, psychosis, right ankle ulcer, and left great toe ulcer that is treated by a visiting nurse twice a day. Mrs Smalls visits her physician every month. On the days of her doctor's appointment, her regular worker is assigned in the afternoon to accompany Mrs Smalls. When Mr Smalls was asked about Cluster Care, he responded, ''It's alright with me because I need someone to assist me with my wife.''

Ms Potts is 68 years of old, lives alone, and would not be a suitable candidate for Cluster Care. She has a history of chronic schizophrenia and is a compulsive smoker. She constantly paces the floor, roams the hallways, and will wander away if left unattended. For safety reasons, Ms Potts needs constant supervision and has a paraprofessional worker or home health aide who provides 24-hour service. Because of her emotional (psychological) status, Ms Potts would not be able to cope with several workers visiting at intervals to care for her.

Because nurses in general are concerned with holistic client care, the nurse must be the stable facilitator or resource among the client, worker, and other team members. In addition to nursing functions, the nurse should encourage and foster on-going communication between the client and the worker, emphasizing the positive aspects of the Cluster Care concept. The nurse and the site coordinator have the responsibility to recognize the change from the Traditional Model to the Cluster Care Model as a potential stressor for the client and should attempt to minimize or alleviate it.

▬SUMMARY

This new home healthcare concept is an alternative to the Traditional Care Model and most likely will be used indefinitely. Community health nurses should assume a more active role in assisting the Cluster Care clients to adjust to the model by educating them to the need and expected outcomes of this new concept. In addition, the nurse should continue to offer the client assurance that services can be adjusted as necessary for the client. This assistance will enable clients to cope with this new service and possibly alleviate stressors that might present in a physical nature.

▬ REFERENCES

1. United Hospital Fund-Home Care Institution. *Making Cluster Care Work*. New York: United Hospital Fund-Home Care Institution, 1993.
2. Stanhope M, Lancaster J. Family Development. *Community Health Nursing: Process and Practice For Promoting Health*, 3rd ed. St Louis: The Mosby-Year Book, Inc, 1992, p 438.
3. Magilvy JK, Brown NJ, Dydyn J. The experience of home health care: Perceptions of older adults. *J Pub Health* 1988; 5(3):140–145.
4. Surpin R, Grumm F. Building the care triangle: Clients and families, paraprofessionals and agencies. *Caring Mag* 1990; 9(4):6–15.
5. Hall H. The definition and role of the paraprofessional in home care. *Caring Mag* 1986; 5(4):8–10.
6. Galten R, Dombi W. *Part-Time or Intermittent Care Explained*. Washington DC: National Association for Home Care, 1990.
7. Visiting Nurse Association of Brooklyn. *Longterm Home Health Care Program Fact Sheet*. New York: Visiting Nurse Association of Brooklyn, 1990.
8. Feldman P. *Report to the New York Human Resources Administration: Background and Baseline Information on the Cluster Care Demonstration*. Boston: Department of Health Policy and Management, Harvard School of Public Health Massachusetts, 1990 (unpublished).
9. Finnerman K. *Cluster Care: A New Approach to Home Care* (ISBN 1-881277-09-7). New York: United Hospital Fund of New York, 1992.
10. Acting Commissioner, New York State Department of Social Services. *Administrative Directive to Commissioners of Social Services, Division of Medical Assistance*. New York: New York State Department of Social Services, 1992 (unpublished).
11. Report from Bureau of New York State Department of Social Services Long Term Care Division of Medical Assistance to Home Care Council of New York City, 1991 (Unpublished).
12. *Your Cluster Care Team — The Team Work Approach to Home Care*. City of New York Human Resources Administration: Income of Medical Assistance Administration, Office of Home Care Services, 1990.

Chapter 23

The Use of the Omaha Information System in a Multidisciplinary Outpatient Rehabilitation Program for Frail Older Persons

RUTH SHUTTLEWORTH-DIAZ

The problem-focused taxonomy of the Omaha Information System is used successfully with frail elderly in a multidisciplinary outpatient rehabilitation program. The system was originally designed for organization of documentation information in the home care setting. The problem-focused classification scheme it uses is more useful with the frail elderly than a diagnoses taxonomy. This is especially true in a rehabilitation program where similar diagnoses may present very different problems in individual clients. A case study is presented to demonstrate the usefulness of the Omaha Information System in outpatient rehabilitation with elders. The use of this system in a setting other than that for which it was originally created may give readers insight into how it may be useful in their clinical settings.

Quality is the ability to achieve desirable objectives using legitimate means. The objective is usually an achievable state of health.[1] Quality of care is the degree to which health services for individuals and populations increase the likelihood of desired health outcomes and are consistent with current professional knowledge.[2] The term *quality of life* is not defined or agreed on, but it is complex because it encompasses health and functional status and it varies with one's age.[3] Quality, quality of care, and quality of life are three concepts that historically have been the concern of health care providers. Quality care positively influences health and quality of life and so there is continued effort to improve the quality of care. More often, a multidisciplinary approach is being used to provide quality care. There is no single profession that has all the skills and expertise needed to provide health services to the older persons, and collaboration among professionals has consistently been shown to be the most effective way to meet the multiple needs of older adults.[4]

From *Topics in Geriatric Rehabilitation* 11(1):67–74, 1995. Reprinted with permission.

DOCUMENTATION

A collaborative approach is used in a multidisciplinary outpatient rehabilitation program to maximize independence, promote health and function, and enhance quality of life for older adults with chronic illness. This multidisciplinary team assesses and intervenes collaboratively so that all of the client's complex needs are met. Because of this thorough process, the client should improve independent functioning and therefore be maintained in the community, thus preventing use of expensive institutional care. Measured and documented improvements in functioning in activities of daily living (ADLs) is a way to show how quality care improves health and quality of life. This is because improving functioning for the frail older person is one of the best ways to improve quality of life. There has been great success for this program in terms of improved client functioning, independence, and life satisfaction. Many of the clients verbally express their appreciation of the staff and their satisfaction with the program. Documentation is often the benchmark by which quality of care is measured.[5] The medical care of the 21st century will require that medical institutions offer data on quality of care, cost-effectiveness, and selection of the appropriate treatment modality.[6]

There is a crucial need for documentation to show progress made toward results for which a plan was designed and initiated.[5] In this multidisciplinary rehabilitation program, staff members from each discipline documented narrative progress notes in their own designated section of the client record, yet this did not reflect their interactive style of providing care. It is difficult to measure client progress and change in function with this method of documentation. One hospital enhanced a collaborative approach among departments by using a computerized documentation system. By incorporating responsibilities of nurses, physicians, and support services within the practice document, the integrated nature of the care provided is reflected more accurately than if each player had a separate document. This documentation system set the stage for continuous quality improvement because it pulled the departments together, reduced duplication, and enhanced collaboration.[7] For effective communication and documentation of care, a standardized language is required.[8] A standardized language becomes essential when a multidisciplinary approach is used because of the different words each discipline uses for similar actions and functions. The challenge of demonstrating that (collaborative) care makes a difference to the public at large and to health policymakers further demands a uniform language that clearly depicts (collaborative) contributions to health care.[8]

THE OMAHA INFORMATION SYSTEM

The Omaha Information System was used to organize documentation information from 100 records of discharged clients. This started as a test to see whether this information system would be applicable to a multidisciplinary outpatient rehabilitation program for older adults. The language is standardized and so it was necessary to see whether this language and information system could capture the problems of the frail older population and the multidisciplinary approach. The Omaha system enabled all of the client's problems and the interventions provided to be organized into a brief summary. Instead of each discipline using its own style of documentation and vocabulary to describe the problems and interventions, data were structured in organization and language was standardized. By using the language provided by this information system, one can see how the client problems and the interventions provided interrelate.

The Omaha Information System was developed for a home care agency, but it was easily used to organize documentation in this outpatient rehabilitation program. It has also been used in a community health needs and utilization survey instrument for the problem identification section. The taxonomy mitigated investigator bias on any preconceptions about the nature of health problems.[9] At Massachusetts General Hospital's Coordinated Care Program for Elderly, the Omaha Information System was added to the COSTAR vocabulary so that the client record met the clinicians' need for flexibility. This program had teams of physicians, social workers, and nurses providing care at satellite health centers. COSTAR is a database developed at Massachusetts General Hospital that is rich with medical diagnoses.[10] It would seem that the Omaha system is not limited to home care, but this may be the first time that it has been applied to a multidisciplinary outpatient rehabilitation program.

The Omaha system is described as a comprehensive schema of nursing diagnoses, client outcomes, and nursing interventions. The three schemata were developed during a series of research studies conducted between 1975 and 1986 by the Visiting Nurses Association of Omaha.[11] The Omaha system offers a method of collecting and analyzing essential client-focused data. It provides a comprehensive, valid, and reliable framework to describe and measure clients' health care requirements and the services provided. It is designed to provide a framework for integrating a clinical practice and a documentation system. It is a method of organizing and entering client data into a manual, partially automated, or automated management information system. Because the language and the organization of the scheme are simple and standardized, it is being used by physical therapists, occupational therapists, social workers, speech pathologists, nutritionists, dentists, physicians, and nurses.[12]

The Omaha Information System has three components. The first is a problem classification scheme that uses problem-focused taxonomy instead of the usual general diagnoses. This is important in an outpatient rehabilitation program because a diagnosis of a stroke does not define the level of rehabilitation required. The problem classification scheme is divided into four domains: (1) environmental, (2) psychosocial, (3) physiologic, and (4) health-related behaviors. This encompasses all of the possible problems that this outpatient program might face. The second component is a problem rating scale for outcomes that consists of a five-point Likert-type assessment of the subscales: (1) knowledge, (2) behavior, and (3) status. This scale allows staff members an opportunity to quantify the severity of the problem. The third component is the intervention scheme, which is divided into four categories: (1) health teaching, guidance, and counseling; (2)

treatment and procedures; (3) case management; and (4) surveillance. There are specific targets or actions to further clarify the interventions. A multidisciplinary team therefore has the ability to describe actual or potential problems, rate the problems, document collaborative interventions, and then rate the problems again to measure the degree of change in knowledge, behavior, and status. The Omaha system measures and documents the impact of the services. Also, because standardized language is used by all of the disciplines, it is clear to see how a multidisciplinary team would be interacting, focusing on the same problems, and collaboratively providing care.

A multidisciplinary team could quickly document client assessments, interventions, and progress using the Omaha system because the system is already numerically coded. Using this information system would standardize language among the several disciplines and enable the team to see how each discipline is addressing the same problems with a different focus. An example would be a client with a problem of pain caused by osteoarthritis. The client can potentially become deconditioned because the pain would have an impact on quality of life. A geriatric nurse practitioner would be intervening by use of medication and case management with the physician. A physical therapist would be using pain-reducing modalities and exercises as the intervention, and an occupational therapist would be focused on managing ADLs around the pain. A geropsychiatric clinical nurse specialist would be dealing with the emotions related to the pain and potential loss of independence. Part or all of the team would become involved in intervening with this one problem. Without this standardized documentation system and language, the interaction of the disciplines addressing this one problem of pain would not be captured. The Omaha system therefore could also provide a check to reduce duplication and fragmentation of services. The team goal could be that the client will be pain free and able to maintain independence in the community, and then each discipline would have more specific goals. The client would be rated according to the problem rating scale for outcomes on admission and at discharge to quantify and measure changes in severity and function as a result of interventions. The client could then be benchmarked against other clients with a similar problem with pain. The purpose of benchmarking derives from the need to establish more credible goals and pursue continuous improvement.[13] There is the potential for internal and external research. The ability to characterize large aggregate populations across different agencies has great potential for future research.[11] A case study has been added to clarify the Omaha system and its use in this outpatient rehabilitation program (see the box).

The Omaha Information System was used to organize discharged client records into quick summaries of the client problems addressed and the multidisciplinary interventions provided. Because this was done retrospectively, the problem rating scale for outcomes was not used. It became clear from the beginning that the Omaha system could be used for more than an improvement in the style of documentation. This information system, with continued use, has the ability to reduce the amount of time spent

CASE STUDY

Mrs H is a 73-year-old female who lives alone in a senior high-rise apartment. She relies on two friends who assist her in higher level ADLs. Her medical diagnoses include polymyositis, right hip inflammation process, hypertension, noninsulin-dependent diabetes mellitus, peptic ulcer disease, and a right kidney mass that was being worked up. She was recently hospitalized for the peptic ulcer disease, and she had recently begun taking Prozac for depression. She complained of a loss of 10 pounds and anorexia. She mostly talked of her fear of being placed in a nursing home, and she expressed concern that she placed too much of a burden on her friends who provide assistance.

Traditionally Mrs H would be assessed by each of the disciplines providing care in this outpatient rehabilitation program, and each discipline would document its assessment and treatment plan in the designated section of the client record. With the use of the Omaha Information System and its standardized language, one can see how the different disciplines identified and addressed the same problems. The organization of the information therefore puts the data into a summary of the patient's problems and the interventions provided by this multidisciplinary team. Ideally, Mrs H would be rated on a scale of 1 to 5 in the areas of knowledge, behavior, and status for each problem by the team on admission and again at discharge for an objective score of severity. Some intervention targets were added to tailor this information system to this program and encompass the typical interventions that would be provided. This is the application of the Omaha Information System to Mrs H's case:

Problem Classification Scheme: 12 Emotional stability, Domain II. Psychosocial

Health Promotion:

Potential Impairment:

Impairment: 01 sadness/hopelessness/worthlessness re: loss of health issues

Problem Rating Scale for Outcomes:

Knowledge

Behavior

Status

Intervention Scheme:

1. Health Teaching, Guidance, and Counseling:
2. Treatments and Procedures: MHNSG — 63 psychotherapy sessions.
3. Case Management: SW — 61 consult/refer to Senior Center. MHNSG — 63 psychotherapy-enc. to continue outpatient therapy; 61 consult/refer with MD for medication treatment.
4. Surveillance:

Problem Classification Scheme: 19 Hearing. Domain III. Physiologic

Health Promotion:

Potential Impairment:

Impairment: 01 difficulty hearing normal speech tones-left ear

Problem Rating Scale for Outcomes:

Knowledge

Behavior

Status

Intervention Scheme:

1. Health Teaching, Guidance, and Counseling: SLP — 09 coping skills-compensatory strategies; 47 signs/symptoms hearing loss right ear.
2. Treatments and Procedures:
3. Case Management:
4. Surveillance:

Problem Classification Scheme: 24 Pain, Domain III. Physiologic

Health Promotion:

Potential Impairment:

Impairment: #1.01 expresses discomfort/pain in right hip

#2.03 compensated movements/guarding

Problem Rating Scale for Outcomes:

Knowledge

Behavior

Status

Intervention Scheme:

1. Health Teaching, Guidance, and Counseling:
2. Treatments and Procedures: PT — 18 exercises using lower extremity therapeutic exercise program.
3. Case Management: NSG — 61 consult/refer with rheumatologist and psychiatrist; 60 obtained MRI results.
4. Surveillance:

Problem Classification Scheme: 27 Neuromusculoskeletal function, Domain III. Physiologic

Health Promotion:

Potential Impairment:

Impairment: #1. 09 difficulties in managing ADLs

#2. 02 decreased muscle strength

Problem Rating Scale for Outcomes:

Knowledge

Behavior

Status

Intervention Scheme:

1. Health Teaching, Guidance, and Counseling: OT — 60 energy conservation; 34 mobility/exercise for body mechanics and joint protection; 42 relaxation/breathing techniques. PT — 18 exercises for home exercise program.
2. Treatments and Procedures: PT — 23 gait training; 18 exercises for endurance. OT — 18 exercises using upper extremity therapeutic exercises.
3. Case Management: OT — 55 supplies of adaptive equipment obtained. SW — 57 support system obtained in-home services.
4. Surveillance: OT — 39 personal care.

Problem Classification Scheme: 29 circulation, Domain III. Physiologic

Health Promotion:

Potential Impairment: 08 abnormal blood pressure readings

Impairment:

Problem Rating Scale for Outcomes:

Knowledge

Behavior

Status

Intervention Scheme:

1. Health Teaching, Guidance, and Counseling:
2. Treatments and Procedures:
3. Case Management:
4. Surveillance: NSG — 62 monitor BP closely and report to primary MD.

Problem Classification Scheme: 35 Nutrition, Domain IV. Health Related Behaviors

Health Promotion:

Potential Impairment:

Impairment: 08 recent loss of 10 lbs, anorexia

Problem Rating Scale for Outcomes:

Knowledge

Behavior

Status

Intervention Scheme:

1. Health Teaching, Guidance, and Counseling: NSG — 36 nutrition regarding food pyramid and diabetes exchange list diet.
2. Treatments and Procedures:
3. Case Management: NSG — 37 nutritionist, 36 nutrition — refer to cheaper product usage.
4. Surveillance: NSG — 36 nutrition — diet recall, weight checks, and monitor blood sugars.

Based on the fact that Mrs H met the goals established by the multidisciplinary team and improved her ability to function independently, a positive change in the Problem Rating Scale for Outcomes scores would be expected. Mrs H was able to verbalize her satisfaction with the program in terms of how much better she felt. Her problems, in this form of data organization, could be compared with other similar problems seen by the multidisciplinary team to benchmark the process and outcome of care for similar problems in similar clients. Also, she could be monitored for a specific time after discharge for maintenance of functioning by scoring the client again according to the Problem Rating Scale for Outcomes. This allows for a way to measure quality of care and its effect on quality of life. Similarly, an aggregate of clients can be compared with another population for further external research on the common problems frail older people face and the benefits of attending an outpatient multidisciplinary rehabilitation program.

documenting and increase efficiency because the client record could become data for future research. A universal goal of administrators and clinicians is to improve practice and streamline documentation. This information system can replace lengthy and disorganized progress notes. Also, by using the problem rating scale for outcomes, assessments are objective because problems are numerically scored; this could be used as an indicator for internal and external quality research. The purpose of such a documentation and data management model is to help staff practice more efficiently and increase the quality of client services.[12]

Structure, process, and outcome are three avenues to judge quality.[1] The structure of the Omaha system has already been proven comprehensive, reliable, and valid, and the ease of organizing client records with this information system shows its appropriateness in this program. By using the change in the method of documentation to a standardized information system, such as the Omaha Information System, the quality of the process of care and outcome of care can be measured for quality improvement. Outcomes have a time dimension incorporated in them. Certain modifications in health status are temporary, whereas others are of a longer duration. It is necessary to include these differences in any accounting of the consequences of care.[14] Using the problem rating scale for outcomes allows the professional to quantify the severity of the problem. This can be done on admission, at discharge, or even after discharge. By being able to measure changes in function as a result of the interventions, the outcomes can then become a benchmark for other clients. There is the potential of using this information system to measure the long-term effects on independence and function.

The intent is to stimulate conceptual development and empirical research to determine what styles and strategies of care are optimal in terms of multiple objectives at the individual and collective levels.[14] The Omaha system pulls all the disciplines together so it is clear how they are integrating their interventions for a common goal. This enables the managers and clinicians to view the process of care for similar types of clients and in a sense map out a plan of reasonable care. These details outline the criteria for further evaluation. This allows for a continuous quality improvement process. Also, now that there is a way to standardize language and pull the disciplines together in one document, it is possible to see what the most common problems being treated are and how the team intervenes. This information could lead to the ability to benchmark these data to other databases. This is how an information system can aid in measuring quality of care and open the door for future research.

Linking patient care standards, documentation, and quality monitoring tools promotes the achievement of quality care and patient outcomes.[15] The selection of the Omaha Information System could provide the opportunity for a rehabilitation program for older adults to monitor quality assurance and quality improvement projects in a different way. The ability is there to improve the current practice and measure the outcomes of the frail older population. This can lead to future research on the most common problems of frail older people and what must be done to improve their functioning in ADLs and their quality of life. To ensure that these methods (of standardized documentation) serve the dual purpose of evaluating the effectiveness of specific technologies on the one hand and continually assessing whether quality of patient care has improved on the other hand, practicing health care providers must be involved in the construction of the data systems and the gathering of information for them.[16]

■ REFERENCES

1. Donabedian A. Quality assessment and assurance: unity of purpose, diversity of means. *Inquiry.* 1988;52:173–192.
2. Lohr KN. Health, health care, and quality of care. In: Lohr K, ed. *Medicare: A Strategy for Quality Assurance.* Washington, DC: National Academy Press; 1990;1:19–44.
3. Faden R, German P. Quality of life considerations in geriatrics. *Clin Geriatr Med.* 1994;10(3):541–551.
4. Pulliam L. Client satisfaction with a nurse managed clinic. *J Commun Health Nurs.* 1991;8(2):97–112.
5. Quigley P, Mathis A, Nodhturft V. Improving clinical documentation quality. *J Nurs Care Qual.* 1994;8(4):66–73.
6. Riddick FA. The role of the multispecialty clinic in health care delivery in the twenty-first century. *Med Clin North Am.* 1992;76(5):1,015–1,020.
7. Krueger NE, Mazuzan JE. A collaborative approach to standards, practices. *AORN J.* 1993;57(2):467, 470–475, 478–480.
8. Moorhead SA, McCloskey JC, Bulechek G. Nursing interventions classification. A comparison with the Omaha system and the home health care classification. *J Nurs Admin.* 1993;23(10):23–29.
9. Lundeen SP. Health needs of a suburban community: a nursing assessment approach. *J Commun Health Nurs.* 1992;9(4):235–244.
10. Zielstorff RD, Jette AM, Barnett GO. Issues in designing an automated record system for clinical care and research. *Adv Nurs Sci.* 1990;13(2):75–88.
11. Martin KS, Scheet NJ, Stegman MR. Home health clients: characteristics, outcomes of care, and nursing interventions. *Am J Public Health.* 1993;83(12):1,730–1,734.
12. Martin K, Leek G, Aden C. The Omaha system. A research-based model for decision making. *J Nurs Admin.* 1992;22(11):47–52.
13. Camp RC, Tweet AG. Benchmarking applied to health care. *Jt Comm J Qual Improve.* 1994;20(5):229–238.
14. Donabedian A. Some basic issues in evaluating the quality of health care. In: *Issues in Evaluation Research.* Kansas City, Mo: American Nurses Association; 1976:3–28.
15. Weiss ME, Teplick FN. Linking perinatal standards, documentation, and quality monitoring. *J Perinat Neonatal Nurs.* 1993;7(2):18–27.
16. Greenfield S. The state of outcome research: are we on target? *N Engl J Med.* 1989;320(17):1,142–1,143.

■ FURTHER READINGS

Catanzano F. Nursing information/documentation system increases quality care, shortens stay at Desert Samaritan Medical Center. *Comput Nurs.* 1994;12(4):184–185.

Lang NM. Quality assurance review in nursing. *Am J Matern Child Nurs.* 1976;1(2):75–79.

Langel BC, Brewer SG, Olszewski C. Developing quality documentation. *Nurs Manage.* 1991;20(11):48–50, 52.

Martin KS, Scheet NJ. *The Omaha System, Applications for Community Health Nursing.* Philadelphia, Pa: WB Saunders; 1992.

McCloskey JC. Implications of costing out nursing services for reimbursement. *Nurs Manage.* 1989;20(1):44–49.

Chapter 24

Cardiac Specialty Program for Home Health Care: A Model for Implementation

MARGALINE LAZARRE   SALLY AX

The unique feature of this chapter is that it presents a cardiac specialty program for home health care that can be adapted for any specialty program in any setting. Lazarre and Ax present a blueprint for developing a specialty program that meets the needs of clients with similar diagnoses. They present a conceptual model, program goals and structure, role delineation, and various other aspects of program development that need to be considered in order to have successful results. In many agencies there are nurses who have identified a specific population with needs that the nurse is prepared to meet or needs with which the nurse is particularly interested in meeting. Combining a nurse's interest and skills with the model presented here, can prepare the caregiver to effectively plan a specialty program that may be needed.

The home care industry has grown tremendously during the past 20 years. Limited resources, coupled with an increasingly educated consumer market, have forced the home care industry to become increasingly innovative while providing the very services it is intended to offer: basic health services in the home. The authors' home care agency implemented a cardiac specialty program in the fall of 1993 that focuses on the specific needs of the cardiac patient. Although the program is relatively in its infancy, the benefits to both patients and staff have been tangible. What follows is a blueprint of how such a program can be implemented in any home health agency.

Health care providers and practitioners have been aware for some time of what is now called the paradigm shift, the trend toward shifting the delivery of the most basic health care services back to the home. Patients are being discharged home earlier. The home care agency that bridges the gap between the acute care and the home provides a continuum of care that is essential in the recovery process. Although the authors' program is

From *Journal of Home Health Care Practice* 8(1):11–18, 1995. Reprinted with permission.

intended for patients with cardiac illnesses, it can be duplicated to serve any patient population. One home health agency in central Florida has implemented a cardiac specialty program to meet the needs of an ever-increasing cardiac population.

The number of people over 65 years of age is rapidly growing to an estimated 13% of the total population. That is about 30 million older adults. It is estimated that by the year 2030, 20% of the total US population will be over 65 years.[1] With such statistics, it makes sense to have programs in place that meet the needs of this large segment of the population. Specialty programs in home care bring advanced skills into the home while caring for specific groups of individuals with similar, but complex needs.

Where does one start when developing a specialty program? The following is a blueprint of steps that must be undertaken when considering the implementation of a specialty program for home care (see Fig. 24-1).

▬ NEEDS ASSESSMENT

The first step is to identify a need for the program. Who would benefit? What is the targeted population? Are there data supporting the identified need? In doing a needs assessment, one must be careful to differentiate

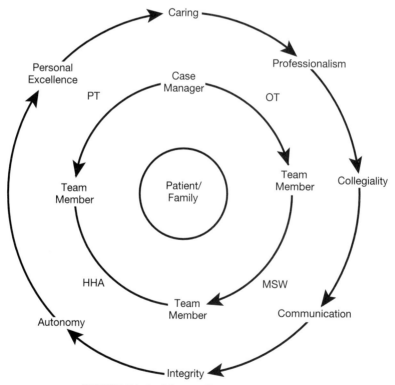

FIGURE 24-1   The cardiac program model.

between a wish and a need. A specialty program must be targeted to a specific population or group. Demographics and funding sources are vital assessment parameters. A program may sound wonderful, but if it does not meet the needs of the population being served, it is not needed. In the authors' case a need was identified by several nurses with critical care backgrounds who were doing home care visits on post-coronary artery bypass grafting (CABG) patients, postmyocardial infarction (MI) patients, and heart failure patients. They identified a knowledge deficit as cause of many exacerbations and hospitalizations within this group. This is true of various groups. A survey of 100 home cardiac patients revealed that on the first visit, patients correctly answered a cardiac health questionnaire only 58% of the time. The same patients correctly responded to the same survey 90% of the time after receiving home health services using cardiac nurses.[2] In the authors' agency it was decided that nurses with in-depth knowledge of cardiovascular disease were needed to care for and to educate this patient population. The client population was identified as elderly, with a mean age of 69 years.

▬GOALS AND OBJECTIVES

Defining goals and objectives [Box 24-1] for the program provides guidance and helps reduce confusion about the purpose of the project. It is important that set goals be measurable with a time line. Achievement of goals may be measured yearly or quarterly, for example. The authors' goals at the agency are to bring the cardiac patient to a level where he or she can effectively manage the disease; to decrease hospitalizations and exacerbations, thereby reducing costs; to attract competent critical care nurses to the program; and to educate the community about heart disease.

▬ACTION PLAN

An action plan sets time limits for achieving certain goals in the implementation process. This may include funding, software, secretarial help, policy development, hiring, educational activities, and marketing activities up to full implementation. In the authors' agency, once the project was approved, the program coordinator spent 3 months developing, for example, objectives, standards, policies and procedures, and protocols of care. She spent

---

BOX 24-1   *Cardiac Program Goals*

- To empower the cardiac patient to effectively manage his or her disease
- To reduce hospitalizations and exacerbations and ultimately health care costs
- To attract and retain highly skilled critical care nurses
- To educate the community about heart disease

another 3 months educating the staff about the specifics of the program. Full implementation was begun at the end of 6 months. Time lines will vary depending on the size of the organization and on the type of program being developed.

MULTIDISCIPLINARY INVOLVEMENT

The success of a specialty program requires the support of all the domains within the organization. The program coordinator must do a good job of educating the different individuals who will have some part in the running of the program, no matter how insignificant their involvement. Management, clerical staff, and medical personnel will be more open and supportive if they know what the program is about and what their role is in the implementation process.

PROGRAM STRUCTURE

Structuring is important as it determines how the program will run (Table 24-1). Is the program going to use a case-management or team-management model? What are the funding sources? In the authors' agency management responded to the authors' proposal by allocating funds to hire specialty staff and to acquire equipment. The program structure was designed as follows:

- Standards of care were developed with emphasis on disease entities, staff credentials, continuing education requirements, continuous quality improvement (CQI) activities, and admission/discharge criteria.
- Goals and objectives were stated.
- Case management was chosen as the model for the delivery of care with a multidisciplinary team approach.
- Job descriptions and performance evaluations were developed for cardiac specialty staff.
- Initial and ongoing competencies were developed to ensure the staff's continued competence.
- CQI activities with identified important aspects of care were developed to assess quality of care and to monitor for trends.
- Patient/staff and physician satisfaction surveys were developed to be an ongoing and integral part of the program.
- Community education presentations that focus on heart disease and healthy lifestyles were developed; they too are ongoing, essential components of the cardiac program.
- Teaching materials (i.e., patient teaching booklet, drug information sheets) were developed to help both the nurses and the patients optimize teaching sessions.
- In addition to basic teaching, specialty nurses were identified as being able to perform ECGs in the home using portable ECG machines.
- Patients with end-stage heart disease were identified as candidates for home intravenous (IV) Lasix (furosemide) or cardiac drug infusions (i.e., dobutamine).

TABLE 24-1   Cardiac Program Structure

MAJOR COMPONENTS	MAJOR OBJECTIVES
Needs assessment	Provides rationale for program development
Targeted population	Identifies population to be served, including physicians
Goals and objectives	Verbalizes overall mission of the program; may be short-term and long-term; must be measurable and specific
Standards of practice	Make up the backbone of the program; must include parameters for measuring outcomes
Care delivery model	Describes how and by whom care is provided using case management, team management, or primary nursing
Financial assessment	Part of strategic planning. Start-up and ongoing costs are part of submitted proposal, including cost of hiring specialized personnel, acquisition of new equipment, if any, and printing of teaching materials
Specialty staff	Advanced practice personnel with clinical expertise and strong credentials make up the specialty team
Specialty paperwork	Includes protocol of care, critical paths—all paperwork pertaining to the program
Satisfaction surveys	Essential to the ongoing assessment of the program; must be done at regular intervals and include patient, staff, and physicians
Special equipment	Enhances any specialty programs; may include portable ECG machine, ECG monitors, pulse oximeters, fetal monitors
CQI activities	Important aspects of care monitored periodically to assess the quality of care being delivered
Program evaluation plan	Part of the strategic plan; may be done yearly or biannually

ROLE DELINEATION

Specialty programs may be headed by clinical nurse specialists or by a clinician with a strong background in the respective specialty. The specialty program coordinator must be an expert with strong credentials. The authors' cardiac program consists of the program coordinator and the cardiac team members. Team members are designated as level I through level III practitioners based on their clinical expertise and years of practice, level III being the most experienced.

The program coordinator coordinates the program throughout the agency. This individual sets up the program in the various branches, interviews prospective cardiac team members, and makes recommendations for hire to each area branch manager. He or she also oversees the quality of the program through random chart audits and staff competency evaluations and provides educational classes to help team members maintain clinical competence.

Critical care experience is a must for prospective team members. Coronary care unit (CCU) experience is preferred. The American Association of Critical Care Nurses (AACN) recognizes the role of the critical care nurse in home health. The November 1994 issue of *AACN News* discusses the transition of two critical care nurses into home health care and the specific characteristics of critical care nurses that make them ideal for nursing in the home.[3] Critical care nurses are independent and very focused, which is important for resolving problems encountered in the home. Their critical thinking abilities and physical assessment skills make them ideal home care nurses.

In addition to the program coordinator and team members, a good working relationship with the branch managers and medical supervisors is essential. Prior cardiac or CCU experience is an asset for the supervisor in charge of cardiac patients. The supervisor plays a major role in screening calls, evaluating referrals, and acting as a link between the program coordinator and the cardiac program staff.

▬ STAFF COMPETENCE

Staff competence is evaluated initially via good preemployment screening. Newly hired cardiac nurses must take an assessment examination and a rhythm interpretation examination. The following competencies are required annually for all cardiac nurses: cardiac and respiratory assessment, identification and administration of cardiovascular drugs, electrocardiogram (ECG) rhythm strip interpretation, care of the patient with congestive heart failure (CHF)/cardiomyopathy (Table 24-2), case management, and group dynamics and principles of teaching/learning theory. Equipment competencies include 12-lead ECG and pulse oximetry. Each cardiac Case Manager is evaluated in the field by the Program Coordinator semi-annually. Ongoing staff competency evaluation is a major component of any specialty program.

TABLE 24-2   Care of the Patient with CHF

PROBLEM	EXPECTED OUTCOMES	NURSING INTERVENTIONS	DATE ACCOMPLISHED

Fluid volume excess	Standard
	  Normal body weight
	  Daily weight log kept
	Criteria
	  Balanced intake and output
	  Peripheral edema absent
	  Patient/caregiver keeps daily weight log
		Instruct
		  Importance of daily weights: same time, same clothing, same scale
		  Fluid restriction
		  Daily weight log	

▬COMMUNITY EDUCATION

Community education is an integral part of the cardiac program, and team members are encouraged to participate in such presentations. The authors' program coordinator has provided a series of lectures titled "Health Heart Living" to various community groups in the program's service areas. Some team members have participated in various blood pressure (BP) screenings for senior groups and in presentations to various physicians' offices. Community activities are a valuable way of providing needed information and of making the public aware of the services provided by the cardiac team.

▬CLIENT MIX

The authors' cardiac clientele primarily consists of geriatric patients whose primary health care provider is Medicare. Diagnoses range from acute MI, to conditions requiring interventional therapies such as angioplasties, to CHF, with the latter being the most common. More aggressive therapies have also been administered in the elderly population, which indicates the existence of an increasing number of seniors who have undergone open heart surgery. Occasionally staff members have cared for patients requiring IV dobutamine or furosemide for intractable heart failure.

▬REFERRAL SOURCE

All patients with a primary cardiac diagnosis are referred to the cardiac program. Patients are usually under the care of an internist with a cardiologist on consult. Referrals are received from area hospitals, physicians' offices, patients or family members, and occasionally from extended care facilities. Patient care coordinators are encouraged to tell potential clients and providers about the program's special features and services.

▬CUSTOMER SATISFACTION

The specialty program is currently sending a customer satisfaction survey to all patients discharged from service. Cardiac patients are identified through personal comments on the returned surveys. Results of 3 months' data have revealed no negative responses. Whenever possible, surveys must target specific patient and client groups.

▬STAFF SATISFACTION

A satisfaction survey questionnaire is given to each cardiac team member after 6 months of employment. Survey content assesses the following: patient/nurse ratio, paperwork, scheduling, job expectations, communication, salary incentives, recognition, case management, teaching materials, and overall job satisfaction. The program is generally viewed positively by the cardiac staff.

■ SALARY INCENTIVES

Specialty programs must present an attractive compensation package to lure experienced critical care nurses from the acute care setting. In addition to outstanding program features, the organization must offer good benefits and attractive salaries. In the authors' case the program coordinator has set some salary guidelines for branch managers to use when hiring cardiac specialty nurses. Salaries are based on years of experience, advanced degrees, and certifications. Ongoing market analyses ensure that the home care agency remains competitive with area hospitals.

■ PROS AND CONS

Implementing a specialty program for home care is a challenging and exciting endeavor. The concept of bringing critical care skills into the home is revolutionary. In addition, specialty programs add a new edge to any organization and make it more competitive in today's market. The challenge will be to remain competitive by changing specialty programs to meet the ever-changing needs of the population they are designed to serve. Another challenge is to attract and retain qualified personnel. Organizations must create an environment where employees feel valued and nurtured.

The health care industry is in a state of turmoil. The delivery of health care services is shifting away from the acute care setting into the home. Health care providers must become innovative in the face of shrinking resources. Specialty programs in home care attempt to provide specialized care using specialty staff for better and shorter outcomes. The cardiac program model described here can be duplicated to serve any patient population. The basics are the same. As these programs become more common, they will have to validate their usefulness to survive, mainly by validating improved patient outcomes and cost-effectiveness.

■ REFERENCES

1. U.S. Department of Commerce. *Statistical Abstract of the United States.* 110th ed. Washington, DC: Bureau of the Census; 1990.
2. Frantz A. *Cardiac Recovery: Home Care's New Horizons: Book of Abstracts.* Ann Arbor, Mich: University of Michigan School of Nursing, Ninth National Nursing Symposium on Home Health Care; 1994.
3. A visit inside home health care. *AACN NEWS.* November 1994: 1.

Chapter 25

Coming Together for Change: Workshops for Women in the Nursing Home

JANET LEE   MARYLEA BENWARE CARR

The authors of this chapter present the innovative idea of developing a series of workshops for residents of nursing homes in surrounding communities in one area of South Central Minnesota. One site served as a host facility, and 10 to 50 women participated in the two consecutive morning workshops. An afternoon workshop was developed with similar topics for the combined staff. The therapeutic and educational workshops were conducted with the twin goals of improving self-esteem and self-reliance and facilitating community building and networking. The workshop content included aging and ageism, self-esteem, choices, and reminiscence through the use of poetry, films, and discussion. Creative nursing and activity staff, along with resident council members, can use the concept presented here to develop a similar program in rehabilitation centers, retirement communities, assisted living centers, and in other skilled nursing facilities.

We share insights from a project aimed at improving the mental health of nursing home resident women through a series of therapeutic and educational workshops. The first project goal involved workshop activities to enhance resident women's self-esteem, self-assertion, and morale, encouraging the individual sharing of experiences to reveal how individual problems might have structural causes and be shared by others. Our second project goal involved networking among women nursing home residents, aiming to foster community and peer advocacy. The final goal included staff education, training, and networking. We hoped to provide a context whereby staff could articulate their needs and those of resident women, as well as learn about strategies for the creation of an environment that would meet the residents' psychosocial needs for dignity and self-respect. The workshops were made possible by monies from a nonrecurring grant, and they were offered on a one-time basis only.

From *The Gerontologist* 34(2):261–266, 1994. Reprinted with permission.

As there was no formal evaluation of the workshops' effectiveness in terms of residents' development, a major limitation of this report is that we cannot present data to support "success." However, our objective here is to offer the workshop model as something practitioners might want to consider using or adapting, in order to improve the quality of life of old women in the nursing home and elsewhere.

■ RATIONALE

The issues and concerns of old women as a group tend to have been neglected by clinicians and academics who are otherwise committed to improving women's status (MacDonald & Rich, 1983; Russell, 1987), and the rich knowledge, experiences, and needs of women in nursing homes have largely been ignored (Doress & Siegal, 1987; Smyer, 1989). Since the nursing home environment tends to be custodial rather than therapeutic, the routines and loss of personal space and possessions can exacerbate a feeling of loss of personal control and can promote psychological and physiological deterioration (Weisberg, 1983). This is also complicated by the fact that nursing homes are currently serving an older and more disabled population (Wells and Singer, 1985). Studies have shown that when nursing home residents experience autonomy and a sense of their personal power, self-esteem and motivation are enhanced, mental clarity and activity levels increase, and depression and mortality rates decrease (McDermott, 1989).

Much research has been done on the effects of life review or reminiscence on increasing cognitive and affective abilities, reducing depression, and improving self esteem (Butler, 1963; Cook, 1984; Merriam, 1989; Rattenbury and Stones, 1989; Romaniuk, 1983). Providing the context where women can review their life experiences, choices and lack of choices, their strengths and achievements can be crucial in overcoming the learned passivity and helplessness of the nursing home environment (Brody, 1990).

Studies have shown that many of the needs of institutionalized elders for emotional support, companionship, advice, and guidance can be met by informal social support networks that buffer the various stresses of aging and decrease the risk of illness and depression (Ell, 1984; Gallo, 1982; Pilisuk & Minkler, 1980). While there has been much research on the positive aspects of intergenerational contacts and friendships, kin generally, and even pets, on nursing home residents' life satisfactions (Hendy, 1987; Kocarnik and Ponzetti, 1991; Seefeldt, 1987), there is less being done on friendship patterns within the institution itself. Gutheil (1991) found that although nursing home friendships tended to lack in depth and intimacy, they provided companionship and support and played an important role in residents' emotional well-being. Similarly, studies by Bitzan and Kruzich (1990) and Retsinas and Garrity (1985) emphasized the importance of a close friend for resident participation in activities and satisfaction with life and the importance of social contacts for physical and mental well-being.

Finally, current literature emphasizes the critical role of nursing home staff development in the maintenance of a healthy institution (Burgio & Burgio, 1990; Hepler, 1987; Safford, 1989). Staff attitudes and ideological orientations to aging and the aged have been found to be especially important in predicting levels of care for the institutionalized elderly (Bagshaw & Adams, 1986; Chandler, Rachal, & Kazelskis, 1986; Cohen-Marshfield, Rabinovich, & Marx, 1991; Tellis-Nayak and Tellis-Nayak, 1989).

▬WORKSHOP ORGANIZATION

The project involved two workshops at each of five different sites throughout a 9-county region of South Central Minnesota. A nursing home located centrally in the county (or counties) acted as host, and residents and staff from surrounding homes traveled to this site. The first workshop for resident women met from 9 a.m. to noon on two consecutive mornings with no staff present, to allow as much freedom of expression as possible (see Table 25-1). Participants varied in age from early 60s to more than 100 years, with most women in their mid 80s. While workshop size ranged from 10 to almost 50 women, the ideal group size was about 15, which allowed for individual sharing but was not too small to distract from our networking goals. Racial and ethnic diversity was very low, reflecting the homogeneity of the nursing home population in this part of Minnesota, a region settled mostly by Scandinavians and Germans. Almost all participants were white women, and more than two-thirds had been living in rural communities. They had been in the nursing home anywhere from a few weeks to seven years, with the average residency about one year.

The staff of each nursing home (primarily activity directors) selected participants on the basis of residents' cognitive and emotional functioning and general levels of health. The higher the functioning of residents, the better able we were to move productively through the workshop, although each individual site involved a range of women with varying degrees of participation and function. The biggest drawback we encountered was hearing impairment, and we found the use of a microphone to be essential. Residents received printed invitations, and on arriving were given a colorful folder with information and handouts (large-print), a name tag, pad of paper, and pen. At the close of the workshop, participants received certificates of attendance. We felt that these details were important in establishing the credibility of the event and in recognizing the value of each woman's personal participation. Refreshments were available during breaks, and breakfast and lunch were also served. These meals provided the opportunity for networking and visiting as well as helping visiting residents feel more comfortable in new surroundings. Finally, we chose music with mature women's voices and empowering lyrics as background music during breaks and registration.

The local Area Agency on Aging was the immediate sponsor of this project, and the director of the Senior Leadership Development Project communicated with nursing home administrators and activity directors to plan and coordinate the workshop on important issues of space, transportation, food, and the availability of audiovisual equipment. A crucial step in

TABLE 25-1 Schedule for Resident and Staff Workshops

RESIDENT WORKSHOP

Morning 1

8:30–9:00	Breakfast and Registration
9:00–9:10	Introduction of project and workshop presenters
9:10–9:30	Residents introduce selves
9:30–10:00	Self-esteem (discussion and poetry)
	Aging and ageism
	Choices
10:00–10:15	Affirmations
10:15–10:30	Break
10:30–11:15	Film: "Ruth Stout's Garden" and discussion
11:15–11:45	Small groups (positive/negative aspects of nursing homes)
11:45–12:00	Poetry reading
	Closure
12:00–1:00	Lunch and Visiting

Morning 2

8:30–9:00	Breakfast and visiting
9:00–9:30	Affirmations
9:30–10:15	Life review—reminiscence
10:15–10:30	Break
10:30–11:00	Small groups: (vision "ideal" nursing home) (identify changes to work toward "ideal")
11:00–11:15	Large group discussion of visions and changes
11:15–11:30	Video: "One Fine Day" and poetry on women's strengths and diversity.
11:30–11:45	Large group—evaluation and sharing
11:45–12:00	Slide show on intergenerational friendships
	Closure
12:00–1:00	Lunch and visiting

STAFF WORKSHOP

1:00–1:15	Introduction of project and workshop presenters
1:15–1:30	Our working perspective
1:30–2:15	Aging and ageism
	Sexism and the double standard of aging
	Small groups: What kinds of an old woman/man do I want to be?
	What societal changes necessary to realize this?
	Large group sharing
2:15–2:30	Break
2:30–3:15	What we did and what we found/questions and discussion
3:15–3:55	Small groups: Identification of barriers to women residents' empowerment
	Staff role in overcoming barriers
	Identification of staff needs
	Large group sharing
3:55–4:20	Film: "Ruth Stout's Garden"
4:20–4:30	Closure

the planning was the communication with activity personnel and the gaining of their enthusiasm and cooperation, since they played the key role in the selection and motivation of participants. We found most nursing home personnel to be enthusiastic, and we appreciated the extra touches they created with flowers on the table, balloons, and other simple festive decorations. We brought a gift to each site in appreciation of their commitment to the project.

A 3-hour workshop was conducted for staff on the afternoon of the second day, following the completion of the residents' morning workshop (see Table 25-1). Staff attendance at the trainings ranged from 12 to 100 participants including nursing, administrative, and housekeeping staff. The smaller group worked best for open sharing and dialogue; as the group got larger, participation and open discussion were hampered, although the small groups worked relatively well to break through this. About 90% of staff participants were female, with a few male administrators and orderlies. Attendance was voluntary, although the option of earning continuing education credits provided motivation for many staff members. Again, negotiations with nursing home administrators were crucial in advertising and providing time for staff to attend. Arranging to have the staff session videotaped and made available to persons who were unable to attend was a way of making the workshop more accessible.

Finally, since the Area Agency on Aging and the local director of the Senior Leadership Development Project organized and set up the workshops, and we were hired as workshop presenters only, the issue of evaluation for short- and long-term effectiveness of the workshops for resident women was not included in the general format. Obviously this is a serious limitation now, because any discussion of "success" is highly subjective and rests on face validity only. Staff evaluations completed at the end of the workshop consisted of Likert scale items indicating levels of agreement to certain statements. They reported an overwhelming agreement to statements that the workshop was useful and that they hoped to consider utilizing the ideas in their own practice. In the "further comments" part, many responded with enthusiasm and found it "interesting" and "thought-provoking"; a few said it was too "idealistic" and "not relevant." For the most part, at least on a short-term basis, the staff workshops were successful.

▬WORKSHOP STRATEGIES
Self-Esteem Work
We began the residents' workshop with introductions of ourselves and participants in order to build the familiarity and trust necessary for any self-esteem or assertiveness-training work. The women were asked to share something special about themselves that they would like others to know, something which made them unique. The women needed considerable and constant encouragement from us and each other to be able to articulate their strengths and achievements. For example, many began their introductions with such statements as, ". . . oh, I don't know, I'm just ordinary, I

don't know about being special. . . ." Then others would jump in and say such as, "but you crochet and paint, you should see her paintings. . . ." Such interactions built trust, recognized women's strengths, and helped them feel at ease with each other. From this we then went on to talk about self-esteem and encouraged the women in a dialogue on aging, ageism, and the double standard of aging. Being able to name these processes can be useful in giving words to generalized emotions. We used affirmations and found them to be effective and useful as self-esteem builders since they were tangible and accessible statements, that, in changing our thoughts, can change our emotions. We had an "affirmation bag" which contained slips of paper with such messages as: "I am a beautiful person"; "I can disagree without being disagreeable"; and "I have choices that I can make and I have the right to make them." The women picked out an affirmation and read it aloud to the group. This was usually accompanied by cheers of encouragement and support by the other women.

We also used poetry with positive results. For example, we shared the poem "Warning" (Joseph, 1987, p. 1), which included a repetition of "when I am an old woman I shall wear purple" as a metaphor for autonomy, self-reliance, and self-control. We were delighted to see several women proudly wearing shades of purple on the second day of the workshops, visibly affected by the poem and talking with each other about how they searched their drawers for something of this color to wear. We also shared several poems from the *Women and Aging* anthology (Alexander, Berrow, Domitrovich, Donnelly, & McLean, 1986), which depicted positive and creative images of old women, emphasizing their strengths and power.

We also used some audiovisuals — one 23-minute film entitled "Ruth Stout's Garden" was especially well-received. It told the story of Ruth Stout, an independent, free-thinking woman in her 80s. Her garden and the way she plants and harvests were metaphors for the way she leads her life as a caring, autonomous, and self-reliant old woman. Another video, "One Fine Day" — a 6-minute, up-beat representation of women's contributions from a historical perspective — gave strong visual effects of the strengths of diverse women. Initially we were concerned that the use of poetry and audiovisuals that symbolize bold declarations of independence might highlight the lack of autonomy available to nursing home residents, and, in accentuating the restrictive nature of their situation, possibly lead to feelings of helplessness and despair. What we found tended to be the opposite; the residents talked about these autonomous women with admiration and respect and tended to see them as role models. Finally, we incorporated a slide show of cross-generational friendship, another aspect built into the goals of the workshop to help women remember an important source of support, each other, no matter what age.

Reminiscence

An important component of the workshop was our use of reminiscence, or life review strategies, to articulate and celebrate the uniqueness and strength of individual women. The specific reminiscence themes we chose involved leadership roles in community work, church, or family; memories of important strong women in their lives who are remembered with special fondness as role models, mentors, or guides; and recognizing, accepting, and celebrating diversity. We chose these themes in order to help participants articulate, value, and celebrate strengths, achievements, and skills which they or other women had and/or still have. Our hope was that they would not only see those skills as valuable, but might potentially be able to transfer them to their present living situation. We used guided imagery techniques to help the women ground themselves and feel relaxed enough to start remembering. An exciting component of reminiscence in this context was the way women responded to each other as they started to talk about their lives, facilitating networking and enhancing self-esteem. For example: "Oh, you lived there?" several would say in response to someone's life history, "Did you know such-and-such a person?" Others would remember the strengths of past role models: "I haven't thought about her in a long time, yes, she really changed my life, I'm who I am because of her," or "It's my mother I'm thinking of . . . now she was quite a woman, I'm like her in lots of ways." Again, an understatedness permeated the dialogue, but women were encouraged by us and each other to recognize their achievements and share memories of personal successes.

Changes in Daily Living

The workshops were set up to provide opportunities for resident women to identify their feelings about their living situations and suggest ideas (however small) for change. They were asked to discuss the positive and negative aspects of their living situation and envision the ideal nursing home, talking about what rules, if any, they would like to change. We told them that we would be sharing their suggestions (anonymously) with the staff in the afternoon staff training. The women worked in small groups with a designated notetaker and spokeswoman. We organized the groups so that there were opportunities for women from the same nursing homes to be together as well as mixing different women from different nursing homes. While for many the very idea of talking about "challenging" rules was a little improper, for others it provided an opportunity to articulate frustrations and feelings they already had. Either way, they chuckled in mock horror at the thought of being asked to challenge rules and envision ideal nursing homes, yet at the same time they started to think about the choices they might have in certain situations. For example, one woman was upset because she felt she was unable to attend the second day of the workshop because her bath was scheduled at this time, and the possibility of changing it seemed remote. She was encouraged by her peers to negotiate this scheduling change and was successful. Her demeanor the next day was remarkably different due to this personal success in the ordering of her everyday life.

Working with Staff

In our attempt to help make the nursing homes a more supportive and hospitable environment for the growth of resident women's self-reliance, and in the hopes of facilitating social change in the institution, we conducted 3-hour staff workshops at each site. As academics who were not in the nursing home on a daily basis, we were aware of being seen as out-of-touch "experts," and thus dismissed. With this in mind we spoke honestly of our respect for their work, and the complexities and difficulties they might experience, and asked them to identify problem areas related to work as well as the kinds of support they needed in order to be effective in these roles.

In terms of our goals for staff development, we focused on the social construction of age and aging in Western society. We explored the sources and consequences of ageism as a system that discriminates and affects people of all ages, and the different contexts such as class, race, and gender that affect these experiences. We asked the participants to imagine "what kind of an old woman/man they wanted to be," and then to consider the barriers to this vision as well as the changes that needed to happen in society in order for them to achieve the kind of experience they had described. This exercise attempted to get participants talking about how ageism is internalized, and how this might affect their relationships with the elderly people in their care. We hoped to foster an empathy and understanding toward residents, their "choices," and the need for change in society generally.

In small groups we asked staff to talk about their perceptions of the barriers to resident women's self-reliance, how they might play a role in overcoming these barriers, and what kind of support they as staff needed in the process. We discussed our experiences of the residents' workshops, insights and techniques, and residents' ideas for changes. Since several ideas were met with some resistance on the part of the staff, we attempted to highlight how institutional structures create parameters for interaction between staff and residents and institutionalize certain ways of doing things. For example, many residents said they would love to be able to choose their roommates so that they could spend time with people they enjoyed and with whom they had developed friendships. Obviously this posed an organizational nightmare as far as many of the staff were concerned, and their valid resistance to the idea stemmed from this realization. We were able to talk with them about how there are institutional structures that prevent such changes from occurring; these are independent of both the idea itself, which stemmed from a valid desire to improve the quality of residents' lives, and from any opinion on the part of the immediate nursing home staff. We talked about wider systemic changes in the organization of health and nursing home services that needed to occur to increase autonomy for all. Staff generally were aware of roadblocks inherent in the nursing home system. Many voiced frustrations which were not unlike the residents' own reactions. These often centered on the day-to-day routine that locked them into certain practices, took up inordinate amounts of time, and often prevented meaningful interaction with residents. Other frustrations (especially by lower-level staff and always in the larger nursing homes) included a general feeling of alienation, of being an anonymous worker within the system. Both resident and staff morale could be improved by a stronger sense of community built into the everyday practices of nursing home life. Pointing to these similarities gave the staff another bridge to those in their care.

■CONCLUSION

Minnesota has a two-decade history of active resident councils as well as family councils in the nursing home. This participation in both everyday running of the institution and in the creation of local policy provides a context whereby such educational and therapeutic workshops as the one described are more likely to be accepted and perhaps encouraged by nursing home personnel and residents. Where such consumer councils are in place, nursing home staff are more used to resident self-expression and participation, thus smoothing the way for a successful intervention of the kind we describe. In areas of the country where consumer councils are relatively unknown, such workshops might meet with much more resistance. In this case, it may be useful to provide some information and education as to the benefits of such resident participation, citing the successes of this model in other states, in the written proposal and/or oral presentation to administrators and other personnel in the negotiating stages. Networking with interested personnel may also need to occur at this initiation stage to "market" the idea.

As discussed above, a serious limitation of the project is the lack of evidence to assess the workshops' consequences for old women in the nursing home setting. On a subjective basis, we felt that the workshops were "successful" in that women told us informally how much they enjoyed them, their affect improved and became more alert, and they became more communicative, interactive, assertive, and interested, hoping to have more of such workshops. The long-term effects are also unknown. One anonymous reviewer made the astute comment that residents might experience "post-workshop depression" having been "teased with this enrichment." We suggest that this needs to be kept in mind, yet also would hate to see such fears prevent the development of programs aimed at resident empowerment, and thus bypass potential positive impact for old women in nursing homes. The general point we wish to make is that while we think these workshops have great merit and would like to see them replicated, we caution practitioners to think through these issues and attempt a longer-term project that has sufficient evaluations built in.

As educators and clinicians we can work with resident women and staff to help them articulate their needs, and recognize and celebrate their strengths and contributions. Providing opportunities, however small, for participation in the ordering of their everyday lives can increase women's psychological well-being and morale. We hope that other professionals and practitioners will attempt projects such as the one shared here, or adapt it for their specific needs, with the goal of increasing the self-esteem and self-reliance of resident women, reducing depression, and increasing the mental clarity and activity levels which so often deteriorate in the nursing home setting.

■REFERENCES

Alexander, J., Berrow, D., Domitrovich, L., Donnelly, M., & McLean, C. (1986). *Women and aging; an anthology by women.* Corvallis, OR: Calyx Books.

Bagshaw, M., & Adams, M. (1986). Nursing home nurses' attitudes, empathy, and ideologic orientation. *International Journal of Aging and Human Development, 22,* 235–246.

Bitzan, J. E., & Kruzich, J. M. (1990). Interpersonal relationships of nursing home residents. *The Gerontologist, 30,* 385–390.

Brody, C. M. (1990). Women in a nursing home. *Psychology of Women Quarterly, 14,* 579–592.

Burgio, L. D., & Burgio, K. L. (1990). Institutional staff training and management: a review of the literature and a model for geriatric, long-term care facilities. *International Journal of Aging and Human Development, 30,* 287–302.

Butler, R. (1963). The life-review: an interpretation of reminiscence in the aged. *Psychiatry, 26,* 65–76.

Chandler, J. T., Rachal, J. R., & Kazelskis, R. (1986). Attitudes of long-term care nursing personnel toward the elderly. *The Gerontologist, 26,* 551–555.

Cohen-Mansfield, J., Rabinovich, B. A., & Marx, M. C. (1991). Nurses' and social workers' perceptions of elderly nursing home residents' well-being. *Journal of Gerontological Social Work, 16* (3, 4), 135–147.

Cook, J. B. (1984). Reminiscing: How can it help confused nursing home residents? *Social Casework, 65,* 90–03.

Doress, P. B., & Siegal, D. L. (1987). *Ourselves growing older: Women aging with knowledge and power.* New York: Simon and Schuster.

Ell, K. (1984). Social networks, social support and health status: A review. *Social Service Review, 58,* 133–149.

Gallo, F. (1982). The effect of social support networks on the health of the elderly. *Social Work in Health Care, 8,* 65–74.

Gutheil, I. A. (1991). Intimacy in nursing home friendships. *Journal of Gerontological Social Work, 17* (1/2), 59–73.

Hendy, H. M. (1987). Effects of pet and/or people visits on nursing home residents. *International Journal of Aging and Human Development, 25,* 279–291.

Hepler, S. E. (1987). Assessing training needs for nursing home personnel. *Journal of Gerontological Social Work, 11,* (1/2), 71–79.

Joseph, J. (1987). Warning. In Martz, S. (Ed.), *When I am an old woman I shall wear purple* (p. 1). Manhattan Beach, CA: Papier-Mache Press.

Kocarnik, R. A., & Ponzetti, J. J. (1991). The advantages and challenges of intergenerational programs in long term facilities. *Journal of Gerontological Social Work, 16* (1/2), 97–107.

McDermott, C. J. (1989). Empowering the elderly nursing home resident: The resident rights campaign. *Social Work, 34,* 155–157.

MacDonald, B., & Rich, C. (1983). *Look me in the eye.* San Francisco: Spinsters/Aunt Lute.

Merriam, S. B. (1989). The structure of simple reminiscence. *The Gerontologist, 29,* 761–767.

One Fine Day (film). (1984). Produced by Martha Wheelock and Kay Weaver, distributed by Circe Records, 256 S. Robertson Blvd., Beverly Hills, CA 90211 and Ishtar Films, Rt. 311, Patterson, NY 12563.

Pilisuk, M., & Minkler, M. (1980). Supportive networks: Life ties for the elderly. *Journal of Social Issues, 3,* 95–116.

Rattenbury, C., & Stones, M. J. (1989). A controlled evaluation of reminiscences and current topics discussion groups in a nursing home context. *The Gerontologist, 29,* 68–71.

Retsinas, J., & Garrity, P. (1985). Nursing home friendships. *The Gerontologist, 25,* 376–381.

Romaniuk, M. R. (1983). The application of reminiscence to the clinical interview. *Clinical Gerontology, 1,* 39–43.

Russell, C. (1987). Aging as a feminist issue. *Women's Studies International Forum, 10,* 125–132.

Ruth Stout's Garden (film). (1976). Arthur Mokin Productions. Distributed by Arthur Mokin, Santa Rosa, CA.

Safford, F. (1989). "If you don't like the care, why don't you take your mother home?" Obstacles to family/staff partnerships in the institutional care of the aged. *Journal of Gerontological Social Work, 13* (3/4), 1–7.

Seefeldt, C. (1987). The effects of preschoolers' visits to a nursing home. *The Gerontologist, 27,* 228–232.

Smyer, M. A. (1989). Nursing homes as a setting for psychological practice: public policy perspectives. *American Psychologist, 44,* 1307–1314.

Tellis-Nayak, V., & Tellis-Nayak, M. (1989). Quality of care and the burden of two cultures: when the world of the nurses' aide enters the world of the nursing home. *The Gerontologist, 29,* 307–313.

Weisberg, J. (1983). Raising self-esteem of mentally impaired nursing home residents. *Social Work, 28,* 163–164.

Wells, L. M., & Singer, C. (1985). A model for linking networks in social work practice with the institutionalized elderly. *Social Work, 30,* 318–322.

Chapter 26

A Center on Ethics in Long-Term Care

ELLEN OLSON   EILEEN R. CHICHIN   LESLIE S. LIBOW

THERESA MARTICO-GREENFIELD   RICHARD R. NEUFELD

MICHAEL MULVIHILL

For over 10 years the Jewish Home and Hospital of Aged (JHHA) has employed an innovative mechanism to deal with ethical issues in long-term care. The Center on Ethics in Long-term Care developed by JHHA incorporates direct service, education, and research in ethics. They conduct "ethics rounds" that are open to residents, families, and staff — similar to clinical grand rounds. Ethics education occurs through the "Decisions" Program, where 600 interprofessional staff members have been educated. Day-to-day ethical issues are dealt with by an Ethics Consult Team. Finally, research in ethics is conducted in this teaching nursing home jointly with the Research Center at JHHA. These authors also present the problems and pitfalls with such a broad program and discuss how effective it can be with internal and external support for such a center.

The growing awareness of the multiplicity of ethical issues facing those who live and work in long-term care settings has encouraged nursing homes to develop mechanisms to address ethical dilemmas. Most long-term care institutions have followed their acute care colleagues and created ethics committees whose primary responsibilities are the provision of direct service and staff education. The Jewish Home and Hospital for Aged (JHHA) in New York City has taken a somewhat different route. In its pioneering Center on Ethics in Long-term Care, it provides direct service and case review via ethics rounds and an ethics consult team. In addition, ethics rounds and another ongoing educational program provide education in ethics. And finally, it actively involves its research department in ethical issues.

■ THE SITE

JHHA is the teaching nursing home affiliated with Mount Sinai Medical Center. Its numerous programs, on a given day, serve approximately 3,000 well and frail elderly. Among its programs are residential housing, three

---

From *The Gerontologist* 33(2):269–274, 1993. Reprinted with permission.

inpatient long-term care facilities, and a short-term inpatient rehabilitation unit. Also under JHHA auspices are a number of community-based services, including adult day care for the frail elderly and for Alzheimer's patients, a geriatric day center for the visually impaired, a long-term home health program, a geriatric outreach program, and the Alzheimer's Disease At-Home Emergency Respite Program.

Each of these groups and settings presents its own set of ethical dilemmas. Among them are issues of how people are placed, the allocation of scarce nursing home resources, and how to move people from one level of care to another while still protecting autonomy. Primary concerns of administration and staff center on the difficulties associated with obtaining informed consent, and how confidentiality and privacy can be preserved once people are in an institutional setting. Dilemmas around end-of-life treatment issues surface regularly. In our experience, the three-pronged approach using direct practice, research, and education encourages the optimal resolution of dilemmas associated with all of these issues.

▄ HISTORY

The Center was created in 1987 as an outgrowth of both the monthly ethics rounds that had been in place for some time at JHHA and several research projects that were being conducted at the Home. The medical leadership at JHHA saw the need to expand the facility's ethics education and case review beyond the monthly rounds and to formalize a research agenda. A unified Center on Ethics that would guide these efforts was formalized in 1990. Physically located at the Home's main campus, the Center was developed to address the ethical issues and concerns that exist throughout the varied settings and programs at JHHA. The specifics of how each of its three components — education, case review, and research — evolved with the Center are described below.

▄ ETHICS ROUNDS: A MECHANISM FOR DIRECT SERVICE AND EDUCATION

The Center on Ethics addresses a substantial number of its direct service and educational concerns via monthly ethics rounds. (See Libow et al., 1992, for a fuller description of ethics rounds.) This format was initiated at JHHA in 1985 to address the need and desire by staff for a forum in which to discuss ethical dilemmas affecting end-of-life decision making. These issues included tube feedings, the impact of religious beliefs on how medical decisions are made, surrogate decision making, restraints, and attempts to determine who should speak for a demented patient. Similar to clinical grand rounds, the usual format of ethics rounds includes a case presentation, with comments and a formal presentation by a guest speaker. Participants, numbering between 50 and 75, include professionals from medicine, nursing, social service, administration, dietary, and physical and occupational therapy. Paraprofessional staff members also attend, and nursing home residents and their families are invited.

The greatest advantage of this format is its ability to expose a wide variety of staff members to end-of-life ethical issues and the mechanisms to guide their resolution. Decisions are not made in ethics rounds; these are left to the team responsible for the care of the resident in question, in concert with the family, the resident (if able to participate), and legal assistance if needed. However, rounds provide guidance and structure to assist the caregiving team in coming to some conclusions regarding care and treatment and encourage dialogue across disciplines. All staff are encouraged to voice their feelings and concerns regarding the case and its resolution and, despite the presence of their coworkers and superiors, speak relatively freely about these issues.

Of particular note is the inclusion of both nursing aides and orderlies, whose participation is encouraged, and of residents and families. Paraprofessionals know a great deal about the residents to whom they render care and are markedly affected by decisions about the medical treatment of these residents. Their involvement in rounds enhances the quality of care delivered to residents. Additionally, it is a statement of the facility's recognition of the inherent value of those workers who provide the bulk of hands-on care to nursing home residents.

Inviting residents and their families to ethics rounds serves three purposes. First, because residents are the focus of the discussion, their insights are particularly useful. Second, observing the interdisciplinary interaction of the professionals and paraprofessionals responsible for their care illustrates to residents and their families the Home's concern for their autonomy and well-being. And attendance at ethics rounds affords family members and residents an important educational opportunity. In our experience to date, residents and families have been active participants in the meetings they have attended.

ETHICS EDUCATION: THE "DECISIONS" PROGRAM

Although ethics rounds are open to residents, their families, and a wide variety of staff, scheduling difficulties prevented a number of staff members from attending. Of concern was the fact that these individuals were line staff who, in many cases, were directly involved in ethical dilemmas. An awareness of the needs of these staff members served as an impetus for the Jewish Home and Hospital to supplement its rounds with another opportunity for staff education.

The first major effort of the Center was to implement a facility-wide educational program in the area of ethics. This was undertaken collaboratively with The Hastings Center, which is known for its research, education, consultation, and publications in the field of bioethics, and the Education Development Center (EDC), an international nonprofit research and development organization that applies educational strategies to address a wide range of health, education, and social problems. JHHA was among eight institutions selected to collaborate with these two groups in the design and development of a three-part educational program titled "Decisions Near the End of Life." The curriculum for this program was developed by The

Hastings Center and EDC with support from the W. K. Kellogg Foundation to educate professional staff in acute and long-term care settings. In the Jewish Home, approximately 600 professional staff members from medicine, nursing, rehabilitation, social work, pharmacy, recreation, and administration participated in the program, and one of the Center's codirectors served as site coordinator for this program.

The "Decisions" program included a training session for those staff members who served as faculty, a before-and-after questionnaire assessing knowledge and attitudes about ethics and identifying areas of concern, and a three-tiered on-site program that began in the fall of 1989 and is ongoing. The first two tiers of the program consisted of a total of six modules that incorporated an overview of the program, discussed the legal implications of ethical dilemmas, and addressed at length the specific issues of planning with patients, learning to weigh burdens and benefits, dealing with the decisionally impaired, and problem solving in particularly difficult cases. The techniques used to address these issues included both grand rounds and small-group discussions. Videotapes were a part of the program, as was a lecture and question-and-answer session with an attorney with expertise in medical care issues at the end of life.

Tier Three of the "Decisions" program is an ongoing process that utilizes working groups to analyze problems and revise policies. In addition, it stimulates ideals for research and provides a basis to plan educational programs for those not reached by the educational efforts already undertaken. JHHA is awaiting the results of a follow-up survey that will measure changes in knowledge and attitudes as a result of the program and identify continued areas of concern.

Additional educational efforts are presently being directed toward the paraprofessional staff. What is different for ancillary staff, perhaps, is their perceived role when ethical dilemmas arise, and an underlying sense of powerlessness stemming from their position vis-a-vis the position of professional staff. Unfortunately, nursing aide education in general does not address the needs of these workers with regard to ethical issues. In an attempt to remedy this, an educational program was developed primarily for nursing aides and orderlies, and the Center coordinator and a codirector have worked closely with nursing administration to design and implement this program.

Prior to initiating this program, focus groups were held with small numbers of nursing assistants, a representative from nursing administration, and the coordinator of the Center on Ethics to discuss some of their ethical concerns and what they would like to see in an educational program. A before-and-after questionnaire was also developed to assess nursing assistants' knowledge and attitudes about ethical issues in long-term care. The formal educational program incorporates a variety of techniques, including lectures, videos, reading material, and small-group discussions to provide nursing assistants opportunities to understand ethical issues and the application of ethical principles in their work.

Although still in its early stages, this program has been met with enthusiasm by the first groups of paraprofessional workers who have participated.

In addition, it has resulted in increased awareness within the facility of the needs of these workers, who are as likely as their professional counterparts to experience ethical dilemmas.

■ THE ROLE OF THE ETHICS CONSULT TEAM

Ethics rounds provide a useful forum for education and to assist in the resolution of ethical issues that are not acute in nature. However, the formally scheduled once-a-month structure precludes the ability to deal with the ethical dilemmas that arise on a day-to-day basis. Thus, a mechanism is needed to address more cases and to do so in a timely fashion. As an outgrowth of ethics rounds, an ethics consult team was developed.

The staff members who volunteered to participate on the consult team were the same individuals involved in the planning and implementation of the "Decisions" program, and include representation from administration, medicine, nursing, and social work. The entire consult team consists of eight to nine individuals who meet regularly to review cases. However, only two or three members of the team work on a rotating basis as needed with the resident's health care team to resolve the particular problem through the application of ethical principles, within the confines of the law and sound medical practice. For example, if the family of a resident without decision-making capacity requests that life-sustaining treatment be withheld or withdrawn, a key issue is respect for the resident's autonomy. Accordingly, the consult team and the primary care team together determine whether the resident is unable to make a decision and whether the resident had stipulated at some earlier time that he or she would not want a particular treatment used to prolong life in the situation in question. (In order for a treatment to be withheld or withdrawn from a decisionally impaired person in New York State, there must be "clear and convincing evidence" of that person's wishes in the form of written or oral statements.)

Key to the resolution of such an ethical dilemma is the gathering of all information relevant to the situation. Here, flexibility and portability of the ethics consult team approach works to great advantage. The consult team is able to come together promptly when a problem is brought to its attention. Since most ethical dilemmas involve a resident, the consult team members assigned to the case begin by collecting information from him or her. Assigning only two or three team members to each case facilitates a bedside evaluation. Typically, the first undertaking of the consult team members is an evaluation of the resident's overall status (including physical and mental condition), any documentation of the resident's wishes, and the availability of family or friends who can and should assist in the decision-making process. The family and/or friends are then contacted, as well as any others connected with a particular case. The consult team members then share all information with the resident's primary care team and make themselves available to initiate and guide a discussion in an attempt to resolve the dilemma.

Thus, the consult team approach supports the resident, the family, and the primary care staff in the process of resolving ethical dilemmas. Particular attention is paid to nursing aides and orderlies who also play a vital role in the resolution of the ethical issues referred to the consult team. They often hear things or know things that other staff may not, such as the resident's attitude toward certain life-prolonging treatments when there is no hope of recovery. They experience firsthand the consequences of whatever decision has been made. This is especially difficult when a treatment is being withheld or withdrawn. For example, when a decision is made to withdraw a feeding tube or discontinue some other life-prolonging treatment, nursing aides and orderlies provide the bulk of comfort care to the patient during the dying process. At the same time, they must deal with whatever personal conflicts they may have about the decision not to treat. Accordingly, their involvement in and understanding of treatment decisions enables them, at least to some extent, to accept these decisions and to continue to provide good care.

■ THE ROLE OF RESEARCH IN ETHICS

A teaching nursing home may be an optimal site to conduct research. Research efforts can be ongoing, with very little interruption in the day-to-day functioning of the facility. The research staff works cooperatively with other staff members in the Home, not only to their mutual advantage, but also to the benefit of residents and their families.

JHHA has conducted research in the area of ethical issues for a number of years prior to the establishment of an Ethics Center. This research has focused on the use of feeding tubes, living wills, the preference of nursing home residents for life-sustaining treatment, and the concordance between nursing home residents and their surrogates regarding end-of-life treatment decisions. Since 1990, the Research Center at JHHA has worked collaboratively with the Ethics Center to develop a research agenda. Projects include attitudes toward life-sustaining treatment and health care decision making for the decisionally impaired. Evaluations of current and future educational and direct service programs will also be undertaken. Among these are plans to study the work of our ethics consult team. Specifically, we hope to identify the ethical issues in each case, determine exactly what the conflicts are, what values are involved, what are the perceived options, who are the principal decision makers, and how the decision is finally realized. Decisions will be studied over time to see whether values of those served by JHHA change and how individual decisions affect the parties involved on an ongoing basis. In doing this, we hope not only to develop a systematic way to address problems but also a mechanism for identifying future areas of research.

Other areas for potential research include the differentiation of ethical and legal rights in medical decision making, especially in regard to families. More research is needed about the use of advance directives among the elderly, especially in light of the federal Patient Self-Determination Act with its emphasis on patient autonomy and advance planning. Quality of life issues demand research attention, as does the concept of institutionalization: what makes an institution excel? What kinds of ethical values do the best institutions support? Finally, a comparison of ethics consult teams and ethics committees should be undertaken to determine the relative effectiveness of each.

■ DEVELOPING A CENTER ON ETHICS: PROBLEMS AND PITFALLS

While ethical issues are and will continue to be an integral part of everyday life in long-term care facilities, mechanisms developed to address them will not always function smoothly. The overarching issues affecting the successful development and implementation of an ethics program are financial, logistical, and philosophical in nature.

With regard to financial issues, there are clearly numerous costs imbedded in many aspects of a Center on Ethics. And, with issues of cost-containment paramount in all aspects of our health care system, a program of this kind may appear nonessential. However, with the growing incidence of ethical dilemmas in long-term care, as well as changing legislation and regulation, all facilities will need to develop mechanisms to address them. In the future some variation of this program may become the norm in many long-term care settings.

Logistically, problems arise when busy individuals in clinical settings have yet another task assigned to them. With one exception, all members of the ethics consult team have responsibilities in other departments. Asking members of an interdisciplinary staff to invest their time and energy in an ethics consult team takes them away from numerous primary responsibilities. Understanding the need to make ethical decisions, in addition to recognizing the importance of the work of the consult team, may encourage reluctant staff members to participate. The consult team members must see their ethics role as important to the functioning and well-being of the facility, just like their other professional responsibilities.

Additional logistical problems occur when one attempts to undertake formal educational programs in an applied setting. Attending seminars and lectures — even those as brief as an hour — takes time away from the bedside. Obviously, not every staff member is able to attend every program, and skill is required to insure that most staff members are able to attend at least on occasion. (This issue also argues for the utilization of a variety of educational efforts, and, as noted earlier, resulted in the use of both ethics rounds and the "Decisions" program to provide ethics education.) A technique that has proven particularly useful is incorporating ethics programs into preexisting educational forums. For example, ethics education has become part of the regular inservice program for nursing assistants.

Philosophically, interdisciplinary teams have traditionally had to cope with the somewhat overlapping but occasionally disparate value systems of their members. The different values of individual staff members involved in long-term care and the residents they serve may present even more problems. The emphasis needs to be on the people who are having the problem, and working with them to determine the appropriate solution. For example, in a case in which several members of a resident's team were distressed by the dying process resulting from termination of treatment, an expert on death and dying provided a great source of comfort and closure to staff. Clergy and social workers with training in group process and interaction are often helpful in resolving these value differences.

Finally, two issues for replication of this model must be addressed. First is the recognition by the institution and its key staff members that sound ethical practice is integral to the work of the institution. Accordingly, any efforts to integrate ethics into education, research, and enhanced direct service benefit the institution as a whole and the individuals who live or work in it. Once the value of an ethics program is accepted, then logistics seem to fall into place.

Second, much of this is uncharted territory. We are in the early stages of evaluating the outcomes of several activities (e.g., staff perception of the work of the ethics consult team; family satisfaction with our decision-making process; and assessment of changes in staff members' knowledge and attitudes about ethical issues). Regular evaluation of the direction and quality of ethics rounds is in process, and the work of the ethics consult team is being monitored by the JHHA Quality Assurance Committee. Clearly, this is an ongoing process in which "learning by doing" is key.

■ A CENTER ON ETHICS: IS IT FOR EVERYONE?

Questions arise about the extent to which a Center on Ethics can be used by other institutions. Clearly, the overall structure mandates the availability of substantial financial backing and capabilities in a variety of areas. Of no less importance is an institutional commitment to the necessity of such a program. At JHHA, there was a strong commitment to ethics education and the development of mechanisms for case review and consultation. Accordingly, ethics rounds were in place, as well as a developing ethics consult team, prior to receiving any formal funding. However, the development of the Center on Ethics, which necessitated hiring personnel to conduct research and to facilitate the coordination of increasing demands for case review and new education programs for a large staff and community-based population, would not have been possible without additional financial support and administrative recognition of the need for such a program.

Can a Center on Ethics be developed in smaller facilities with markedly fewer human and financial resources? And is such a center always necessary? A negative response to this second question does not negate the fact that certainly much of what is undertaken in larger facilities with sophisticated resources is transferable with success to smaller institutions, even if a formal center is not created. For example, ethics rounds provide a useful format for both education and direct service. Extending an invitation to a guest speaker to address the staff, residents, and families on an ethical issue and comment upon an appropriate case is possible in most facilities, if only periodically. Local clergy and college and university faculty with expertise in this area are particularly well suited to speak at ethics rounds. This approach permits residents and their families to observe the facility's respect and concern for those it serves. Further, ethics rounds provide guidance to staff members in the resolution of ethical dilemmas.

Additional educational tools are widely available. Videos dealing with ethical issues can easily be shown to staff members in small groups within a facility. Conferences on ethics occur regularly, where a few staff members can be educated and then share material. In addition, national, regional, and local conferences for most professional groups frequently focus on ethical issues.

We found the use of an ethics consult team to be an especially effective mechanism in a long-term care setting. Its flexibility and portability allows a smaller number of individuals to go to the bedside, collect information, and work with a resident's health care team to resolve an ethical dilemma. A large group of consultants is not necessary for the daily functioning of the team; any number of people with varied expertise may be called upon when needed. Building on the collective wisdom within a facility, in concert with what is available in the community, will effectively address most ethical dilemmas. Further, the primary mechanism for the resolution of ethical conflicts is already in place in most long-term care settings in the form of the interdisciplinary team responsible for resident care. This team can often resolve ethical dilemmas on its own; in those cases in which it cannot, the ethics consult team can come to its assistance.

The ethics consult team is a useful mechanism not only for educating staff in small groups, but also for identifying problems that can be addressed in a larger educational forum. As previously mentioned, members of the consult team at JHHA were also instrumental in the implementation of the "Decisions" program; in other facilities, they could be utilized for a variety of educational efforts.

The desire and ability to do research in long-term care settings is often precluded by time, money, interest, and the necessary personnel. Accordingly, many facilities may not see conducting research as appropriate or necessary. However, the importance of research on ethical issues should not be underestimated.

Bioethical research focusing on later life is a relatively new phenomenon. Nonetheless, a number of studies have focused on end-of-life issues. Examined have been health care decision making in the event of decisional incapacity (Diamond et al., 1989; Molloy et al., 1991; Ouslander, Tymchuck, & Rahbar, 1989; Uhlmann, Pearlman, & Cain, 1988; Zweibel & Cassel, 1989); preferences for surrogate decision makers (High, 1988); views on life prolongation (Kohn & Menon, 1988); the use of advance directives in nursing homes (Danis et al., 1991) and the preferences for (Michelson et al., 1991) and participation in (Wetle et al., 1988) medical treatment. In addition to these empirical studies, the ethical issues inherent in everyday life in nursing homes have been addressed in "case and commentary" format by Kane and Caplan (1990) in their comprehensive discussion of the "everyday ethics" in nursing home life.

Although every long-term care facility need not conduct research, those who work in them should be familiar with research findings. It may be useful to designate a committee if possible (or an individual, if not) to familiarize the staff of a facility with current literature in ethics and long-term care to enhance practice.

A number of factors will help to ensure the success of this kind of program. Among these are a strong administrative commitment to it, and one or more individuals who keep the program on track. Over time at JHHA, numerous individuals from several departments contributed to the conceptualization of the Center. When it became a reality, the two physicians who were responsible for its development sought the assistance of an individual with an interest in ethics and a clinical background in either nursing or social work to coordinate the Center's day-to-day activities. At the present time, the Center's staff consists of two physician codirectors (both of whom have other institutional responsibilities outside the Center) and a full-time coordinator who is a registered nurse with a doctorate in gerontological social work. A part-time secretary assists on an as-needed basis. Clearly, it may be possible for one person both to be the visionary of the program and to assume responsibility for its ongoing work. However, due to the large size of the facility and our desire to address a variety of issues and tasks and to focus on education, research, and direct service, we have found a collaborative, interdisciplinary effort among individuals with different but complementary skills and knowledge to be the most effective model.

In summary, there are three intertwined areas with regard to ethical issues in long-term care: practice, education, and research. Addressing one or more of these areas can usually result in improvements in all of them and can enhance a facility's ability to meet the needs of residents, families, and staff. For example, we have noted an increased institution-wide awareness of the primacy of patient autonomy in health care decision-making and a "consciousness-raising" regarding the everyday issues related to resident self-determination — what Caplan (1990) has referred to as "the morality of the mundane."

Equally important, we have seen an intensified recognition and understanding of interdisciplinary value perspectives. There is evidence of an augmented sensitivity on the part of the Home's professional and administrative leadership to the needs of nursing home staff and a recognition of the vital role they play in the lives of residents. At present, this is anecdotal and reflected in individual team discussions. Efforts are underway to study the changing awareness and the factors contributing to this in a more formal manner.

In conclusion, in long-term care settings with the capability to institute a center on ethics, such a center can serve many purposes for its residents, families, staff, the community, and the field of aging. Institutions with neither the desire nor necessary resources to develop such a program can utilize many components of it and adapt them to their own settings.

▬ REFERENCES

Caplan, A. L. (1990). The morality of the mundane: Ethical issues arising in the daily lives of nursing home residents. In R. A. Kane & A. L. Caplan (Eds.). *Everyday ethics: Resolving dilemmas in nursing home life* (pp. 37–50). New York: Springer.

Danis, M., Southerland, L. I., Garrett, J. M., Smith, J. L., Hielema, F., Pickard, C. G., Egner, D. M., & Patrick, D. L. (1991). A prospective study of advance directives for life-sustaining care. *New England Journal of Medicine, 324*(13), 882–888.

Diamond, E. L., Jernigan, J. A., Mosely, R. A., Messina, V., & McKeown, R. A. (1989). Decision-making ability and advance directive preference in nursing home patients and proxies. *The Gerontologist, 29,* 622–626.

High, D. (1988). All in the family: Extended autonomy and expectations in surrogate health care decision-making. *The Gerontologist, 28(Suppl.),* 46–51.

Kane, R. A., & Caplan, A. L. (Eds.). (1990). *Everyday ethics: Resolving dilemmas in nursing home life.* New York: Springer.

Kohn, M., & Menon, G. (1988). Life prolongation: Views of elderly outpatients and health care professionals. *Journal of the American Geriatrics Society, 36,* 840–844.

Libow, L. S., Olson, E., Neufeld, R. R., Martico-Greenfield, T., Meyers, H., Gordon, N., & Barnett, P. (1992). Ethics rounds at the nursing home: An alternative to ethics committees. *Journal of the American Geriatrics Society, 40,* 92–97.

Michelson, C., Mulvihill, M., Hsu, M., & Olson, E. (1991). Eliciting medical care preferences from nursing home patients. *The Gerontologist, 31,* 358–363.

Molloy, D. W., Clarnette, R. N., Braun, E. A., Eisemann, M. R., & Schneiderman, B. (1991). The "Daughter from California Syndrome." *Journal of the American Geriatrics Society, 39,* 396–399.

Ouslander, J. G., Tymchuck, A. J., & Rahbar, B. (1989). Health care decision-making among elderly long-term care residents and their potential proxies. *Archives of Internal Medicine, 149,* 1367–1372.

Uhlmann, R. F., Pearlman, R. A., & Cain, K. C. (1988). Physicians' and spouses' predictions of elderly patients' resuscitation preferences. *Journal of Gerontology, 43*(5), M115–M121.

Wetle, T., Levkoff, S., Cwikel, J., & Rosen, A. (1988). Nursing home resident participation in medical decisions: Perceptions and preferences. *The Gerontologist, 28(Suppl.),* 32–38.

Zweibel, N. R., & Cassel, C. K. (1989). Treatment choices at the end of life: A comparison of decisions by older patients and their physician-selected proxies. *The Gerontologist, 29,* 615–621.

SELECTED BIBLIOGRAPHY

Abbey, C., Didion, J., Durbin, M. B., Perzynski, K., & Zechman, R. (November 1994). Neighborhood wellness centers: Collaboration between home care and nursing education. *CARING Magazine* 26–31.

Carty, A. E. S. & Day, S. S. (1993). Interdisciplinary care: Effect in acute hospital setting. *Journal of Gerontological Nursing* 19(3): 22–32.

Hunter, K. A., Florio, E. R., & Langberg, R. G. (1996). Pharmaceutical care for home-dwelling elderly persons: A determination of need and program description. *The Gerontologist* 36(4): 543–548.

Hyde-Robertson, B., Pirnie, S. M., & Freeze, C. (November, 1994). A strategy against elderly mistreatment. *CARING Magazine* 40–44.

Mahmud, K. & LeSage, K. (May 1995). Telemedicine: A new idea for home care. *CARING Magazine* 48–50.

Pallett-Hehn, P. & Lucas, M. (1994). LIFE: Learning informally from elders. *The Gerontologist* 34(2): 267–270.

Penning, M. & Wasyliw, D. (1992). Homebound learning opportunities: Reaching out to older shut-ins and their caregivers. *The Gerontologist* 32(5): 704–707.

Petit, J. M. (1994). Continuing care retirement communities and the role of the wellness nurse. *Geriatric Nursing* 15(1): 38–31.

Post, J. A. (1996). Internet resources on aging: Data sets and statistics. *The Gerontologist* 36(4): 425–429.

Schank, M. J., Weis, D., & Matheus, R. (1996). Parish nursing: Ministry of Healing. *Geriatric Nursing* 17(1): 11–13.

Wolf, R. S. & Pillemer, K. (1994). What's new in elder abuse programming? Four bright ideas. *The Gerontologist* 34(1): 126–129.

Unit 5

If I Live to Be 102, Will I Be Able to Tie My Shoes? Theory Development and Research With Older Adults

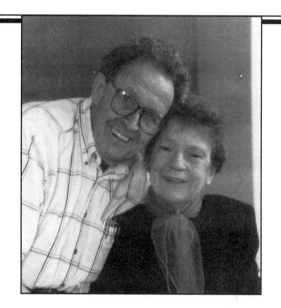

I n nursing it is important to be able to describe, explain, and predict phenomena. In many ways, the wisdom of old age is based on lived experiences that, if fully understood, help us to more accurately forecast later human reactions to similar situations. This reflects the importance of theories or conceptual frameworks. They can better assist us in explaining and anticipating our clients' responses to a wide variety of experiences, such as grief, caregiving, or the ravages of Alzheimer's dementia. They can also help us better understand our clients' need to relive the past and put their lives into greater perspective, for example.

Theory and research go hand in hand, both feeding and being fed by the other. Research substantiates theory, and theory guides research. To obtain a clearer picture of our older clients' needs or concerns, it is vital to have a wide base of empirical research on which to base our assessments and subsequent interventions. Further, it is important to be actively engaged in solid, pertinent research to further enhance knowledge in the field of gerontological nursing. Funding for research with older adults is provided by many government and private entities. Major governmental funders include the National Institute on Aging, the Health Care Financing Administration, the Agency for Health Care Policy and Research, the National Center for Health Statistics, the Centers for Disease Control and Prevention, and the Administration on Aging. The Robert Wood Johnson Foundation, the American Association of Retired Persons (AARP), and the Retirement Research Foundation are commonly cited private funding sources.

Research with older adults runs the gamut from large-scale public health studies, focusing on epidemiological methodologies, to smaller, qualitative approaches that involve face-to-face interviews with only a handful of subjects. Elegant multivariate statistical studies, emphasizing solely quantitative research techniques, as well as single case studies of elders' experiences, are helpful in discovering the "true picture."

In this unit, the chapters are organized to move from application of theories or models in predicting client needs and designing meaningful interventions to recommendations on the use of qualitative research methodologies in gerontological nursing and suggestions for overcoming validity threats when interviewing institutionalized elders. The unit concludes with examples of various research methodologies (i.e., grounded theory, ethnography, evaluation research) utilized in current research with older adults. Research studies are also included throughout other units of this book. In Unit III, for example, grounded theory methods were utilized in the chapter on Chinese American elders, and two other chapters in that unit describe studies using quantitative methods.

By using the tools of theory and research in their practice, nurses can become better practitioners and design more appropriately targeted interventions for their clients.

Chapter 27

Integrality as a Holistic Framework for the Life-Review Process

GLORIA BLACK   BARBARA KAVANAGH HAIGHT

> Older adults are often accused of "living in the past" and "reminiscing about the good old days." As nurses who work with this age group know, life review is a necessary developmental task — an important step in making sense of one's life and gaining a truer perspective of one's accomplishments and conflicts. However, can this process also be a therapeutic intervention? These authors advise gerontological nurses to work within Martha Rogers' framework of repatterning in order to reintegrate older adults' past conflicts or "disorganization" into a greater sense of meaning or "organization." This chapter also includes a set of structured life review questions.

Life-span developmental psychologists assign tasks or stepping stones to each stage of life.[1] Perhaps the most well known of these psychologists is Erikson.[2] He links societal values to each task as he describes the infant's need to establish trust in others and the adolescent's search for a stable identity. He further states that as people travel on through life, they must learn to form intimate relationships and become productive and creative. Finally, the task of late life is to develop a sense of integrity while transcending life's experiences.

More recent and popular psychologists, such as Gail Sheehy, use this same approach to discuss life's passages.[3] Sheehy makes her approach more applicable to modern-day women, but like those of other developmental psychologists, Sheehy's last task is a form of integrity. Sheehy describes a need to find a personal feeling of achievement and success, a need to find a meaning for the way the life occurred.[4] She and others state that when one examines the past, there is a gestalt, and finally the life becomes whole. This examination may be called soul searching or looking for life's meaning, and as such is facilitated through memory and recalling the past. Perhaps this soul searching is best described as a life review.

From *Holistic Nursing Practice* 7(1):7–15, 1992. Reprinted with permission.

■LIFE REVIEW

Life review is one of the developmental tasks of the last stage of life. Older people urgently need to share their life stories, and the past-scanning function of a life review allows them to reclaim their past while sharing their memories. Memory allows them to hold fast to their identity while shaping and interpreting it in new ways. Through memory, connections are made, and people discover patterns and meaning in the past that they had not truly recognized at an earlier stage. As in a tapestry, the underside is a mass of tangled threads without patterns or picture. But when the tapestry is turned over, a picture emerges. Each color, each thread, has a purpose and meaning, and together they are necessary to weave the tapestry of a life, to create the colorful, orderly patterns and pictures on the front of the tapestry. So the life review is like the weaver; it is the instrument that helps to form the pattern, to find the meaning, and to arrive at a complete sense of oneself.

Butler was the first to describe life review as a spontaneous and universal occurrence in older people in which life events were surveyed and reintegrated.[5] Butler noted the common phenomenon among older persons of repeatedly bringing up past events in reminiscence or life review.[6] He considered life review a necessary part of successful aging and said that life review is a means of deriving meaning from past experiences and resolving old conflicts.

Butler's notion of life review puts events in their proper place. With life's events evaluated and accepted, one could then be at peace. Butler proposed that this process accounted for the increased reminiscence in the aged. He defined the life review as a naturally occurring universal mental process characterized by the progressive return to consciousness of past experiences. He particularly thought it was necessary for unresolved conflicts to be surveyed and reintegrated during the life-review process.

Though Butler experienced the power of the life review, he did not attempt to explain and put the phenomenon into operation for others to use. As a result, researchers and clinicians talked about the processes of life review and reminiscing interchangeably. Thus, the adaptive role of life review became clouded, and the process as a therapeutic intervention became unclear. Eighty-five published articles in the last 20 years, testing and talking about reminiscing, have further clouded the concept, leaving the practitioner with little direction for using life review as an intervention.[7]

■LIFE REVIEW AS INTERVENTION

Though scholars use the terms life *review* and *reminiscing* interchangeably, they are two separate modalities and should be discussed individually. Life review is only one type of reminiscing. Under that same umbrella one can find oral history, autobiography, and storytelling, to name a few. Certainly reminiscing is a part of the life-review process, but a true life review is more complicated than simple reminiscing.[8] To use life review as an intervention, researchers must first clarify the concept of life review and differentiate it from reminiscing. With the differentiation in mind, practitioners must establish a goal for life review, which is to reach integrity. To reach integrity, the practitioner must then provide structure to the recall of memories.

Coleman was one of the first researchers to find a difference between life-review reminiscing and simple reminiscing.[9] He reported that those people who received therapeutic benefits from the process were those who had participated in an evaluative and insightful process of reminiscing. The process he described was similar to the process experienced in therapeutic groups by Butler.

Wong and Watt differentiated different types of reminiscing and selected those that contributed the most to successful aging.[10] They found that successful agers used more instrumental and integrative types of reminiscing. Instrumental reminiscing talked about past plans and the attainment of goals, whereas integrative reminiscing involved achieving a sense of self-worth, coherence, and reconciliation with regard to one's past. Wong and Watt[10] stated that integrative reminiscence was very similar to Butler's life review.

Thus, a true life review must be a thoughtful process aimed toward achieving the goal of integrity. Life review is not a random sharing of pleasurable past events, but rather a structured process containing a component of self-evaluation. Haight used a structured process of life review as a nursing intervention, first to raise life satisfaction and then to prevent depression.[11,12] Instead of reminiscence occurring naturally, Haight instigated the process using a Life Review and Experiencing Form (LREF) (see Appendix 27-A). She described life review as a facilitator of integrity and suggested it as a potentially useful and powerful nursing intervention for improving the psychological well-being of older people.

In a further study, Haight[13] examined different reminiscing interventions to determine the ones that were most therapeutic. Specifically, she tested the concepts of evaluation, structure, and individuality to evaluate their contribution to therapy. The findings pointed to evaluation as the most important component of therapeutic life review, followed by individuality and structure. Hence, a therapeutic life review should cover the entire life span, analyze, evaluate, and synthesize life's events, and be conducted individually with one other therapeutic person acting as a guide and a sounding board. Combining these components into the reminiscing intervention will facilitate reaching the goal of integrity, the measure of success.[13]

Practitioners and researchers continue to be interested in the use of life review as an intervention. Groups such as the American Association of Retired Persons (AARP) sponsor reminiscing programs on a national level and encourage volunteers to reminisce with older people who are homebound.[14] At a recent National Institute of Mental Health (NIMH) presentation, reminiscing was listed as a potential intervention for treating depression.[15] Practitioners are adopting the good in the process without really knowing how it works and without the strong support of a theoretical framework.

Both researchers and clinicians need to know why a life review is sometimes effective and sometimes not. Only recently have researchers begun to describe what actually happens in the reminiscing process.[9,13,16] If used as an intervention, it is essential for gerontological nurses to understand life review and its use in practice, and to examine the effects of life review in aging people. Perhaps the notion of life review as a facilitator of integrity is more acceptable if framed within a nursing model that provides a framework for the future growth of the older person while valuing the whole person. One such model is Martha Rogers' model that examines human development over time.[17] Rogers' principle of integrality may well provide a holistic framework for conducting the life review process.

Rogers' Model

The notion of life review as an intervention to enhance the developmental task of conflict integration fits within Martha Rogers' conceptual framework. Rogers' framework holds that the human energy fields continuously repattern; thus, aging is viewed as a developmental process.[17] Rogers' model of unitary human beings is built on four fundamental precepts:

1. Unitary human beings are energy fields, and each has a corresponding, contiguous, environmental energy field. The person and environment *are* these fields, rather than *having* these fields.
2. These energy fields are open and infinite.
3. The fields can be identified by their patterns, which continuously change, becoming more complex and diverse.
4. The fields are four-dimensional, and as such, are nonlinear, without characteristics bounded by space or time.[18]

Rogers also developed three principles of homeodynamics within her framework of unitary human beings. The first, the principle of helicy, states that the interaction between the human and environmental fields is continually changing in a nondirectional and increasingly differentiated manner. The second, the principle of resonancy, asserts that the energy-field patterns of person and environment are identified by the pattern and organization of their wave frequencies, which undergo constant change. The third, the principle of integrality, alleges that the human and environmental field mutually and simultaneously interact in a continuous manner.[18]

The integrality of the human and environment fields means that these fields through constant interaction have increasing heterogeneity, differentiation, diversity, and complexity of pattern.[18] Mutual repatterning between person and environment is constantly occurring and people are active participants in the developmental process.[19] Repatterning with the nurse as facilitator is the basis for nursing intervention.

Rogers' paradigm holds that persons cannot be understood in relation to their parts.[20] They are more than and different from a sum of their parts. Human beings must be understood from their field-pattern interactions, and they must be understood as a whole. Consequently, Rogers' model of human development lends itself to the holistic study of older people as they have developed over time. Rogers' model is particularly applicable to the change engendered through the use of life review as a therapeutic nursing intervention.

Rogers' Model and Life Review

There is a reasonable, logical fit of Butler and Haight's vision of life review within Rogers' model.[21] The reports of Butler and Haight indicate that the evaluative component of the life review is a significant factor. Butler indicates that finding meaning through integration of conflict from one's past is the purpose and therapeutic benefit of life review.[6] Whereas Haight states the goal of the structured process is integrity, Rogers states, in turn, that the meaning of health and sickness is "derived out of an understanding of the life process in its totality."[20(p85)]

Rogers' definition of helicy applied to aging emphasizes that the pattern and organization of the human field becomes more diverse as it develops over time.[18] As a person progresses through life, both the person field and the corresponding environmental field become more complex and diverse. In any person's life there is unresolved conflict, which can be viewed as disorganized patterns in the human–environment fields. With integrality we see that the basis for intervention lies within the repatterning and reorganization of these fields.[21] Haight states that the life review must cover the entire life span. The life review reintegrates past conflict by adding organization to the older person's increased complexity of experience, thereby fostering ego integrity. Lewis and Butler view the therapeutic role in life review as facilitating the reintegration of experiences and conflict with the client.[22]

Butler suggests that a reexamination of the past and its meaning can lead to expanded understanding.[5] Butler states that finding meaning and usefulness from an examination of the past serves a developmental function for older people.[6] Haight reinforces Butler's view by identifying evaluation as one of the three important constants necessary for therapeutic reminiscing. The systematic examination of the past undertaken by older people helps them reinforce their resources and strengths by reintegrating conflict and increasing the organization of the individual field pattern. Logically, life review is seen as supportive of health maintenance and health promotion and therefore functional well-being.

Within Rogers' model, the therapeutic role is to assist the human field to repattern toward increasing complexity. Nurses can use life review to assist repatterning to reintegrate conflict and to facilitate the older person's pattern reorganization and the developmental process of aging. The reintegration of the conflicts that have arisen during this interaction uses the older person's ability to find his or her meaning in life. The usefulness of life review as a nursing intervention is supported by nursing's view of persons as wholes. By facilitating the developmental process for aging persons, nurses can assist them in maintaining functional well-being. If personal development (increased organization of the human field) occurs as a result of life review, the benefits should not be transient.[21,23]

Thus, a model for conflict reintegration is offered. The Conflict Reintegration Model shows a holistic concept in which, as the person resolves

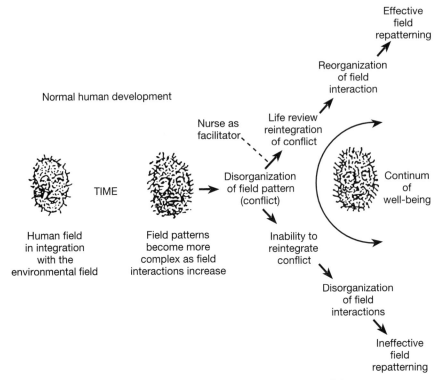

FIGURE 27-1   The Conflict Reintegration Model.

conflict and achieves personal development, functional well-being can be maintained. This model shows both ends of a continuum with neither extreme reflecting an actual human condition (Fig. 27-1).

Rogers holds a positive view of the changes that occur with aging in her description of unitary human beings.[20] Unitary human beings are open, infinite energy fields whose identifying wave patterns are continuously changing in an increasingly differentiated manner. The older person has not simply deteriorated with age, but has become more complex as a result of lifelong interaction with his or her corresponding contiguous environmental energy field. As a person ages, additional life experiences yield a more complex energy field. Yet, not all persons perceive aging as a positive experience. Many are caught up in conflicts and losses and cannot view aging as another type of growth.

An evaluative life review allows older persons to reintegrate past conflicts by adding organization and meaning to their increased complexity of experience. A model of reintegrative life review places Butler's view of this common need of older persons within Rogers' framework of unitary human beings. In this model, the wave patterns of the human field in interaction with its integral environmental field become more complex over time. This complexity makes it more difficult for an older person to organize his or her experiences and to find meaning from that life as it was lived. Unresolved conflict may cause the older person to persistently reminisce about one or two distressful events from the past. An evaluative life review can, through conflict reintegration, assist the older person to find meaning from life's experiences and to organize them within the human–environmental field patterns.

■REFERENCES

1. Spier BE. Life changes experienced by the aged. In: Yunick AG, Spier BE, Robb SS, Ebert NJ, eds. *The Aged Person and the Nursing Process.* East Norwalk, Conn: Appleton & Lange; 1989.
2. Erikson E. *Childhood and Society.* New York, NY: W.W. Norton, 1950.
3. Sheehy G. *Passages.* New York, NY: Bantam Books; 1974.
4. Sheehy G. *Pathfinders.* New York, NY: Bantam Books; 1981.
5. Butler RN. The life review: an interpretation of reminiscence in the aged. *Psychiatry.* 1983;26(1):65–76.
6. Butler RN. Successful aging and the role of life review. *Journal of the American Geriatrics Society.* 1974;22(12):529–535.
7. Haight BK. Reminiscing: the state of the art as a basis for practice. *International Journal of Aging and Human Development.* 1991;33(1):1–32.
8. Haight BK. Psychological illness in aging. In: Baines E, ed. *Perspectives in Gerontological Nursing.* Newbury Park, Calif: Sage; 1991.
9. Coleman PG. *Aging and Reminiscence Processes: Social and Clinical Implications.* New York, NY: Wiley; 1986.
10. Wong PTP, Watt LM. What types of reminiscence are associated with successful aging? *Psychology and Aging.* 1991;6(2):272–279.
11. Haight BK. Life review: a report of the effectiveness of a structured life-review process: part II. *Journal of Religion and Aging.* 1989;5(3):31–41.
12. Haight BK. The therapeutic role of the life review in homebound elderly subjects. *Journal of Gerontology.* 1988;43(2):40–44.
13. Haight BK, Dias J. Examining the variables of life review. *International Journal of Psychogeriatrics.* 1992. In press.
14. AARP Training Manual. *Reminiscence: Finding Meaning in Memories.* Washington, DC: American Association of Retired Persons; 1989.
15. Report of the NIMH Invitational Conference on Depression. Forty-fourth annual scientific meeting: New knowledge: the key to meeting the challenges of aging. *The Gerontologist.* 1990;31(SI1):108.
16. Merriam SB. The structure of simple reminiscence. *The Gerontological Society of America.* 1989;29(6):761–767.
17. Rogers ME. Nursing: a science of unitary man. In: Riehl J, Roy L, eds. *Conceptual Models for Nursing Practice.* 2d ed. New York, NY: Appleton-Century-Crofts; 1980.
18. Rogers ME. *Science of Unitary Human Beings: A Paradigm for Nursing.* Clemson, SC: Clemson University; 1984. Unpublished paper.
19. Rogers ME: Beyond the horizon. In: Chaska NL, ed. *The Nursing Profession: A Time to Speak.* New York, NY: McGraw-Hill; 1982.
20. Rogers ME. *An Introduction to the Theoretical Basis of Nursing.* Philadelphia, Penn: F.A. Davis; 1970.
21. Black GA. *Life Review and the Maintenance of Functional Well-Being among Homebound Older Persons.* Columbus, SC: University of South Carolina; 1986. Thesis.
22. Lewis MI, Butler RN. Life-review therapy: putting memories to work in individual and group psychotherapy. *Geriatrics.* 1974;29(1):165–173.
23. Haight BK. The long-term effects of a structured life-review process. *The Gerontologist.* 1987;27:5.

■APPENDIX 27-A
Haight's Life Review and Experiencing Form

Childhood

1. What is the very first thing you can remember in your life? Go as far back as you can.
2. What other things can you remember about when you were very young?
3. What was life like for you as a child?
4. What were your parents like? What were their weaknesses, strengths?
5. Did you have any brothers or sisters? Tell me what each was like.
6. Did someone close to you die when you were growing up?
7. Did someone important to you go away?
8. Do you ever remember being very sick?
9. Do you remember having an accident?
10. Do you remember being in a very dangerous situation?
11. Was there anything that was important to you that was lost or destroyed?
12. Was church a large part of your life?
13. Did you enjoy being a boy/girl?

Adolescence

1. When you think about yourself and your life as a teenager, what is the first thing you can remember about that time?
2. What other things stand out in your memory about being a teenager?
3. Who were the important people for you? Tell me about them — parents, brothers, sisters, friends, teachers, those you were especially close to, those you admired, those you wanted to be like.
4. Did you attend church and youth groups?
5. Did you go to school? What was the meaning for you?
6. Did you work during these years?
7. Tell me of any hardships you experienced at this time.
8. Do you remember feeling that there wasn't enough food or necessities of life as a child or adolescent?
9. Do you remember feeling left alone, abandoned, not having enough love or care as a child or adolescent?
10. What were the pleasant things about your adolescence?
11. What was the most unpleasant thing about your adolescence?
12. All things considered, would you say you were happy or unhappy as a teenager?
13. Do you remember your first attraction to another person?
14. How did you feel about sexual activities and your own sexual identity?

Family and Home

1. How did your parents get along?
2. How did other people in your home get along?
3. What was the atmosphere in your home?
4. Were you punished as a child? For what? Who did the punishing? Who was "boss"?

(continued)

▬ APPENDIX 27-A
Haight's Life Review and Experiencing Form (*continued*)

5. When you wanted something from your parents, how did you go about getting it?
6. What kind of person did your parents like the most? The least?
7. Who were you closest to in your family?
8. Who in your family were you most like? In what way?

Adulthood

1. What place did religion play in your life?
2. Now I'd like to talk to you about your life as an adult, starting when you were in your twenties up to today. Tell me of the most important events that happened in your adulthood.
3. What was life like for you in your twenties and thirties?
4. What kind of person were you? What did you enjoy?
5. Tell me about your work. Did you enjoy your work? Did you earn an adequate living? Did you work hard during those years? Were you appreciated?
6. Did you form significant relationships with other people?
7. Did you marry?
   (yes) What kind of person was your spouse?
   (no) Why not?
8. Do you think marriages get better or worse over time? Were you married more than once?
9. On the whole, would you say you had a happy or unhappy marriage?
10. Was sexual intimacy important to you?
11. What were some of the main difficulties you encountered during your adult years?
    a. Did someone close to you die? Go away?
    b. Were you ever sick? Have an accident?
    c. Did you move often? Change jobs?
    d. Did you ever feel alone? Abandoned?
    e. Did you ever feel needed?

Summary

1. On the whole, what kind of life do you think you've had?
2. If everything were to be the same would you like to live your life over again?
3. If you were going to live your life over again, what would you change? Leave unchanged?
4. We've been talking about your life for quite some time now. Let's discuss your over-all feelings and ideas about your life. What would you say the main satisfactions in your life have been? *Try for three. Why were they satisfying?*
5. Everyone has had disappointments. What have been the main disappointments in your life?

(*continued*)

■ APPENDIX 27-A
Haight's Life Review and Experiencing Form (*continued*)

6. What was the hardest thing you had to face in your life? Please describe it.
7. What was the happiest period of your life? What about it made it the happiest period? Why is your life less happy now?
8. What was the unhappiest period of your life? Why is your life more happy now?
9. What was the proudest moment in your life?
10. If you could stay the same age all your life, what age would you choose? Why?
11. How do you think you've made out in life? Better or worse than what you hoped for?
12. Let's talk a little about you as you are now. What are the best things about the age you are now?
13. What are the worst things about being the age you are now?
14. What are the most important things to you in your life today?
15. What do you hope will happen to you as you grow older?
16. What do you fear will happen to you as you grow older?
17. Have you enjoyed participating in this review of your life?

Note: Derived from new questions and two unpublished dissertations

Gomey J. (1968). *Experiencing and Age: Patterns of Reminiscence among the Elderly.* (Unpublished doctoral dissertation, University of Chicago).

Falk J. (1969). *The Organization of Remembered Life Experience of Older People: Its Relation to Anticipated Stress, to Subsequent Adaptation, and to Age.* (Unpublished doctoral dissertation, University of Chicago).

Chapter 28

Cognitive Developmental Approach to Dementia

MARY ANN MATTESON   ADRIANNE D. LINTON

SUSAN J. BARNES

Combining Piagetian theory with a systematic review of observational research findings of older adults diagnosed with Dementia of the Alzheimer's type (DAT), the authors have synthesized a cognitive developmental approach that helps to explain stages of dementia behavior and predict possible caregiver needs and interventions. This chapter demonstrates how gerontological nursing practice can be guided by the use of pertinent theory and research.

Dementia associated with Alzheimer's disease has been defined as the development of multiple cognitive deficits manifested by both memory impairment and one or more of the following cognitive disturbances: aphasia (language disturbance), apraxia (impaired ability to carry out motor activities despite intact motor function), agnosia (failure to identify objects despite intact sensory function), and disturbance in planning, organizing, sequencing, and abstracting. The cognitive deficits cause significant impairment in social or occupational functioning, and represent a significant decline from a previous level of functioning (American Psychiatric Association, 1994). The loss of functional abilities and disappearance of learned behaviors is progressive and generally irreversible. These losses appear to be predictable and related to the cognitive and sensorimotor changes that occur with dementia.

Research findings may provide information about alleviation of some of the frustration and hopelessness associated with care of dementia patients. Caregivers contend with agitation, wandering, resisting care, sleep problems, and impaired activities of daily living. Insight into behavior associated with Alzheimer's disease may help prevent unrealistic expectations (Thornbury, 1992) that include both over- and under-estimations of performance. The problem of overestimation of performance abilities usually arises in long-term relationships in which the afflicted individual had been fully

From *Image: Journal of Nursing Scholarship* 28(3):233–240, 1996. Reprinted with permission.

functional; underestimation can lead to excess disability and exaggerated helplessness (Beck, Heacock, Mercer, Walton, & Shook, 1991).

Systematic empirical observation of people suffering from dementia of the Alzheimer's type (DAT) has repeatedly revealed evidence that patients regress in behavior and become childlike (Farran & Kean-Hagerty, 1989; Gugel, 1988; Haight, 1989; Trocchio, 1989). These observations have led to structuring clinical research and therapeutic interventions. However, no concise theoretical framework has been developed from research (Maas & Buckwalter, 1991; Thornbury, 1993). Models for care exist but many lack an adequate conceptual framework for the long-term care of a person with DAT (Adams, 1988; Bell & McGregor, 1991; Fitzgerald, 1988; Mayeux, 1990; Schwab, Rader, & Doan, 1985).

▆ THE COGNITIVE DEVELOPMENTAL APPROACH (CDA)

In the CDA loss of cognitive abilities follows a reverse order to the acquisition of those abilities. The cognitive developmental theory of Piaget serves as a guide to understanding the acquisition of thinking skills and therefore an understanding of the order of loss of those skills. Research on DAT based on Piagetian theory of cognitive development was originally begun because of anecdotal observations: Caregivers of Alzheimer's patients consistently noted that patients seem to "go backward" during the course of the disease. Once regression occurs at each stage, there is no reversal of the process.

A specific order of cognitive decline has been identified in patients with DAT (Reisberg et al., 1989). Reisberg (1984) has likened seven stages of Alzheimer's disease to the reverse stages of childhood, moving from adolescence to infancy. The changes appear to be developmentally congruent and loss of skills appears to take place in reverse order of acquisition (Nolen, 1988; Sclan, Foster, Reisberg, Franssen, & Welkowitz, 1990).

In a study conducted on 12 community-residing patients with DAT with varying levels of cognitive impairment, findings confirmed that key functional abilities such as bathing, dressing, and toileting are lost in reverse order of the acquisition of these abilities in children. In addition, approximately the same amount of time is needed to learn a skill as to lose it (Reisberg, 1985, 1986; Turkington, 1985). Nolen (1988) found similar results with a sample of institutionalized older adults with late-stage dementias.

▆ PIAGET THEORY

Jean Piaget's (1952) theory of intellectual development identified four major stages. Major features of each stage follow:

1. Sensorimotor (0 to 24 months): Children move from neonatal birth reflexes to symbolic images. There is an effort to reproduce behavior that was first achieved by chance and development of habits begins. Rudimentary trial and error occurs; imitation begins. There is interest in producing new behavior and novel events.

2. Preoperational (2 to 7 years): Children develop the ability to use symbols. This period is characterized by egocentric thought but children gradually display progressively more socialized behavior as they steadily move away from egocentric thought. Most play is parallel. Children take instructions literally and therefore need specific instruction in behaviors to be carried out.

3. Concrete Operations (7 to 12 years): Children think and reason with inductive logic first, deductive later. They understand the value of rules and base judgements on reason.

4. Formal Operations (age 12 years and older): There is development of logical reasoning and ability to think about the hypothetical and abstract. Human beings progress through each stage in a systematic manner although the rate of progression varies with each individual (Ginsberg & Opper, 1979).

The theory is useful in describing how one changes as a result of repeated interactions with the environment (Flavell, 1977). There is emphasis on the interactive relationship between internal operations and the environment in the acquisition of knowledge.

Cognition and behavior in children and in people with DAT are remarkably similar. People with DAT appear to experience cognitive decline in a predictable, progressive manner. Behaviors are often described as childlike and include memory impairment, declining language and computational skills, poor judgement, and inappropriate social behavior (Haight, 1989). Similarities in the behaviors and underlying cognitive processes that might reflect sensorimotor and preoperational stages in an infant or child and in reverse order of the stages of a person with DAT (Table 28-1), are as follows.

1. The world of an infant is described as "a series of unstable and unconnected 'pictures'" (Ginsberg & Opper, 1979). It has been said that having Alzheimer's disease is like walking in in the middle of a movie, not aware of what has already transpired.

2. Children actively seek out new stimulation. They are most attentive to events that are moderately novel, complex, unanticipated, or puzzling (Flavell, 1977; Ginsberg & Opper, 1979). Patients with DAT seem drawn to similar types of events.

3. Infants and children test the effect of their actions on the environment (Ginsberg & Opper, 1979). Perhaps DAT patients' "purposeless" wanderings and manipulations reflect a similar kind of testing.

4. Events that cannot be assimilated produce cognitive uncertainty. A person engages in cognitive activity to rectify the situation (Flavell, 1977). One could ask how patients with DAT react when they encounter situations that they cannot comprehend. What behaviors might result from cognitive uncertainty? How are they adaptive?

5. According to Ginsberg and Opper (1979), patients with DAT are observed to repeat well-rehearsed behaviors. Some behaviors seen as purposeless may actually reflect available schemes as defined by Piaget

TABLE 28-1 Piaget's Developmental Levels and Stages of Alzheimer's Disease

PIAGET DEVELOPMENTAL LEVEL	ALZHEIMER'S STAGE
1. Sensorimotor Period (*first 2 years of life*):	**Late Dementia:**
Substage 1 — Use of Reflexes Automatic innate or reflex responses to external stimuli	Speech and motor dysfunction; few words spoken; inability to walk; incontinence; inability to eat
Substage 2 — Primary Circular Reactions Effort to reproduce behavior that was first achieved by chance; development of habits	
Substage 3 — Secondary Circular Reactions Beginning association of events that occur close together; dawning recognition of symbols; beginning recognition of causality; object permanence	**Middle Dementia** (moderately severe Alzheimer's disease): Recall own name; recent memory loss; little remote memory; disturbed diurnal rhythm; generally unaware of surroundings; personal hygiene dysfunction; fear of bathing — requires assistance; difficulty putting clothes on properly; inability to handle mechanics of toileting; urinary incontinence; fecal incontinence; agitation, wandering; obsessive symptoms; loss of willpower; difficulty counting to 10
Substage 4 — Coordination of Secondary Circular Reactions Simple problem-solving using behaviors that have already been mastered; anticipatory behavior; object permanence	
Substage 5 — Tertiary Circular Reactions Rudimentary trial and error; manipulation of objects; object permanence	
Substage 6 — Invention of New Means through Deduction Well developed understanding of the nature of objects; concept of causality; use of mental symbols and words to refer to absent objects; ability to remember, plan and imitate someone else's previous actions; object permanence	
2. Preoperational Period (*age 2 to 7 years*):	**Early Dementia** (moderate Alzheimer's disease): Unable to recall phone number; can recall own name and names of spouse and children; no assistance required with eating or toileting; difficulty choosing proper clothing; coaxing required for bathing; difficulty substracting 3s from 20
Stage 1 – Preconceptual Stage Formation of mental images (symbolic thought); imitation of previously viewed activities; parallel play; instructions taken literally	
Stage 2 — Perceptual or Intuitive Stage Prelogical reasoning; experiences and objects judged by outside appearances and results; selective attention (centration) — can only concentrate upon one characteristic of an object at a time; beginning use of words; but thoughts still acted out; more social; transductive reasoning	

(*continued*)

TABLE 28-1 Piaget's Developmental Levels and Stages of Alzheimer's Disease (*continued*)

PIAGET DEVELOPMENTAL LEVEL	ALZHEIMER'S STAGE
3. Concrete Operational Period (*age 7 to 12 years*): Think and reason with inductive logic at beginning, deductive later; conservation and reversibility; capable of decentration (ability to focus on multiple aspects of an object, event or situation at the same time); understand the value of rules; judgement based on reason; inability to comprehend the future and the abstract	**Early and Late Confusional** (borderline to mild Alzheimer's disease): Decreased ability to perform in demanding employment and social interactions; deficit in memory and ability to concentrate; difficulty with serial 7s
4. Formal Operational Period (*age 12 onward*): Logical reasoning and ability to think about hypothetical and abstract	**Normal Forgetfulness:** No impairment but subjective concern about memory loss

when he described a scheme as an organized pattern of behavior that may be innate or based on experience.

6. Children explore problems unsystematically or systematically, depending on the stage of development (Flavell, 1977). As a DAT patient's abilities diminish, exploration may switch from systematic to unsystematic.

7. Children gradually become less egocentric as they grow older (Ginsberg & Opper, 1979); patients with DAT seem to become more egocentric as they regress.

8. Imitation is an important aspect of infant behavior (Ginsberg & Opper, 1979). This behavior often is seen in patients with DAT and provides a basis for many interventions.

9. Children's language and thoughts are different from adults. To understand children, we need to understand their cognitive function (Ginsberg & Opper, 1979). The same principle may be applied to patients with DAT.

These similarities suggest that patients in the later stages of DAT function at sensorimotor and preoperational stages described by Piaget. Knowledge of these stages can guide caregivers in selecting appropriate interventions according to patients' abilities.

Piaget's theory provides a useful theoretical model of cognitive impairment even though it has generated some controversy (Ginsberg & Opper, 1979; LaFrancois, 1982; Musser, Conger, & Kagen, 1974). One criticism is that Piaget's initial work was based on naturalistic observations of his own children; other criticisms are based on controversy about the best way to explain developmental changes in a child's thinking (Cohen, 1983; Musser et al., 1974). However, in recent years, more rigorous studies have supported most of Piaget's findings and many sources agree that his observations of sequences appear to be essentially correct. Despite the criticism, the theory has proven useful in understanding how children think and behave (LaFrancois, 1982). Furthermore, Piaget's theory provides direction for appropriate activities to foster development of cognitive skills at various ages.

▰ASSESSMENT AND STAGING

Accurate assessment and staging of cognitive levels and dementia are critical for developing appropriate interventions for problem behaviors (Mayeux, 1990; McDougall, 1990; Reisburg, Franssen, Sclan, Kluger, & Ferris, 1989; Sloan & Matthew, 1991). Use of a medical model in staging methods has predominated until recently (Absher & Cummings, 1992; Flicker, Ferris, Crook, & Bartus, 1987; Johnson & Keller, 1989; Kettle, 1993; Mira, Hart, & Terry, 1993; Ninos & Makohon, 1985; Rubin et al., 1993). Attempts to clearly categorize dementia patients can be traced to the 19th century; and until the 1980s, no method listed more than four stages (Reisberg et al., 1993). The limited number of stages contributed to errors in diagnosis concerning treatable conditions such as depression, drug toxicity, and allergic reactions that produce behavioral problems in older adults that are similar to DAT.

The need for a reliable method of measuring pathological cognitive changes generated many screening and diagnostic tests; 52 such instruments are cited by Ritchie (1988).

Functional Assessment Staging Test (FAST) (Reisberg, 1988; Reisberg, Ferris, & Franssen, 1985; Sclan & Reisberg, 1992) has proven particularly useful for a cognitive developmental approach and has undergone thorough testing for reliability and validity. In addition, the framework behind the instrument incorporates the latitude to encourage further observation in the area of the cognitive developmental approach (Reisberg, 1988). Research associated with development of the FAST has subsequently become significant in the development of the conceptual model under scrutiny.

Staging and Piagetian Instrumentation and the Elderly

Piaget developed standard tests or tasks that have been used widely to test infants, children, and adolescents in order to determine their cognitive level of development. Examples of these tasks are 4-digit test and color combinations (formal operations); tests of conservation and complementary classes (concrete operations); reproduction of figures and seriation or reversibility (preoperational); and imitation, figurative versus non-figurative concepts, and object permanence (sensorimotor). The tests have been used extensively to evaluate children.

Although methods for ascertaining cognitive functioning of children and adolescents are well established, a review of the literature suggests that the depth of experience in using these instruments in an aging population does not exist. Research studies using a reverse Piagetian framework have been limited in that most studies examined only one stage of cognitive development.

A study of linguistic loss in dementia patients included a Piagetian component (Emery, 1985; Emergy & Breslau, 1987). The study used one Piaget test consisting of five tasks that determined concrete operations. A significant difference ($p < .001$) existed between test scores for the well elderly and the demented elderly. Mean scores for well elderly were 2.9 out of five compared to .79 for people with DAT. Measurement 1 year later showed a predictable pattern of regression reflecting the reverse order of Piaget's theory. It also was observed that not all the well elderly subjects were able to complete all of the tasks in the concrete operational level. This deficit indicated the presence of a normal decline in ability to perform the tests, a factor to be considered in future research.

Thornbury (1993) assessed community-dwelling elders for Piaget levels using Infant Psychological Development Scale (IPDS) (Uzgiris & Hunt, 1975) and the Concrete Operational Test (COT) (Emergy & Breslau, 1987). The investigator made several noteworthy instrument modifications including the following: First, one of six scales was omitted from the ISPD because it was not appropriate for older adults. Second, the requirement for a verbal explanation for actions in the COT was omitted because of verbal deterioration present in patients with DAT. This omission would most likely be questioned by scholars associated with pure Piagetian theory because verbal explanation is required for successful completion of the test items when performed in children. The result of this study confirmed a significant relationship between cognitive loss and Piaget level.

The Ordinal Scales of Psychological Development (OSPD) (Uzgiris & Hunt, 1975) was also used in an attempt to deal with the uniformly zero scores obtained by other traditional measurements in patients in advanced stages of DAT (Sclan et al., 1990). A modified OSPD revealed information regarding cognition in severely demented patients. In addition, reliability of the OSPD ranged from .94 to .99. Validity was $r = .58$ with a $p < .01$. These results suggest potential usefulness of the measurement scales.

The Hierarchical Dementia Scale (HDS) (Cole, Dastoor, & Koszycki, 1983) was developed based on the successive nature of cognitive decline observed in dementia. This scale was based on work done in the 1960s that documented that functional decline approximated Piaget's developmental stages in reverse. Specifically reversed concepts included dissociation of ideation of weight and volume, which precedes impairment of conservation of weight, which precedes impairment of conservation of the horizontal, which in turn precedes impairment of conservation of the vertical. Investigators using the scale found it helpful in longitudinal study of an individual's decline but the measure falls short of the original purpose of displaying optimal concordance across categories (Cole & Dastoor, 1987; Reisberg, Ferris, et al., 1989).

Preliminary analysis of results from a recently completed study have been promising in regard to congruence between Piaget levels and cognitive levels. Investigators attempted to develop strategies for managing problem behaviors associated with dementia based on Piagetian cognitive developmental levels (Matteson, Linton, Cleary, & Lichtenstein, 1993). The instrument used was developed specifically for the study and is the first to include all levels of cognitive functioning. Multiple regression analysis revealed that Piaget levels were significantly correlated with scores on the Mini-Mental State Exam (MMSE) (Folstein, Folstein, & McHugh, 1975) (R^2 = .8195, p < .001). Analysis of variance showed significant differences in mean MMSE scores among the Piaget levels (p < .0001). Only five of the 93 institutionalized subjects scored in the formal operations while 26 scored in the concrete operations' categories, which is thought to be congruent with scoring in the general population regardless of age. Indications for further research are to refine the Piaget instrument to more clearly stage early and late phases of sensorimotor and preoperational stages.

▄ IDENTIFICATION AND MANAGEMENT OF PROBLEM BEHAVIORS

Behavioral symptoms that emerge during the evolution of DAT are related to psychological losses accompanying cognitive decline (Reisberg et al., 1986). The inability to follow directions and to conceptualize, abstract, comprehend, reason, or learn new information are factors in the development of behavioral problems (Gugel, 1988). Research foci on behavioral problems have taken two slants: (a) identifying behaviors peculiar to DAT and (b) determining how to best manage the problems.

Identification of Problem Behaviors

Identification of problem behaviors related to DAT has been accomplished to a significant degree through research. Problems identified include paranoid and delusional ideation, hallucinations, activity disturbances, aggressiveness, diurnal rhythm disturbance, affective disturbance, and anxieties (Ray, Taylor, Lichtenstein, & Meador, 1992; Ray, Taylor, Lichtenstein, & Meador, et al., 1991; Reisberg, Franssen, Sclan, Kluger, & Ferris, 1989). The appearance of certain behaviors has also been related to specific stages of Alzheimer's disease (Reisberg et al., 1993).

Problem behaviors have been identified not only by researchers and licensed practitioners but also by paraprofessionals who provide most of the direct care (Beck, Baldwin, Modlin, & Lewis, 1990; Bjorkheim, Olsson, Hallberg, & Norberg, 1992; Gwyther & Matteson, 1983; Haight, 1992; Rossby, Beck, Heacock, 1992).

Behavioral Management

In the past, management approaches to problem behaviors have frequently followed the medical model or assumptions based on anecdotal observations (Hall & Buckwalter, 1987; Hall & Buckwalter, 1990; Maas & Buckwalter, 1991). Physical and chemical restraints have often been used to control unwanted behaviors (Beardsley, Larson, Burns, Thompson, & Kamerow, 1989; Beers et al., 1988; Kahn & Stoudemire, 1990; Travis & Moore, 1991; Wragg & Jeste, 1988).

Behavioral interventions have been attempted for increasing independence in activities of daily living, decreasing agitated and wandering behaviors, and preventing catastrophic reactions (Maas, 1988; Beck & Heacock, 1988). Unfortunately these interventions for symptom management have been based largely on trial and error with no theoretical basis. Additionally, while there is clinical information related to symptom management, few controlled studies have been carried out to test behavioral interventions. One recent study (Beck, Heacock, Mercer, & Walton, 1991; Beck, Heacock, Mercer, Walton, & Shook, 1991) was conducted to decrease demented older adults' need for assistance with dressing. Subjects were assessed for cognitive decline and performance ability and were taught to dress using simple commands and modeling. The level of caregiver assistance decreased significantly ($p < .002$) after the treatment period; however, not all subjects were able to dress themselves. The cognitive developmental approach provides a theoretical model explaining that the subjects who were able to perform had not regressed past the Piaget stages where modeling and simple commands were effective and those who were unable to perform had regressed to the point where these strategies were of little use.

Environmental measures including carpeting, colorful furniture, and noise reduction for coping with difficult behaviors have been suggested by many (Cox, 1985; Hussian & Brown, 1987; Lemke & Moos, 1987; Mathew & Sloane, 1990; Namazi, Rosned, & Calkins, 1989; Schafer, 1985; Roberts & Algase, 1988). Physical cues, such as colors, pictures, and words have been suggested for orientation. Social cues, such as the use of gestures and touch have been suggested for promoting interaction and socialization.

The few studies carried out in relationship to the environment usually have involved use of visual barriers to prevent wandering away from a nursing-home unit. Hussian and Brown (1987) in a small sample of eight demented male patients found that tape in a two-dimensional grid pattern limited exiting from the unit by 42%. Namazi et al. (1989) tested seven different visual barrier conditions for reducing patient exits from a dementia unit. Their findings indicated that exiting was eliminated with the use of cloth to conceal the doorknob. The findings could support the proposition that the Piaget sensorimotor stage of cognitive development is similar to cognitive ability in moderately severe Alzheimer's disease because people at the sensorimotor level of cognitive development do not look behind a cloth to see what is there.

Scrutiny of such practices by researchers has demonstrated that the use of physical and chemical restraints has not only had less than desirable effects in patient therapeutics but has been associated with increased injuries accompanying falls, agitation, and disorientation (Blazer, 1993; Miles & Irvine, 1992; Morse & McHutchion, 1991; Strumpf & Evans, 1988; Werner, Cohen-Mansfield, Braun, & Marx, 1989). Overuse of pharmacologic restraint agents created sufficient concern that regulations regarding their use in nursing homes were established by the Health Care Financing Administration through the Omnibus Budget Regulatory Act in 1988 (Matteson, Linton, Lichtenstein, & Cleary, 1991).

Constraints on effectively measuring effects of pharmacological and behavioral interventions led Beck, Heacock, Rapp, & Mercer (1993) to develop the Disruptive Behavior Scale. The operational definition of the term disruptive behaviors was "behaviors that negatively affect quality of life, quality of care, and resource efficiency." A multi-stage research process was used to develop the items, test interrater agreement, and to define and validate severity weights. This effort is considered a hallmark in nursing research with dementia patients in its quality and usefulness.

Several studies by occupational therapists have revealed positive results in management of problems between dementia patients and their caregivers (Corcoran, 1992; Corcoran & Gitlin, 1992; MacDonald, 1986). These studies were adequate in research design but lacking in a theoretical framework and each was isolated in relationship to other studies, indicating a need for corroborating investigations.

Other studies from nonmedical models are often without corroboration and are questionable to the extent results derived in one setting (home or institution) can be generalized to other settings. The development of a theory based, holistic, patient-oriented approach to understanding the DAT patient could greatly influence progress in managing behavioral problems.

Approaches to Activities of Daily Living (ADL)

These activities serve as focal points for promoting independence and preventing excess disability in a cognitively-impaired individual. Research has shown that most disabilities related to performance of ADL belong to one of four specific areas including attention deficits, language impairment, sequencing problems, and impaired judgment. Behavioral assistance for ADL deficits consists of caregiver actions that have the potential to promote independent behaviors in a client (Beck, Heacock, Mercer, Walton, & Shook, 1991). Seven levels of assistance have been delineated: (a) stimulus control, (b) initial verbal prompt, (c) repeated verbal prompt, (d) gestures or modeling, (e) occasional physical guidance, (f) complete physical guidance, and (g) complete assistance (Beck, et al., 1993).

Several studies have focused on the interaction between caregivers and patients with DAT. Exploratory research in the activity of feeding patients with dementia has revealed the complex nature of the act (Ort & Phillips, 1992). Researchers found that patients previously judged "not able to feed themselves" were actually able to do so given the right circumstances. With adequate caregiver support, a "hidden" capability was revealed, indicating that it is important for nursing staff to distinguish between partial and total dependence to avoid creating excess disability (Osborn & Marshall, 1992, 1993). Another study on feeding a person with DAT confirmed that the relationship of the caregiver to the patient is an integral part of the feeding process (Athlin & Norberg, 1987). A study on the effects of language on successfully performing ADL indicated that caregivers respond negatively to people with more severe language impairment (Ekman, Norberg, Vitanen, & Winblad, 1991). It can be concluded that all DAT clients require recognition as individuals despite outcomes of functional assessment (Burgener, Shimer, & Murrell, 1993).

■ COGNITIVE FUNCTIONAL AGE APPROACH:
A PIAGETIAN BASE

The Piagetian theory of cognitive development provides a model for understanding cognition throughout the life span (Matteson, et al., 1993). Early psychological inquiries into specific conservation abilities of older adults using Piagetian theory did not continue (Hooper, Fitzgerald, & Paplia, 1971; Hornblum & Overton, 1976; Hughston & Protinsky, 1978; Rubin, 1976). A reemergence of reports regarding the presence of childlike behavior in DAT clients has stimulated renewed interest in the usefulness of Piagetian principles (Farran & Keane-Hagerty, 1989; Gugel, 1988; Trocchio, 1989). Specific inquiries into the use of a concept of cognitive decline occurring in reverse order of acquisition include researchers in nursing, psychology, and medicine (Emery, 1985; Emery & Breslau, 1987; Flicker, et al., 1987; Matteson, et al., 1993; Reisburg, Ferris, Torossian, Kluger, & Monteiro, 1992; Thornbury, 1993).

Research correlating mental status to Piagetian tests of cognitive functions have been positive (Matteson, et al., 1993; Thornbury, 1992). People in more advanced stages of DAT appear to be in earlier preoperational and sensorimotor stages of cognitive function (Emery, 1985; Emery & Breslow, 1987; Matteson, et al., 1993; Thornbury, 1992). Changes in cognitive functioning appear to be developmentally congruent and skills are lost in reverse order of acquisition (Nolen, 1988; Reisberg, Ferris, et al., 1989). Consistency of the order of loss is high (Reisberg, Ferris, et al., 1989). Researchers have identified the reappearance of neonatal or release signs (cortical or frontal disinhibition signs) adding impetus to the use of reverse order Piagetian model (Franssen, Kluger, Torossian, & Reisberg, 1993; Reisberg, Pattschull-Furlan, et al., 1992).

Studies applying a cognitive behavioral approach to clinical management of behavioral symptoms and ADL functioning have not been published thus far. Matteson and associates (1995) are completing a 3-year federally funded study to determine the effect of a cognitive developmental approach to the management of behavioral symptoms associated with DAT. The purposes of this study were to determine the relationship between Piaget's levels of cognitive development and levels of cognitive impairment in people with dementia, and to develop and test behavioral interventions for institutionalized people in various stages of Alzheimer's disease using Piaget's stages of cognitive development as a theoretical model for cognitive dysfunction. The ultimate goal was to reduce the number of problem behaviors and the number of psychotropic medications taken to manage behavior. Individualized care plans based on Piaget levels were studied for behavioral interventions while subjects were systematically withdrawn from psychotropic medications. In addition, environmental modifications (symbols, music, activities) were introduced during the last year of the study. Preliminary results indicate that it was possible to manage problem behaviors while reducing the number of psychotropic medications (Matteson, Linton, Barnes, Cleary, & Lichtenstein, 1995; Matteson, Linton, Cleary, Barnes, & Lichtenstein, 1995).

▬CONCLUSION

There is a need for the development of theory-based practice in dealing with DAT (Duffy, Hepburn, Christensen, Brugge-Wiger, 1989). Clinical progression of the malady has not been studied sufficiently to understand the disease from the patient's viewpoint. As research is conducted, theory should be consistently developed (Fawcett & Downs, 1993). The most meaningful interventions and interactions on the part of the caregiver can only be structured when an appropriate conceptualization can take place regarding a client's cognitive status. Efficacy of environmental structure could be greatly enhanced if an understanding of a client's cognitive developmental level were incorporated into design. Ways must be developed to address the skill of caregivers and their ability to implement interventions based on cognitive developmental theory.

This state-of-the-science chapter has demonstrated that there is growing evidence to support a cognitive functional age approach to dementia. The Piagetian model for assessment of cognitive functioning has proven useful when used in conjunction with other existing staging and assessment models. But there is a need for developing an instrument that is more sensitive to the earlier periods of cognitive functioning because DAT patients have been typically misclassified as sensorimotor or preoperational. Use of a cognitive developmental approach to qualitatively and quantitatively characterize impaired cognition in DAT patients can contribute to a better understanding of caregiving practices, education, and the world of dementia patients (Thornbury, 1993).

▬REFERENCES

Absher, J. R., & Cummings, J. L. (1992). Dementia diagnosis and therapy in the elderly. Comprehensive Therapy, 5, 28–33.

Adams, T. (1988). A model example. Geriatric Nursing and Home Care, 3, 24–5.

American Psychiatric Association. (1994). Diagnostic and statistical manual of mental disorders. (4th ed.). Washington, DC: Author.

Athlin, E., & Norberg, A. (1987). Caregivers' attitudes to and interpretations of the behavior of severely demented patients during feeding in a patient assignment care system. International Journal of Nursing Studies, 24, 145–153.

Beardsley, R. S., Larson, D. B., Burns, B. J., Thompson, J. W., & Kamerow, D. B. (1989). Prescribing of psychotropics in elderly nursing home patients. Journal of the American Geriatrics Society, 37, 327–330.

Beck, C., Baldwin, B., Modlin, T., & Lewis, S. (1990). Caregiver's perception of aggressive behavior in cognitively impaired nursing home residents. Journal of Neuroscience Nursing, 6, (22), 169–172.

Beck, C., & Heacock, P. (1988). Nursing interventions for patients with Alzheimer's disease. Nursing Clinics of North America, 23, 95–124.

Beck, C., Heacock, P., Mercer, S., & Walton, C. (1991). Decreasing demented older adults' need for assistance with dressing. Third National Conference on Research for Clinical Practice: Key Aspects of elder care: Managing falls, incontinence and cognitive impairment. The University of North Carolina, Chapel Hill, NC.

Beck, C., Heacock, P., Mercer, S., Walton, C. G., & Shook, J. (1991). Dressing for success: Prompting independence among cognitively impaired elderly. Journal of Psychosocial Nursing, 29, (7), 30–40.

Beck, C., Heacock, P., Rapp, C. G., & Mercer. (1993). How much help will it take? Assisting cognitively impaired elders with activities of daily living. Unpublished manuscript, College of Medicine, University of Arkansas of Medical Sciences, Little Rock, AR.

Beers, M., Avorn, J., Soumerai, S. B., Daniel, E. E., Sherman, D. S., & Salem, S. (1988). Psychoactive medication use in intermediate-care facility residents. Journal of the American Medical Association, 260, 3016–3020.

Bell, J., & McGregor, I. (1991). Living for the moment. Nursing Times, 87, (18), 45–47.

Bjorkheim, K., Olsson, A., Hallberg, I. R., & Norberg, A. (1992). Caregivers' experience of providing care for demented persons living at home. Scandinavian Journal of Primary Health Care, 10, 53–59.

Blazer, D. (1993). Reducing antipsychotic drug use in nursing homes. Archives of Internal Medicine, 153, 713–721.

Burgener, S. C., Shimer, R., & Murrell, L. (1993). Expressions of individuality in cognitively impaired elders: Need for individual assessment and care. Journal of Gerontological Nursing, 4, 13–22.

Cohen, D. (1983). Piaget: Critique and reassessment. New York: St. Martin's Press.

Cole, M. G., Dastoor, D. P., & Koszycki, D. (1983). The hierarchic dementia scale. Journal of Clinical and Experimental Gerontology, 5, 219–234.

Corcoran, M. A. (1992). Gender differences in dementia management plans of spousal caregivers: implications for occupational therapy. American Journal of Occupational Therapy, 46, 1006–1012.

Corcoran, M. A., & Gitlin, L. N. (1992). Dementia management: An occuparional therapy home-based intervention for caregivers. The American Journal of Occupational Therapy, 46, 801–807.

Cox, K. (1985). Milieu therapy. Geriatric Nursing, 6, 152–156.

Duffy, L. M., Hepburn, K., Christensen, R., & Brugge-Wiger, P. (1989). A research agenda in care for patients with Alzheimer's disease. Image: Journal of Nursing Scholarship, 22, 254–257.

Ekman, S. L., Norberg, A., Vitanen, M., & Winblad, B. (1991). Care of demented patients with severe communication problems. Scandinavian Journal of Caring Sciences, 5, 163–170.

Emery, O. B. (1985). Language and aging. Experimental Aging Research, 11, 3–60.

Emery, O. B., & Breslau, L. (1987). The acceleration process in Alzheimer's disease: Thought dissolution in Alzheimer's disease early onset and senile dementia Alzheimer's type. The American Journal of Alzheimer's Care and Related Disorders & Research, 9/10, 24–30.

Farran, C. J., & Keane-Hagerty, E. (1989). Communicating effectively with dementia patients. Journal of Psychosocial Nursing, 27, 13–16.

Fawcett, J., & Downs, F. (1993). The Relationship of Theory and Research (2nd ed.). Philadelphia: F.A. Davis.

Fitzgerald, J. (1988). Nothing but the truth. Nursing Times, 84, 48–9.

Flavell, J. H. (1977). Cognitive Development. Englewood Cliffs, NJ: Prentice-Hall.

Flicker, C., Ferris, S. H., Crook, T., & Bartus, R. T. (1987). A visual recognition memory test for the assessment of cognitive function in aging and dementia. Experimental Aging Research, 13, 127–132.

Folstein, M., Folstein, S., & McHugh, P. (1975). "Mini-mental state:" A practical method for grading the cognitive state of patients for the clinician. Journal of Psychiatric Research, 12, 189.

Franssen, E. H., Kluger, A., Torossian, C. L., & Reisberg, B. (1993). The neurologic syndrome of severe Alzheimer's disease: Relationship to functional decline. Archives of Neurology, 50, 1029–1039.

Ginsberg, H., & Opper, S. (1979). Piaget's Theory of Intellectual Development (2nd ed.). Englewood Cliffs, NJ: Prentice-Hall.

Gugel, R. N. (1988). Managing the problematic behaviors of the Alzheimer's victim. American Journal of Alzheimer's Care and Related Disorders & Research, 5/6, 12–15.

Gwyther, L., & Matteson, M. A. (1983). Care for the caregivers. Journal of Gerontological Nursing, 9, 92–95, 110.

Haight, B. K. (1992). Focusing on dementia. Journal of Gerontological Nursing, 7, 39–48.

Haight, B. K. (1989). Nursing research in long-term care facilities (1984–1988). Nursing and Health Care, 10, 147–150.

Hall, G. R., & Buckwalter, K. C. (1987). Progressively lowered stress threshold: A conceptual model for care of adults with Alzheimer's disease. Archives of Psychiatric Nursing, 1, 399–406.

Hall, G. R., & Buckwalter, K. C. (1990). From almshouse to dedicated unit: Care of institutionalized elderly with behavioral problems. Archives of Psychiatric Nursing, 9, 3–11.

Hooper, F. H., Fitzgerald, J., & Papalia, D. (1971). Piagetian theory and the aging process: Extensions and speculations. Aging and Human Development, 2, 3–20.

Hornblum, J. N., & Overton, W. (1976). Area and volume conservation among the elderly: Assessment and training. Developmental Psychology, 12, 68–74.

Hughston, G. A., & Protinsky, H. O. (1978). Conservation abilities of elderly men and women: A comparative investigation. The Journal of Psychology, 98, 23–26.

Hussian, R. A., & Brown, D. C. (1987). Use of two-dimensional grid patterns to limit hazardous ambulation in demented patients. Journal of Gerontology, 42, 558–560.

Johnson, L., & Keller, K. L. (1989). Staging Alzheimer's disease. Geriatric Nursing, 7/8, 196–197.

Kahn, N., & Stoudemire, A. (1990). Behavioral and pharmacologic management of patients with Alzheimer's disease. Journal of Medical Association of Georgia, 79, 287–294.

Kettle, P. A. (1993). Ten basic rules for managing dementia. Patient Care, 1, 79–86.

LaFrancois, G. R. (1982). Psychology for Teaching (4th ed.). Belmont, CA: Wadsworth Publishing.

Lemke, S., & Moos, R. H. (1987). Measuring the social climate of congregate residences for older people: The sheltered care environment scale. Psychology and Aging, 2, 20–29.

Maas, M. (1988). Management of patients with Alzheimer's disease in long-term care facilities. Nursing Clinics of North America, 23, 57–64.

Maas, M. L., & Buckwalter, K. C. (1991). Alzheimer's disease. Annual Review of Nursing Research, 9, 19–55.

MacDonald, K. C. (1986). Occupational therapy approaches to treatment of dementia patients. Physical & Occupational Therapy in Geriatrics, 4, 61–72.

Mathew, L. J., & Sloane, P. J. (1990). Applying knowledge gained through the special care unit concept to improve care for all demented residents. Gerontologist, 30, 260A.

Matteson, M. A., Linton, A., Cleary, B. L., & Lichtenstein, M. J. (1993). The relationship between Piaget levels of cognitive development and cognitive impairment in persons with dementia. The Gerontologist, 33, 207.

Matteson, M. A., Linton, A., Barnes, S. J., Cleary, B. L., & Lichtenstein, M. J. (1996). The relationship between Piaget and cognitive levels in persons with Alzheimer's disease and related disorders. Aging: Clinical and Experimental Research, 8, 61–69.

Matteson, M. A., Linton, A., Cleary, B. L., Barnes, S. J., & Lichtenstein, M. J. (1995). Management of behavioral symptoms of dementia. Unpublished manuscript, University of Texas Health Science Center, School of Nursing, San Antonio, TX.

Mayeux, R. (1990). Therapeutic strategies in Alzheimer's disease. Neurology, 40, 175–189.

McDougall, G. J. (1990). A review of screening instruments for assessing cognition and mental status in older adults. Nurse Practitioner, 15, 18–28.

Miles, S. H., & Irvine, P. (1992). Deaths caused by physical restraints. Gerontologist, 32, 762–766.

Mira, S. S., Hart, M. N., & Terry, R. D. (1993). Making the diagnosis of Alzheimer's disease: A primer for practicing pathologists. Archives of Pathological Laboratory Medicine, 117, 132–144.

Morse, J. M., & McHutchion, E. (1991). Releasing restraints: Providing safe care for the elderly. Research in Nursing & Health, 14, 187–96.

Musser, P. H., Conger, J. J., & Kagen, J. (1974). Child development and personality (4th ed.). New York: Harper & Row.

Namazi, K. H., Rosner, T. T., & Calkins, M. P. (1989). Visual barriers to prevent Alzheimer's patients from exiting through an emergency door. Gerontologist, 29, 699–702.

Ninos, M., & Makohon, R. (1985). Functional assessment of the patient. Geriatric Nursing, 5/6, 139–142.

Nolen, N. R. (1988). Functional skill regression in late-stage dementias. American Journal of Occupational Therapy, 42, 666–669.

Ort, S. V., & Phillips, L. (1992). Feeding nursing home residents with Alzheimer's disease. Geriatric Nursing, 9/10, 249–253.

Osborn, C. L., & Marshall, M. J. (1992). Promoting mealtime independence. Geriatric Nursing, 9/10, 254–256.

Osborn, C. L., & Marshall, M. J. (1993). Self-feeding performance in nursing home residents. Journal of Gerontological Nursing, 4, 7–14.

Piaget, J. (1952). The Origins of intelligence in children. (M. Cook, trans.) New York: International Universities Press.

Ray, W. A., Taylor, J. A., Lichtenstein, M. J., & Meador, K. G. (1992). The nursing home behavior problem scale. Journal of Gerontology: Medical Sciences, 47, M9–16.

Ray, W. A., Taylor, J. A., Lichtenstein, M. J., & Meador, K. et al. (1991). Managing behavior problems in nursing home residents. Geriatric Medicine, 1, 71–112.

Reisberg, B. (1984). Stages of cognitive decline. American Journal of Nursing, 84, 225–228.

Reisberg, B. (1985). Assessment tool for Alzheimer's type dementia. Hospital and Community Psychiatry, 6, 593–595.

Reisberg, B. (1986). Dementia: A systematic approach to identifying reversible causes. Geriatrics, 4, 30–46.

Reisberg, B. (1988). Functional assessment staging (FAST). Psychopharmacology Bulletin, 24, 653–655.

Reisberg, B., Borenstein, J., Franssen, E., Shulman, E., Steinberg, & Ferris, S. H. (1986). Remedial behavioral symptomatology in Alzheimer's disease. Hospital and Community Psychiatry, 37, 1199–1201.

Reisberg, B., Ferris, S. H., & Franssen, E. (1985). An ordinal functional assessment tool for Alzheimer's-type dementia. Hospital and Community Psychiatry, 36, 593–595.

Reisberg, B., Ferris, S. H., Kluger, A., Franseen, E., de Leon, M. J., Mittelman, M., Borenstein, J., Rameshwar, K., & Alba, R. (1989). Symptomatic changes in CNS aging and dementia of the Alzheimer type: Cross-sectional, temporal and remedial concomitants. In Bergener & B. Reisberg (Eds.), Diagnosis and treatment of senile dementia (193–223). Verlag, Germany: Springer.

Reisberg, B., Ferris, S. H., Torossian, C., Kluger, A., & Monteiro, I. (1992). Pharmacologic treatment of Alzheimer's disease: A methodologic critique based upon current knowledge of symptomatology and relevance for drug trials. International Psychogeriatrics, 4, 9–42.

Reisberg, B., Franssen, E., Sclan, S., Kluger, A., & Ferris, S. H. (1989). Stage specific incidence of potentially remediable behavioral symptoms in aging and Alzheimer disease: A study of 120 patients using the BEHAVE-AD. Bulletin of Clinical Neurosciences, 54, 85–112.

Reisberg, B., Pattschull-Furlan, A., Franssen, E., Sclan, S. G., Kluger, A., Dingcong, L., & Ferris, S. H. (1992). Dementia of the Alzheimer type recapitulates ontogeny inversely on specific ordinal and temporal parameters. In M. T. Rostovic, S. Knezezic, H. Siwniewski, & G. Spilich (Eds.), Neurodevelopment, aging, and cognition (345–369). Boston: Birkhauser.

Reisberg, B., Sclan, S. G., Franssen, E., de Leon, M. J., Kluger, A., Torossian, C., Shulman, E., Steinberg, G., Monteiro, I., McRae, T., Boksay, I., Mackell, J., & Ferris, S. H. (1993). Clinical stages of normal aging and Alzheimer's disease: The GDS staging system. Neuroscience Research Communications, 13, S51–S54.

Ritchie, K. (1988). The screening of cognitive impairment in the elderly: A critical review of current methods. Journal of Clinical Epidemiology, 41, 635–643.

Roberts, B. L., & Algase, D. L. (1988). Victims of Alzheimer's disease and the environment. Nursing Clinics of North America, 23, 83–93.

Rossby, L., Beck, C., & Heacock, P. (1992). Disruptive behaviors of a cognitively impaired nursing home resident. Archives of Psychiatric Nursing, 6, 98–107.

Rubin, E. H., Storandt, M., Miller, J. P., Grant, E. A., Kinscherf, D. A., Morris, J. C., & Berg, L. (1993). Influence of age on clinical and psychometric assessment of subjects with very mild dementia of the Alzheimer type. Archives of Neurology, 50, 380–383.

Rubin, K. H. (1976). Extinction of conservation: A life span investigation. Developmental Psychology, 12, 51–56.

Schafer, S. C. (1985). Modifying the environment. Geriatric Nursing, 6, 157–159.

Schwab, M., Rader, J., & Doan, J. (1985). Relieving the anxiety and fear in dementia. Journal of Gerontological Nursing, 11, 8–15.

Sclan, S. G., Foster, J. R., Reisberg, B., Franssen, E., & Welkowitz, J. (1990). Application of Piagetian measures of cognition in severe Alzheimer's disease. Psychiatric Journal of the University of Ottawa, 15, 223–228.

Sclan, S. G., & Reisberg, B. (1992). Functional assessment staging (FAST) in Alzheimer's disease: Reliability, validity, and ordinality. International Psychogeriatrics, 4, 55–69.

Sloan, P. D., & Mathew, L. J. (1991). An assessment and care planning strategy for nursing home residents with dementia. Gerontologist, 31, 128–131.

Strumpf, N. E., & Evans, L. K. (1988). Physical restraint of the hospitalized elderly: Perceptions of patients and nurses. Nursing Research, 37, 132–137.

Thornbury, J. M. (1992). Cognitive performance on Piagetian tasks by Alzheimer's disease patients. Research in Nursing & Health, 15, 11–18.

Thornbury, J. M. (1993). The use of Piaget's theory in Alzheimer's disease. The American Journal of Alzheimer's Care and Related Disorders & Research, 7/8, 16–21.

Travis, S. S., & Moore, S. R. (1991). Nursing and medical care of primary dementia patients in a community hospital setting. Applied Nursing Research, 4, 14–18.

Trocchio, J. (1989). Life is a bell-shaped curve. Geriatric Nursing, 10, 71.

Turkington, C. (1985). Alzheimer's losses reverse child's gains. American Psychological Association Monitor, 11, 17.

Uzgiris, I. C., & Hunt, J. McV. (1975). Assessment in infancy: Ordinal scales of psychological development. Chicago: University of Illinois Press.

Werner, P., Cohen-Mansfield, J., Braun, J., & Marx, M. S. (1989). Physical restraints and agitation in nursing home residents. Journal of the American Geriatrics Society, 37, 1122–1126.

Wragg, R. E., & Jeste, D. V. (1988). Neuroleptics and alternative treatments. Psychiatric Clinics of North America, 11, 195–213.

Chapter 29

Gerontological Nursing: Application of Ethnography and Grounded Theory

LOIS M. BRANDRIET

Qualitative research methods have long been important to nursing research. This chapter explains the basic principles of two qualitative methods, ethnography and grounded theory, and suggests ways that these methods can enhance nursing knowledge in areas related to care of elders. This author believes that some of the most crucial questions facing us can best be answered through participant observation and interview methods, rather than more standard quantitative approaches.

Immigration, decreasing death rates in infants and children, and the postwar baby boom are contributing to an increasing elder population and will create a gerontological boom following the turn of the century (Schmidt, 1994). Moreover, scientific advances and modern technology have extended the average life span, promulgating chronic disease in elders (Robb, 1984). Increasing health care needs of elders have led to a focus on gerontological research for investigation and funding on a national level; specific areas identified for development include technology assessment, continuity of care, and longterm institutional care (Haight, 1989; Hinshaw, 1988).

The purpose of this chapter is to explicate areas in which ethnography and grounded theory — two qualitative research methods — can be used to advance gerontological nursing research. The basic principles of ethnography and grounded theory are reviewed, and specific research content areas and questions that are amenable to exploration by these methods are addressed.

Whereas quantitative research methods are deductive and intended to test theory, qualitative methods are inductive and generate theory through analyses of rich, detailed data (Lincoln, 1985). Qualitative research is naturalistic in that investigations typically are done in natural field settings, without manipulation of the external environment (Patton, 1987).

Qualitative methods are ideal for exploring when little is known about a phenomenon and for building or generating a theory when a theoretical

From *Journal of Gerontological Nursing* 33–40, July, 1994. Reprinted with permission.

297

framework does not exist (Morse, 1991). Qualitative research is empiric and independent from other studies; however, results also may represent a preliminary step to experimental designs (Patton, 1987). Existing theories, frameworks, or routines also may be questioned by qualitative investigations.

Dogma (received knowledge) has had a great impact on nursing knowledge and requires critical analysis to facilitate productive inquiry (Rodgers, 1991). An example of dogma affecting nursing practice is the provision of nursing care in a manner consistent with institutional routines (versus patient needs) because it is the standard or "known" way to provide care. Thus, qualitative inquiry is used to question or challenge nursing dogma.

In a review of gerontological journals during a 2-year period, the quantity of gerontological nursing and multidisciplinary research was found to be limited, suggesting the need for qualitative exploration of the aging process (O'Leary, 1990). Using qualitative methods also will bypass methodologic limitations inherent with quantitative research of elders, such as the need for large samples, and the lack of valid and reliable instruments specific for elderly populations (Burns, 1987; Engle, 1990).

Without preconceived notions (from nursing dogma/received knowledge), qualitative exploration elicits data from elders' perspectives, without investigator-imposed boundaries. The need to understand elders in relation to cultures and social processes makes ethnography and grounded theory ideal approaches for the study of the aged. Characteristics of these qualitative methods are described below and summarized in Table 29-1.

TABLE 29-1   Ethnography and Grounded Theory: Similarities and Differences

	ETHNOGRAPHY	GROUNDED THEORY
Features	Empirical	Empirical
	Inductive	Inductive
	Holistic	Holistic
	Descriptive	Exploratory
	Discovery oriented	Discovery oriented
	Seeks to understand people of a culture	Seeks to understand social processes
Data Collection	Fieldwork	Fieldwork
	In-depth interviews	In-depth interviews
	Participant observation	Participant observation
	Key informants	Purposive sampling
	Immersion in cultural environment	Immersion in social environment
Data Analysis	Rich description	Patterns/Themes
	Interpretation from emic view	Constant comparative analysis
	Explanatory theories of culture	Interactional processes conceptualized
	Data grounded in cultural experiences	Data grounded in social processes
	Theory generation	Theory generation

Ethnography

Ethnography is a qualitative research method that is used to understand the people of a culture/cultural system to discover meaning and experiences as perceived by its inhabitants. Characterized by inductive, empirical exploration, ethnography is the descriptive fieldwork traditionally used by anthropologists and sociologists (Leininger, 1985). A foreign culture/cultural system, such as a health care institution, may be studied (Leininger, 1970). Appreciation of ethnographic research has been realized by nurses in recent years; it is viewed as a research strategy that emphasizes the holism of nursing.

The ethnographic researcher gains entrance into the culture and becomes immersed with the people and ways of living in order to understand the meanings that cultural participants attach to behaviors, rituals, knowledge, and other experiences. Key informants within the culture/cultural system assist the researcher with translation and understanding of cultural ways of life.

Data collection consists of intentive, in-depth interviewing of key informants and participant observation (Knapp, 1979; Munhall, 1986). Data analysis includes rich description and interpretation from an "emic" point of view; that is, the perspective derived directly from study participants (Leininger, 1988). Description and analysis lead to the products of ethnography, which are descriptive and explanatory theories of a culture. Rich depiction and vivid detail comprise the final ethnography, so that the reader senses what it is like to be part of that culture (Cameron, 1990; Munhall, 1986).

Grounded Theory

Grounded theory is an exploratory qualitative research method developed by sociologists Glaser and Strauss (1967) that is gaining popularity in nursing. Like ethnographers, grounded theorists perceive the world through the eyes of informants, and discover/generate theory by inductive, holistic, and empirical analyses. Unlike ethnographers, grounded theorists seek to understand social processes by immersion in social environments.

In-depth interviewing and participant observation are used to collect data in a naturalistic setting. Purposive sampling ensures that subjects possess the phenomenon of interest. Due to the voluminous data generation of in-depth interviews, sample size is typically small. Actual sample size is generally not predetermined; rather, data are collected until no new information surfaces (data saturation). Through constant comparative analyses, grounded theorists look for common themes and patterns in the development of theoretical constructs, and complex interactional processes are conceptualized (Glaser, 1967; Hutchinson, 1986).

▬RESEARCH DEVELOPMENT AND FUNDING PRIORITY CONTENT AREAS

Qualitative exploration has unlimited potential for studying gerontological content areas that are targeted for research development and funding. Technology, continuity of care, and long-term care are research development and funding priority areas that will be described in relation to specific issues and questions, and are amenable to ethnographic or grounded theory inquiry.

Technology Assessment

Due to increased chronic disease and institutionalization, elders are mass consumers of modern technology. Artificial devices, computers, and invasive/obtrusive equipment for patient monitoring, maintenance, and diagnosis are examples of "hardware" technology. Increasingly complex technology has a tremendous impact on nurses and provision of patient care, creating a more stressful machine-oriented environment — and less time for personalized, empathic patient care. Individual/family response to technology dependence is a research development priority, yet few studies have assessed the impact of technology on the elder, nurse, nursing practice, or quality of care (Leininger, 1988; Pillar, 1990).

Studying technology from an ethnographic perspective would contribute to an understanding of elders' (foreign and/or native) reluctance or refusal to consent to procedures or equipment (hardware technology) (Leininger, 1988). Environments immersed in invasive or obtrusive equipment would be ideal for studying the impact of technology on elders and nurses. Such environments are no longer limited to intensive care units or acute care settings. Computers, ventilators, and intravenous equipment are but a few of the technologic advances in long-term care settings today.

Potential research questions for ethnographic or grounded theory study are numerous and include moral, ethical, legal, social, and human components of care (Pillar, 1990). How does technology influence empathic patient care? What are elder/family responses to invasive or obtrusive equipment when the elder is technologically dependent or terminally ill? How is it morally and ethically determined when not to employ or when to remove life-sustaining devices? Moral and ethical issues involving basic human needs also should be addressed. For example, how is it determined if and when a terminally ill elder should be hydrated with intravenous fluid?

Resolving such issues is especially problematic with institutionalized elders due to their perceived vulnerability and inability to make decisions (Coulton, 1982; Ryden, 1984). Although often thought of in terms of its "hardware" orientation, technology also includes "software," such as laws, work patterns, and information systems. An example of technology software affecting elders is the prospective payment system of 1983 (Pillar, 1990). Its promotion of early hospital discharges for Medicare recipients raised continuity of care issues.

Continuity of Care

A form of software technology and research development priority area, the Medicare prospective payment system promotes early hospital discharge, reduces planning time, and increases complexity of discharge planning for hospitalized elders (Blumenfield, 1987). The advantage of timely hospital discharge is that acute health care costs are reduced; however, elders often need to complete their recovery in nursing homes or at home with caregiver or professional nursing assistance (Smith, 1985).

Quality assessment of discharge planning programs has become crucial because of these challenges. In a quantitative study examining discharge planning programs for positive outcomes in elders, no relation was found between the process used for discharge planning and positive patient outcomes (Haddock, 1991). A relation may exist between the variables that could not be identified quantitatively. The "process" of discharge planning may be better discerned by qualitative methods. A qualitative research method to evaluate program processes has been explicated (Patton, 1987).

Discharge planning programs are multifactorial and give rise to many research questions that could be assessed by using grounded theory. How is patient referral made to a discharge planner? What step-by-step processes does an elder receiving discharge planning encounter from pre-admission to post-discharge? Hospital discharge planning also should be examined in terms of its impact outside the acute care setting. For example, how have early hospital discharges affected elders, caregivers, and nurses in long-term and home health care?

One aspect of continuity of care about which little is understood is decision-making involvement of hospitalized elders in planning their post-discharge care (Cameron, 1990). In a correlational study of institutionalized elders, Brandriet (1991) found no relation between decision-making involvement in hospital discharge planning and acceptance of change to nursing home placement. Brandriet's assumption, based on dogma/received knowledge, was that hospitalized elders would want to be involved in their discharge decisions. To the contrary, elders' comments consistently indicated that they had no desire to be involved in the decision-making process.

The incongruence between Brandriet's (1991) and elders' perceptions of decision making suggests that exploration is required to discover the emic meaning of making decisions. What led to elder passivity in making decisions — that is, the decision to discharge to a nursing home? An ethnographic study would identify the emic meaning of active or passive decision making of elders within an acute care setting, and thereby clarify the construct. Grounded theory would further clarify the construct by explicating processes involved in active or passive discharge decisions.

Institutional Long-Term Care

Escalating numbers of elders, longevity, chronic diseases, and early hospital discharges have increased occupancy rates and patient acuity in long-term care facilities (Institute of Medicine, 1986). As a consequence, more elders are in need of highly complex, skilled, quality long-term care than ever before (Ambrogi, 1990; Rantz, 1990). Increasing complexity of care for greater numbers of elders has resulted in new directions for research specific to long-term care. Quality of care, health promotion, self-care agency, and elder dependence are research funding priority areas that will be discussed in relation to elders in long-term care facilities.

QUALITY OF LONG-TERM CARE. In addition to increasing patient care needs, recent government regulations have placed quality of care issues at the forefront of long-term care (Ammentorp, 1991). Although long required for accreditation standards by hospitals, formal quality assurance programs have been mandated in nursing homes only recently. The Omnibus Budget Reconciliation Act (OBRA) (1987), a legislative response to long-standing quality of care issues in long-term care facilities, was enacted on October 1, 1990. Among other factors, the law stipulates quality assurance requirements in detail. The reality that quality assurance had to be mandated gives credence to the enormity of quality issues and the need for evaluative research in long-term care.

Quality assurance programs in long-term care should have a direct impact on quality of patient care as opposed to merely representing written standards for accreditation purposes. Exploratory research is necessary to evaluate these newly implemented programs, particularly in regard to actual patient outcomes. Quality assurance research also should evaluate the cost-effectiveness of resources/nursing interventions, program operations, process, and documentation of patient benefits and associated costs. A broad research question to evaluate a quality assurance program should elicit whether the program does what it is intended to do.

For example, two patient care areas that quality assurance programs are required (by OBRA) to address are psychosocial functioning and activities of daily living. Is assessment and maintenance of psychosocial functioning in long-term care elders a reality to elders, nurses, and administrators? The reality of nurses and administrators may differ greatly from the reality of patients (emic view), which ethnographers seek to understand. Ways in which independence is promoted in activities of daily living could be assessed by using grounded theory to explicate the process.

A grounded theorist also might study the social system of long-term care to discover behavior problems contributing to poor quality care. System subgroups strive to gain rewards, recognition, and power within the system. This process may lead to decreased staff morale and increased staff turnover, chronic problems in long-term care (Leininger, 1970; Tellis-Nayak, 1989). Explicating staff behavior patterns would guide leaders in long-term care regarding counseling and conflict resolution needs of staff members. Enhancing staff morale would likely have a positive impact on quality care.

Program evaluation researchers examine data for recurring themes and patterns in comprehending the day-to-day reality of program functioning. Grounded theory offers an ideal way to study programs, both as process and product. The process reveals how the program came to do what it does; the product explicates a model or theory of program outcomes.

HEALTH PROMOTION IN LONG-TERM CARE. Provision of nursing care to promote health in long-term care is largely based on institutional policies and routines (dogma), although little is known about health and illness from elders' perspectives. Thus, ethnographic study is needed to elicit the emic view of health, illness, and care needs (as opposed to the nursing or institutional view). For instance, what does health promotion or disease prevention mean to the institutionalized elder? Health may be perceived differently by the elder residing in the community than by the institutionalized elder. Grounded theorists could explain practices/processes by which elders meet their health care needs.

A medical model of care predominates in long-term care, which supports patient dependency on health care personnel (Ambrogi, 1990). In contrast, gerontological nursing models promote independence in activities of daily living, prevention of disease, and health promotion and maintenance (American Nurses Association, 1986). In addition to understanding elders' view of health, seeking in-depth knowledge about health meaning and experiences may have a broader impact on nursing practice in two ways. First, emerging theories, grounded in data from ethnography or grounded theory, may refine and expand nursing practice models to promote health and independence in long-term care elders. Secondly, theory development may guide the design and initiation of formal health promotion programs.

SELF-CARE AGENCY/INDEPENDENCE IN LONG-TERM CARE. Qualitative inquiry can be used to question nursing dogma (i.e., a concept within an existing theory). To illustrate, Orem's (1971) self-care theory assumes that the concept of independence is a requisite for health and is desired by health care recipients (Munhall, 1986). Eliciting meanings and processes of self-care inductively would serve to clarify and/or question the concept of independence.

Little is known about patterns of self-care in long-term care elders, although shifting health care values from curing to disease prevention has initiated an interest in the phenomenon. Acquiring knowledge of self-care practices is important for health promotion purposes and to reduce health care costs. Exercising self-care agency promotes psychosocial health by increasing satisfaction and self-confidence; costs of care decrease as independent elders reduce nursing care needs (Davidson, 1988; Kearney, 1979; Lakin, 1988).

Several instruments have been developed to measure self-care (Denyes, 1980; Hanson, 1985; Kearney, 1979). As a consequence, many investigations have used quantitative data and analysis. Unfortunately, no self-care instruments were identified that had been designed for and validated on elderly populations, making quantitative studies of self-care in elders prone to measurement error.

Findings from an ethnograph or grounded theory could be used to develop a self-care instrument for institutionalized elders. Because data are grounded in elders' reality, instrument items would be relevant to this population (Mishel, 1990). Qualitative data, then, also can be used to enhance quantitative measurement.

ELDER DEPENDENCE IN LONG-TERM CARE. Instead of self-care or independence, dependent behavior frequently is observed in institutionalized elders. Similar to acute care settings and consistent with the medical model of care, the long-term care environment fosters the sick role and, hence, the dependent-patient role (Ammentorp, 1991).

Exploration of the concept *dependence* is needed in long-term care to assess whether dependent behavior is due to functional disabilities/limitations or environmental factors (iatrogenic dependence). Long-term care elders may become iatrogenically dependent as a consequence of nurses and nurse aides "doing" tasks to expedite their completion, regardless of elder ability (Miller, 1985).

Elder independence in feeding or bathing often is not encouraged or tolerated because tasks may be performed at a slower pace. Expedience in carrying out tasks may be supported and rewarded by administrative personnel to maintain institutional routines, reduce staff time, and thereby reduce costs.

In the long run, however, a nurse will likely spend more time "doing" tasks than facilitating or guiding self-care behavior. Moreover, promotion or encouragement of dependent behavior may decrease elder control, autonomy and self-worth, thereby promulgating psychosocial and physical problems (Jirovec, 1990).

Ethnographic study would identify the meaning of dependence within the long-term care arena as a cultural system. Grounded theory would explore processes leading to dependent behavior, such as the social and environmental impact on patient dependence.

Specific questions should elicit opportunities for patient decision-making and control within the nursing home (social system). By what process are elders (who are capable of performing activities of daily living) encouraged and/or allowed to independently perform these activities? What aspects of elders' lives are most important for them to control? Is a resident council established and functioning so that elders have involvement in decisions regarding patient care and services?

Participant observation would enable the researcher to observe and record behaviors of elders and nursing staff members and interactions among them. Interviewing elders, nurses, and administrative staff members would elicit various perspectives of dependence and factors involved with its evolution.

▬LIMITATIONS/STRENGTHS OF ETHNOGRAPHY AND GROUNDED THEORY IN ELDERLY POPULATIONS

Interviewing institutionalized elders may pose threats to internal validity. In an ethnographic study of nursing home elders, validity threats were imposed by physical, cognitive, affective and personal characteristics of elders, which led to unclear, insufficient interviews (West, 1991). The authors recommended several strategies for countering interview validity threats. Both ethnography and grounded theory use indepth interviews as a primary data collection tool and could be plagued by similar interviewing difficulties.

Strengths of using ethnography and grounded theory include eliciting data from elders' perspectives without preconceived hypotheses. Provided that interviewing difficulties are overcome, elders, with their history of experiences, have much to share. Data are rich in individualistic and cultural experiences. Moreover, data are grounded in the understanding of cultural beliefs, social systems, and program evaluations. For this reason, nursing practices designed as a result of these data are likely to be useful.

▬ NURSING PRACTICE IMPLICATIONS

Ethnography and grounded theory are viable research approaches to examine many aspects of elder care. Ethnography focuses on understanding elders in relation to their culture or cultural system (i.e., health care institution); grounded theory explores basic social processes. Both methods elicit data rich in detail and grounded in the reality of elders.

Gerontological content areas with research development and funding priority on a national level include technology, continuity of care, and institutional long-term care. These content areas are prime investigative domains, in part, because of their national attention. However, technology, continuity of care, and longterm care also represent areas of significance to the clinical practice of gerontological nurses.

Although advancements in technology may supplement and strengthen nursing interventions, they may simultaneously pose moral/legal dilemmas, affecting the ability of a nurse to care for patients (versus machines) in an empathic manner. Assessing/maintaining quality of discharge planning programs may prevent premature patient discharge and smooth the transition to a post-discharge setting.

To meet the needs of increasing numbers of elders in need of complex care in long-term care facilities, enhancing quality of care, promoting health and independence, and minimizing iatrogenic elder dependence are not luxuries. Rather, they are necessities — not only to provide and improve care, but also to reduce long-term health care costs. Answering research questions specific to these content areas may contribute understanding to issues about which little is known — but must be known — by practicing gerontological nurses.

▬ REFERENCES

Ambrogi, D.M. Legal issues in nursing home admissions. *Law, Medicine, and Health Care* 1990; 18(3):254–262.

American Nurses Association. *ANA Statement on minimal professional staffing in nursing homes.* Kansas City, MO: Author, 1986.

Ammentorp, W., Gossett, K.D., Euchner, N.P. *Quality assurance for long-term care providers.* Newbury Park, CA: Sage, 1991.

Blumenfield, S., Lowe, J.I. A template for analyzing ethical dilemmas in discharge planning. *Health Soc Work* 1987; 12(1):47–56.

Brandriet, L.M. Decision-making involvement related to acceptance of the elderly to nursing home placement. *Clinical Gerontologist: The Journal of Aging and Mental Health* 1991; 11(1):77–79.

Burns, N., Grove, S.K. *The practice of nursing research: Conduct, critique, and utilization.* Philadelphia: W. B. Saunders, 1987.

Cameron, C. The ethnographic approach: Characteristics and uses in gerontological nursing. *Journal of Gerontological Nursing* 1990; 16(9):5–7.

Coulton, C.J., Dunkle, R.E., Goode, R.A., MacKintosh, J. Discharge planning and decision making. *Health Soc Work* 1982; 7(4):253–261.

Davidson, J.D.U. *Health embodiment: The relationship between self-care agency and health promoting behaviors.* Unpublished doctoral dissertation, Texas Women's University, Denton, 1988.

Denyes, M. Development of an instrument to measure self-care agency in adolescents (Doctoral dissertation, University of Michigan, 1980). *Dissertation Abstracts International* 1980; 80:25672.

Engle, V.F., Graney, M.J. Meta-analysis for the refinement of gerontological nursing research and theory. *Journal of Gerontological Nursing* 1990; 16(9):12–15.

Glaser, B.G., Strauss, A.L. *The discovery of grounded theory.* Chicago: Aldine, 1967.

Haddock, K.S. Characteristics of effective discharge planning programs for the frail elderly. *Journal of Gerontological Nursing* 1991; 17(7):10–14.

Haight, B.K. Nursing research in long-term care facilities (1984–1988). *Nursing and Health Care* 1989; 10(3):147–150.

Hanson, B.R., Bickel, L. Development and testing of the questionnaire on the perception of self-care agency. In J. Riehl-Sisca (Ed.), *The science and art of self-care.* Norwalk, CT: Appleton-Century-Crofts, 1985, pp. 271–278.

Hinshaw, A.S., Heinrich, J., Bloch, D. Evolving clinical nursing research priorities: A national endeavor. *J Prof Nurs* 1988; 4(6):398,458–459.

Hutchinson, S. Grounded theory: The method. In P.L. Munhall, C.J. Oiler (Eds.), *Nursing research: A qualitative perspective.* Norwalk, CT: Appleton-Century-Crofts, 1986, pp. 113–130.

Institute of Medicine, Committee on Nursing Home Regulation. *Improving the quality of care in nursing homes.* Washington, DC: National Academy Press, 1986.

Jirovec, M.M., Kasno, J. Self-care agency as a function of patient-environmental factors among nursing home residents. *Res Nurs Health* 1990; 13:303–309.

Kearney, B.Y., Fleischer, B.J. Development of an instrument to measure exercise of self-care agency. *Res Nurs Health* 1979; 2(1):25–34.

Knapp, M.S. Ethnographic contributions to evaluation research. In T.D. Cook, C.S. Reichardt (Eds.), *Qualitative and quantitative methods in evaluation research.* Beverly Hills, CA: Sage, 1979, pp. 118–139.

Lakin, J.A. Self-care, health locus of control, and health value among faculty women. *Public Health Nurs* 1988; 5(1):37–44.

Leininger, M.M. *Nursing and anthropology: Two worlds to blend.* New York: John Wiley and Sons, 1970.

Leininger, M.M. *Qualitative research methods in nursing.* Orlando, FL: Grune & Stratton, 1985.

Leininger, M.M. History, issues, and trends in the discovery and uses of care in nursing. In M.M. Leininger (Ed.), *CARE: Discovery and uses in clinical and community nursing.* Detroit: Wayne State University, 1988, pp. 11–28.

Lincoln, Y.S., Guba, E.G. *Naturalistic inquiry.* Newbury Park, CA: Sage, 1985.

Miller, A. Nurse/patient dependency — is it iatrogenic? *J Adv Nurs* 1985; 10(1):63–69.

Mishel, M. Methodological studies: Instrument development. In P. Brink, M.J. Wood (Eds.), *Advanced design in nursing research.* New York: Sage, 1990, pp. 238–284.

Morse, J.M. *Qualitative nursing research: A contemporary dialogue.* Newbury Park, CA: Sage, 1991.

Munhall, P.L., Oiler, C.J. *Nursing research: A qualitative perspective.* Norwalk, CT: Appleton-Century-Crofts, 1986.

O'Leary, P.A., McGill, J.S., Jones, K.E., Paul, P.B. Gerontological research: Is it useful for nursing practice? *Journal of Gerontological Nursing* 1990; 16(5):28–32.

Omnibus Budget Reconciliation Act of 1987. Public Law 100-203, Subtitle C, 1819(c)(5) & 1919(c)(5).

Orem, D.E. *Nursing: Concepts in practice.* New York: McGraw-Hill, 1971.

Patton, M.Q. *How to use qualitative methods in evaluation.* Newbury Park, CA: Sage, 1987.

Pillar, B., Jacox, A.K., Redman, B.K. Technology, its assessment, and nursing. *Nurs Outlook* 1990; 38(1):16–19.

Rantz, J. Inadequate reimbursement for longterm care. *Nursing and Health Care* 1990; 11(9):470–472.

Robb, S. The elderly in the United States: Numbers, proportions, health status, and use of health services. In A.G. Yurich, B.E. Spier, S.S. Robb, N.J. Ebert (Eds.), *The aged person and the nursing process.* Norwalk, CT: Appleton-Century-Crofts, 1984, pp. 33–61.

Rodgers, B.L. Deconstructing the dogma in nursing knowledge and practice. *Image: Journal of Nursing Scholarship* 1991; 23(3):177–181.

Ryden, M.B. Morale and perceived control in the institutionalized elderly. *Nurs Res* 1984; 33(3):130–136.

Schmidt, M.G., Burnside, I. Demographic and psychosocial aspects of aging. In I. Burnside, M.G. Schmidt (Eds.), *Working with older adults: Group process and techniques.* Boston: Jones and Bartlett, 1994, pp. 8–23.

Smith, D.S., Coleman, J.R., Lebeda, J.R. Capturing savings from system design. *Nursing Management* 1985; 16(5):25–33.

Tellis-Nayak, V., Tellis-Nayak, M. Quality of care and the burden of two cultures: When the world of the nurse's aide enters the world of the nursing home. *Gerontologist* 1989; 29(3):307–313.

West, M., Bondy, E., Hutchinson, S. Interviewing institutionalized elders: Threats to validity. *Image: Journal of Nursing Scholarship* 1991; 23(3):171–176.

Chapter 30

Interviewing Institutionalized Elders: Threats to Validity

MARY WEST   ELIZABETH BONDY   SALLY HUTCHINSON

As the previous chapter espouses, qualitative research methods can provide us with wonderful data, but there are inherent problems with validity — especially when interviewing institutionalized elders. Is it possible to increase the validity of our data when we interview cognitively or physically impaired older adults? These authors encountered many problems while doing ethnographic research in a nursing home setting. Based on this experience, they analyze the most common threats to validity, and delineate effective strategies that worked for them.

A fundamental assumption of qualitative research is that reality is "a multiple set of mental constructions" (Lincoln & Guba, 1985, p. 295). The researcher's goal is to represent reality as it has been constructed by the individuals being studied. In short, the researcher strives for valid findings, which means "to understand a situation as it is seen by the participants" (Dobbert, 1982, p. 260). Although people being studied may not be aware of their mental constructions of reality, the constructions are expressed in what they say and do. By observing and talking with individuals, a researcher can gain access to their reality. However, observing and interviewing pose problems for researchers who are concerned with the validity of their findings, and these problems have been widely discussed (LeCompte & Goetz, 1982; McCall & Simmons, 1969; Schwartz & Jacobs, 1979). Dobbert (1982) summarized the following characteristics of "good" informants; that is, those participants who are likely to provide valid data:

> They appear comfortable and unstrained in interactions with the researcher; they are generally open and truthful although they may have certain areas about which they will not speak or where they will cover up; they provide solid answers with good detail; they stay on the topic on related important issues; they are thoughtful and willing to reflect on what they say. (p. 263)

From *Image: Journal of Nursing Scholarship* 23(3):171–176, 1991. Reprinted with permission.

When studying the institutionalized elderly, few informants can be found who display Dobbert's characteristics of good informants. In fact, the characteristics of impaired, institutionalized elders threatens the validity of studies which seek to uncover elders' views of reality. The purpose of this paper is to explicate the difficulties encountered when interviewing institutionalized elders and to recommend strategies for overcoming these difficulties.

■BACKGROUND AND LITERATURE REVIEW

The preponderance of research on institutionalized elders has relied on quantitative methods of study. In an exhaustive review of elders' responses to instruments used in quantitative studies of social functioning of elders, Kane and Kane (1981) conclude: "The consistently positive responses of institutionalized patients to a wide range of experimental interventions suggest that the attention and stimulation itself may produce the change as much as the specific independent variable" (p. 139). This summary of the state of research on institutionalized elders underscores the need to adopt alternative approaches to learn about this population.

Qualitative research methods provide an alternative approach by offering institutionalized elders the opportunity to define their feelings about interventions designed to affect their lives; unhappily, these same methods introduce major problems for the researcher. With informant interviewing and participant observation the major data collection tools, qualitative researchers face significant challenges when studying frail, impaired elders in institutional settings, a fact recently discovered in the course of an ethnographic study of an intergenerational Geriatric Remotivation Program in a Southeastern U.S. nursing home.

The program under study involved 15 volunteer, middle-school children who were transported by van after school for twice-weekly, one-hour sessions in the nursing home. Each child was paired with an elder who became his or her "Pal." In many cases these partnerships continued for two or three years. Activities planned by program coordinators were games and crafts chosen to promote certain outcomes in the elders such as physical stimulation or reminiscence. Occasionally, there were special programs, such as picnics, nursing home festivities or visits to the school. In all cases, the elder-child partners participated together during activities. The research questions relevant to the present paper were:

How do elders experience the program? Do they value the program? Do they hear, see and understand program activities? Do they actively participate in the program and value their participation? Do they find their relationships with their middle-school partners satisfying? Does the child-elder relationship contribute positively to the life satisfaction of the elders? Are these relationships satisfying to children?

Data were collected during three week periods in the fall, winter and spring of two consecutive school years. The three methods of data collection were audio-visual documentation, participant observation and informant interviewing. Many interviews were taped; others were hand-written and dictated into a tape recorder immediately after the interview. We took field notes and later dictated our notes into a tape recorder. This paper focuses on difficulties with interviewing the elder.

We approached this study of social interaction between institutionalized elders and middle-school children in fundamentally the same way we would approach the study of subjects of other ages in other settings. Literature that provides direction for qualitative study, such as Spradley's (1979, 1980) texts on ethnographic methodology, did not prepare us for the particular problems of interviewing impaired elders with multiple functional disabilities: hearing loss, memory impairment or communication deficits. Furthermore, methodologists provided no strategies for decoding impaired elders' behavior during participant observation. Profound poverty of movement, gesture or expression was the rule. Low volume voices, difficult to hear in close proximity, let alone on videotape, were the norm. We came to expect "thin" data and were overjoyed when snippets of rich data emerged from time to time.

A search of the literature for reports of methodology difficulties encountered by other investigators conducting similar studies was non-productive. Powers (1988) used participant observation and informant interviews in a study of institutionalized elders' social networks; however, no mention was made of methodologic difficulties. The investigator acknowledged that elders with physical, cognitive or communication deficits were excluded from the study — the very subjects least able to muster or sustain social support and presumably most in need of being studied. The recently released *Qualitative Research Methods Series* and *Applied Social Research Methods Series* (Sage Publications, 1989) suggest that differences exist in populations at the extremes of the life cycle by including a volume about problems using qualitative methods to study children (Fine & Sandstrom, 1988). Yet no author in these 33 volumes contributed a similar perspective about elders, in particular those who reside in institutions.

The bulk of the literature addresses issues about quantitative methodology in aging research. One problem discussed extensively in the medical and sociological literature is the validity and reliability of elders' responses to data collection instruments (Jackson, Ramsdell, Renvall, Swart, and Ward, 1989; Perry, 1982; Ebrahim, Morgan, Dallosso, Bassey, Harries, and Terry, 1987). Another methodology problem described by a number of authors (Berkowitz, 1978; Butler, Vestal, Lawton, et al. 1977; Duffy, Wyble, Wilson, and Miles, 1989; Herzog and Rodgers, 1988; Hoffman, Marron, Fillit, and Libow, 1983; Mercer and Butler, 1967; Norris, 1985; Robb, 1983; Todd, Davis and Cafferty, 1984) is getting and keeping elders in studies; that is, obtaining informed consent, avoiding recruitment bias and recognizing the causes for and outcomes of subject attrition.

Although the abundant literature about recruitment and retention of elderly subjects focused solely on the entry or exit point of the research process, the problems described by these authors mirror those we experienced during data collection. Hoffman et al. (1983) enumerated these obstacles in an article about obtaining informed consent from elderly subjects: time-consuming interviews; need for repetition; vision and hearing deficits; memory and cognitive impairment; aphasias and language barriers; limited education; poor vocabulary skills; and the lonely elder's desire to chat with a captive listener.

Sample and Method
Nursing home staff identified elders in need of social stimulation and referred them to the therapeutic program under study. In order to understand whether the therapy worked, all elders in the program were studied. Consequently, our sample included elders with varying degrees of psychological and physical impairment. Diagnoses included Parkinson's disease, stroke and a variety of dementias. The all-male sample ranged in age from 58 to 100.

▬FINDINGS
Our findings came from a search of our field notes that documented our difficulties in interviewing these men. Four main clusters of elder characteristics threatened the validity of interview data: (1) physical characteristics; (2) cognitive characteristics; (3) affective characteristics; and (4) personal characteristics. Essentially, elders' impairments often made it difficult for us to collect and interpret data.

Physical characteristics included such things as being in pain; being unable to see and hear; urinary urgency; and being unable to move small and large muscles. All of these factors affected elders' ability to communicate clearly. Although all the elders did not experience all of these conditions, many of them experienced several. Elders frequently were difficult to understand because they spoke so quietly and/or did not articulate clearly. The meaning of their restricted movements was often difficult to interpret. And, data often were nonexistent due to an elder's physical condition; that is, an elder in extreme pain or suffering from a distressing physical ailment was likely to remain in bed or leave a program session early.

Cognitive factors also threatened the validity of data gathered from some elders. A number of the men were frequently disoriented to time and place, had difficulty remembering people and events (long and short term memory deficits) and failed to recognize others. Often elders could not remember what happened only a few minutes earlier. Because some of the elders were disoriented during the sessions, we had difficulty interpreting their actions or lack of activity.

Affective characteristics of elders refer to the ways in which elders expressed their feelings. Generally, elders displayed flat affect — blank faces and unexpressive eyes. For some this was due to a physical condition, such as Parkinson's Disease. Others appeared to be depressed or unhappy with their circumstances at the nursing home. Although facial expression and body language normally provide a researcher with clues to participants' thoughts and feelings, these clues were unavailable from a number of participants.

Finally, elders' personal characteristics threatened data validity. The elders in this institution represented a range of socioeconomic, educational, career and ethnic backgrounds. As a result, although they all spoke English, their language reflected their backgrounds and life experience. In attempting to understand the elders, we had to tune in to many dialects spoken in the nursing home. Differences phonological, syntactic and semantic features of language were evident. For instance, often we were not sure what an elder meant when he used familiar words in ways which were unfamiliar to us. Attempts to clarify meaning were frequently unsuccessful, due to the elder's cognitive and physical impairments.

The four main characteristics — physical, cognitive, affective, and personal — directly affected interview data. We categorized problematic data as *insufficient, unclear, nice* and *emotionally charged.* Recommendations for researchers studying institutionalized elders follow a presentation of types of problematic data.

Insufficient or "thin" data were the norm. Many elders responded to standardized, open-ended, evaluative questions about the program with patterned, minimized responses.

> *Int:* What do you talk to your pal about?
> *Elder:* Different things.
> *Int:* Like what?
> *Elder:* Different things.
> *Int:* Are the kids coming today?
> *Elder:* Yeah.
> *Int:* What do you think you'll be doing?
> *Elder:* I don't know what they'll be doing today.
> *Int:* What do they do most times?
> *Elder:* Different things.
> *Int:* Do you remember what those things are?
> *Elder:* Not off hand.

After numerous difficult interviews like the ones above, we erroneously concluded that the length of time between the end of that day's activity and the interview itself directly affected the quality of the data. However, *altering the time of the interview,* as in the following example of an interview done less than 10 minutes after the activity had ended, often proved unsuccessful.

> *Int:* Were the kids here today?
> *Elder:* The boy was, I know. (His partner was a girl)
> *Int:* The boy was. Un-huh.
> *Elder:* Uh-huh.
> *Int:* What does the boy look like?
> *Elder:* I couldn't tell you, he's a little dark skinned boy. (Partner was fair with very light brown hair)
> *Int:* A little dark skinned boy. Were you at the program today?
> *Elder:* I was there.
> *Int:* What did they do?
> *Elder:* I don't know. I don't pay them too much attention cause it wasn't so hot to me.

Although we had been schooled in the use of open-ended questions, our lack of success in acquiring meaningful data led us by trial and error to use probing questions. As the following example demonstrates, this too did not guarantee success.

Int: When you were talking about autumn with the children, I'd like to know whether you had any memories about autumn and what you used to do when you were younger.

Elder: No

Int: When you think about it right now, when you think about the fall of the year, do you have any memories of what you used to do as a young man during the fall?

Elder: No. I don't remember anything particular.

Int: If you had a choice, let's say between spending an hour the way you did yesterday when you saw baby pictures and made some crafts, or spending an hour just talking with your pal, what do you think that you would enjoy the best of those two activities?

Elder: I just can't say, I just don't know.

Int: I guess what I'm getting at, is there anything you would rather be doing with the children than what you are presently doing?

Elder: I can't think of nothing.

For some elders, *waiting for the response* for several minutes occasionally paid off.

Int: What do you like about the program?

Elder: Everything, everything.

Int: Tell me what you like. (several minutes of silence elapsed)

Elder: It brings us much closer together.

Unclear data refers to data that simply did not make sense to the interviewer. Sometimes the answer did not fit the question being asked. Note the following examples:

Int: Are there other things here in the nursing home that make you laugh, or is the kid's program the most laughable one?

Elder: Well, laughable one. It is not foolish though.

Int: I don't understand.

Elder: A lot of them school show that senior citizens can take up.

Int: Tell me about that.

Elder: Well, like you shouldn't throw them away.

Int: Hmm?

Elder: You shouldn't throw those things away. Keep them in the back of the noodle.

Int: Throw what things away?

Elder: What the kids do and what they say. I should only said some of them.

Int: I don't think I understood what you said.

Elder: Well, there is a lot of senior citizens that don't follow the rules and they stay in a group.

Int: They stay where?

Elder: They stay in one place. They are afraid to move from one place to another and they don't say really what they mean.

In other examples, of unclear data elders used words and syntax that required *translation* by the investigator.

"Not really they can't talk the past far enough for me." (translation: The kids are too young to be able to talk about the old days or historical events.)

"She doesn't put up any conversation." (translation: My pal doesn't talk to me.)

"I've sat at the Judge's Bench and don't know what a child or children might construe." (translation: I don't talk to my pal because she might misunderstand me.)

(When asked if he thought the kids were the right age for this type of program) "They can say all the conversations when they are a bit smaller, but to get meaning on it should be 10 until 12." (translation: Younger kids can talk but they have to be older to really carry on a good conversation.)

"It's hard for me to say, because this one will say one thing and another one another, and you got it hard to get it together to where you understand it yourself. (translation: Sometimes it's hard for me to follow the kid's conversations.)

(When asked how he knows his pal doesn't like to be corrected) "It takes her breath away from her." (translation: She acts surprised.)

In other situations, *listening for a theme, interpreting it, and stating it in the form of a question* helped the researchers understand the elder's meaning:

Int: What about the older men? What do they get out of the Program?
Elder: They get to, with the children, younger children, every, they won't ever, they have somebody, some old man, some like me or somebody else, they have a pal and they, whatever . . . ah, I don't know.
Int: So you think the men get friendships out of it?
Elder: Yeah. Friendships. They have somebody to, the little girls, they have little girls and the little girls have the person and when they come and she does talks to him in that way.

Nice data refer to socially acceptable comments that appear interview after interview, contributing little to the purpose of evaluating the program. Elders who provided nice data did not seem to be actively involved in the conversation with the researcher. *Probing questions* or *waiting for responses* were unsuccessful in acquiring rich data. Following is an example of nice data:

Int: Hi. I'm interested in knowing how you felt about the program and finding out if you have any suggestions about how we might be able to improve it.
Elder: Oh, I can't tell you, I like it so well.

Emotionally charged refer to data gathered during interviews in which the elder expressed strong emotions such as sadness, anger, fear, or pain.

Sadness:

Int: What would be your general analysis of the kid's program?
Res W: Well, I think it's a great thing.

Int: And why do you think that?
Res W: Well, it does us good and the kids good. (Starts to cry).
Int: Does you good.
Res W: (still crying) Yeah.
Int: Tell me why it does you good or how would you describe the good it does you.
Res W: (still crying) Well, being around kids.
Int: What about being around kids is good?
Res W: It just makes me feel good.
Int: Happiness.
Res W: Yeah.
Int: Huh. Well that's great. So you think being around 'us old folks' isn't near as much fun, huh?
Res W: (laughs through tears) No, it ain't.

Anger:

Int: Un-huh. What do you do with Debbie?
Elder: We just talk and converse back and forth and do things together.
Int: Can you tell me what you talk about?
Elder: Well, about school and activities and . . .
Int: So what she's doing you talk about.
Elder: What she's doing and I tell her what I'm doing.
Int: Un-huh. What are you doing?
Elder: Well, what I'm doing every day, like now talking to you and . . .
Int: Um-hum. So you might tell her about that, today.
Elder: Yeah. And what I make in OT, occupational therapy, and then I make her things.
Int: Oh, you do. Great.
Elder: Yeah, well, keep her interested in me.
Int: That keeps her interested in you by giving her gifts. Is that right?
Elder: Yeah . . . Not exactly, I'm not buying . . . You're kinda irritating me.
Int: I'm so sorry.
Elder: I'm not buying her friendship.
Int: No, I'm sorry. That isn't, I thought I was repeating back what you said. I didn't mean to read anything into that. Okay. I apologize. Would . . .
Elder: I'm kinda irrational, I . . .
Int: Would you like to, would you rather that I not interview you, because I don't want to make you uncomfortable.
Elder: Well, yes, I would rather that you wouldn't interview me.
Int: Okay. That's just fine. I'm glad that you told me that.
Elder: I'm kinda touchy on a couple subjects.

Fear:

Int: What do you think of the program?
Elder: I'd rather not talk about it.
Int: You're uncomfortable talking about it?
Elder: Yes.

Int: Do you mind telling me why?

Elder: I just can't talk about it.

Int: Are you afraid if you tell me you might get in trouble?

Elder: Yes. (shakes his head yes.)

Pain:

Int: What do you think about while the program is going on?

Elder: Well, I'll tell ya, I hurt so bad I don't know. I don't know what's going on. I'm hurting right now so bad I can hardly stand it.

Int: Do you think that the more active you are or the more involved you are with life around you, do you think it makes you feel better if you can get involved?

Elder: No. I tell ya, like I've tole ya before, if I didn't suffer all the time like I do, I'd enjoy it a whole lot better. I'd enjoy those kids better being with them, but I hurt all the time and suffer. I don't enjoy nothing much.

Insufficient, unclear, nice, and *emotionally charged* data were problematic for us since we were trying to determine how elders perceived the geriatric remotivation program. These data were the direct result of elders' physical, cognitive, affective and personal characteristics. Elders who could not hear well or who were in constant pain (physical characteristics), had memory deficits or were disoriented (cognitive characteristics), displayed flat affect (affective characteristics) and used language unfamiliar to researchers (personal characteristics) provided data which were difficult to interpret.

■ STRATEGIES FOR INCREASING VALIDITY IN STUDIES OF IMPAIRED INSTITUTIONALIZED ELDERLY

Our experience working with this population provided some clues to strategies which can improve a researcher's chances of drawing valid conclusions about elders' sense of reality.

Increase Sample Size

Due to the difficulties inherent in collecting data from this population, researchers should consider focusing on a larger sample than they might in a different population. With a larger sample the researcher is more likely to get enough data to be able to piece together an interpretation of elders' perspectives. It is difficult to reach saturation when studying impaired elders; that is, patterns do not emerge and repeat themselves quickly as they can in an unimpaired population. By increasing the sample size, researchers increase their chances of achieving saturation, thereby increasing their confidence that their findings are valid.

Return to Setting Frequently

The purpose of this strategy is to insure that a researcher gets enough rich data on which to base interpretations. Although qualitative researchers typically spend a lot of time in the setting they are studying, they should allow for even more visits to a nursing home. Because data are hard to get and interpret, many opportunities to collect data are necessary. Also, if researchers hope to build rapport with elderly participants, they must make frequent contact with them. Although some elders are quick to respond to strangers, others are very guarded. Finally, frequent visits are necessary to overcome the problems posed by elders' memory deficits and disorientation. It is common for impaired elders to forget people and events or to be confused about time and place.

Lengthen Observation Periods

Researchers hoping to get useful data from impaired elders must be prepared to spend time with those elders. It is common for elders to fall asleep, become disoriented, cry, and have to leave for therapy sessions while researchers are interviewing and/or observing them. In order to gain insight into elders' views, researchers need flexible schedules and long blocks of time for "hanging around."

Recognize the Value of Stories

Frequently, impaired elders do not seem to provide a direct answer to an interviewer's question. In fact, at first glance it appears that many elders go on to talk about an entirely different subject than that presented to them. Rather than dismissing these apparently irrelevant stories, we recommend that researchers tune in to elders' stories. While they may appear to be off the subject, they often provide insight into the elders' opinions and concerns. In addition, elders are grateful to have someone listen to their stories. By listening patiently, researchers may receive helpful data while providing reciprocity.

Recognize the Value of Socializing

In many settings participant observers achieve insights into the view of the people under study through casual socializing. This is true for researchers studying the institutionalized elderly, too. We found that by chatting with the elders on the floors, in their rooms, in the television room, in the lobby, and in the dining room we were able to gather data that helped us understand their views. Restricting data collection to the remotivation therapy sessions and the periods directly preceding and following those sessions resulted in a much "thinner" body of data.

Use Videotapes

Because elders' movements are often restricted, their behavior can be difficult to detect and interpret. Note the following example:

> *An elder was videotaped ramming the table with his wheelchair while awaiting the arrival of the children for the program. Under other circumstances this behavior might have been interpreted as confused, antisocial or even belligerent. Because the incident was captured on videotape, we were able to discover that the elder was actually trying to move the table to allow a table mate to negotiate his wheelchair around a table leg — a very sociable act indeed!*

Videotapes capture the details of elder behavior and preserve them for repeated analysis. We found that it was essential to have videotapes to study elders' participation in and responses to remotivation therapy sessions. There are, of course, difficulties inherent in using videotapes. Although a stationary camera is less obtrusive than a roving camera, it captures activity within a narrow range. The researcher is not guaranteed to capture all of the activity, even among a small group of participants. The quality of the audio recording is also a concern, particularly for elders with low volume voices. We addressed these problems by using two stationary cameras and conference microphones. In addition, at least one researcher recorded field notes during remotivation therapy sessions.

Collect Interview and Observation Data

We are not the first to recommend that qualitative researchers should collect more than one kind of data. Because the elders' words and actions can be so difficult to interpret, it is essential to have a large quantity of data and more than one kind of data. Although the videotapes and the field notes helped capture elders' actions, the interviews provided insight into meaning behind those actions. Interviews alone, however, would have been difficult to interpret without observations to ground them in specific events. Looked at together, then, observation and interview data create a more thorough and interpretable picture of the phenomenon under investigation than either of the data sources alone. Also, each source of data provides a means of checking the meaning and validity of data collected via the other method.

Have Elders View and Respond to Videotaped Recordings

Many impaired elders cannot remember events for more than a few minutes. To enable elders to talk about their experiences in an earlier activity, researchers should consider showing them a videotape of the activity. While we do not have extensive experience with this technique, we found some success in conducting interviews while elders viewed themselves participating in a remotivation therapy session. Although use of videotape addresses the elders' memory problems, it can pose other problems. For instance, elders can become confused by what they see on the screen. Additionally, some elders have trouble seeing the screen at all. Despite the problems this strategy can present, we think it is worth the attention of researchers who are wrestling with the problem of elders' memory deficits.

All qualitative researchers must take steps to insure that their findings represent the world as seen through the eyes of the participants. Researchers interested in studying the elderly should be alerted to the special challenges involved in gathering and interpreting data from this population. It is important for researchers to spend a lot of time with elders, to value their stories and to collect different kinds of data. By adjusting research methods to be sensitive to the characteristics of the elderly, researchers can address the many threats to validity inherent in studying this population.

■REFERENCES

Applied social research methods series. (1989). Newbury Park, CA: Sage Publications, Inc.

Berkowitz, S. (1978). Informed consent, research, and the elderly. The Gerontologist, 18, 237–243.

Butler, R., Vestal, R., Lawton, M., Chalkley, D., Mishkin, B., Kelty, M., & Reich, W. (1977). In Protection of elderly research subjects. Summary of the National Institute on Aging Conference. DHEW No. (NIH) 79-1801: Government Printing Office.

Dobbert, M. (1982). Ethnographic research. New York: Praeger.

Duffy, L., Wyble, S., Wilson, B., & Miles S. (1989). Obtaining geriatric patient consent. Journal of Gerontological Nursing, 15, 21–24.

Ebrahim, S., Morgan, K., Dallosso, H., Bassey, J., Harries, U., & Terry, A. (1987). Interviewing the elderly about their health: Validity and effects on family doctor contact. Age and Ageing, 16, 52–57.

Fine, G. & Sandstrom, K. (1988). Knowing children. Participant observation with minors. Qualitative Research Methods, 15, Newbury Park, CA: Sage Publications, Inc.

Herzog, A. & Rodgers, W. (1988). Age and response rates to interview sample surveys. Journal of Gerontology, 43, S200–S205.

Hoffman, P., Marron, K., Fillit, H., & Libow, L. (1983). Obtaining informed consent in the teaching nursing home. Journal of the American Geriatric Society, 31, 565–569.

Jackson, J., Ramsdell, J., Renvall, M., Swart, J., & Ward, H. (1989). Reliability of drug histories in a specialized geriatric outpatient clinic. Journal of General Internal Medicine, 4, 39–43.

Kane, R. & Kane, R. (1981). Assessing the elderly. Lexington, MA: D.C. Heath and Company.

LeCompte, M. & Goetz, J. (1982). Problems of reliability and validity in ethnographic research. Review of Educational Research, 52, 31–60.

Lincoln, Y. & Guba, E. (1985). Naturalistic inquiry. Beverly Hills: Sage.

McCall, G. & Simmons, J. (1969). Issues in participant observation: A text and reader. Reading, MA: Addison-Wesley.

Mercer, J. & Butler, E. (1967). Disengagement of the aged population and response differentials in survey research. Social Forces, 46, 89–96.

Norris, F. (1985). Characteristics of older non-respondents over five waves of a panel study. Journal of Gerontology, 40, 627–636.

Perry, B. (1982). Validity and reliability of responses of the aged to surveys and questionnaires. The Journal of Family Practice, 15, 182–183.

Powers, B. (1988). Social networks, social support and elderly institutionalized people. Advances in Nursing Science, 10, 40–58.

Qualitative research methods series. (1989). Newbury Park, CA: Sage Publications, Inc.

Robb, S. (1983). Beware the informed consent. Guest Editorial. Nursing Research, 32 (3), 132.

Schwartz, H. & Jacobs, J. (1979). Qualitative sociology. New York: Free Press.

Spradley, J. (1979). The Ethnographic Interview. New York: Holt, Rinehart & Winston.

Spradley, J. (1980). Participant Observation. New York: Holt, Rinehart & Winston.

Todd, M., Davis, K. & Cafferty, T. (1984). Who volunteers for adult development research?: Research findings and practical steps to reach low volunteering groups. International Aging and Human Development, 18, 177–184.

Chapter 31

Older Adults' Experience of Health Promotion: A Theory for Nursing Practice

MARILYN FRENN

Understanding how older adults promote their health, and the factors that motivate or discourage them, is important to controlling health care expenditures in this rapidly growing population. This grounded theory-based study includes participant observation techniques and semistructured interviews with elderly clients of a community-based nursing clinic that led to the development of a theory of health promotion for this age group. The major constructs and components of "Going About Health" are delineated and compared with other recent research in this area. What factors most influence our patients' health promotion, and how can we become more effective at motivating them?

This is a time when exploding health care costs threaten health care benefits on which many older adults have come to depend. Health care professionals, therefore, must understand and capitalize on clients' way of promoting their own health. Leveille, LaCroix, Hecht, Gorthaus, and Wagner (1992) stated that we can meet the health care needs of an increasingly older population at 62% of the current cost if we preserve functional independence and prevent disability.

Improved community health is defined by the community, not the professional (Schroeder, 1994). Qualitative methods offer greater utility and power for the examination of health concepts and the subsequent development of consumer-sensitive interventions than do conventional approaches (Lincoln, 1992). Munhall (1993) described qualitative approaches as being a means to develop initial levels of theory within the domain of nursing. Problems that occur when theories are borrowed from other disciplines such as dependence on deducing hypotheses from unrelated contexts or populations were cited. The purpose of this study was to examine older adults' experience of health promotion as a basis for developing the factor-

From *Public Health Nursing* 13(1):65–71, 1996. Reprinted with permission.

isolating and factor-relating steps of theory that might guide nursing practice in promoting health with this important group of clients.

▬METHOD

A simultaneous process of collecting, coding, and analyzing data congruent with grounded theory (Chenitz & Swanson, 1986; Glaser & Strauss, 1967; Strauss, 1987) was used in the collection and analysis of the data. Schulz (1987) stated that the use of an instrument as well as qualitative sources of data may provide a more holistic view of the phenomena of concern to nursing. Therefore, the Health Self Determinism Index (HSDI) (Cox, Miller, & Mull, 1987) was used to gather client perspectives related to intrinsic motivation for health. Intrinsic motivation for health is defined as the human need to be competent and self-determining with respect to the environment (Deci, 1980).

The HSDI was used within the "emergent fit" mode of grounded theory (Artinian, 1986). This means that the investigator considered prior research, but pursued the present inquiry with openness to perspectives offered by older adults.

Three research questions were used to focus the inquiry concerning older adults' experience of health promotion: 1) How do older adults go about maintaining or promoting their health? 2) What influences older adults' health promotion efforts? and 3) What aspects of the environment, or contexts, do older adults describe as relevant to promoting their health?

▬SETTING AND SAMPLE

An assumption of qualitative research incorporated in this study was that reality is socially as well as personally constructed, and the context of the inquiry is of special importance (Riley, 1992). An urban midwestern community center that housed a nursing clinic where older adults gathered for a federally subsidized meal program was selected. A nurse practitioner in the clinic provided care for about 25 elderly clients each day. There were 70–80 individuals seen on a regular basis.

Demographic data were not available for all of the persons included in participant observation. Respondents participating in semistructured interviews included 18 men and 13 women with a mean age of 73 years. Twenty-two interviewees lived with their spouses, seven lived alone, and two lived with persons other than a spouse. Thirty interviewees were Caucasian and one was African American. Fourteen of the interviewees' household incomes were at or below $10,000, 14 were between $10,000 and $30,000, and three interviewees stated their income was greater than $30,000 per year. Eleven interviewees completed high school; of these two had additional education but did not receive college degrees. The remaining 18 interviewees' education ranged between the 6th- and 11th-grade levels.

▬APPARATUS

Qualitative and quantitative data in this study were collected in 5 months of data collection through semistructured and structured client interviews. Field notes were taken in and around the community center, ranging from 1–3 hours per day, 3–5 days per week when older adults were present, prior to and during their meal. Demographic data including age, income, ethnicity, education, and medical problems were collected at the end of the interview to better describe the respondent sample.

Semistructured Interview Guide

A semistructured interview guide was constructed by the investigator to elicit what older adults experienced as helpful in maintaining or improving their health. The interview guide had been previously developed based on review of the literature related to wellness/health promotion. This was used to understand client experience in this study and was reported by a group of middle-aged and older adult clients during a cardiac rehabilitation program (Frenn, Borgeson, Lee, & Simandl, 1989).

As in the Frenn et al. (1989) study, respondents were asked to describe their health, what they thought was important in staying healthy, and what they actually were doing to promote their health. They were also asked to give examples of how they began to promote their health, what helped or hindered them in promoting their health, and to share any other thoughts they thought were important in maintaining or promoting their health.

Interviews were conducted individually and usually lasted 30–45 minutes. Interviews were not repeated, but participant observation data were used to confirm or disconfirm and to expand on data gathered in the interviews. The 31 respondents who were interviewed constituted the older adults willing to share information in that format. Other elders expressed willingness for the investigator to join them during their meal, because they did not want to miss the opportunity to relate to others. Insights shared by older adults gathered at their tables were recorded in field notes.

Health Self-Determinism Index (HSDI)

The HSDI statements were used as qualitative probes regarding health motivation. The HSDI, a 17–item, Likert-type scale instrument, had been used with older adults living in the community. Acceptable internal consistency (alpha = 0.78) was demonstrated and 56% of the variance in factor analysis was accounted for (Cox et al., 1987). Chronbach's alpha coefficient in the present study was 0.67 (N = 31). Although triangulation among qualitative and quantitative data was originally intended, quantitative data from the HSDI were not included in this report because of the low alpha.

Field Notes

Participant observation data collected in the community center were recorded in field notes. Observational, methodological, and theoretical notes (Glaser & Strauss, 1967; Mariano, 1995) were taken in the community center, during the interviews, and throughout analysis. These notes guided further interview probes and data analysis. Rodgers and Cowles (1993) described the necessity of synthesizing the three types of notes to produce dense description and ultimate trustworthiness of the emerging theory.

▬ PROCEDURES

Following institutional review for protection of human subjects, a description of the study was placed in the meal program room and on the outer door of the nursing clinic. The study also was explained verbally to potential respondents during participant observation. To enhance sampling validity as identified by Krippendorf (1980), members of each of the naturally occurring conversation groups in the meal program were asked if they would be willing to share their perspectives about health in a tape-recorded interview. Written permission was requested prior to the interviews.

The semistructured interview questions were asked first, followed by additional questions that emerged from previous interviews or participant observation. The HSDI then was verbally administered and the respondent invited to comment as the questions were asked.

Copies of the typed transcripts containing the semistructured interview and verbal HSDI data were independently coded by the investigator, and three masters prepared nurse cocoders to enhance reproducibility and consensus of the coding categories. Interrater agreement, without discussion, was 50%–75%. When codes were discussed, agreement was 100%. The investigator recoded the first three interviews after completion of all interviews to examine stability in coding. A 90% agreement was found between the first and second coding.

The codes generated from line-by-line analysis of the interviews were noted on an evolving outline of roughly ordered concepts. Semantic validity, as identified by Krippendorf (1980), was enhanced through respondent verification of the data, during participant observation, and by reporting samples of data using respondents' own words.

To enhance product validity (Krippendorf, 1980), perceptions shared by respondents were further explored with subsequent respondents after they completed the semistructured interview. Data obtained through interviews, participant observation, and extant literature were compared using the constant comparative method (Glaser & Strauss, 1967). The patterns ultimately discovered were then compared with analogous patterns reported in the literature for the purpose of enhancing the process-oriented validity (Krippendorf, 1980). Process oriented validity is the degree to which the categories of analysis are supported by valid theory.

▬ RESULTS

Grounded theory leads to the discovery of a basic social process (Strauss, 1987). A process called Going about Health emerged from the present analysis (Fig. 31-1). Older adults' statements and observed behaviors of what they actually did to promote their health constituted the major patterns of Going about Health. Older adults' statements and observed behaviors that

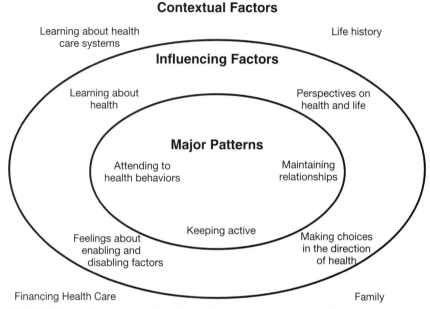

FIGURE 31-1   Going about Health: A theory for nursing practice.

led to and affected the maintenance of the behaviors they saw as promoting their health were called influencing patterns. Aspects of the older adults' experience that formed the context for what they actually did to maintain their health were called contextual factors.

▬MAJOR PATTERNS

For purposes of this study, patterns were defined as the naturally occurring configurations of relationships among elements of the phenomena being studied. Major patterns, components, and constructs are shown in Fig. 31-2.

Interview and participant observation data led to discovery of constructs that in turn led to discovery of larger components and finally the major patterns. Major patterns included maintaining relationships, attending to health behaviors, and staying active. For example, a number of respondents described walking as something they did to promote their health. An 87-year-old man said, "I attribute my long life to walking. . . . I go all over. I love to go down to the river, walk the falls and listen to the birds."

Respondents also identified going somewhere to exercise, personal exercise at home, dancing, work at home, purposeful work, and sports as promoting their health. These theory constructs led to naming exercise as the first component of the emerging pattern Staying Active (see Fig. 31-2).

Although exercise might have been part of the pattern Attending to Health Behaviors (see Fig. 31-1), respondents also described social activity

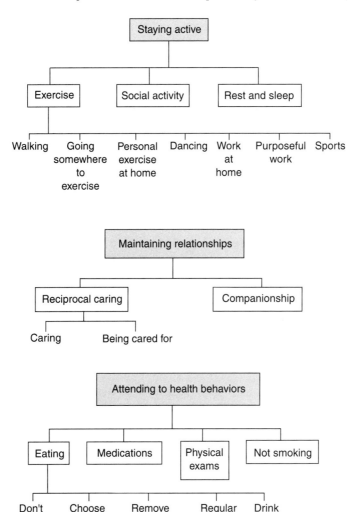

FIGURE 31-2 Major patterns, components, and constructs.

as a way to promote their health. The following observational note taken during participant observation is illustrative of data leading to development of this theory construct:

A 76-year-old man said, "If you stay active you don't need a doctor." He stays active by fixing toys for the younger children, building cabinets for the teens' video equipment, volunteering in the meal program when the paid coordinator was on vacation, doing errands in the afternoon, and watching baseball in the evenings.

Similarly, respondents described balance between staying active and sufficient rest and sleep as being important to staying healthy. Moving from the factor-isolating to the factor-relating stage of theoretical development, the three components Exercise, Social Activity, and Rest and Sleep formed the pattern Staying Active (see Fig. 31-2).

The other two major patterns, Maintaining Relationships and Attending to Health Behaviors (see Fig. 31-2), similarly were formulated from the data. For example, a 67-year-old woman said, "I think when you give to somebody else you get back twice as much." These data, along with those provided by other respondents, led to the component Reciprocal Caring (see Fig. 31-2). Reciprocal Caring, along with Companionship, formed the major pattern Maintaining Relationships (see Fig. 31-2).

Another woman provided an example of the relationship between the major patterns Maintaining Relationships and Attending to Health Behaviors when she said, "I think these centers are great, because we get to talk to other people, even if it's only for an hour. Because we come here to eat, it's just enough to get out of the house and talk to someone else." The meal program functioned for these urban older adults in much the same way as Bonder (1994) described the social support networks functioning for rural elders around grocery stores, post offices, and banks.

The patterns Staying Active, Maintaining Relationships, and Attending to Health Behaviors were central in that they pattern consistently were experienced by older adults as promoting their health. Lack of these major patterns was similarly related to ill health.

Hansson and Carpenter (1994) suggest that we understand the role relationships play in health by studying their consequences. In the current study, a man who had a pattern of poor relationships throughout his life experienced a myocardial infarction. Nurses helped him reconnect with essential services to support his recovery, and listened as he grieved the fact that few, if any, people came to visit him during his hospitalization. This is not to say that poor relationships and myocardial infarctions are always connected experiences, but that regaining relationships was essential for this man to pursue health.

■ INFLUENCING PATTERNS

Influencing patterns (shown in Fig. 31-1) included Making Choices in the Direction of Health, Learning about Health, Perspectives on Health and Life, and Feelings about Enabling and Disabling Factors. The first influencing pattern, Making Choices in the Direction of Health (see Fig. 31-1), included Motivation, Moderation, and Coping with Chronic Health Problems. In addition to the constructs of intrinsic motivation, which were Self-Determination and Perceived Competence, older adults shared three important components of motivation: External Forces, the Way They Were Raised, and New Awareness. A 77-year-old man described his "new awareness": "Once I found out it wasn't good to eat organ meats. Well, I quit them. And that was a little bit hard too. But not anymore. Today I think it would repulse me, I'm not sure. But I know it isn't good for you, so I wouldn't eat it."

Older adults learned by reading, watching others, and teaching themselves. For example, a respondent reported that he learned from watching his uncle who had not stayed active, become ill, "and now he's pushing up daisies." Respondents also reported teaching themselves: "I am (sic) into the doctor about 25 years ago," said an 87-year-old man. "He said, I should use this Metamucil. I did for a little while, but just by chance, I ate an apple about 7 P.M., and that settled my stomach much better than Metamucil. And, from that time on I eat apples — two or three every evening around 7 P.M."

Health and life were very intertwined in older adults' experience. The respondents mainly described their health as being good despite chronic illness and "okay for my age."

As a group, respondents' views on what was important for staying healthy were much the same as what they reported they actually did to stay healthy. However, individual respondents surprised themselves upon discovering differences between what they said was important and what they were actually doing. For example, having said that staying active was important to health, chagrin spread over the face of a 77-year-old man when he was asked to describe what he was doing to stay active. He said, "I really need to walk more."

Feelings about Enabling and Disabling Factors (see Fig. 31-1) constituted the last pattern influencing health. Enabling factors included spouse, life history, and health professionals. Disabling factors included illness, that health behaviors were hard to accomplish, spouse, previous patterns, and societal disablers. The issue was how the older adult in this study felt about the enabling and disabling factors, rather than the factors themselves; respondents' spouses, for example, were described both as enabling and disabling.

■ THE CONTEXT OF GOING ABOUT HEALTH

Contextual factors (see Fig. 31-1) were important to Going about Health in that they formed the environment in which the process occurred. They included Life History, Family, Relationship with Health Care System, and Financing Health Care.

Respondents described Going about Health as being very intertwined with their life. As one 65-year-old woman said, "I've been a widow for 26 years. I raised my children through high school and college myself. That's why I live in the (housing) project, because without the project I couldn't have done it. But, all three of them went to high school and college, and graduated, and all three holding down good jobs, and have their own homes, so my work is done. I finally can put my head on the pillow and sleep." The respondents' families of origin, as well as their current family relationships, provided a context through which they enacted the process of Going about Health (see Fig. 31-1). Said a 67-year-old man about his wife, "Yeah, I think we're good for each other, you know. And we'll just have to get out and walk and watch our diet."

Respondents identified health care systems, the nursing clinic in the community center, and relationships with physicians as major components of their context of good health practices. The major client responses concerning the nursing clinic were that the nurses took their blood pressure, were good listeners, and were nice people. Respondents stated they were glad to be able to see physicians when they were sick even though physician services were not available at the community center clinic. Relationships, trust, and making choices about their own health were described as important.

Older adults with low income identified finances as a contextual factor more readily than did those with greater income. Differences in the patterns of Going about Health were not apparent by respondents' incomes. Rather, dealing with life challenges and low income was described as an additional burden that had to be addressed before health promotion could be pursued. Cutler and Coward (1992) noted similar problems in that urban elders tend to have low incomes and inadequate housing when compared to their rural and suburban counterparts.

The overall process of Going about Health was summarized by what a 65-year-old woman said, "Childhood, don't leave you. Because it's there, the whole pattern. ... When you're raised up like that you don't change it." Another 65-year-old woman elaborated, "The coming and going, you know, the process, and it's unavoidable for everybody. You're born, you live, and you die. And, therefore, if you make it to old age, it's beautiful, and you're very lucky."

■ DISCUSSION

The view that the generation of knowledge in nursing evolves through analysis of constancy or inconstancy patterns in different situations, age groups, or cultures over time (Stevenson, 1988) was central to the present study. In accordance with the grounded theory approach (Strauss, 1987), other theories were first analyzed for areas of convergence (see Table 31-1).

Kolanowski and Gunter's (1985) qualitative study with older women resulted in patterns that were very similar to those reported in the present study. Boyle and Counts (1988) found patterns similar to Attending to Health Behaviors and Staying Active in their study of Appalachian elders, but did not find maintaining relationships to be central to health in that context.

In contrast, Craig (1994) found extensive support for the centrality of maintaining relationships among rural Great Plains elders, but did not describe the patterns Attending to Health Behaviors or Staying Active as central to residents' health. Similarly, Ruffing-Rahal (1989) identified core themes of well-being among 27 midwestern, independently living elders as including activity, affirmation, and synthesis. Ruffing-Rahal's categories of affirmation and synthesis were similar to the influencing pattern subcomponents Motivation and Values by which Elders Live, identified in the present

TABLE 31-1   Areas of Convergence of Extant Research-based Theories
with Major Patterns

EXTANT RESEARCH	MAINTAINING RELATIONSHIPS	ATTENDING TO HEALTH BEHAVIORS	STAYING ACTIVE
Kolanowski & Gunter (1985)	X	X	X
Boyle & Counts (1988)		X	X
Craig (1994)	X		
Brown and McCreedy (1986)		X	X
Walker et al. (1988)	X	X	X
Pender (1990)	X	X	X
NANDA (1994)	X	X	X
Omaha System (Martin & Scheet, 1992)	X	X	X

study. Thus, cultural and regional differences may lead to some variance in centrality of the major patterns, but the three patterns consistently were reported in other qualitative studies (Craig, 1994; Ruffing-Rahal, 1989).

Day (1991), in a qualitative study of a subsample of 20 aging women taken from a longitudinal, national quantitative study, recommended that health professionals address the meaning of individual goals, and plan health interventions specifically to enable older women to achieve them. Day also identified the growing consensus among researchers that strategies for successful aging must be sought not only in individual biological and psychological potential, but also in broader social influences and opportunities for health and well-being.

Because this was a study focused on developing theory to guide nursing practice, classification systems relevant to health promotion phenomena also were examined relative to the major patterns. Among such systems, Pender (1990) developed a taxonomy of expressions of health. The North American Nursing Diagnosis Association (NANDA) Taxonomy I Revised (Carroll-Johnson, 1991) and Omaha Classification Systems (Martin & Scheet, 1992) also were used for comparison with major patterns in the present study.

The major patterns were closely analogous to Pender's classification, the NANDA patterns Moving, Relating, and Exchanging, and categories within the Omaha System. The influencing patterns and contextual factors identified by older adults in Going about Health (see Fig. 31-1) were not identified in the previously cited research and classification systems. Although each influencing pattern and contextual factor had also been reported in other extant research, the relationships among the patterns discovered in Going about Health had not been previously reported.

As a great deal of congruity was found between major patterns in Going about Health and in extant research and classification systems, these patterns may be useful in health promotion practice among older adults. With further study, constructs within the major patterns may be useful additions to ongoing taxonomic development.

Further research is needed to examine influencing patterns and contextual factors related to health promotion among older adults from other ethnic and socioeconomic groups. Differences between "young old" and "old old" have been reported (Hazan, 1994). However, the focus of the present study did not elicit such differences, nor were gender-specific differences found. Further research is planned to explicate context specific factors as well as age-related patterns of promoting health.

■ REFERENCES

Artinian, B. M. (1986). The research process in grounded theory. In W. C. Chenitz & J. M. Swanson (Eds.). *From practice to grounded theory: qualitative research in nursing* (pp. 16–23). Menlo Park, Calif.: Addison-Wesley.

Bonder, B. R. (1994). Growing old in the United States. In B. R. Bonder & M. B. Wagner (Eds.). *Functional performance in older adults* (pp. 4–11). Philadelphia: F. A. Davis.

Boyle, J. S., & Counts, M. M. (1988). Toward healthy aging: a theory for community health nursing. *Public Health Nursing, 5*(1), 45–51.

Brown, J. S. & McCready, M. (1986). The hale elderly: health behavior and its correlates. *Research in Nursing & Health, 9,* 317–329.

Carroll-Johnson, R. M. (1991). *Classification of nursing diagnoses: proceedings of the ninth conference.* Philadelphia: J. B. Lippincott.

Chenitz, W. C., & Swanson, J. M. (1986). Qualitative research using grounded theory. In W. C. Chenitz & J. M. Swanson (Eds.). *From practice to grounded theory: qualitative research in nursing* (pp. 3–15). Menlo Park, Calif.: Addison-Wesley.

Cox, C. L., Miller, E. H., & Mull, C. S. (1987). Motivation in health behavior: measurement, antecedents, and correlates. *Advances in Nursing Science, 9,* 1–15.

Craig, C. (1994). Community determinants of health for rural elderly. *Public Health Nursing, 11*(4), 242–246.

Cutler, S. J., & Coward, R. T. (1992). Availability of personal transportation in households of elders: age, gender and residence differences. *Gerontologist, 32,* 77.

Day, A. T. (1991). *Remarkable survivors: insights into successful aging among women.* Washington, D.C.: Urban Institute Press.

Deci, E. (1980). *The psychology of self-determinism.* Lexington, Mass.: Lexington Books.

Frenn, M., Borgeson, D., Lee, H., & Simandl, G. (1989). Lifestyle changes in a cardiac rehabilitation program: the client perspective. *Journal of Cardiovascular Nursing, 3,* 43–55.

Glaser, B. G., & Strauss, A. L. (1967). *The discovery of grounded theory: strategies for qualitative research.* Chicago: Aldine.

Hansson, R. O., & Carpenter, B. N. (1994). *Relationships in old age: Coping with the challenge of transition.* New York: Guilford Press.

Hazan, H. (1994). *Old age: constructions and deconstructions.* Cambridge, England: Cambridge University Press.

Kolanowski, A., & Gunter, L. M. (1985). What are the health practices of retired career women? *Journal of Gerontological Nursing, 11*(12), 22–30.

Krippendorf, K. (1980). *Content analysis — an introduction to its methodology.* Beverly Hills, Calif.: Sage Publications.

Leveille, S. G., LaCroix, A. Z., Hecht, J. A., Gorthaus, L. C., & Wagner, E. H. (1992). The cost of disability in older women and opportunities for prevention. *Journal of Women's Health, 1,* 53–61.

Lincoln, Y. S. (1992). Sympathetic connections between qualitative methods and health research. *Qualitative Health Research, 2,* 375–391.

Mariano, C. (1995). The qualitative research process. In L. A. Talbot (Ed.). *Principles and practice of nursing research* (pp. 463–491). St. Louis, Mo.: Mosby.

Martin, K. S., & Scheet, N. J. (1992). *The Omaha system: applications for community health nursing.* Philadelphia: W. B. Saunders.

Munhall, P. L. (1993). Language and nursing research. In P. L. Munhall & C. O. Boyd (Eds.). *Nursing research: a qualitative perspective* (2nd ed. pp. 5–38). New York: National League for Nursing.

NANDA (1994). *Nursing diagnoses: definitions & classification.* Philadelphia: North American Nursing Diagnosis Association.

Pender, N. J. (1990). Expressing health through lifestyle patterns. *Nursing Science Quarterly; 3,* 115–122.

Riley, M. W. (1992). Forward. In M. G. Ory, R. P. Abeles, and P. D. Lipman (Eds.). *Aging, health, and behavior.* London: Sage Publications.

Rodgers, B. L., & Cowles, K. V. (1993). The qualitative research audit trail: a complex collection of documentation. *Research in Nursing and Health, 16,* 219–226.

Ruffing-Rahal, M. A. (1989). Ecological well-being: a study of community-dwelling older adults. *Health Values, 13*(1), 10–19.

Schroeder, C. (1994). Community partnerships and medical models of health? I don't think so. . . *Public Health Nursing, 11*(5), 283–284.

Schulz, P. R. (1987). Toward holistic inquiry in nursing: a proposal for synthesis of patterns and methods. *Scholarly Inquiry for Nursing Practice, 1*(2), 135–146.

Stevenson, J. S. (1988). Nursing knowledge development: into era II. *Journal of Professional Nursing, 4,* 152–162.

Strauss, A. L. (1987). *Qualitative analysis for social scientists.* Cambridge, England: Cambridge University Press.

Walker, S. N., Volkan, K., Sechrist, K. R., & Pender, N. J. (1988). Health-promoting life styles of older adults: comparisons with young and middle-aged adults, correlates and patterns. *Advances in Nursing Science, 11*(1), 76–90.

Chapter 32

Successful Aging of the Oldest Old Women in the Northeast Kingdom of Vermont

RITA H. LAFERRIERE   BRENDA P. HAMEL-BISSELL

In this miniethnography, the health lifeways of six elderly women over the age of 85 are described. How did these remarkable women manage to outlive their husbands and remain independent, living alone in their own homes with minimal assistance? Delightful vignettes exemplify the hardiness and resiliency underlying their life stories. Gerontological nurses may avoid promoting dependence and helplessness in their aging clients by working with them to problem solve ways to increase their self-reliance and commitment to independence.

In the northeast corner of Vermont near the Canadian border are the counties of Caledonia, Essex, and Orleans, popularly called the "Northeast Kingdom" (Brown & Lindbergh, 1987). This 2,000-square-mile area is the most sparsely populated region in the state (Vermont Department of Employment and Training, 1990). The people who live here are viewed by many to have a distinct set of values and way of life (Brown & Lindbergh, 1987).

Currently, the Northeast Kingdom has a population of women over 85 years of age who seem to age with remarkable success. This age group, the "oldest old", is one of the fastest growing in Vermont. In this age group, women outnumber men with widows representing a high percentage of this older population (Department of Aging and Disabilities, 1991). Community health nurses have noted that, in spite of many health problems, declining physical strength, altered family relationships, and declining mobility, some of these women maintain a high level of morale and adjust successfully to the problems of aging.

From *Image: Journal of Nursing Scholarship* 26(4):319–323, 1994. Reprinted with permission.

▬SUCCESSFUL AGING AND HEALTH IN RURAL SETTINGS

Rowe and Kahn (1987) distinguish between usual and successful aging. In usual aging, physiologic, psychosocial, and sociologic factors contribute to normal aging, but in successful aging extrinsic factors such as autonomy, social support, and control affect aging either in a positive or negative manner. Rowe and Kahn (1987) state that "providing help, care, and assistance may be directly health protective" (p. 147). These authors suggest that strong psychosocial influences may contribute to enhanced health-promoting behaviors and can directly effect the reduction of morbidity and passivity.

Anthropologists have provided nursing with important research to further understand successful aging. Two classic studies are Underhill's (1936) life history of a 90-year-old Papago woman and Hart and Pilling's (1960) study of the Tiwi of North Australia. These studies portray societies in which power and influence are built by successful gerontocrats where individual personality influences life achievements. Simic's (1978) study of aging Yugoslavians in a changing world used the life history method and depicted successful aging as building a lasting structure of relationships, accomplishments, and respect to give meaning to life. These three components of successful aging were explored in the life histories of the Vermont women.

Nursing studies exploring hardiness and resilience have also contributed to knowledge about successful aging. Kobasa (1979) hypothesized that hardy people with the greatest control over what occurs in their lives will remain healthier than those who feel powerless. Hardiness consists of the desire to remain active, the belief one has influence over the course of life events, and the belief that change can be a stimulus for growth.

Wagnild and Young (1990) describe resilience as an important element of "successful psychosocial adjustment" (p. 252). The concept, resilience, connotes emotional stamina and has been used to describe people who display courage and adaptability in the wake of life's misfortunes (Wagnild and Young, p. 254). Rural health practices and lifeways have been explored in several nursing studies. Leininger's (1984) description of southern rural black and white American lifeways exemplifies the importance of identifying care and health values of cultures from an "emic" perspective. In an Australian cross-cultural ethnographic study using Leininger's (1985) life history protocol, King (1989) identified hardiness and keenness for learning. Long and Weinert (1989), in their 6-year ethnographic study of the culture of rural Montana, found that health is assessed by rural people in relation to their work roles and activities. Self-reliance and independence of rural people are also seen as key. A desire to do and care for oneself was strong among self-reliant and independent rural Montanans.

The U.S. population continues to age and the size of the oldest old population continues to increase, yet little is known about rural oldest old women. A literature review revealed no published studies on successful aging or health lifeways of elderly people in rural New England and in particular, in northeastern Vermont, one of the most rural regions of America. Two studies (King, 1990; Berman, 1986) were found in which life history was used to identify characteristics of successful aging in this group. Research is needed to discover the factors contributing to successful aging in the rural oldest old. Long and Weinert (1989) maintain that further research about the health practices and values of rural populations is necessary to develop a "sound theory base for rural nursing practice" (p. 123).

▄ METHODS

Mini-ethnography is a "a small-scale ethnography focused on a specific or narrow area of inquiry" (Leininger, p. 35). Although a limited focus of inquiry is used, this type of nursing research examines the general lifeways of informants in their own environments. A mini-ethnographic approach was used in this study to explore and describe the health lifeways and beliefs of six elderly women. Participant observation and intensive interviewing were used as was life review. Leininger (1985) states that in obtaining an oral life health care history the researcher gains a longitudinal personalized perspective of an informant's life-time health, care behaviors, and illness patterns.

Purposive sampling was done of six oldest old women over age 85 who had lived in the Northeast Kingdom for at least 20 years. They were willing participants with relatively good hearing who spoke English. Referrals were provided by local home health agencies, community leaders, neighbors, and area aging advocates. This sample included those oldest old women who were perceived by the referral sources as having successfully adjusted to their aging and exhibited a high level of morale. Informants also had a reputation in the community as reliable historians.

The researchers spent time with the women to establish an understanding of the project's purpose and to develop a trusting relationship before beginning interviews and observation in each informant's home. Four to five individual interviews, lasting an average of 2 hours, were conducted with each woman using open-ended questioning and active listening as described by Spradley (1979). An interview guide was developed using the guidelines described in Leininger's (1985, pp. 126–127), life history protocol with protocol additions suggested by King (1989). Questions were phrased in language that was understandable to the informants. For example, the women were asked: What do you do to stay healthy? What remedies, if any, do you practice that have been handed down in your family or among neighbors? What characteristics do you value in people who take care of you? All interviews were audio-taped. After analysis of each interview, new questions were generated and follow-up interviews were scheduled. Photographing of the informants and their home environments added an important dimension. The camera captured germane scenes of the informants and their environments. Data were analyzed using content analysis to identify domains of meaning, organize these domains into categories, and then to describe the evolving cultural themes.

Validity and reliability were enhanced by carefully selecting informants who were willing to accurately present their personal histories. Validity and reliability were further supported by the researchers checking and cross-checking data content with the informants. Informants reviewed the written transcriptions of the audio-taped interviews for accuracy. The use of consensus provided pragmatic validity as data obtained in interviews with one informant were verified through interview or observation with another informant. The protocol for this study, the interview guide, and informed consent forms were approved by The University of Vermont Committee on Human Research-Behavioral Studies.

The six women, whose ages ranged from 87 to 93, were all widowed and Caucasian. Four described themselves as "true" Vermonters with a "plain old English-Yankee" background. Two were of French-Canadian descent and although not born in the Kingdom, they have lived there at least 70 years. The women, married at least once, were widowed for an average of 18 years. All but one have living children or grandchildren, many of whom live in Vermont. Although most of the women grew up on farms, only two were married to farmers. One was a teacher and housewife, another a housewife helping her husband run a grain store, two were housewives and seamstresses working in garment shops or making quilts at home. All but one participated actively, for as long as their health permitted, in various civic or community organizations such as church groups, the American Legion, or the Daughters of Isabella.

These six women, however, all suffer from various chronic illnesses. All have some form of arthritis. Other chronic problems include multiple hospitalizations for heart disease, hypertension, pernicious anemia, diabetes, back pain, and fractures caused by falls. Despite these problems, all remain in their own homes, living alone, with assistance from family or friends. Three receive home health services that include only skilled nursing visits.

Four dominant themes of health lifeways are, "Being a Woman With Family and Friends", "Living Off the Land", "Dealing With the Difficult Times", and "Working Hard and Staying Active."

▬ BEING A WOMAN WITH FAMILY AND FRIENDS

The most rewarding and necessary aspect of the women's lives is their close and supportive relationships with others. The rural environment and busy day-to-day work isolate them from large numbers of people. Their intimate relationships are with family members and a few close neighbors. They connected with larger groups of people during the occasional market days, church meetings, fairs, dances, and school years. Their primary roles have been that of wife, mother, housewife, teacher, and caretaker. The following reports exemplify the women's experiences of "Being a Woman with Family and Friends,"

Spending time together as family and friends helped to keep us healthy. We went on picnics, looked at old mills and went brook fishing.

We weren't very faithful church-goers. I'm not a member, but I've always worked for the church and in the church society. I always worked on the suppers and everything pertaining to the church, but I never joined. There used to be more community activities than there is now.

My greatest rewards in life were my husband, father, mother and being a teacher in school with children.

I went to dances where all the other families went. We would gather in the evenings at our house to peel apples, play card games, and play the phonograph.

I think women in the neighborhood were a great help to one another. When we were sewing we shared patterns and ideas and talked. We were a community. It wasn't any one person, but many.

▰LIVING OFF THE LAND

The informants also enjoyed the outdoors and described the importance of living in a quiet and clean environment. With their families, they participated in daily routines to earn a living and to grow and prepare food. Several said,

We helped with the farm work and ate potatoes, millet, milk gravy and all kinds of garden vegetables. We made all our own food; raised chickens, beef, and went berrying.

We had an awful lot of fruits and vegetables year around. We grew all our own vegetables and fruit such as potatoes, beans, corn, apples, strawberries, raspberries. They weren't polluted or full of preservatives. We loved dandelion greens better than anything. There was no smoking or drinking although my father would smoke a pipe and take a drink of liquor socially once in a while.

Dad said, "Never take anything that don't belong to you; always keep your credit good." My mother worked hard for us; she loved to pick berries and work outside. I picked a lot of berries.

Daily routines began at dawn and ended late in the evening. Twelve-hour days were usual. The routines the women described are ongoing and repetitive, however, varying with the seasons. Tasks that were accomplished during these routines were described by some as monotonous yet achievable.

▰DEALING WITH THE DIFFICULT TIMES

The women viewed their lives as a series of ups and downs. In spite of a number of serious losses, they described their life accomplishments as positive. They dealt with the hardships of death, injury, disease, miscarriages, suicide, economic insecurity, bankruptcy, and loss of home and the family farm in a practical, self-reliant manner. "You do what you have to do and make do." They did not mourn for their lack of greater worldly materials or resources.

The women lacked easy access to healthcare. They dealt with the problem of access by being self-reliant and using home remedies. One said,

My mother was always stewing up things for sore throat, canker sores, colds, or tummy aches. Camphor, camphor bag and all those funny things for a cold, peppermint for a tummy ache, hot cloths for the tummy, or a mustard plaster if you had a back ache.

They believed in facing their difficulties and persevering in the search for solutions. They displayed a stoic acceptance of hardship as part of life's reality. They also displayed quiet defiance: "You do not allow these hard times to get you down. You go on." The future was always visible and they were hopeful. The women described dealing with the difficult times as follows:

My advice to others is learn to cope with something as it comes along. Learn to age gracefully. I am not a worrier. Having a positive outlook makes you a lot happier while you live life. I get through each day by my determination and trying to get around.

The worst times was when we lost our farm and had to auction off everything. I got through it by praying a lot. This gave me faith that things will get better. Prayer is one of my greatest strengths.

Stressors never worried me too much. I tried to calm down and not let things bother me too much. You get through each day by handling things as they arise.

My daughter's death was a hard time but I kept busy with my oil painting and I made quilts. Just like I always have. I kept busy on the farm, working outdoors. I did things I enjoyed like working outdoors with my husband. Keeping busy helped.

▬WORKING HARD AND STAYING ACTIVE

Another prominent theme was "Working hard" to live off the land. The women enjoyed working hard and staying active and came by this sentiment through family expectations. They managed their households, gardens, farms, and businesses; they painted, quilted, baked, and read. Their routines kept them physically, emotionally, and spiritually active. Work and activity gave them a reason for being and brought meaning to their lives. Although unending, their work could be successfully done. It provided a sense of control over their lives. They stated,

Stick to whatever you like to do. Keep busy, keep working, be gritty.

With me, I've never lost the desire to learn and to be curious; maybe that keeps me living longer.

I believe and have lived by that you should do for yourself; you should not be waited on. One should get out and do things; one should not dwell on the [losses] of life.

My assets are the way I am now . . . able to take care of myself. Be the labor great or small, do it well or not at all.

When I was 85, I made one quilt every month. . . . Quilt making has kept my spirits up. I'm happy when I'm making quilts and I think it helped my life a lot.

▬DISCUSSION

The life histories of these women reflect that, in spite of significant loss and illness, they have approached aging with success. For these women, successful aging is "dealing with the difficult times," "working hard and staying active," "being a woman with family and friends," and "living off the land."

Kobasa (1979) defines the dimensions of hardiness as challenge, commitment, and control. Hardiness was exhibited by all the women in their life histories. Their hardiness is manifest in their desire to remain active in life events, in a belief that one has influence over the course of events, and by recognizing that change is normal and can be a stimulus for growth. Challenge was a reoccurring characteristic in "Dealing with the difficult times" and "Working hard and staying active". One commented,

It was a terrible thing when I thought I wasn't going to be able to read. Twenty-three years ago I had surgery on my eyes in Burlington and the doctor told me that in a year or so I'd only have 5% to 10% eyesight. It didn't feel very good to feel that way, but oh well, if that's the way it is — that's the way it is. I came home and began to organize everything in the house so I'd know right where it was. It (eyesight) never did get that bad. It was a miracle that I appreciate it so, I read every spare minute I can.

Control was reflected in their traits of self-reliance and independence required to live off the land in a rural community. Examples of self-reliance and independence described by the women are:

Oh my goodness — a hospital — my word! We were a farm family. We never heard the word hospital and the doctor was 12 miles away by horse and buggy, a half-day trip with a wagon. If you cut your finger, you didn't go to the doctor. My mother had typhoid and we did have a doctor once for her. Then my father got a woman who had had it to come and take care of her. If we got sick, we either got well or died.

I was tough but I don't know that we were any more tough than other folks living in rural communities at that time. Don't know what made us tough. We had to be tough to survive. Tough means that you survived; that you were stubborn and persistent.

All the women described a commitment to life in their stories of relationships within their rural communities, strength of ties to family, friends and neighbors, and continuing involvement and interest in the activities of daily living. Commitment was evident in the themes of "Being a women with family and friends" and "Working hard and staying active."

If we tried to make something or do something he (father) wouldn't let us give up. We got to do it again, so we could do it. That was his belief. Don't give up. This is a value I've carried with me all through my life.

"The concept, resilience, connotes emotional stamina and has been used to describe persons who display courage and adaptability in the wake of life's misfortunes" (Wagnild & Young, 1990, p. 254). This term accurately describes the Vermont women. Life histories revealed that in spite of personal losses, tragedy, and increasing physical illness, these women have continued to exhibit courage, enthusiasm, and a positive outlook. These rural women discuss health beliefs and practices that have contributed to their making it through difficult times or enabling them to stay well even when their access to health services are often limited. Knowledge, self-care, and self-reliance are contributing factors in their enjoyment of a perceived high level of wellness.

Blaney and Ganellen (1990) assume a relationship exists between the elements of hardiness — challenge, commitment, and control — and physical and psychological well-being. This premise was supported by these women of the Kingdom. One said,

> *My grandchildren have helped to keep me healthy all these years. They cheer me up. They tell me I'm doing good. They praise me up. That means a lot to me. More than anything else it's my family that's kept me going. My neighbors have helped too. I have a sign for every neighbor. I put a light in my window if I want anything. They (neighbors) are so good to me. I hope God will give them someone to look after them.*

Together the characteristics of challenge, commitment, and control combined with resiliency and blended with an adequate social support system have afforded these very old women with the ingredients for successful aging. This study indicates that strong health values and adherence to health practices have influenced their health. Although more research is needed to discover the factors contributing to successful aging in oldest old rural populations, these research findings can be used to improve rural nursing practice.

Findings from this research suggest that nursing care and health promotion for the oldest old needs to focus on maximizing a person's desire for independence while promoting self-reliance rather than dependency or learned helplessness. Early identification of cultural values, personal characteristics, health beliefs, and health practices is essential in offering appropriate health care that can assist this population to achieve their highest level of function and maximum quality of life.

The importance and value of strong social support systems need to be recognized. People need to be encouraged to strengthen informal relationships within their families and communities. Health policy making and program planning should be directed toward addressing not only the healthcare needs but also the health promotional needs and desires of the oldest old.

■ REFERENCES

Berman, H. J. (1986). To flame with a wild life: Florida Scott-Maxwell's experience of old age. The Gerontologist, 26, 321–324.

Blaney, P. H., & Ganellen, R. J. (1990). Hardiness and social support. In B. R. Sarason, I. G. Sarason, & G. R. Pierce, Social support: An interactional view (197–318). New York: John Wiley & Sons.

Brown, R. & Lindberg, R. (1987). The view from the Kingdom. New York: Harcourt, Brace, Javanovich Publishers.

Department of Aging and Disabilities. (1991). Long term care in Vermont. Waterbury, VT: Agency of Human Services.

Hart, C. W. M., & Pilling, A. R. (1960). The Tiwi of North Australia. New York: Holt, Rinehart, & Winston, Inc.

King, P. A. (1989). A woman of the land. Image: Journal of Nursing Scholarship, 21, 19–22.

Kobasa, S. (1979). Stressful life events, personality, and health: An inquiry into hardiness. Journal of Personality and Social Psychology, 37(1), 1–11.

Leininger, M. M. (1984). Southern rural black and white American lifeways with focus on care and health phenomena. In Care: The essence of nursing and health (133–160). Thorafare, NJ: Charles B. Slack.

Leininger, M. M. (1985). Qualitative research methods in nursing. Orlando, FL: Grune & Stratton, Inc.

Long, K. A., & Weinert, C. (1989). Rural nursing: Developing the theory base. Scholarly Inquiry for Nursing Practice: An International Journal, 3, 113–127.

Simic, A. (1978). Winners and losers: Aging Yugoslavs in a changing world. In B. G. Myerhoff & A. Simic (Eds.), Life's career — aging: Cultural variations on growing old (77–103). Beverly Hills, CA: Sage Publications.

Rowe, J. W., & Kahn, R. L. (1987). Human aging: Usual and Successful. Science, 237(7), 143–149.

Spradley, J. P. (1979). The ethnographic interview. New York: Holt, Rinehart, & Winston.

Underhill, R. (1936). The autobiography of a Papago woman. Menasha, WI: The American Anthropological Association.

Vermont Department of Employment and Training. (April 1990). Vermont an economic-demographic profile series: Northeastern Vermont. Montpelier, VT: Department of Employment & Training.

Wagnild, G., & Young, H. M. (1990). Resilience among older women. Image: Journal of Nursing Scholarship, 22, 252–255.

Weinert, C., & Long, K. A. (1991). The theory and research base for rural nursing practice. In A. Bushy (Ed.), Rural nursing (vol. 1, 21–38). Newbury Park, CA: Sage Publications.

Chapter 33

Gaps in Discharge Planning

MARGARET J. BULL   ROBERT L. KANE

Evaluation research is important for ensuring quality outcomes and assessing potential problem areas in caregiving systems. As elders are discharged from acute care hospitals, many opportunities for miscommunication and gaps in service can occur. How can we better plan for smooth transitions for our patients? Robert Kane, a noted gerontological researcher, and Margaret Bull, a nursing professor and researcher, did secondary analysis of qualitative data from two separate studies to pinpoint where system weaknesses most often occurred. If nurses are to be effective in improving patient outcomes and cutting costs, we must be ready to assume client advocate and case manager roles to avoid these gaps in planning and care.

Continuity of care is vital for frail, older persons. Not all older persons discharged from acute care hospitals need follow-up care, but those who do often have serious problems. Discharge planning, a key component in continuity of care, has been defined as an interdisciplinary process that assesses need for follow-up care and arranges for that care, whether the care is self-care, care from family, care provided by paid providers, or a combination of these options (Beatty, 1980; McKeehan, 1981). Medicare's DRG-based prospective payment system and managed care environments provide incentives for shortened hospital stays, thereby compressing the planning process (Gerety, Soderholm-Difatte, & Winograd, 1989; Gornick & Hall, 1988; Randall, 1994).

Despite attempts to improve discharge planning by employing various mechanisms to identify elders' needs (Berkman, Millar, Holmos, & Bonander, 1990; Coulton, 1992; U.S. Department of Health and Human Services, 1992), for over a quarter of a century the process has rarely gone smoothly (Berkman & Abrams, 1980; Proctor & Morrow-Howell, 1990). Experts have rated the quality of discharge planning in the United States as very poor (Fink, Siu, & Brook, 1987). Studies reporting unmet needs of elders, difficulties in managing care, and hospital readmissions indicate that problems persist (Bull, 1992; McWilliam & Sangster, 1994; Wolock,

From *The Journal of Applied Gerontology* 15(4):486–500, 1996. Reprinted with permission.

Schlesinger, Dinerman, & Seaton, 1987). In fact, the findings from one study indicated that 97% of elders reported one or more needs postdischarge and approximately one third of the elders indicated that their needs were not met (Mamon et al., 1992). The persistence of the problem coupled with the observation that 38.5% of elders in one study (Bull, Maruyama, & Luo, 1995), all of whom had family caregivers, were readmitted within 2 months of discharge led us to conduct secondary analysis on qualitative data gathered in two studies.

One purpose of qualitative data is to provide insights on the nature of problems, rather than produce generalizations based on a representative sample. These insights can generate possible solutions. The purpose of the secondary analysis was to (a) describe the nature of the difficulties encountered by elders and family caregivers following hospitalization, and (b) identify the system constraints encountered in planning for discharge.

■METHOD

Qualitative designs were selected to obtain health professionals', elders', and family caregivers' perspectives about discharge planning and posthospital transitions. Because discharge planning and posthospital transitions are dynamic processes, qualitative approaches were selected for identifying the nature of the system constraints and families' posthospital experiences. Qualitative methods are particularly appropriate for understanding processes from the perspectives of the persons involved in a particular situation (Glaser, 1978; Morse & Field, 1995).

The data reported here were limited to interview data, in which participants could choose how much information they wished to share. Validity and reliability of the data from interviews with elders and family members, however, were enhanced by having contact with the same interviewer over time (predischarge, 2 weeks postdischarge, and 2 months postdischarge). In other words, there was time to build a trusting relationship, which is critical for credibility (validity) of qualitative data (Lincoln & Guba, 1985; Sandelowski, 1986). Triangulation of data sources (e.g., interviews with nurses, social workers, and physicians) within and across units enhanced validity and reliability of interview data from health professionals.

Sources of Data

STUDY 1: DISCHARGE PLANNING. The original intent of this study was to identify factors professionals and elders considered important in planning for discharge and their perspectives on quality in discharge planning (Bull, 1994). The purpose of the secondary analysis was to identify the nature of the problems encountered by professionals and elders. Data were collected via semistructured interviews with health care professionals and elders recently discharged from an acute care hospital using a grounded theory approach. Professionals were asked to describe discharge planning at the hospital with which they were affiliated. Elders were asked what they considered important in planning to leave the hospital and how things had been going since they left the hospital. Interviews ranged from 25 minutes to

90 minutes, were audiotaped, and transcribed verbatim. The interviews with professionals and patients yielded 1,100 single-spaced pages of transcribed interview data.

McBee sort cards were used to facilitate retrieval of categories in analyzing the data. Content analysis and the constant comparison approach described by Glaser and Strauss (1967) were used in analyzing the data. Initially, substantive codes, reflecting the words of the participants, were developed by having the investigator and research assistants read and independently code the data. Substantive categories were later collapsed into broader categories. For instance, health care professionals referred to lack of communication among health care providers; both elders and health care professionals mentioned patients' receipt of conflicting messages about how to manage their care. These categories were collapsed in the broader category, inadequate communication.

The purposive sample consisted of 38 health care professionals (19 nurses, 11 physicians, 8 social workers) and 25 elders. The health professionals were affiliated with one of three hospitals (two community hospitals and a large university hospital) located in a metropolitan area of a midwestern state with a population of approximately 2 million. All of the health professionals worked with elders who were hospitalized for chronic illnesses and were involved in planning for discharge. Although few of the physicians specialized in geriatrics, all of them indicated that they cared for high volumes of elders in their practice. The elders ranged in age from 68 to 90 years, with a mean age of 78.2 years. All had been hospitalized for an acute episode of a chronic condition, such as congestive heart failure, chronic obstructive lung disease, or diabetes mellitus. The majority (84%) were discharged to their home.

STUDY 2: POSTHOSPITAL TRANSITIONS. The primary goal of the original project was to test a structural equation model of factors influencing family caregiver burden and health following an elder's hospitalization (Bull et al., 1995). Participants were recruited from six community hospitals in a midwest metropolitan area that has a population of approximately 2 million. Qualitative data were collected to illustrate the nature of situations encountered by elders and their family caregivers postdischarge. Semistructured interviews were conducted with 253 family caregivers for elders 2 weeks and 2 months following the elders' hospitalization. Participants were asked how things had been going since their family member left the hospital, about any concerns they had about themselves or the elder, and what difficulties, if any, were encountered. Although the intended focus of the interview was on the posthospital experience, all family members included their experiences in planning for discharge.

Family caregivers ranged from 20–86 years with a mean of 62 years; their elders ranged in age from 55–97 with a mean of 73 years. The majority of family members were White (96.3%), female (75.1%), and spouses (63.6%) of the elder. Content analysis was used in analyzing the data. Categories were developed by having the investigator and research assistants independently review the interview data. Initial categories used the words of participants.

For instance, problems with diet or medications were each assigned separate codes and were designated as problems either because the caregiver defined it as a concern or because it was an area in which they had questions that had not been answered. Later, these categories were collapsed into a broader category, problems managing care. After categories were developed and coded, data were entered in SPSS, a computer software package, so that frequencies could be obtained (Miles & Huberman, 1984).

▄▀FINDINGS

The findings from the two studies provided insights on the system constraints that impede discharge planning and on the problems encountered by elders and family caregivers. Systems problems such as inadequate communication, insufficient time for planning, and inadequate resources manifested themselves for elders and family caregivers in the form of premature discharge, insufficient information about how to manage the elder's care and lack of access to resources. Table 33-1 summarizes information on the frequency of the major problems identified by health professionals, elders, and family caregivers.

Inadequate Communication

Inadequate communication was a fundamental source of discontinuity in discharge planning. Data from elders, health care professionals, and family caregivers consistently indicated gaps in information transfer. Inadequate communication referred to gaps in information transfer and impediments in the system of care. Lapses in information transfer occurred at several levels. First, communication gaps between health care providers in hospitals and those external to the hospital (e.g., home health care agencies, equipment vendors) impeded care coordination. The problems that ensued generally involved equipment and personnel that did not arrive, or home

TABLE 33-1   Frequency with Which Health Professionals, Elders, and Family Caregivers Identified Problems

PROBLEM OR CONSTRAINT	STUDY 1				STUDY 2
	MDs ($n = 11$)	Nurses ($n = 19$)	Social Workers ($n = 8$)	Elders ($n = 25$)	Family Caregivers ($n = 253$)
Communication	8 (73)[a]	19 (100)	8 (100)	20 (80)	159 (63)
Time	10 (90)	19 (100)	8 (100)	0 (0)	0 (0)
Ageism	0 (0)	0 (0)	0 (0)	16 (4)	41 (16)
Premature discharge	3 (27)	0 (0)	1 (13)	3 (12)	48 (19)
Access to resources	6 (55)	17 (89)	8 (100)	5 (20)	122 (48)

[a] Numbers in parentheses are in percentages.

care personnel that did not understand the treatments ordered. For example, one family was told that a visiting nurse and physical therapist would be coming to the home for follow-up care. Two weeks later neither the nurse or therapist had come out to visit. When the family caregiver called the agency that was supposed to provide care, he was told that they never received any orders. Gaps in communication occurred even when the home care agencies received the orders. The following quote from a hospital nurse illustrates this type of problem:

> *One home care nurse called the hospital and asked to speak with me regarding the care the patient was to receive. I explained what we were doing for the patient, but this nurse wasn't comprehending this kind of care and what had to be done. She called me again the next day and said she didn't understand what we were doing. Obviously she was not familiar with the terminology we used and it caused a problem.*

Problems with information transfer also were apparent among patients, physicians, nurses, and social workers in the hospital. Conflicting information, a problem for more than half the elders in Study 1 and nearly 30% of family caregivers in Study 2, was more likely to occur when more than one physician was working with a patient. For instance, a primary physician might order one therapy for a patient and a specialist might order something different. Nurses and social workers needed to spend time calling physicians to inform them about what specialists had told the patient and what the patient wanted. If the nurses and social workers did not have time to go between the patients and their doctors, confusion ensued for patients and their families. Patients reported receiving contradictory information, especially with respect to medications and how to manage their care following discharge. For instance, one physician gave instructions to take a specific medication; another physician came in and said they were discontinuing the same pill. The following family caregiver's quote illustrates this problem:

> *Her family practice doctor doesn't encourage her to exercise. In fact, he discourages it. He makes her feel there isn't much use to it. Her heart doctor doesn't feel that way. He wants her to exercise.*

These situations were complicated further when family members, who planned to assist elders with managing their care, received different information and had a different understanding of the medications than the elder.

Approximately one fourth of the nurses and social workers noted that communication was facilitated when someone took time to ask questions and advocate for the elder. A nurse recounted the following situation in which a family member coordinated the planning:

> *The daughter knew the right questions to ask and she was willing to stick her neck out and keep bugging the doctor saying, "This is what we need to do, we need to do something to get Mom independent." At first the doctor just wanted to stick her mother in a nursing home because the insurance company wanted to get her out of the hospital real quick. But the daughter really facilitated communication*

among everyone. The physical therapist told us what they planned to do and we tried to cooperate as much as possible. It was a good team effort and her mother is totally independent again.

The gaps in communication described here led to elders and their family members receiving insufficient information about how to manage the elder's care. Insufficient information about the elder's condition and treatment referred to situations in which elders and family members had questions about care that had not been addressed. Approximately one third of participants in Study 2 lacked information about medications, special diets, or treatment; 56.4% did not know how to discern whether symptoms were a reaction to medication or a complication of the medical condition. One elder summarized this difficulty by stating, "We've spent over a hundred dollars on medication and don't know what any of these pills are for." Lack of information and insufficient understanding of medications and therapeutic diets was likely to result in poor management of the condition at home and for some elders it led to readmission to the hospital. Although elders stated that they expected health care professionals to provide information automatically, approximately one fourth of the physicians and social workers indicated that it was the elders' and families' responsibility to ask for information.

Time

Time often constrained the communication process. Insufficient lead time to plan for discharge impeded coordination of care. Hospital nurses frequently indicated that they might not know ahead of time when a patient was going to be discharged. The attending physician might make rounds at 10 A.M. and write orders to discharge a patient on that day. On the other hand, physicians were reluctant to commit themselves too soon on a discharge date because the patient's condition might change and necessitate a longer stay. In many systems, utilization review personnel would require further explanation from the physician for keeping the patient in the hospital longer than originally projected. Nonetheless, the effect of waiting until the day of discharge to inform nurses and social workers of the discharge affected care coordination. A social worker shared the following situation:

A patient was transferred from another floor and he had an HMO (health maintenance organization) that tends to push people out. The doctor wrote an order to "discharge to nursing home today." The doctor never told the family. Then I had to be the one to tell the family and arrange for nursing home care. . . . It's difficult to arrange nursing home care in one day.

The majority of physicians affirmed that time constrained planning. Physicians stated that they have limited time with each patient, and as a result left discharge planning to the nurses and social workers. The scope of hospital nurses' and social workers' responsibilities for planning often ended with discharge as these professionals did not follow patients after they left the hospital. In fact, they reported that they did not receive feedback on the discharge plan unless a patient or family called to complain or if the patient was readmitted. Limited time in which to coordinate care became more critical when system boundaries did not extend beyond discharge.

Elders and family members did not express concern about time constraints in planning for follow-up care. Because family members indicated that they were left out of the information loop in planning for aftercare, they might not have experienced the time constraints in the same way as the health care professionals. Elders stated that doctors and nurses told them what had been arranged and their family members "took care of things for them" after they left the hospital. Elders' and family members' lack of involvement in discharge planning might account for their lack of concern about time constraints.

Ageism

Health care professionals' ageism also impeded care coordination. Elders and family members who identified ageism as a problem tended to have higher education (i.e., education beyond high school) and higher income than those who did not mention it. These elders and family members reported instances in which physicians and nurses conveyed negative attitudes toward elders. For instance, elders reported that some nurses argued with them when they questioned the medications they were given and treated them like children. Physicians talked about patients instead of talking with them. Primary care physicians refused requests to see a specialist by saying "We're doing all we can, a specialist wouldn't do anything different. After all, she's 84 years old." None of the health care professionals identified ageism as a problem. Health care professionals might not have been aware of the problem because family members and elders voiced dissatisfaction to each other, rather than confronting health care professionals on this issue.

Premature Discharge

Premature discharge referred to situations in which family caregivers or health professionals felt the elder was discharged too early and was too sick to be at home. Often family members indicated that they were surprised to find the elder was being discharged so soon. These sorts of situations tended to be stressful and evoked worry for both the elder and family caregiver. Elders were still feeling weak when they left the hospital and required more assistance from family than anticipated. The majority of the elders, however, indicated that they were happy to leave the hospital and viewed discharge as a sign that they were getting better.

Of the health care professionals interviewed for Study 1, 27% of the physicians and 13% of the social workers expressed concern that elders were discharged prematurely. Physicians indicated that they felt pressure from health insurance companies to discharge patients quickly. Social workers attributed the premature discharges to pressures from health insurance companies and utilization review personnel. Although health care professionals acknowledged that the managed care environment and particularly pressures from insurance companies led to early discharge, nearly 19% of the family caregivers stated premature discharge was a problem for them. The following wife's comment illustrates the difficulty:

> *It was upsetting that he came home and then went back to the emergency room. We called 911. He had a reaction. . . . I feel they sent him home too soon. He was put on some new medicines and maybe those interacted with his diabetes to bring on the reaction. They should have kept him in the hospital longer to see how his body tolerated the medicine.*

Access to Resources

Another system problem was availability of, and access to, resources. In rural areas (i.e., located outside the metropolitan area) nursing home care and home health services were not as prevalent as in urban centers. With fewer resources available in rural areas health care providers needed to expend extra effort in developing and coordinating informal resources. In both rural and urban areas, elders without insurance or financial resources to pay for follow-up care encountered access problems. The following social worker's statement illustrates this sort of problem:

> *If an HMO does not want to do a home nursing visit, or if they think a patient who just had an acute stroke should go to a nursing home instead of acute rehab, then things don't go well. It's a problem.*

Health care professionals charged with the responsibility of coordinating care needed to know about insurance coverage, the nuances of how to state things in such a way that services were more apt to be covered, and what resources existed in the patient's community.

Difficulties with access to resources included both situations in which elders were not referred to services and those in which access was limited by what their insurance would cover. The following wife's quote illustrates the nature of problems that occurred when insurance limited access:

> *I was upset that the doctor wrote a prescription for Isordil 30 mg. three times a day instead of 10 mg., which he meant my husband to have. With the large dose, my husband became faint and dizzy. I wonder if this didn't contribute to the bleeding and heart attack he had (referring to readmission). When I tried to call the cardiologist to question the difference in dosage the nurse said I couldn't see the doctor without a referral from the HMO.*

Approximately 20% of elders indicated that they could have used some type of home care service but did not receive any information about what might be available. In addition, nearly 16% indicated they had sought information on services on their own. One family member indicated "I'm on a paper chase. . . . I wish they could make it easier to find out what's available and what's covered by insurance."

In summary, the gaps in care coordination affected elders and their families. Two weeks following discharge, 91% of the families were having difficulties managing the elder's care; 63% reported having questions about the elder's condition, medications, diet, activities, or all of these. The major difficulties elders and family members encountered were premature discharge, insufficient information on how to manage the elder's condition and treatment, and lack of access to resources.

▄POSSIBLE SOLUTIONS

Although Jackson (1994) noted that there is little evidence to support that discharge planning influences the patient's health status, our findings suggest that the gaps in care coordination may be costly. Gaps are costly not only in terms of hospital readmissions but also in terms of the stress experienced by elders and their family caregivers in trying to manage care with inadequate preparation for the task. As noted previously, the major problems included premature discharge, inadequate access to resources, ageism, lack of communication, and time constraints. The problems encountered in planning for discharge as well as suggestions from participants indicate that several factors need to be addressed to improve overall coordination.

Difficulties with premature discharge and access to care might be addressed by structural reform. Nurses and social workers who participated in Study 1 suggested that our current third-party reimbursement be replaced by some type of national health insurance.

Some form of national health insurance might lead to more equitable access to care. Even under such an arrangement, however, problems with premature discharge might persist unless more time is provided to plan for care. Although time for discharge planning could come from extended hospital stays, the costs might be prohibitive. Managed competition may create managed greed as the needs of patients become secondary to profits. Shaughnessy, Schlenker, and Hittle (1994) found that home health care supplied by HMOs provided fewer services and had poorer outcomes than that offered by fee-for-service (FFS) plans. Their findings suggest that HMOs have a different philosophy about use of home care services than FFS plans. Currently, managed care is being proposed as a solution to control cost and improve efficiency. Bringing all services under a single aegis could rationalize incentives and improve continuity, but early observations raise serious concerns about the outcomes of care.

Alternatively, special subacute units in hospitals might be developed for posthospital care planning. Discharge planning might be delegated to postacute care centers in which more time could be spent on planning for, and arranging follow-up care, as well as providing time for a more thorough discussion of the options for care. Although some subacute care units that initially developed in response to Medicare's Prospective Payment System experienced financial losses, others were successful in structuring their programs to correspond with existing reimbursement limits and generated revenue (Balsano & Fowler, 1993; Fowler, 1992). Financial losses or gains were assessed from the perspective of the hospital, without attention to the overall societal impact. Further systematic evaluation is needed on the effectiveness of subacute care units.

Another alternative might be to begin discharge planning prior to admission. An educational program to prepare elders to think about options for their care might be offered as part of preadmission workup for elective cases. This approach, however, would only work for elective admissions. Elders admitted for an emergency would require a different approach. The latter group might benefit from some type of case management or from transfer to subacute care units to allow time to consider options for postdischarge care.

Education of health care professionals might address difficulties related to ageism and care coordination. Ageism might be addressed by exposing health care professionals to models of successful aging to counter negative stereotypes. Care coordination necessitates addressing not only the patient's needs, but also the family context, the community resources, and the payment systems for care. Clinical training programs give little attention to how one coordinates care across systems, assesses resources in the community in which the elder resides, or negotiates systems of care. Although physicians may have limited time to invest in discharge planning, one might expect medical education to place greater emphasis on personalized care and treating elders in a manner that maximizes functioning and independence. Training needs also include information on options available postdischarge and how to assist families with decision making. More effective use of gerontological nurse practitioners in providing primary care to elderly persons might include special discharge planning services. Both nurses and physicians need information on advantages and disadvantages of home care, nursing home placement, and rehabilitation. Because the available options for nursing home, home health care, rehabilitation, ancillary services, and supports for family caregivers are likely to vary by community, physicians need some background in assessing communities and their resources. Listening to patient and family preferences, incorporating these preferences in the plans, providing information on the options available, and facilitating decision making are essential components in the discharge planning process. Training is also needed in addressing the non-medical aspects of patient care, such as assessing social and physical environments to which the patient might return. Equally important is that the learning occur in an interdisciplinary environment so the various professionals can learn how each discipline can contribute to the planning process and thereby avoid duplication of effort.

Another option to improve care coordination might be some form of case management. Case management is a system of care that focuses on the achievement of outcomes within specified time frames. It differs from traditional discharge planning in that some models of case management cross all settings in which the patient receives care (Williams, 1993). There is lack of agreement on who needs case management and ethical dilemmas inherent in models in which the case manager serves as gatekeeper of the resources and provider of patient needs (Clemens, Wetle, Feltes, Crabtree, & Dubitzkyl, 1994). There is also lack of agreement on who should provide case management services, particularly services that include discharge planning. Should case managers replace discharge planners? If not, how might the case manager and discharge planner interface to prevent duplication of services? Whereas case management is a logical function for both nurses and social workers, most curricula for nursing and social work do not provide opportunities to acquire the knowledge and skills needed for case management (Redford, 1992). Although it is possible to integrate content on case management in curricula for both nurses and social workers, it might be more efficient for academic institutions to offer an interdisciplinary minor in case management.

The case manager role is now sometimes filled by a patient's family member. Previous studies indicate that family members wanted to have some control over the way in which services were delivered (Malone-Beach, Zarit, & Spore, 1992). Assuming the role of case manager is one way of maintaining control: Family members take an active role in coordinating posthospital care, have vested interest in the welfare of their loved ones, and are likely to be committed to coordinating care. Although family members do not have formal training in negotiating systems of care, they learn from experience. The learning experience is, however, marked with frustrations (including rehospitalizations) that might be avoided if family were better prepared for the role. Seltzer, Litchfield, Kapust, and Mayer (1992) found that family members who were prepared to function as case managers assumed more tasks on behalf of their elder and did not experience an increase in caregiving burden. If family members assume this role, one might ask whether some form of financial reimbursement or paid leave of absence from their job might be appropriate as this might reduce the stress or burden they experience. In assuming the case manager role they provide a vital service, one that may well save insurance companies dollars spent on hospital readmissions. To fulfill the case manager role, however, family members often give up jobs or take on the additional task while sacrificing personal health and social activities. Providing financial reimbursement for their time might allow family members to maintain their health and lessen the multiple demands.

The pressures of DRG-based prospective reimbursement brought issues of discharge planning to the forefront. Although DRGs provided hospitals with financial incentives for shortening hospital stays, reimbursement to hospitals or physicians for discharge planning was not included. Furthermore, there was less time in which to plan for discharge. The end result is a false sense of economy, particularly when one reflects on the costs associated with Medicare readmissions. There is reason to believe that an investment in discharge planning might produce better results.

Although all patients need to have their needs for follow-up care assessed and are entitled to some degree of discharge planning, not all patients need extensive discharge planning from either the hospital or physician. It might be reasonable to pay for discharge planning for only a "high risk" subset of the population. Medicare is a logical source of payment because discharge planning might save costs associated with readmissions. Hospitals that provide these services might receive payments above the DRG allowances or discharge planning costs could be incorporated into selected DRGs. Use of criteria such as age, functional status, and living arrangements to identify persons at risk have resulted in both false negatives (persons need care and are not referred) and false positives (persons receive care who do not need it) (Berkman et al., 1990). Further research is needed on how to identify persons at risk and whether an investment in discharge planning leads to improved patient outcomes and lower costs. Studies such as the following might provide insights on the benefits of discharge planning: (a) a randomized clinical trial examining the effects of structured discharge planning on outcomes, (b) the effects on outcomes of using swing beds or short-term stays in nursing homes for discharge planning, and (c) the effects of bundling hospital and posthospital care payments on delivery of health services and on outcomes of care. The latter is currently being examined by the Health Care Financing Administration.

There are no quick and easy answers to the problem of providing continuity of care. No single solution will meet the diverse needs of different cultural groups. In fact, state laws create unique environments that can enhance or inhibit different approaches to coordinating care and need to be considered in developing a system to address continuity of care. We need to investigate which systems of care coordination are most effective, and under what conditions. What is effective in a university teaching hospital may not work, or even be needed in a rural community hospital. Educating health care professionals to key aspects of care coordination and how to work effectively in interdisciplinary teams, however, is critical if any of the solutions are to work.

▬REFERENCES

Balsano, A., & Fowler, F. (1993). Subacute care as a new source of revenue. *Healthcare Financial Management, 47*(7), 56–62.

Beatty, S. R. (1980). An overview of continuity of care. In S. Beatty (Ed.), *Continuity of care: The Hospital and the community* (pp. 3–12). New York: Grune and Stratton.

Berkman, B., & Abrams, R. (1980). Factors relating to hospital readmission of elderly patients. *Social Work, 33,* 99–103.

Berkman, B., Millar, S., Holmos, W., & Bonander, E. (1990). Screening elder cardiac patients to identify need for social work services. *Health and Social Work, 15*(1), 64–72.

Bull, M. J. (1992). Managing the transition from hospital to home. *Qualitative Health Research, 2*(1), 27–41.

Bull, M. J. (1994). Patients' and professionals' perceptions of quality in discharge planning. *Journal of Nursing Care Quality, 8*(2), 47–61.

Bull, M. J., Maruyama, G., & Luo, D. (1995). Testing a model for posthospital transition of family caregivers for elders. *Nursing Research, 44*(3), 131–138.

Clemens, E., Wetle, T., Feltes, M., Crabtree, B., & Dubitzky, D. (1994). Contradictions in case management: Client-centered theory and directive practice with frail elderly. *Journal of Aging and Health, 6*(1), 70–88.

Coulton, C. (1992). Evaluating screening and early intervention: A puzzle with many pieces. *Social Work and Health Care, 13*(3), 65–72.

Fink, A., Siu, A., & Brook, R. (1987). Assuring the quality of health care for older persons. *Journal of the American Medical Association, 258,* 1905–1908.

Fowler, F. (1992). Subacute care offers flexibility, revenue. *Modern Healthcare, 22*(43), 50.

Gerety, M., Soderholm-Difatte, V., & Winograd, C. (1989). Impact of prospective payment and discharge location on the outcome of hip fracture. *Journal of General Internal Medicine, 4,* 388–391.

Glaser, B. (1978). *Theoretical sensitivity.* Mill Valley, CA: Sociology Press.

Glaser, B., & Strauss, A. (1967). *The discovery of grounded theory.* Chicago: Aldine.

Gornick, M., & Hall, M. (1988). Trends in Medicare use of posthospital care. *Health Care Financing Review, 9,* 27–38.

Jackson, M. (1994). Discharge planning: Issues and challenges for gerontological nursing. *Journal of Advanced Nursing, 19,* 492–502.

Lincoln, Y., & Guba, E. (1985). *Naturalistic inquiry.* Beverly Hills, CA: Sage.

Malone-Beach, E., Zarit, S., & Spore, D. (1992). Caregivers' perceptions of case management and community-based services: Barriers to service use. *Journal of Applied Gerontology, 11*(2), 146–159.

Mamon, J., Steinwachs, D., Fahey, M., Bone, L., Okay, J., & Klein, L. (1992). Impact of hospital discharge planning on meeting patient needs after returning home. *Health Services Reaserch, 27*(2), 155–175.

McKeehan, K. M. (1981). *Continuing care. A multidisciplinary approch to discharge planning.* St. Louis, MO: C. V. Mosby.

McWilliam, C., & Sangster, J. (1994). Managing patient discharge to home: The challenges of achieving quality of care. *International Journal for Quality in Health Care, 6*(2), 147–161.

Miles, M., & Huberman, A. M. (1984). *Qualitative data analysis.* Beverly Hills, CA: Sage.

Morse, J., & Field, P. (1995). *Qualitative research methods for health care professionals.* Thousand Oaks, CA: Sage.

Proctor, E., & Morrow-Howell, N. (1990). Complications in discharge planning with Medicare patients. *Health and Social Work, 15,* 45–54.

Randall, V. (1994). Impact of managed care organizations on ethnic Americans and underserved populations. *Journal of Health Care for the Poor and Underserved, 5*(3), 224–237.

Redford, L. (1992). Case management the wave of the future. *Journal of Case Management, 1*(1), 5–8.

Sandelowki, M. (1986). The problem of rigor in qualitative research, *Advances in Nursing Science, 8,* 27–37.

Seltzer, M., Litchfield, L., Kapust, L., & Mayer, J. (1992). Professional and family collaboration in case management: A hospital-based replication of a community-based study. *Social Work in Health Care, 17*(1), 1–22.

Shaughnessy, P., Schlenker, R. E., & Hittle, D. F. (1994). Home health outcomes under capitated and fee-for-service payment. *Health Care Financing Review, 16*(1), 187–222.

U.S. Department of Health and Human Services, Health Care Financing Administration. (1992). *Report of the secretary's advisory panel on the development of a uniform needs assessment instrument.* Washington, DC: U.S. Government Printing Office.

Williams, J. (1993). Case management: Opportunities for service providers. *Home Health Care Services Quarterly, 14*(1), 5–40.

Wolock, I., Schlesinger, E., Dinerman, M., & Seaton, R. (1987). The posthospital needs and care of patients: Implications for discharge planning. *Social Work and Health Care, 12*(4), 61–76.

SELECTED BIBLIOGRAPHY

Achenbaum, W. A. & Bengtson, V. L. (1994). Re-engaging the Disengagement Theory of Aging: On the history and assessment of theory development in gerontology. *The Gerontologist* 34(6): 756–763.

Badger, T. A. (1993). Physical health impairment and depression among older adults. *Image: Journal of Nursing Scholarship* 25(4): 325–330.

Boult, C., Altmann, M., Gilbertson, D., Yu, C., & Kane, R. (1996). Decreasing disability in the 21st century: The future effects of controlling six fatal and nonfatal conditions. *American Journal of Public Health* 86(10): 1388–1393.

Brink, C. A., Sampselle, C. M., Wells, T. J., Diokno, A. C., & Gillis, G. L. (1989). A digital test for pelvic muscle strength in older women with urinary incontinence. *Nursing Research* 38(4): 196–199.

Courneya, K. S. (1995). Understanding readiness for regular physical activity in older individuals: An application of the Theory of Planned Behavior. *Health Psychology* 14(1): 80–87.

Duffy, M. E. (1993). Determinants of health-promoting lifestyles in older persons. *Image: Journal of Nursing Scholarship* 25(1): 23–28.

Hendricks, J. (1994). Revisiting the Kansas City study of adult life: Roots of the Disengagement Model in social gerontology. *The Gerontologist* 34(6): 753–755.

Hoffman, R. (1991). Medication-taking by the frail elderly in two groups. *Nursing Forum* 26(4): 19–24.

LaVeist, R. A. (1995). Data sources for aging research on racial and ethnic groups. *The Gerontologist* 35(3): 328–339.

Logan, J. R., & Spitze, G. (1994). Informal support and the use of formal services by older Americans. *Journal of Gerontology: Social Sciences* 49(1): 525–534.

Pohl, J. M. & Boyd, C. J. (1993). Ageism within feminism. *Image: Journal of Nursing Scholarship* 25(3): 199–203.

Preston, D. B. & Bucher, J. A. (1996). The effects of community differences on health status, health stress, and helping networks in a sample of 900 elderly. *Public Health Nursing* 13(1): 72–79.

Resnick, B. (1995). Measurement tools: Do they apply equally to older adults? *Journal of Gerontological Nursing* 21(7): 18–22.

Sayles-Cross, S. (1993). Perceptions of familial caregivers of elder adults. *Image: Journal of Nursing Scholarship* 25(2): 88–92.

Strumpf, N. E., Evans, L. K., Wagner, J., & Patterson, J. (1992). Reducing physical restraints: Developing an educational program. *Journal of Gerontological Nursing* 18(11): 21–27.

Unit 6

From Malnutrition to Sleep Problems: Assessing Older Adults

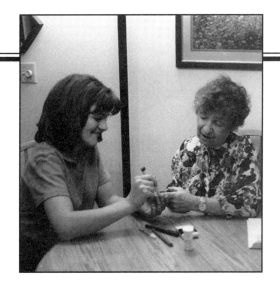

C areful, diligent assessment of older adults is necessary before effective nursing interventions can be designed. An atmosphere of trust is generally regarded as a precursor to the gathering of data, or assessment. This is generally accomplished by developing rapport and engagement with older adults — taking an interest in their concerns and symptoms, treating them with respect and dignity, and using effective communication strategies such as reflective listening. The sometimes vague symptom complaints or concerns about deterioration of functional abilities can be important clues to the gerontological nurse. New or changing concerns may indicate a need for further assessment and intervention.

Gerontological nurses may work individually with clients, or as part of an interdisciplinary assessment team. Because of the diverse problems many frail elderly clients possess, a team approach is considered best by many experts in the field of aging. Nursing brings a holistic, family systems approach to team assessment, and a rich history of client advocacy.

The unique health problems that many elders face require special assessment skills of the nurses who work with them. Cognitive impairment, malnutrition, depression and suicide, along with heart disease and hypertension, are problems commonly associated with older clients.

Although textbooks offer explicit information on a wide variety of assessment skills, this unit attempts to highlight selected areas of interest for nurses and other health care professionals working with geriatric clients. This unit focuses on several areas of assessment specific to the elderly client. Chapters in this unit cover interdisciplinary teamwork in regard to quality of life; nutrition; sleep disturbances; protocols for cognitive assessment; and assessment of elder abuse.

Through careful assessment of elderly patients, gerontological nurses can gain greater insight into the needs of their clients and better protect their safety and health.

Chapter 34

Quality of Life, Values, and Teamwork in Geriatric Care: Do We Communicate What We Mean?

PHILLIP G. CLARK

What does "quality of life" truly mean to our older clients? Is it the same for everyone, or does it have a uniquely individual interpretation? If it is based solely on measures of functional independence, what does that mean for our aging disabled clients? This author explains that we, as service providers, must individually and jointly, as team members, clarify our thoughts and biases on this issue — for they may shade our definition of client problems as well as our suggested interventions. And, to complicate matters further, each member of an interdisciplinary team may have disparate definitions because of unique professional paradigms and training methods. He recommends developing an "empowering and reflective ethic" and joining with our aging clients in a spirit of mutual respect, and proposes that this will enable health care team members to better discover the true meaning of this oft-repeated phrase.

The expression "adding life to years rather than years to life" captures the changing direction in the care of the frail elderly over the last decade. From a past emphasizing of the "heroic" model of medicine extending life at any cost is emerging a more "humanistic" model of care, focusing on individual quality of life. As acute illness has increasingly given way to chronic disease as the major health challenge facing Western societies — mirrored in greater numbers of the elderly at risk for chronic illness and its associated disabling conditions — a gradual shift from curing to caring is occurring within our health care system. This transformation is still in process, however, creating conflicts and communication problems between health care providers, as well as between these professionals and the frail elderly and their families.

From *The Gerontologist* 35(3):402–411, 1995. Reprinted with permission.

Solving these problems hinges on the continued theoretical development and practical application of new concepts to guide geriatric care, such as quality of life. However, this concept means different things to different people, whether providers or consumers of care. In assessing these differences, it is important that we carefully examine our thought and language, and ask the question: "Do we understand and communicate what we really mean?" in clinical practice and decision-making settings involving frail older persons — whether institutionalized or living in the community. In particular, individual and cultural values play an important role in defining and operationalizing the concept of quality of life. For example, families may differ considerably in their definition of the burden of care created by a frail, impaired member and their resultant assessment of the quality of that life (Kayser-Jones, 1986). Similarly, a poor quality of life for one person may be a rich life for another: What we might consider to be a life full of sickness, frailty, and dependence might provide another person with new insights into the existential nature of human life and its continual conditionality and precariousness (Gadow, 1983). Importantly, over-emphasis on individual independence in constructing a definition of quality of life may neglect the values of community, collectivism, and interdependence that are equally important in human existence (Clark, 1991a). Clearly, the concept of quality of life is at once crucial and confusing, important and intangible, clinically central and conceptually elusive.

In order to respond to this challenge of relating quality of life to communication patterns in geriatric care, the purpose of this discussion is multifaceted. First, it outlines a framework for understanding the different dimensions of the concept of quality of life for elderly persons with functional disabilities — particularly as it is used in communication among health care providers, and between them and their frail elderly patients and families. By examining the differing assumptions and values underlying this concept, we may achieve a better understanding of differences in its use and thereby improve communication about it in the future. Second, this article examines and summarizes empirical research on: (1) professional communication involving elderly patients and their families, with respect to the barriers to effective dialogue around the concept of life quality; and (2) interprofessional communication patterns, particularly those involving physicians, nurses, and social workers. This discussion provides concrete examples of how quality of life notions can be interpreted very differently by different persons. Third, a conceptual framework — based on emerging medical, nursing, and social work models — is proposed for more effectively involving the concerns, goals, and values of the frail elderly individual in the dialogue with health care providers over issues of quality of life. Finally, the conclusion explores methods for achieving more effective overall communication to reveal the essential dimensions of quality of life and how it may be operationalized in clinical practice, a process I will term "developing an empowering and reflective ethic."

▬ THINKING ABOUT QUALITY OF LIFE FOR THE FRAIL ELDERLY

Discussions of such concepts as quality of life are fraught with major conceptual and practical challenges. Not the least of these relates to clarifying its different foundations and dimensions. The concept of life quality is seen both as deeply personal and subjective, and as a kind of general intuitive yardstick with which to make clinical decisions about the wisdom of pursuing various types of treatments for very frail older persons. The purpose of this section is not to provide an exhaustive examination of all the facets of this concept, but rather to explore it in sufficient detail to highlight some major developments in the fields of gerontology and geriatrics that may help us to think more clearly about what it really means in the lives of older persons with disabling conditions. The three themes which I wish particularly to discuss are: (1) the growing attraction of the level of personal functional ability as a proxy for the more slippery concept of life quality; (2) the relationship between autonomy and quality of life in the gerontological literature; and (3) lessons to be learned about quality of life from the independent living movement.

Accompanying changes in the focus on health care outcomes for the elderly are new measurement methodologies that seem to be intuitively related to quality of life. For example, the long-used indicator of *life expectancy* has recently been replaced by Katz et al.'s (1983) and Katz, Greer, Beck, Branch, and Spector's (1985) concept of *functional life expectancy*, defined as simple survival in the former but by independence of personal function in the latter. Growth of interest in individual functional ability is apparent in the increasing emphasis on functional assessment of elderly persons, advocated by such official groups as the American College of Physicians (Almy, 1988) and the Society of General Internal Medicine (Rubenstein et al., 1989). Assessment methodologies are typically multidimensional, reflecting the multifaceted nature of the health problems of older persons, and they incorporate biological, psychological, and social aspects of an individual's life — further reinforcing their appeal. Moreover, this expansion of clinical concerns beyond the realm of a narrow medical model has helped to support the growth of interprofessional health care teams in assessing and managing the health problems of the elderly with disabilities, based on the simple recognition that not any one health discipline "owns" an in-depth understanding of them (Tsukuda, 1990; Zeiss & Steffen, in press).

There are major potentials and pitfalls in equating functional independence with quality of life. This is seen clearly in the growing literature on autonomy and aging. For example, research has linked personal control or autonomy to the concept of successful aging in particular (Rowe & Kahn, 1987) and more generally to positive health outcomes (e.g., Langer & Rodin, 1976; Rodin, 1986; Rodin & Langer, 1977). Others have seen quality of life and autonomy critically linked to health care decision making for older persons (Clark, 1987; 1988) and to their empowerment in the health care system (Clark, 1989). Indeed, entire issues of major gerontological journals have been devoted to the central importance of preserving auton-omy in frail, at-risk elderly populations — for example, supplements to *The Gerontologist* in 1988 and to *Generations* in 1990.

Two important caveats to this heavy reliance of quality of life language on measures related to functional independence and autonomy must be mentioned. First, over-reliance on simple individual autonomy ignores the critical contributions made to life by a sense of community. Certainly the important contribution of social supports in maintaining independence is a major theme in gerontology that nicely captures the paradox in our thinking about autonomy. Even in long-term care settings in which auton-omy has traditionally been emphasized the most, other voices are being raised that question its perceived domination. For example, although Kane and Caplan (1990) underscore the importance of autonomy for the nursing home resident, they also explore the situational complexities of over-emphasis on this single concept in an institutional context. Similarly, Agich (1990) suggests the need to consider the complex interrelationship between dependence and independence in long-term care. Collopy, Boyle, and Jennings (1991) explore the limitations that traditional individualistic con-ceptions of autonomy impose on the nursing home setting, and they call for the development of the notion of "autonomy within community" as an appropriate expression of this insight. In the community long-term care setting as well, authors such as Collopy, Dubler, and Zuckerman (1990) suggest that the simplistic dichotomy between independence and depen-dence no longer accurately describes the complexities facing elderly, frail individuals, and their families in the struggle to provide care and support to loved ones.

A second caveat is to be found in the expanding literature on disability and aging. Minkler (1990), for example, warns that the growing reliance on the concept of "successful aging" may reinforce the prejudice against elders with disabilities — the "elderly mystique" explored earlier by Cohen (1988). Calling for the development of a unified, dialectical approach to aging instead of the bipolar, "successful" versus "unsuccessful" dichotomy, she draws on the independent living movement for inspiration and guid-ance concerning the abilities and capabilities of the disabled. Older persons themselves may fall victim to the elderly mystique stereotype, assuming that the onset of disability associated with chronic health problems marks the beginning of inevitable decline and the end of control over their lives — their perceived "failure" in growing older. Even worse, prac-titioners, program planners, and policy makers may unwittingly reinforce this message by fashioning programs based on the success/failure dichot-omy (Cohen, 1992).

The growing conjunction between the aging and the disabilities fields (e.g., Ansello, 1992; Ansello & Eustis, 1992; Ansello & Rose, 1989) provides an important insight into the interrelationships among autonomy, disabil-ity, and human services that has implications for our thinking about quality of life. As Cohen (1992) observes for the independent living movement, autonomy relates to the achievement of individual consumer goals; services are seen less as compensating for physical and psychological deficits than as enhancing or limiting independence. Importantly, services are evaluated on the basis of whether they are controlled by the consumer or by the agency; they should be directed at goals that enhance the meaning of life by encouraging involvement and engagement — not simply assuring survival and postponing institutionalization. This important distinction is captured conceptually by Collopy's (1988) exploration of the polarity in decisional versus executional autonomy: Decisional autonomy consists in the freedom to make decisions without external coercion, whereas executional autonomy is the ability to carry out and implement these personal choices. Giving individuals with disabilities power to control their use of services to act on their own goals in life becomes an essential element linked to their perceived control — not whether or not they have a disability. Moreover, the control of services needed to operationalize choice must rest with the consumer, not the agency. This way of framing autonomy and the use of services is very different from that traditionally prevailing in the aging service network, and it can give us an important insight into the social construction of aging and disability to clarify our thinking about quality of life for the frail elderly.

■ COMMUNICATION ABOUT THE MEANING OF QUALITY OF LIFE AMONG PROVIDERS AND CONSUMERS

Issues relating to assumptions, concepts, and values surrounding the meaning of quality of life for the frail elderly are not simply "academic" — they have major implications for how providers and consumers communicate with each other in making health care decisions, and for how professionals communicate with each other in collaborative or interprofessional contexts.

Dimensions of Meaning of Health and Life Quality for Providers and Consumers

As discussed earlier, service providers may dichotomize aging into positive and negative (healthy and disabled) categories, and develop and offer services for the frail elderly based on a deficit model. Under these conditions, services may be "packaged" by providers in response to their definition of what is the elderly individual's particular disability. The communication problem here is that a major conceptual gap exists between professionals and laypersons with regard to their construction of the meaning of health and health-related problems. Providers and consumers approach health issues from different perspectives — with the former reflecting the professional and organizational concepts and patterns of practice in which they have been trained, and the latter embodying different influences from their personal experiences, familial contexts, and cultural backgrounds (Dill, 1993). Providers and consumers speak different languages, though they may use the same words.

Moreover, because of differentials in power between the professional and the patient, the professional's definition of need, or the "problem" to be "solved," usually takes precedence over that of the client. The person who controls the definition of the problem simultaneously defines the range of options available to solve it (Clark, 1993) — an insight having both clinical (Dill, 1993) and public policy relevance (Aronson, 1992; 1993). In other words, recipients of clinical care and public policies must have genuine input into the basic construction of need and the concepts used to describe it, or else consumers will be prevented from effective dialogue and discussion regarding the important outcomes of the needs assessment process. Unfortunately, frail older persons may not even be aware that their needs are being defined by others, and they may have to be empowered to break out of this pattern — as the independent living movement has accomplished for younger persons with disabilities.

This definitional difference is especially apparent in the perceptions of health by the elderly. For example, research (Mangione et al., 1993) has shown that the elderly have a greater gap between their objectively and subjectively assessed health status than younger age groups. In particular, they report similar overall health perceptions to younger persons even when they are "objectively" assessed as having poorer role function, lower energy levels, and less physical function. This difference between subjective and objective measures of health status in the elderly has been recognized for some time by researchers who were puzzled by high self-reported global health assessments and low objectively defined health scores.

Even taxonomies of quality of life that are broadly defined to include the comprehensive categories of *functioning* (social, physical, emotional, and intellectual) and *perceptions* (life satisfaction and health status) may not necessarily guarantee that professionals will understand quality of life of the elderly with disabilities, because they were not derived with input from patient populations themselves (e.g., Pearlman & Uhlmann, 1988). This lack illustrates the crucial importance of involving client populations in the development of frameworks defining need.

Indeed, research into the perceptions of quality of life among elderly persons with chronic diseases found a disparity between how the concept was interpreted by physicians and their patients. Generally, elderly patients considered their quality of life to be "good enough" if they had no major complaints, regardless of the degree of severity of their illness. In contrast, physicians rated their patients' quality of life as significantly worse. In this same research, in their responses to open-ended questions patients emphasized medical care, health-related problems, and interpersonal relationships (involving family and friends) as factors affecting quality of life (Pearlman & Uhlmann, 1988). Importantly, subsequent research by these same authors (Uhlmann & Pearlman, 1991) has shown that physicians' estimations of quality of patient life are significantly associated with their attitudes toward life-sustaining treatment for their patients. This demonstrates the important clinical decision-making implications of differences in interpretations of life quality, given that patients' perceived quality of life was *not* found to be associated with their preferences for life-sustaining treatment.

A similar disparity between professionals on the one hand and frail, elderly patients and their families on the other is echoed in the research to map values in long-term care decision making (McCullough, Wilson, Teasdale, Kolpakchi, & Skelly, 1993). Recognizing that major differences exist between acute and long-term care settings with regard to the clarity of clinical problem definitions, the authors nevertheless noted that autonomy-related issues still seem central in both types of settings. More importantly, the researchers discovered major differences among the "value maps" of individuals, families, and professionals. For example, professionals identi-fied the values of care (quality care, adequate supervision), physical health (medical care, safety from health threats), interpersonal relationships (so-cialization and companionship), and psychological well-being (emotional and mental health) to be of greatest importance. For the frail elderly, environmental factors (privacy, pleasant living conditions), self-identity (in-dependence and self-sufficiency), and interpersonal relationships (having company and acquaintances) were preeminent. In contrast, for family and friends the researchers determined that the three major areas of value importance were: care (meeting needs and having supervision), security (safety), and psychological well-being (happiness and activities).

Based on these findings, the authors' conclusions were that ". . . elders may have values and priorities of values for themselves other than health-related values. Elders expressed values related to self-identity . . . more often than values concerned with physical and mental health — in contrast to the frequency of health-related generic values expressed by the profes-sionals" (pp. 330–331). A major implication of this disparity is the impact of these different values and priorities on the type and quality of communi-cation between health professionals and their patients and families, particu-larly with regard to what different aspects of quality of life each selectively emphasizes. How can both sides in this dialogue be assured that each party understands the other, that "what they are saying" is truly understood by the other in an ongoing attempt to make the difficult decisions embedded in the constantly shifting settings of long-term care, where quality of life considerations figure prominently in how decisions are made? More im-portantly, how can professionals develop the kind of inner moral reflectivity and sensitivity needed to detect and understand these important value dif-ferences?

Some commentators suggest that the development of a "communicative ethic" may overcome these problems. For example, empirical research (Miller, Coe, & Hyers, 1992) documents that some physicians take into account the concept of "patient wishes" as a central, organizing theme in initially attempting to reach consensus among patients and their families on withdrawing or withholding care for critically ill patients. Physicians were judged in most cases to provide direct and unambiguous *introductions* to the concept of limiting treatment and to encourage a participatory style of decision making to balance the competing goals of extending life, providing high quality life, fostering patient autonomy, and maximizing social justice (i.e., balancing competing obligations). Unfortunately and importantly, however, this research also showed that by the *end* of the discussion, many physicians had shifted to a shaded presentation of out-comes reflective of their own biases.

The philosophical basis for open communication in the long-term care decision-making context has been developed by Moody (1988) in his concept of the "communicative ethic" emphasizing the "three Cs" of "communication, clarification, and consensus-building" in negotiating the shifting shoals of client autonomy and professional paternalism in long-term care decision making for the frail elderly. Although recognizing its imperfections, Moody suggests that such a procedural ethic based on communication is preferable to a static, principled approach that is frequently unattainable in professional practice. Moreover, when dealing with particularly thorny quality of life considerations, it should be obvious by now that the various professional parties in this discussion need to examine the concepts, assumptions, and values underlying their various approaches to defining the clinical problem and seeking its solution. Hence, we must now turn to issues relating to communication among different health care professionals.

Communication among Professionals: Do We Say What We Mean on the Interprofessional Team?

Due to the multifaceted nature of the chronic health problems of the frail elderly, the need for teams of professionals from different disciplines to work together in creating and coordinating necessary care has become widely recognized (e.g., Clark, Spence, & Sheehan, 1987; Tsukuda, 1990; Zeiss & Steffen, in press). However, simply assembling professionals into a group falls far short of developing an effective team in which patterns of communication are at the level necessary for true interdisciplinary functioning (Clark, Spence, & Sheehan, 1986). This fact is evident in a widely quoted definition of the interdisciplinary team (Luszki, 1958; cited in Given & Simmons, 1977, p. 16):

> *The interdisciplinary team is a group of persons who are trained in the use of different tools and concepts, among whom there is an organized division of labor around a common problem with each member using his own tools, with continuous intercommunication and re-examination of postulates in terms of the limitations provided by the work of the other members and often with group responsibility for the final product.*

The development of a truly interdisciplinary team requires recognition of the importance of both knowledge- and value-related dimensions of professional practice (Clark, 1991b). Values, in particular, are a major source of conflicting and competing communication patterns among health professionals, who are educated and trained in very different modes and methods of practice with regard to their relationships with each other, as well as with the client or patient (Clark, 1994). The concept of quality of life is fraught with divergent interpretations precisely because of these differences in how health care professionals are socialized into differing systems of care.

For example, Qualls & Czirr (1988) suggest that professionals may differ in their logic of geriatric clinical assessment; that is, how to define the problem. This difference may be characterized by two different styles of practice, one emphasizing "ruling out problems" by systematically eliminating possibilities until only one problem and a corresponding solution are discovered. In contrast, the other approach of "ruling in problems" relies on expanding the range of professional view to encompass an increasingly long list of potential factors. For example, physicians are trained in diagnostic techniques that narrow down the range of options, relying heavily on "objective" data such as laboratory tests in the process. Social workers, on the other hand, are taught to go beyond the narrow presenting problem to encompass larger psychosocial issues, such as income, family relationships, and environment. In this process, they tend to rely on "subjective" data collected by interviews that are heavily interpreted by clinical judgment and experience. Nurses, depending on their background and training, may fall somewhere between these two extremes. Such differences in delimiting the domain of inquiry in clinical practice have major implications for communication over such conceptually slippery concepts as quality of life.

For example, empirical research in nursing homes has found that physicians and nursing assistants (whom we may consider to be aligned generally with nursing practice models) differ considerably on their feelings about the basis for life-extending treatment and the meaning of care (Kayser-Jones, 1986):

> *To the nursing assistants, caring is a more important factor than mental and physical status of the patient. "We are here to take care of these patients," they repeatedly stressed. Physicians, they believe, are oriented toward curing illness, and when a cure cannot be achieved their interest in caring for the patient may tend to decline. A 65-year-old physician confirmed the nursing staff's observation: "The more untreatable the condition, the more disinterest there is on the part of younger physicians in treating the patient."... One doctor confided that in some cases he would prefer to withhold treatment but, because the nurses were so pro-life, he would be in trouble if he did not treat the patient (pp. 1282–1283).*

Additional findings from this research revealed that differing interpretations of the concept of quality of life underlay these differences in approaches to care. For most physicians, quality of life was related to mental status or freedom from mental impairment; by contrast, quality of life for nurses was more relative. Physical strength, even in the presence of mental impairment, was considered a key determinant of life quality. This contrast can be seen in typical comments about quality of life. One doctor said: "Quality of life is being mentally unimpaired, being continent of urine and feces, being able to talk, and knowing who you are." When nursing assistants were asked to define quality of life, they responded: "Being able to see and hear, good health, having friends, and having someone to love you" (Kayser-Jones, 1986, p. 1284).

These differences in defining quality of life may be understood within the larger framework of disparities in the perception of ethical problems by physicians and nurses. Divergence between these two professions with regard to the recognition of moral dilemmas in practice suggests that such differences are crucial to understanding why communication about such value-laden concepts as "quality of life" can be so difficult. For example, Gramelspacher, Howell, and Young (1986) found that physicians and nurses differed significantly within each group with regard to how often they perceived ethical dilemmas, and that nurses were much more often to report conflicts with physicians over ethical dilemmas than were physicians to recognize disagreements with nurses. Subsequent research by Walker, Miles, Stocking, and Siegler (1991) also found significant differences between nurses and physicians with regard to the ethical problems they identified. For example, three-quarters of the problems centering on a patient's quality of life were described by physicians rather than nurses. The authors explained the disagreement over ethics problems as a function of professional orientation and socialization, with nurses increasingly oriented toward patient-centered issues — such as patient preferences, family issues, pain control, implementing treatments, and discharge planning. By contrast, physicians were directed more toward problems embodying increased concern about the cost of care and the proper use of medical resources — such as quality of life, economic factors, and inappropriate admissions. Importantly, physicians' concerns about quality of life were interpreted as consistent with previous research (summarized earlier) linking life quality considerations to decisions to withhold therapy, and to the tendency of physicians to rate the life quality of chronically ill elderly more negatively than do their patients.

In addition to medicine and nursing, social work affords us another perspective on the differences underlying the health professions regarding life quality interpretations involving the frail elderly. Social work has traditionally represented the broader psychosocial perspective on quality of life concerns in health and illness (e.g., Sharp, 1993). This view entails the involvement of several relevant dimensions, including: (1) an assessment of the social environment (including family, social support, economic and cultural factors, and the physical setting); (2) the right of the individual to make his or her own decisions (autonomy); (3) the identification and mobilization of resources in the family and the community; and (4) mediation among the major professional and institutional "players" in defining and solving the elderly individual's "problem" (Jones, Meredith, Wadas, Watt, & Weisz, 1991). This philosophical orientation ensures that the individual's perspective on, and definition of, quality of life will be incorporated into the ongoing discussion among other health professionals, the patient or client, and the social worker — an important principle discussed earlier. However, the very skills that social workers employ to make certain that individuals have a voice in decision making about their own lives may not serve them well in working with other health professionals. Indeed, some observers (such as Kane, 1975) suggest that social workers' ability to communicate on the interprofessional team may be impaired by their socialization and professional orientation. Given the central importance of including in clinical decision-making processes individuals' values and personal perspectives on what constitutes quality of life *for them* (Cassel, 1992), it seems imperative that this essential orientation not be lost in the dialogue among the different professions represented on the interdisciplinary team. New models of health care may be required to address this communication-related need.

■NEW MODELS FOR CARE AND COMMUNICATION

It is significant that along with the dual emphasis on the concepts of quality of life and the interdisciplinary team in clinical geriatric practice have emerged new theoretical frameworks to integrate into the care model the values of the individual client or patient that shape his or her definition of quality of life. These new approaches promise to break down the barriers separating patients from care providers, and the providers from each other; and they are suggestive of ways to change forever how health professionals conceptualize their roles and goals in caring for the frail elderly with disabling conditions. Importantly, the principle of empowerment of the consumer, client, or patient in defining quality of life is a central organizing theme of these approaches.

Beyond Biomedical Nursing

Theories of nursing reflect different emphases and assumptions, with some clearly tied to the prevailing biomedical model which tends to be "problem-based," with an emphasis on functional abilities, problems, deficits, and special needs determined by assessment methodologies and evaluations by "experts." Some observers (e.g., Mitchell, 1992) have noted that the compartmentalization of the individual into such categories lends itself well to the interprofessional team, with each specialist "owning" a particular part of the patient or client. In contrast to this model, however, is a more holistic one, such as that developed by Parse (1987; 1992), which emphasizes the unity of the individual — who is not known simply as the sum of various parts. Rooted in a humanistic ethic, this theoretical perspective emphasizes quality of life as *perceived by the individual* and his or her family. According to Mitchell (1992), ". . . health is not defined according to the biological, psychological, and social norms established by experts. Rather, health is a process of living what is important in daily life according to each individual's value priorities, meanings, hopes, and dreams" (p. 104).

The emphasis on the lived experience and personal history of the elderly individual, embodying his or her own values and life goals, becomes the center-piece of this model of caring; and different professionals on the interdisciplinary team are challenged to recognize that their caring must be directed to the concerns and goals of this person — not their own agendas, needs, and problem definitions. In particular, the old modes of thought and practice of health care disciplines, founded on problem-based methodologies of assessment and care plan development controlled by the professional, must give way to a new mode of practice driven by an ethic of communication about the goals and concerns of the individual. In summary:

> *The values of traditional nursing direct nurses to focus on assessment, prediction, and control of problems. This approach is enacted with the misguided belief that reverence for the person and ethical decisionmaking can then be "added on." But ethics is not a separate way of knowing. All knowledge is already rooted in an ethic, and practice related to that knowledge reflects the ethic (Mitchell, 1992, p. 105).*

Goal-Oriented Medical Practice

Theoreticians in geriatric medicine have also developed a new conceptual framework, "goal-oriented health care," which embodies some of the same principles already discussed for nursing. Suggesting that the old model of problem-based care — founded on a biomedical model emphasizing the detection of problems, their correction, and the return of individual functioning to "normal limits" — is no longer suitable for geriatric practice, observers such as Mold, Blake, and Becker (1991) have offered a new vision of what medical care for the frail elderly should be. This model represents a revolutionary way to reconceptualize both health and health care. In brief, the old *problem-based model* is based on the following premises (Mold, 1995):

- There exists an ideal "health" state that each person should achieve and maintain. Any significant deviation from this state represents a problem, disease, or disorder.
- Each problem has one or more identifiable causes, whose correction will resolve the problem and restore health.
- Health professionals, because of their scientific understanding, are the best judges of the causes and appropriate treatments of problems.
- Clients/patients are expected to concur with health professionals' assessments and comply with their recommendations.
- The success of health interventions is measured by the degree to which individual problems have been identified and appropriate techniques/technologies applied to solve them.

Although there are still relevant applications of the problem-based model, such as in treating an elderly person with an acute medical condition, it loses currency when dealing with the chronic, disabling conditions found in many elderly. Importantly, the issue is not only how the problem is described, but also who controls how the problem is defined and subsequently treated.

In contrast, the *goal-oriented model* embodies fundamentally different assumptions:

- Health must ultimately be defined by each individual, and it may be different for different persons and for the same person at different times.
- An individual's health goals can best be determined through a dialogue involving the individual and his or her health care provider(s), each using the special information they bring to the caring relationship.
- The development of health goals requires assessing the individual's strengths and resources, interests and needs, and personal values — in addition to determining obstacles and challenges.
- Final decisions about health goal priorities, and the amount of effort expended in their achievement, must reside with the individual. Health professionals must decide whether their involvement will be beneficial and how they can participate.
- Success for both the individual and the health professionals is measured by the extent to which the individual's health goals are achieved.

Thus, in the goal-oriented framework, health is defined not as an out-come, but as a process, incorporating the following dimensions: physical maturation and differentiation, self-actualization, development of adaptability and coping skills, and the acquisition of wisdom — all potential aspects of quality of life considerations. In this process, health care professionals must enter into a dialogue with the elderly individual, each expressing the unique contributions of knowledge and skills brought to this relationship. It is through this collaborative process that a broader array of health professionals is brought into the personal health goal attainment of the individual than is generally the case with the problem-based model. With a wider definition of health, the degree of contribution and participation of disciplines beyond the traditional emphasis on medicine is now possible. Importantly, the relative contribution, role, and power of each discipline may vary with the unique goals of the older person with a disability.

In short, a goal-oriented model of health care recasts the traditional relationship between care provider and frail elderly recipient into a collaborative process, in which the values of the individual — as embodied in his or her personal and life goals — take precedence over the traditional control of professionals over the assessment of needs and development of solutions to problems. In this model, professionals will have to learn to listen more carefully not only to the individual, but also to each other. Such a model sets forth a new challenge for communication at all levels in the pursuit of health, in which the understanding of both information and values takes on a new urgency and importance.

Social Work: Empowerment with a History

The field of social work represents a third perspective on the development of innovative models of care incorporating new images of communication and power among providers and consumers of services. In addition to representing the major influence of psychosocial factors in defining health and assessing the origin of health "problems," social workers have traditionally emphasized the rights of their clients to self-determination and acted in such a way as to help them recognize or develop their own skills to help themselves (Kane, 1975), principles that are increasingly relevant to the frail elderly who are at risk of losing control over their lives and the health care decisions affecting them. More recently, a renewed theme in social work has underscored the central importance of client self-determination and empowerment in social work practice (Tower, 1994). Drawing on the concepts represented by the independent living movement within the field of developmental disabilities, this trend embodies the shift from professionally determined problem definitions and solutions to consumer-defined needs and personal processes of discovering or creating ways of meeting them (DeJong, 1984). Thus, social work practice with the elderly is being increasingly influenced by empowerment strategies for persons with disabilities in general.

In this transition, the leadership of the geriatric team shifts from one of professional dominance to one of consumer control and power. Tower

(1994) calls upon practitioners and instructors in social work to develop the basic knowledge and skills necessary to model empowering behaviors to clients and students alike. As Cohen (1988) has counseled gerontologists, we need to adopt a more robust ideological stance to embody new conceptual principles in the design and delivery of services, and he too draws on the inspiration of the independent living movement:

> *Traditional professional views see the consumer as the problem, focusing on the disability and skills deficits. From the independent living movement point of view, the problem is not in skill deficits due to disability, but rather in the dependence that is shaped by traditional service models and a society shaped by the needs, skills, capabilities, and demands of the dominant reference group (p. 26).*

Thus, a shift away from professionally defined needs and toward individually determined goals in social work is dependent upon the empowerment of the frail, elderly health care consumer. Only by changing the underlying conceptualization of need, reflected in the socialization process of professional training, can new models and definitions of services be created.

■CONCLUSION: TOWARD AN EMPOWERING AND REFLECTIVE ETHIC

If our vision of more effective collaboration among members of the health care team and the frail elderly individual over issues of quality of life is to be realized through new conceptual frameworks for clinical practice and communication, we need an innovative set of guiding principles to achieve this goal. Schon's (1987) concept of the "reflective practitioner" is, I believe, a good candidate for this purpose. For Schon, the true professional embodies competency in both the *science* and the *art* of practice; he or she is technically knowledgeable and capable — but, more importantly, is able to grapple with those "gray areas" of professional practice where value conflicts, uncertainty, and uniqueness conspire to undercut the "rationality and objectivity" of scientific practice. This area constitutes the domain of the *artistry* of professional practice, of which the formation of professional judgment is the hallmark. Judgment involves the thought processes involved in selecting and using information, developing intuition, and forming the reflective thinking that we associate with a high degree of professional development.

As I have argued elsewhere (Clark, 1994), collaborative interprofessional teamwork is a powerful method for training the reflective practitioner, because team participants are forced to recognize both the great power and the severe limitations of their own particular ways of generating and using information. In this sense, as Petrie (1976) has suggested, participants must acquire a basic understanding of the *cognitive maps* of other disciplines on the team, as well as that of the individual client or patient. By the term "cognitive map" is meant (a) the conceptual frameworks; (b) modes of inquiry and understanding; (c) problem definitions; (d) and observational, representational, and explanatory methods of other disciplines.

Not only must professionals gain insights into how knowledge is generated, used, and transmitted in professional practice, but — as Schon suggests — they must be able to understand equally well the *value maps* of other professions. These include an understanding of the basic normative assumptions, modes of ethical analysis or moral reasoning, and how value conflicts are resolved in different disciplines. The task of ascertaining the value maps of different professionals and the individual served by the team is the analogue to that of "public ethics," a term coined by Jonsen and Butler (1975) to describe the process of revealing and examining the principal values underlying and guiding the public policy process. In particular, public ethics examines the assumptions in the development of policy "problems" and assists in evaluating the range of alternative "solutions" to them. By extrapolation, the clinical value-mapping process must reveal how and why elderly individuals with disabilities choose different courses of action to address specific issues of concern to them about the quality of their lives. It helps to uncover the values implicit in our everyday lives and decisions, as well as those having professional relevance.

Most importantly, professionals must be open to the empowerment of the elderly individual with disabilities, the recognition that it is he or she who must define the appropriate means and ends of care. Restructuring health care around the unique individual and his or her experience with illness or frailty represents a new countertheme to medical control in traditional clinical practice (Reiser, 1993). A fundamental cornerstone of this emergent perspective is a concentration on the relationship between the consumer and the provider of care, emphasizing an understanding of the basic values and meanings attached by individuals to the health care encounter and its relation to their overall lives and life goals (Delbanco, 1992; Matthews, Suchman, & Branch, 1993). Attention to the nature of communication between care provider and recipient depends on the joint recognition of the need for dialogue, interdependence, and empowerment on both sides (Clark, 1989). Empowerment must include the kinds of reflective processes that underlie an understanding of whose interpretation of facts and whose selection of personal and professional values drives the processes of defining and solving problems. This may mean the unmasking of professional constructions of "need" and their replacement with consumer-developed and inspired visions of what is really important in life. Mutual respect must emerge as the hallmark of this process if it is to be successful in achieving open communication and understanding.

In summary, providers and consumers alike must acquire an "empowering and reflective ethic." This ethic should be an integral part of the artistry of professional practice — incorporating insights into both the knowledge base of professional practice and the normative dimensions of establishing important goals and how to achieve them. It should also be the foundation of what it means to be an empowered consumer. In this process, the term "quality of life" becomes a metaphor that incorporates these two dimensions into geriatric practice, because of necessity it involves both factual and moral aspects of care as perceived by provider and recipient. It is not accidental, I think, that this concept has emerged as important from the vision of a new, more collaborative model of professional practice, in which health and health care are increasingly visualized as a process of mutual exploration and discovery. In addition, we are guided in this conceptual transition by an understanding of empowerment and quality of life informed by both gerontology and the field of developmental disabilities. By meeting the challenges of communication about such important concepts we can gain fresh insights into the development of new ways of thinking and acting as health care professionals, individuals, and family members as we grapple together over what we mean when we say "quality of life" for the frail elderly.

▬ REFERENCES

Agich, G. J. (1990). Reassessing autonomy in long-term care. *Hastings Center Report, 20*(6), 12–31.

Almy, T. P. (1988). Comprehensive functional assessment for elderly patients. *Annals of Internal Medicine, 109*(7), 70–72.

Ansello, E. F. (1992). Seeking common ground between aging and developmental disabilities. *Generations, 16*(1), 9–15.

Ansello, E. F., & Eustis, N. N. (1992). A common stake? Investigating the emerging 'intersection' of aging and disabilities. *Generations, 16*(1), 5–8.

Ansello, E. F., & Rose, T. (1989). *Aging and lifelong disabilities: Partnership for the twenty-first century.* Palm Springs, CA: Elvirita Lewis Foundation.

Aronson, J. (1992). Are we really listening? Beyond the official discourse on needs of old people. *Canadian Social Work Review, 9*(1), 73–87.

Aronson, J. (1993). Giving consumers a say in policy development: Influencing policy or just being heard. *Canadian Public Policy-Analyse de Politiques, XIX,* 367–378.

Cassel, C. K. (1992). Issues of age and chronic care: Another argument for health care reform. *Journal of the American Geriatrics Society, 40,* 404–409.

Clark, P. G. (1987). Individual autonomy, cooperative empowerment, and planning for long-term care decision making. *Journal of Aging Studies, 1,* 65–76.

Clark, P. G. (1988). Autonomy, personal empowerment, and quality of life in long-term care. *Journal of Applied Gerontology, 7,* 279–297.

Clark, P. G. (1989). The philosophical foundation of empowerment: Implications for geriatric health care programs and practice. *Journal of Aging and Health, 1,* 267–285.

Clark, P. G. (1991a). Ethical dimensions of quality of life in aging: Autonomy vs. collectivism in the United States and Canada. *The Gerontologist, 31,* 631–639.

Clark, P. G. (1991b). Toward a conceptual framework for developing interdisciplinary teams in gerontology: Cognitive and ethical dimensions. *Gerontology & Geriatrics Education, 12*(1), 79–96.

Clark, P. G. (1993). Moral discourse and public policy in aging: Framing problems, seeking solutions, and "public ethics." *Canadian Journal on Aging, 12,* 485–508.

Clark, P. G. (1994). Social, professional, and educational values on the interdisciplinary team: Implications for gerontological and geriatric education. *Educational Gerontology, 20,* 35–51.

Clark, P. G., Spence, D. L., & Sheehan, J. L. (1986). A service/learning model for interdisciplinary teamwork in health and aging. *Gerontology & Geriatrics Education, 6*(4), 3–16.

Clark, P. G., Spence, D. L., & Sheehan, J. L. (1987). Challenges and barriers to interdisciplinary gerontological team training in the academic setting. *Gerontological & Geriatrics Education, 7*(3/4), 93–110.

Cohen, E. S. (1988). The elderly mystique: Constraints on the autonomy of the elderly with disabilities. *The Geronaologist, 28*(Suppl.), 24–31.

Cohen, E. S. (1992). What is independence? *Generations, 16*(1), 49–52.

Collopy, B. J. (1988). Autonomy in long-term care: Some crucial distinctions. *The Gerontologist, 28*(Suppl.), 10–17.

Collopy, B., Boyle, P., & Jennings, B. (1991). New directions in nursing home ethics. *Hastings Center Report, 21*(Suppl.), 1–15.

Collopy, B., Dubler, N., & Zuckerman, C. (1990). The ethics of home care: Autonomy and accommodation. *Hastings Center Report, 20*(Suppl.), 1–16.

DeJong, G. (1984). Independent living: From social movement to analytic paradigm. In P. Marinelli & A. Dell Orto (Eds.), *The psychological and social impact of physical disability* (pp. 39–64). New York: Springer.

Delbanco, T. L. (1992). Enriching the doctor-patient relationship by inviting the patient's perspective. *Annals of Internal Medicine, 116*, 414–418.

Dill, A. (1993). Defining needs, defining systems: A critical analysis. *The Gerontologist, 33*, 453–460.

Gadow, S. (1983). Frailty and strength: The dialectic in aging. *The Gerontologist, 23*, 144–147.

Given, B., & Simmons, S. (1977). The interdisciplinary health care team: Fact or fiction? *Nursing Forum, 16*, 165–184.

Gramelspacher, G. P., Howell, J. D., & Young, M. J. (1986). Perceptions of ethical problems by nurses and doctors. *Archives of Internal Medicine, 146*, 577–578.

Jones, J. M., Meredith, S., Wadas, L., Watt, S., & Weisz, E. (1991). The contribution and role of the social worker. In National Advisory Council on Aging (Ed.), *Geriatric assessment and treatment: Members of the team* (pp. 35–52). No. H71-2/1-9-1991E. Ottawa, ON: Minister of Supply and Services Canada.

Jonsen, A. R., & Butler, L. H. (1975). Public ethics and policy making. *Hastings Center Report, 5*(4), 19–31.

Kane, R. A. (1975). *Interprofessional teamwork*. Manpower monograph no. 8. Syracuse, NY: Syracuse University School of Social Work.

Kane, R. A., & Caplan, A. L. (1990). *Everyday ethics: Resolving dilemmas in nursing home life*. New York: Springer.

Katz, S., Branch, L. G., Branson, M. H., Papsidero, J. A., Beck, J. C., & Greer, D. S. (1983). Active life expectancy. *New England Journal of Medicine, 309*, 1218–1224.

Katz, S., Greer, D. S., Beck, J. C., Branch, L. G., & Spector, W. D. (1985). Active life expectancy: Societal implications. In Institute of Medicine, Committee on an Aging Society (Ed.), *America's aging: Health in an older society* (pp. 57–72). Washington, DC: National Academy Press.

Kayser-Jones, J. S. (1986). Distributive justice and the treatment of acute illness in nursing homes. *Social Science in Medicine, 23*, 1279–1286.

Langer, E., & Rodin, J. (1976). The effects of choice and enhanced personal responsibility for the aged: A field experiment in an institutional setting. *Journal of Personality and Social Psychology, 34*, 191–198.

Luszki, M. (1958). *Interdisciplinary team research methods and problems*. New York: National Training Laboratories.

Mangione, C. M., Marcantonio, E. R., Goldman, L., Cook, E. F., Donaldson, M. C., Sugarbaker, D. J., Poss, R., & Lee, T. H. (1993). Influence of age on measurement of health status in patients undergoing elective surgery. *Journal of the American Geriatrics Society, 41*, 377–383.

Matthews, D. A., Suchman, A. L., & Branch, W. T. (1993). Making "connexions": Enhancing the therapeutic potential of patient-clinician relationships. *Annals of Internal Medicine, 118*, 973–977.

McCullough, L. B., Wilson, N. L., Teasdale, T. A., Kolpakchi, A. L., Skelly, J. R. (1993). Mapping personal, familial, and professional values in long-term care decisions. *The Gerontologist, 33*, 324–332.

Miller, D. K., Coe, R. M., & Hyers, T. M. (1992). Achieving consensus on withdrawing or withholding care for critically ill patients. *Journal of General Internal Medicine, 7*, 475–480.

Minkler, M. (1990). Aging and disability: Behind and beyond the stereotypes. *Journal of Aging Studies, 4*, 245–260.

Mitchell, G. J. (1992). Parse's theory and the multidisciplinary team: Clarifying scientific values. *Nursing Science Quarterly, 5*, 104–106.

Mold, J. W. (1995). An alternative conceptionalization of health and health care: Its implications for geriatrics and gerontology. *Educational Gerontology, 21*, 85–101.

Mold, J. W., Blake, G. H., & Becker, L. A. (1991). Goal-oriented medical care. *Family Medicine, 23*, 46–51.

Moody, H. R. (1988). From informed consent to negotiated consent. *The Gerontologist, 28*(Suppl.), 64–70.

Parse, R. R. (1987). *Nursing science: Major paradigms, theories, and critiques.* Philadelphia: Saunders.

Parse, R. R. (1992). Human becoming: Parse's theory of nursing. *Nursing Science Quarterly, 5,* 35–42.

Pearlman, R. A., & Uhlmann, R. F. (1988). Quality of life in chronic diseases: Perceptions of elderly patients. *Journal of Gerontology: Medical Sciences, 43,* M25–M30.

Petrie, H. G. (1976). Do you see what I see? The epistemology of interdisciplinary inquiry. *Journal of Aesthetic Education, 10,* 29–43.

Qualls, S. H., & Czirr, R. (1988). Geriatric health teams: Classifying models of professional and team functioning. *The Gerontologist, 28,* 372–376.

Reiser, S. J. (1993). The era of the patient: Using the experience of illness in shaping the missions of health care. *Journal of the American Medical Association, 269,* 1012–1017.

Rodin, J. (1986). Aging and health: Effects of the sense of control. *Science, 233,* 1271–1276.

Rodin, J., & Langer, E. (1977). Long-term effects of a control-relevant intervention with the institutionalized aged. *Journal of Personality and Social Psychology, 35,* 897–902.

Rowe, J. W., & Kahn, R. L. (1987). Human aging: Usual and successful. *Science, 237,* 143–149.

Rubenstein, L. V., Calkins, D. R., Greenfield, S., Jette, A. M., Meenan, R. F., Nevins, M. A., Rubenstein, L. Z., Wasson, J. H., & Williams, M. E. (1989). Health status assessment for elderly patients. *Journal of the American Geriatrics Society, 37,* 562–569.

Schon, D. A. (1987). *Educating the reflective practitioner.* San Francisco: Jossey-Bass.

Sharp, J. W. (1993). Expanding the definition of quality of life for prostate cancer. *Cancer, 71*(Suppl.), 1078–1082.

Tower, K. D. (1994). Consumer-centered social work practice: Restoring client self-determination. *Social Work, 39,* 191–196.

Tsukuda, R. A. (1990). Interdisciplinary collaboration: Teamwork in geriatrics. In C. K. Cassel, D. E. Riesenberg, L. B. Sorenson, & J. R. Walsh (Eds.), *Geriatric medicine* (2nd ed.) (pp. 668–675). New York: Springer-Verlag.

Uhlmann, R. A., & Pearlman, R. A (1991). Perceived quality of life and preferences for life-sustaining treatment in older adults. *Archives of Internal Medicine, 151,* 495–497.

Walker, R. M., Miles, S. H., Stockling, C. B., & Siegler, M. (1991). Physicians' and nurses' perceptions of ethics problems on general medical services. *Journal of General Internal Medicine, 6,* 424–429.

Zeiss, A. M., & Steffen, A. M. (in press). Interdisciplinary health care teams: The basic unit of geriatric care. In L. L. Carstensen, B. A. Edelstein, & L. Dorbrand (Eds.), *The handbook of clinical gerontology.* Newbury Park, CA: Sage.

Chapter 35

Position of the American Dietetic Association: Nutrition, Aging, and the Continuum of Care

AMERICAN DIATETIC ASSOCIATION

Eating habits are formed over a lifetime. Older adults may need nutrition-related assistance in several areas, including shopping, meal preparation, adequate dietary intake, and special diets. This chapter provides a good overview of nutritional issues related to the elderly population, and discusses potential risk factors for malnutrition, as well as current research findings.

Nutritional well-being is integral to successful aging. Successful aging, in turn, results from a broadly defined continuum of care that promotes quality of life, independence, and health. Medical and other supportive services, including food and nutrition services, that are appropriate to levels of dependency, diseases, conditions, and functional ability are key components of the continuum of are (Fig. 35-1). The burgeoning elder population, changing concepts of aging itself, and dramatic changes in the delivery of health care accentuate the importance of food and nutrition as sustenance as well as in disease prevention and therapy.

▬ POSITION STATEMENT
The American Dietetic Association supports comprehensive food and nutrition services for older adults as an integral component of the continuum of care.

▬ PROFILE OF OLDER ADULTS
This section provides an overview of the current status of the elderly population in the United States. These facts demonstrate the urgency of developing a comprehensive strategy for ensuring the health and well-being of this growing population.

From *Journal of the American Dietetic Association* 96(10):1048–1052, 1996. Reprinted with permission.

Case management A system for assessing, planning treatment for, referring, and monitoring patients to ensure the provision of comprehensive and continuous service and the coordination of payment and reimbursement for cost of care (8).

Continuum of care A coordinated system of settings, services, providers, and care levels in which health, medical, and supportive services are provided in the appropriate care setting (eg, acute, subacute, ambulatory, community, and day care; hospice; respite, retirement, and continuing care communities; and group housing, assisted-living, home care, and traditional nursing home facilities). Ideally, the older person moves according to need to different sites and services with strong continuity of care within the system.

Continuum of health care An integrated delivery system that provides its patients with access to all services needed for health care. The patient is allowed to move to different sites and services in the system to ensure strong continuity of care. The continuum of health care includes physician services, emergency services, acute care, subacute care, skilled nursing facilities, outpatient centers, home care programs, day treatment programs, adult day care, assisted-living facilities, mental health services, and family/community supports (8).

Long-term care Assistance expected to be provided over a long period to people with chronic health conditions and/or physical disabilities who are unable to care for themselves without the help of another person (9).

National Aging Services Network The Administration on Aging administers the Older Americans Act through a network consisting of 216 tribal and native organizations, 57 state agencies on aging, approximately 660 local area agencies on aging, and several thousand organizations that provide direct services to older persons. Institutions of higher education receive funding to provide information, training, and technical assistance to the network as well as to conduct research and build knowledge. The National Aging Services Network is mandated to establish a system and provide comprehensive, coordinated in-home and community-based services (29).

§1115 (a) Medicaid waiver Waiver under the Social Security Act that allows a great deal of flexibility through demonstration projects for designing eligibility standards and arranging reimbursement mechanisms in providing acute-care and long-term care services under Medicaid (9).

§1915 (c) Home and community-based Medicaid waiver Waiver under the Social Security Act that allows states to use Medicaid funds to provide in-home and community-based services, previously not covered by Medicaid, to a specific caseload of persons who are aged or disabled and nursing facility certified (9).

FIGURE 35-1 Definitions and descriptions related to services for older adults.

Demographics

In 1994, more than 33 million adults (13% of the American population) were aged 65 years and older; by 2030, this number will increase to 70 million (20% of the population) as baby boomers age (1). Subgroups of the older adult population are typically categorized as the young-old (65- to 74-year-olds); the old (75- to 84-year-olds); and the oldest old (those aged 85 years and older), which is the most rapidly growing group. Another category often used for comparative purposes is persons approaching the older ages (55- to 64-year-olds) (2). Older minorities will increase from 13% in 1990 to 25% of older adults in 2030. Currently, California, Florida, New York, Pennsylvania, Texas, Ohio, Illinois, Michigan, and New Jersey each have more than 1 million older residents; this number is expected to increase dramatically in the 21st century (1). With life expectancy at 79 years for women and 72 years for men, older women are increasingly outnumbering older men, especially among the oldest old. Older women are three times as likely as men to be widowed, and 8 of 10 of the community-dwelling older persons who live alone are women.

Malnutrition Risk

Many older adults are at risk for malnutrition. Multiple and synergistic factors, including hunger, poverty, and anorexia nervosa or anorexia tardive, frequently precede malnutrition (3,4). Other malnutrition risk factors among older adults include inadequate food intake, social isolation, depression, dementia, dependency, functional disability, oral health and chewing and swallowing problems, presence of acute or chronic diseases or conditions, polypharmacy, and advanced age (5). An evaluation of the Elderly Nutrition Program of the Older Americans Act indicates that 67% to 88% of participants are at moderate to high nutritional risk (6). These community-based programs are finding serious nutrition-related problems among older adults, especially among the frail homebound. Many older adults have two to three diagnosed chronic health conditions; 26% of participants in congregate meal programs and 43% of those who receive home-delivered meals had a hospital or nursing facility stay in the previous year. One survey found that almost two thirds of respondents had a weight outside the healthful range and that 18% to 32% had involuntarily gained or lost 10 lb within the 6 months before the survey (6).

Food Security

Approximately 8% to 16% of older adults (2.5 to 4.9 million) experience food insecurity; in other words, they do not have access at all times to a nutritionally adequate, culturally compatible diet (7). Federal programs to combat hunger and food insecurity reach only one third of needy older adults (7). The Older Americans Act's congregate and home-delivered meal programs and the US Department of Agriculture's Food Stamp Program reach those with the highest rates of food insecurity, but fail to reach many who do not meet the income guidelines for food stamps or who will not accept aid because of its connotation as welfare. Many may be unaware of, are unable to get to, or are uncomfortable attending a congregate meal program, or no programs exist in their area. Additionally, they may fail to qualify or be placed on long waiting lists for home-delivered meals (6,7). To date, older adults have not been a primary focus of hunger advocacy groups, food banks, food pantries, and soup kitchens.

Poverty and Income Resources

Poverty is a strong indicator of malnutrition risk. Almost 20% of older adults are poor or near-poor; older women experience nearly twice the poverty rate of older men (1). Older adults who live alone or with nonrelatives, are from a minority group, reside in the South, did not complete high school, or are too ill or disabled to work are most likely to be poor (1).

Even older adults who are not poor may live on a fixed income. As expenses increase, those older adults may opt to reduce their food intake, thereby placing themselves at risk for malnutrition. For example, when physical/mental impairments interfere with grocery shopping and cooking, elders may balance the resulting increase in food-related costs from delivery charges, use of more costly convenience and other special foods, and the higher price of restaurant meals by eating fewer meals. In addition, many older adults take an extensive number of costly medications; money spent for medications often reduces the amount of money available to purchase food.

Medical Expenditures

Older adults have major economic uncertainties in terms of health expenditures and longevity. Although the majority have access to health care through Medicare, Medicare does not pay all their health care costs. Access to affordable and continuous health care concerns persons approaching retirement as well as Medicare and Medicaid beneficiaries. Third-party payers emphasize use of managed-care delivery systems to contain escalating health care costs for older persons (8). Medicare beneficiaries now have a choice between the traditional fee-for-service option or enrollment in a Medicare-approved health maintenance organization (HMO). In the traditional Medicare option, participants are generally required to pay premiums, copayments, and deductibles and are not reimbursed for prescription drugs, preventive care, dental care, and long-term care. Medicare HMOs must include all the traditional Medicare benefits and, depending on the plan, offer limited or no copayments, coverage of prescription drugs and physician visits, and primary and preventive care (8,9).

Nutrient Needs

Physiologic and functional changes during aging result in changes in nutrient needs (10). Altered ability to taste and smell, poor oral health, dysphagia, and/or failure-to-thrive syndrome (ie, nonspecific symptoms associated with deteriorating mental status and functional ability, social isolation, and decreased food intake) can contribute to decreased nutrient intake, involuntary weight loss, and malnutrition (11–13). The current Recommended Dietary Allowances (RDAs) do not provide separate recommendations for persons older than 51 years and, thus, do not take into account that older adults have special nutrition needs (14). For example, although vitamin A needs decrease with age, which makes toxicity from supplements more common, other nutrient needs may increase. In addition, protein requirements for older adults exceed current RDAs (1.0 to 1.25 vs 0.8 g/kg body weight, respectively) (15). Morbidity and mortality increase with protein-energy undernutrition (ie, no overt clinical signs of malnutrition), low serum levels of albumin and/or thyroid hormones, and hypothermia. Vitamin D serum levels may be reduced even with adequate sunlight exposure, and deficiency may be exacerbated by homebound status, sunblock use, poor dietary intakes, decreased capacity to synthesize cholecalciferol in the skin, and decreased number of gastrointestinal receptors (3,16). Fracture rate increases, especially among older African Americans, when vitamin D levels are low (3). Vitamin D and calcium supplementation may reduce the incidence of hip fractures and increase bone density (17).

Metabolic and physiologic changes that affect the status of vitamin B-12, vitamin B-6, and folate may alter behavior and general health, whereas adequate intake of these nutrients prevents some decline in cognitive function associated with aging (18). Deficiencies of these nutrients, along with insufficient intake of vitamin C and riboflavin, may result in poor memory (18). Very low cholesterol levels (<4.16 mmol/L[1]) may be predictive of mortality (19) and future cognitive dysfunction (3). Although current research does not directly implicate nutrition, there may be an association between unexplained weight loss and Alzheimer's disease (20). The antioxidants α-tocopherol, beta carotene, and ascorbic acid may affect visual capacity, that is, cataract formation (21) and macular degeneration (22). Likewise, immune function affected by nutritional status may be improved by supplementation of protein, vitamin E, zinc, and other micronutrients (10,18,23). Nutritional well-being as well as exercise and resistance weight training affect functional ability of older adults to perform the activities of daily living (24,25).

Dehydration, a major problem in older adults, especially the oldest old, blacks, and men, substantially increases Medicare costs and results in death within a year of admission for nearly half of the elderly hospitalized Medicare patients (26). Dehydration risk increases because of the kidney's decreased ability to concentrate urine, altered thirst sensation, decreased renin activity and aldosterone secretion, relative renal resistance to vasopressin, changes in functional status, delirium and dementia, medication side effects, and mobility disorders (27). Fear of incontinence and increased arthritic pain resulting from numerous trips to the toilet may also interfere with consumption of adequate fluid intake.

▬AGING AND THE CONTINUUM OF CARE

Automatically assuming that advanced age and increased frailty coexist denies the heterogeneity among older adults. Poor health is not as prevalent as many assume; in fact, 75% of the community-dwelling young-old consider

---

[1]To convert mmol/L cholesterol to mg/dL, multiply mmol/L by 38.7. To convert mg/dL cholesterol to mmol/L, multiply mg/dL by 0.026. Cholesterol of 5.00 mmol/L = 193 mg/dL.

their health to be good. Only 1% of the young-old live in nursing facilities compared with about 24% of the oldest old. Among community-dwelling older adults, 9% of the young-old and 50% of the oldest old need assistance with the activities of daily living (1). Today, older adults themselves, the increasing numbers of adult children caregivers, and federal and state agencies want a choice among a variety of long-term-care options because of quality-of-life and cost issues.

The term "aging in place" has many definitions and does not necessarily mean aging in one setting or in one's own home until death. Ideally, aging in place offers choices from a spectrum of living options and services to accommodate those who have no impairments, those who require limited assistance, and those with more severe impairments who require care in a nursing facility. Options that enable an older person to continue to reside in the community include private residences, adult continuing care (or life care) retirement communities, assisted-living facilities, group housing, and adult day care.

An integrated continuum of seamless, coordinated medical and supportive services facilitating movement of older persons among community, acute, and long-term care sites is needed, yet is still uncommon. Routine provision of food and nutrition services across this continuum is incomplete. Currently, medical and social supportive needs are served through two separate parallel systems, resulting in fragmented provision and continuity of care.

Older persons receive medical care for acute and chronic diseases in a variety of settings — acute, subacute, skilled nursing, rehabilitation, community health, home care, adult day care, life care, assisted-living, and nursing facilities — and not necessarily in a particular order (28). Older adults are being discharged earlier from acute-care and long-term-care facilities with the expectation that meals and additional services, such as follow-up care, will be provided in the home and community.

The National Aging Services Network mandated by the Older Americans Act delivers supportive in-home and community-based services to delay or prevent placing persons with impairments in nursing facilities (29, Fig. 35-1). These services, which include home health, personal care, homemaker support, adult day care, respite care, assisted transportation, and home-delivered meals (30), vary nationwide and are usually charged on a sliding fee scale. In-home and community-based services have expanded to include medical and preventive health in addition to supportive services; however, to date, nutrition services, other than congregate and home-delivered meal programs, have not routinely been included. Because medical and social supportive delivery systems frequently function separately, duplication of effort and unmet needs often result.

Many states, burdened by rising Medicaid long-term-care costs, are seeking ways to delay placing elders in nursing facilities by enrolling Medicaid beneficiaries in HMOs (9) and by using Medicaid waivers to provide necessary home- and community-based medical, social, and supportive series (see Figure 35-1). Some states include home-delivered meals and medical nutrition therapy as part of waiver services (30).

To reduce fragmentation, duplication, and costs of care, federal and state initiatives are beginning to integrate acute- and long-term care into a single capitated managed care package that combines medical and supportive services. Federal demonstration projects include the Social Health Maintenance Organizations and the Program of All-inclusive Care for the Elderly programs (9). These alternatives are positive steps toward achieving a seamless continuum of care for older adults. Whether they are less expensive than traditional nursing home placement is presently unknown.

▬COMPREHENSIVE FOOD AND NUTRITION SERVICES ACROSS THE CONTINUUM OF CARE

Food and nutrition services belong in the integrated interdisciplinary continuum of care that is evolving because they are unique in both a medical and a social context. Within this continuum of care, the psychosocial aspects of food and meals must be combined with the preventive/therapeutic aspects of medical nutrition therapy to achieve or maintain nutritional well-being. Nutrition services should be designed to respond to the changing physiologic, mental, functional, and socioeconomic capabilities of older adults. The social and nurturing aspects of food enhance quality of life and become even more important as preventive and therapeutic effects of food and nutrition may begin to diminish with age (31).

The continuum of food and nutrition services needed by older adults includes all assessment and treatment options encompassed by medical nutrition therapy, from screening to in-depth nutrition assessment, from provision of meals to nutrition education and individualized counseling, and from nutrient and texture modifications (at times via medical food and food for special dietary uses) to enteral and parenteral infusion therapy in all settings from home and community to hospitals and long-term-care facilities (32). Medical nutrition therapy, when provided in accordance with practice guidelines, contributes to increased physical mobility, mental alertness, and cognitive function; aids in the management of acute and chronic diseases; reduces medical and surgical complications and infections; promotes faster wound healing; and prevents or delays clinical complications of certain diseases in acute care, rehabilitation, or ambulatory clinics, nursing facilities, and home and community settings (33–35). Food and nutrition are also important in palliative hospice care for persons with a terminal illness (36).

Mirroring the shift of medical service delivery into home and community settings, medical nutrition therapy for older adults with acute and chronic conditions is also moving from hospitals to home and community settings, often before a patient has recovered completely. Today, more needy, frail, and debilitated older adults need medical nutrition therapy outside of hospitals. As a result, an array of intensive services, including requisite medical nutrition therapy, must become more available in home and community settings to facilitate recovery of these nutritionally compromised persons. Such comprehensive clinical, cognitive, social, and nutrition services encompass the management of transition feedings, enteral and parenteral therapies, feeding complications, dysphagia, and hydration (37). The effectiveness of medical nutrition therapy in speeding wound healing related to pressure sores (35) and recovery from hip fractures (38) is documented. Interdisciplinary practice guidelines attest to the importance of nutrition care (35,39–41).

An example of emerging coordination of services is demonstrated by the fact that many older persons who have been recently discharged from acute-care settings receive home-delivered meals, yet at least 41% of Elderly Nutrition Programs have waiting lists for home-delivered meals (6). The cost of providing a nutritious home-delivered meal to a person for 1 year equals the cost of one in-hospital day (34). Therefore, it is important to be aware that many of these older adults are potentially at risk for malnutrition.

Good nutritional status in older adults benefits both the individual and society: health is improved, dependence is decreased, time required to recuperate from illness is reduced, and utilization of health care resources is contained (34,42). Nevertheless, in older adults, improvements in frailty and limitations in one or more of the activities of daily living may not always result in improved economic outcomes (3). There are other ways to measure outcomes besides cost savings, however. Food and nutrition may add an important dimension to quality of life, and improving or maintaining quality of life is a viable outcome especially for older adults (31,43).

Today, continuity of care is provided through interdisciplinary case or care management. Medical nutrition therapy helps improve outcomes most effectively when it is integrated into comprehensive interdisciplinary care management. In case management, costs are overseen and services are coordinated from different funding streams. Case management begins with a comprehensive screening and assessment and draws together information about the medical, nutritional, mental, socioeconomic, and functional activities of daily living as well as the ability to eat, shop, and prepare meals. After a patient's problem is identified, a care plan is developed that coordinates appropriate treatments and maintains continuity of care through periodic review and modification. The interdisciplinary process often uses care conferences and includes older persons themselves, families, and caregivers. Nutrition screening and assessment and food and nutrition services are integrated into the process (44). Cross-functional and/or interdisciplinary teams minimize duplication of tasks and improve decision making, access, delivery of services, and outcomes (37,45).

Although it is not case management per se, discharge planning also coordinates institutional and noninstitutional care. Many interdisciplinary opportunities exist to merge food and nutrition services into continuity of care. Similar to the 1996 Joint Commission on Accreditation of Healthcare Organizations (JCAHO) standards for nutrition services in long-term-care settings (28), the 1995 JCAHO accreditation process for home health agencies that offer nutrition services specifies that nutrition screening of patients must occur before or at admission and that screening must be followed by coordinated food and nutrition services for those at nutritional risk (46).

Nutrition screening and assessment evaluate the multifaceted nature of malnutrition. First, nutrition screening identifies those with poor nutritional status and those at nutritional risk. A comprehensive nutrition assessment is then used to probe further into the patient's anthropometric, biochemical, clinical, dietary, psychosocial, economic, functional, mental health, and oral health status. The complete assessment is the basis for the development of a care plan (32).

The interdisciplinary care plan synthesizes all risk indicators and factors to identify desirable outcomes. Appropriate interventions must be selected, prioritized, and implemented. Potential interventions must be multidisciplinary in scope (5). Food and nutrition interventions include congregate or home-delivered meal programs; nutrition education; diet modification and nutrition counseling; and specialized medical nutrition therapies, including supplementation with medical foods and enteral and parenteral nutrition (34). Period reevaluation of the plan monitors a patient's progress toward the desired outcomes to ensure continuity of care.

■ FUTURE DIRECTIONS
FOR DIETETICS PROFESSIONALS

Dietetics professionals must move forward individually and collectively to position food and nutrition services within the continuum of elder care. Local networks, including every setting and dietetics practice specialty, should share information and make referrals to establish community-institutional linkages and to coordinate improved care for older adults. Data can be collected and used to further demonstrate to policy makers the value of food and nutrition services.

Dietetics professionals can strengthen the continuum of care for older adults in their facilities and communities through proactive involvement, coordination, and debate. Dietetics professionals can enhance the nutritional status of older adults when they:

- implement appropriate elder-centered nutrition practice guidelines and standards of practice for gerontological nutritionists that are matched to the home, community, and/or institutional care setting(s) (35,39–41);
- position nutrition services realistically and flexibly within the rapidly changing delivery of medical, health, and supportive services;
- advocate (and volunteer) to alleviate elder poverty, hunger, and malnutrition in communities and through legislative processes;
- network in their communities across dietetics specialties and practice settings and with colleagues in interdisciplinary fields to bridge gaps in elder care;
- integrate comprehensive coordinated nutrition services for older adults into the care provided in acute, subacute, nursing facility, home, or community settings, aging network programs; and/or managed care organizations;

■ participate as an active essential team member in care management, discharge planning, and/or case management, and

■ document and promote the vital nature and cost-effectiveness of the provision of appropriate nutrition services to quality of life and independence of older adults.

▰ REFERENCES

1. US Census Bureau. Sixty-five plus in the United States, Statistical Brief. http://www.census.gov/ftp/pub/socdemo/www/agebrief.html. June 6, 1996:1–7.
2. National Center for Health Statistics. *Trends in the Health of Older Americans: United States, 1994.* Hyattsville, Md: US Dept of Health and Human Services; 1995.
3. Morley JE, Solomon DH. Major issues in geriatrics over the last five years. *J Am Geriatr Soc.* 1994;42:218–225.
4. Sullivan DH, Walls RC. Impact of nutritional status on morbidity in a population of geriatric rehabilitation patients. *J Am Geriatr Soc.* 1994;42:471–477.
5. *Incorporating Nutrition Screening and Interventions into Medical Practice: A Monograph for Physicians.* Washington, DC: Nutrition Screening Initiative;1994.
6. Ponza M, Ohls JC, Millen BE. *Serving Elders at Risk: The Older Americans Act Nutrition Programs, National Evaluation of the Elderly Nutrition Program, 1993–1995.* Washington, DC: Mathematica Policy Research, Inc; 1996.
7. Burt MR. *Hunger Among the Elderly: Local and National Comparisons.* Washington, DC: Urban Institute;1993.
8. Position of The American Dietetic Association: nutrition services in managed care. *J Am Diet Assoc.* 1996;96:391–395.
9. Kane R, Kane R, Kaye N, Mollica R, Riley T, Saucier P, Snow KI, Starr L. *Managed Care: Handbook for the Aging Network.* Minneapolis, Minn: University of Minnesota; 1996.
10. Morley JE, Miller DK, eds. *Annual Review of Gerontology and Geriatrics: Focus on Nutrition,* vol 15. New York, NY: Springer Publishing Co; 1995.
11. Sullivan DH, Martin W, Flaxman N, Hagen JE. Oral health problems and involuntary weight loss in a population of frail elderly. *J Am Geriatr Soc.* 1993;41:725–731.
12. Johnston BT, Li Q, Castell JA, Castell DO. Swallowing and esophageal function in Parkinson's disease. *Am J Gastroenterol.* 1995;90:1741–1746.
13. Kimball MJ, Williams-Burgess C. Failure to thrive: the silent epidemic of the elderly. *Arch Psych Nurs.* 1995;IX:99–105.
14. Food and Nutrition Board. *Recommended Dietary Allowances.* 10th ed. Washington, DC: National Academy Press; 1989.
15. Campbell WW, Crim MC, Dallal GE, Young VR, Evans WJ. Increased protein requirements in elderly people: new data and retrospective reassessments. *Am J Clin Nutr.* 1994;60:501–509.
16. Gloth MF, Gundberg CM, Hollis BW, Haddad JG, Tobin JD. Vitamin D deficiency in homebound elderly persons. *JAMA.* 1995;274:1683–1686.
17. Chapuy MC, Arlot ME, Duboeuf F, Brun J, Crouzet B, Arnaud S, Delmas PH, Meunier PJ. Vitamin D-3 and calcium to prevent hip fractures in elderly women. *N Engl J Med.* 1992;327:1637–1642.
18. Rosenberg IH, Miller JW. Nutritional factors in physical and cognitive functions of elderly people. *Am J Clin Nutr.* 1992;55 (suppl):1237S–1243S.
19. Rudman D, Mattson DE, Nagraj HS, Caindec N, Rudman I, Jackson DL. Antecedents of death in the men of a Veterans Administration nursing home. *J Am Geriatric Soc.* 1987;35:496–502.
20. Wolf-Klein GP, Silverstone FA. Weight loss in Alzheimer's disease: an international review of the literature. *Int Psychogeriatr.* 1994;6:135–142.
21. Vitale S, West S, Hallfrisch J, Alston C, Wang F, Moorman C, Muller D, Singh V, Taylor HR. Plasma antioxidants and risk of cortical and nuclear cataract. *Epidemiology.* 1993;4:195–203.
22. West S, Vitale S, Hallfrisch J, Munoz B, Muller D, Bressler S, Bressler NM. Are antioxidants or supplements protective for age-related macular degeneration? *Arch Ophthalmol.* 1994;112:222–227.

23. Bogden JD, Bendich A, Kemp FW, Bruening KS, Shurnick JH, Denny T, Baker H, Louria DB. Daily micronutrient supplements enhance delayed-hyposensitivity skin test responses in older people. *Am J Clin Nutr.* 1994;60:437–447.
24. Galanos AN, Pieper CF, Cornoni-Huntley JC, Bales CW, Fillenbaum GG. Nutrition and function: is there a relationship between body mass index and the function capabilities of community-dwelling elderly? *J Am Geriatr Soc.* 1994;42:368–373.
25. Campbell WW, Crim MC, Young VR, Evans WJ. Increased energy requirements and changes in body composition with resistance training in older adults. *Am J Clin Nutr.* 1994;60:167–175.
26. Warren JL, Bacon WE, Harris T, McBean AM, Foley DJ, Phillips C. The burden and outcomes associated with dehydration among U.S. elderly. *Am J Public Health.* 1994; 84:1265–1269.
27. Weinberg AD, Menaker KL. Dehydration: evaluation and management in older adults. Council on Scientific Affairs, American Medical Association. *JAMA.* 1995;274:1552–1556.
28. Robinson GE. Applying the 1996 JCAHO nutrition care standards in a long-term-care setting. *J Am Diet Assoc.* 1996;96:400–403.
29. *Compilation of the Older Americans Act of 1965 and the Native American Programs Act of 1974 as Amended through December 31, 1992.* Washington, DC: US Government Printing Office; 1993.
30. Administration on Aging. *Infrastructure Of Home and Community Based Services For The Functionally Impaired Elderly-State Source Book.* Washington, DC: US Dept of Health and Human Services; 1993.
31. Schlettwein-Gsell D. Nutrition and the quality of life: a measure for the outcome of nutritional intervention? *Am J Clin Nutr.* 1992;55:1263S–1266S.
32. American Dietetic Association Council on Practice Quality Management Committee. ADA's definitions for nutrition screening and nutrition assessment. *J Am Diet Assoc.* 1994;94:838–839.
33. Rudberg MA, Furner SE, Cassel CK. Measurement issues in preventive strategies: past, present, and future. *Am J Clin Nutr.* 1992;55:1253S–1256S.
34. Position of The American Dietetic Association: cost-effectiveness of medical nutrition therapy. *J Am Diet Assoc.* 1995;95:88–91.
35. Bergstrom N, Allman RM, Alvarez OM, Bennett MA, Carlson CE, Frantz RA, Garber SL, Jackson BS, Kaminski MV, Kemp MG, Krouskop TA, Lewis VL, Makelbust J, Margolis DJ, Marvel EM, Reger SI, Rodeheaver GT, Salcido R, Xakellis GL, Yarkeny GM. *Pressure Ulcer Treatment. Clinical Practice Guideline. Quick Reference Guide for Clinicians, No. 15.* Rockville, Md: US Dept of Health and Human Services, Public Health Service, Agency for Health Care Policy and Research; 1994. AHCPR publication No. 95-0653.
36. Gallagher-Allred CR. Nutritional care of the terminally ill. *The Consultant Dietitian.* 1995;20:1,3–4.
37. Arensberg MBF, Schiller MR. Dietitians in home care: a survey of current practice. *J Am Diet Assoc.* 1996;96:347–353.
38. Delmi M, Rapin CH, Bengoa JM, Delmas PD, Vasey H, Bonjour JP. Dietary supplementation in elderly patients with fractured neck of the femur. *Lancet.* 1990;335:1013–1016.
39. Dietetics in Physical Medicine and Rehabilitation dietetic practice group. *Nutrition Practice Guidelines for Dysphagia.* Chicago, Ill: American Dietetic Association;1995.
40. Raymond J. Assessment and nutrition management of the older adult. In: Winkler MF, Lysen LK, eds. *Suggested Guidelines for Nutrition and Metabolic Management of Adult Patients Receiving Nutrition Support.* 2nd ed. Chicago, Ill: American Dietetic Association; 1993: 42–52.
41. Shoaf LR, Bishirjian KO. Standards of practice for gerontological nutritionists: a mandate for action. *J Am Diet Assoc.* 1995;95:1433–1438.
42. Gallagher-Allred CR, Voss AC, Finn SC, McCamish MA. Malnutrition and clinical outcomes: the case for medical nutrition therapy. *J Am Diet Assoc.* 1996;96:361–369.
43. Butler RN. Quality of life: can it be an endpoint? How can it be measured? *Am J Clin Nutr.* 1992;55:1267S–1270S.
44. Saffel-Shrier S, Athas BM. Effective provision of comprehensive nutrition case management for the elderly. *J Am Diet Assoc.* 1993;93:439–44.

45. Ellis JR, Cowles ED. Physician response to dietary recommendations in long-term-care facilities. *J Am Diet Assoc.* 1995;95:1424–1425.
46. Westbrook NH. Applying the 1995 JCAHO standards to dietetics practice in home care. *J Am Diet Assoc.* 1996;96:404–406.

■ ADA Position adopted by the House of Delegates on October 26, 1986, and reaffirmed on October 24, 1991 and September 15, 1995. This position will be in effect until December 31, 1999. The American Dietetic Association authorizes republication of the position statement/support paper, *in its entirety,* provided full and proper credit is given. Requests to use portions of the position must be directed to ADA Headquarters at 800/877-1600, ext 4896.

■ Recognition is given to the following for their contributions:
Authors:
Dian Weddle, PhD, RD, FADA; Nancy S. Wellman, PhD, RD, FADA; Linda R Shoaf, PhD, RD
Reviewers:
Joseph M. Carlin, MS, MA, RD; Connie L. Codispoti, MS, RD; Consultant Dietitians in Health Care Facilities dietetic practice group (Mary Ellen Posthauer, RD; Carlene M. Russell, MS, RD, FADA); Gerontological Nutritionists dietetic practice group (Marilyn M. Abernethy, Dr PH, RD; Sylvia Escott-Stumpl, MA, RD; Eileen Kass Kutnick, MS, RD); Mary F. Tonore, MS, RD, FADA; Jane V. White, PhD, RD.

Chapter 36

Nursing Standard-of-Practice Protocol: Sleep Disturbances in Elderly Patients

MARQUIS D. FOREMAN   MAY WYKLE

It is not uncommon for elderly patients to complain of problems sleeping. But, is this owing to normal aging processes or the numerous medications they are taking? Sorting out the causes for sleep disturbances and determining appropriate interventions can be extremely difficult. The practice protocol presented by these authors provides for a systematic assessment of the problem and lists common medications and their sleep disturbing side effects.

Sleep is a mechanism for restoring the body and its function and maintaining energy and health.[1] It has a renewing and replenishing effect, both physically and emotionally. Sleep is a necessity for survival.[2] When sleep is disrupted, physical, emotional, and behavioral disturbances arise. With severe disruption of sleep, physiologic instability may occur. Thus for everyone adequate sleep is essential. It is particularly essential for older adults who are receiving medical care. This article presents a nursing standard of practice protocol for sleep disturbances in elderly patients. Foundational to this nursing standard-of-practice is a discussion of sleep, the changes in sleep that accompany aging, and an overview of sleep disorders.

▄ REM AND NREM

Sleep, a complex combination of physiologic and behavioral processes, is defined as "a reversible behavioral state of perceptual disengagement from and unresponsiveness to the environment."[3] Within sleep, there are two states: rapid eye movement (REM), or desynchronized, sleep and nonrapid eye movement (NREM), or synchronized, sleep.[3]

NREM sleep accounts for approximately 75% to 80% of total sleep time and is characterized by a minimum of mental activity in a movable body.[3] REM sleep, entered some 60 to 90 minutes into the sleep cycle, accounts for about 20% to 25% of total sleep time and is considered essential for well-being.[2] REM sleep, characterized by an abundance of mental activity,

From *Geriatric Nursing* 16(5):238–243, 1995. Reprinted with permission.

as reflected by electroencephalographic activation, and rapid eye movements, is associated with dreaming. In REM sleep there is muscle atonia; blood pressure, pulse, and respirations increase and fluctuate.[2] Deprivation of REM sleep is associated with anxiety, irritability, inability to concentrate, and, if the deprivation is severe enough, disturbed behavior.[2,4]

The sleep cycle usually progresses from stage 1 NREM sleep, through stages 2, 3, and 4, to REM sleep. REM sleep typically occurs after a change from stage 3 or stage 4 NREM to stage 2 NREM sleep, and continues to alternate between REM and NREM stages in 70- to 120-minute cycles. Typically there are 4 to 6 cycles per night. According to Carskadon and Dement,[3] during the first third of a typical night, stages 3 and 4 NREM sleep predominate, while in the last third, stage 2 NREM and REM sleep predominate and stage 4 NREM sleep may be absent.

Changes in Sleep with Aging

Changes in the way people sleep as they age occur as with other human mechanisms.[5] The changes in sleep observed with aging are listed in Table 36-1; these changes lead to sleep that is lighter, shorter, and interrupted. These changes are for the most part minor, still allowing for sleep to achieve its restorative function. Recent evidence indicates these changes observed in sleep are more likely to be the result of chronic health problems and their treatment than to aging.[6] However, elders are predisposed to poor sleep as a result of heightened autonomic activity and an increased susceptibility to external arousal.[6] In addition to these normal changes in sleep that accompany aging, there are disturbances in the sleep-wake cycle that are not normal.

These alterations in sleep require prompt and appropriate assessment and intervention, as they are associated with increased morbidity, mortality, and a reduction in the quality of life.[1,4,5] These alterations in the sleep-wake cycle have been classified into four major categories, summarized in Table 36-2: (1) dyssomnias, (2) parasomnias, (3) sleep disorders associated

---

TABLE 36-1 Common Changes in Sleep With Aging

- Decrease in actual time asleep
- Increase in total sleep time (i.e., more time in bed but less of it asleep)
- Increase in sleep latency (i.e., more time required to fall asleep)
- Increase in the number of awakenings each night
- REM sleep more interrupted
- Increase in stage 1 sleep
- Stages 3 and 4 sleep less deep
- Decreased sleep efficiency
- More easily disturbed by environmental factors
- More frequent comments about poor quality of sleep
- Increases in daytime sleepiness and napping

**TABLE 36-2 The International Classification
of Sleep Disorders**

Dyssomnias
Intrinsic sleep disorders, e.g.,
  Narcolepsy
  Nocturnal myoclonus
Extrinsic sleep disorders, e.g.,
  Environmental sleep disorder
  Hypnotic-dependent sleep disorder
Circadian rhythm sleep disorders, e.g.,
  Time-zone change (jet lag) sleep disorder
  Shift-work sleep disorder

Parasomnias
Arousal disorders, e.g.,
  Confusional arousals
  Sleepwalking
Sleep-wake transition disorders, e.g.,
  Rhythmic movement disorders
Parasomnias associated with REM sleep, e.g.,
  Nightmares
Other parasomnias, e.g.,
  Sleep enuresis
  Primary snoring

Medical or Psychiatric Disorders
Mental disorders, e.g.,
  Psychoses
  Mood disorders
Neurologic disorders, e.g.,
  Dementia
  Parkinsonism
Other medical disorders, e.g.,
  Chronic obstructive pulmonary disease
  Nocturnal cardiac ischemia

Proposed Sleep Disorders
Menstrual-associated sleep disorder

Adapted from Thorpy[7] and Diagnostic Classification Steering Committee[8]

---

with medical or psychiatric disorders, and (4) proposed sleep disorders.[7,8] Each category is described in greater detail below.

Dyssomnias are disorders of initiating and maintaining sleep (also known as *insomnias*) and those of excessive somnolence.[7,8] The dyssomnias are the primary sleep disorders associated with disturbed nighttime sleep and impaired wakefulness.[7,8] These dyssomnias are further divided into three major groups, based, in part, on pathophysiologic mechanisms: (1) intrinsic sleep disorders, (2) extrinsic sleep disorders, and (3) circadian rhythm sleep disorders. Intrinsic sleep disorders are disorders associated with complaints of insomnia or excessive sleepiness that are caused by pathophysiologic processes within the body. Examples of intrinsic sleep disorders include narcolepsy, sleep apnea syndromes, and nocturnal myoclonus. Conversely, extrinsic sleep disorders are caused by processes external to the body, most frequently environmental in nature. Extrinsic sleep disorders are also characterized by insomnia and excessive sleepiness. Examples include disturbances in sleep resulting from excessive lighting or noise, caffeinated beverages, and hypnotic drug or alcohol dependence.[7,8] Circadian rhythm sleep disorders share a common chronobiologic etiology, and include: jet-lag syndrome, shift-work sleep disorder, and irregular sleep-wake pattern. Treatment of these disorders consists primarily of identifying the underlying pathophysiologic process and correcting, eliminating, or minimizing it.

Parasomnias are manifested by central nervous system activation, autonomic nervous system changes, and skeletal muscle activity.[7,8] They are disorders of arousal, partial arousal, and sleep stage transition, caused not by abnormalities in basic sleep processes but by undesirable physical phenomena that occur during sleep.[7,8] Parasomnias are further subdivided into (1) arousal disorders, disorders associated with impaired arousal from sleep; (2) sleep-wake transition disorders, those that occur during the transition from sleep to wakefulness or in sleep stage transitions; (3) parasomnias associated with REM sleep; and (4) other parasomnias.[7,8] Sleep-wake transition disorders are an exception in that they are considered to be caused from altered physiologic processes rather than from pathophysiologic changes.[7,8]

Medical-psychiatric sleep disorders are those disturbances in sleep and wakefulness associated with a large number of health problems and their treatment. This category is further subdivided into three groups, those sleep disorders associated with (1) mental, (2) neurologic, and (3) medical disorders. These disturbances in sleep, referred to by some as secondary sleep problems, are frequent concomitants of hospitalization for acute illness in older patients and may be remedied by a variety of nursing strategies. These sleep disorders, although common, are associated with poorer outcomes of hospitalization (delayed healing, protracted recuperation, transient states of cognitive impairment, and physiologic instability). Sleep disturbances also are associated with a decreased ability to function and to perform daily activities; therefore these disturbances occasionally result in institutionalization. Despite these negative consequences of sleep disturbances, the sleep of hospitalized patients generally is not carefully assessed by nurses; interventions are predominately pharmacologically based and are more likely to exacerbate the sleep disturbance they were intended to solve (Table 36-4). The practice protocol in Table 36-3 outlines the parameters for the assessment of sleep and the nursing strategies for the prevention and management of sleep disturbances. Central to this practice protocol is the principle that pharmacologically based interventions should be used as a temporary means of last resort. Parameters for the evaluation of these nursing strategies also are included.

Proposed sleep disorders is a category for newly described sleep disorders and those for which there is insufficient or inadequate information.[7] Information for establishing the nature of these sleep disorders is anticipated.

Assessment of Sleep

The underlying causes of sleep disturbances in the elderly population include acute and chronic illness and their treatment, characteristics of the hospital environment, characteristics of the older individual, and disruptions in daily routines. As a result, an assessment of sleep and sleep disturbances should encompass the parameters of (1) usual sleep-wake patterns, (2) bedtime routines/rituals, (3) diet and drug use (not to overlook over-the-counter medications), (4) environmental factors, (5) physiologic factors, and (6) illness factors. Specific areas of questioning are found in the protocol for sleep disturbances in elderly patients. Information elicited should include objective data as well as subjective appraisals of the quality of sleep. Questions of family or significant others also may provide insight into usual patterns and certain aspects of sleep.

This assessment is focused to elicit information relative to indicators, or defining characteristics, of sleep disturbance, which include: verbal comments by the individual of not sleeping well, of not feeling rested, of being tired, of being awakened earlier than usual, or of having interrupted sleep. Changes in behavior or performance also will be observed. For example, the person will be irritable, restless, lethargic, listless, or apathetic.[10] Additionally, the person may be observed to have difficulty concentrating, an increased reaction time, a greater sensitivity to pain, and diminished daytime alertness. If ambulatory, this person may be prone to accidents and falls.

Nursing Strategies

Given the prevalence of sleep disturbances in older hospitalized patients and their association with poorer outcomes of care, it was clear to us that practice guidelines were needed. As part of the John A. Hartford Foundation's Nurses Improving Care of the Hospitalized Elderly (NICHE) Project, a panel of gerontologic nurse experts developed a standard of practice for hospital nurses to follow to prevent and manage sleep disturbances (see Table 36-3). This practice guideline for sleep was developed upon two basic principles. First, for the strategy to be effective, it must be individualized, considering the specific characteristics of the patient and the nature of the sleep disturbance as determined by means of the sleep assessment. Second, pharmacologic treatment (e.g., prescription and administration of a sedative or hypnotic agent) should be considered an intervention of last resort. Additionally, when pharmacologic treatment is considered appropriate, only a short-acting, low-dose medication with a wide margin of safety is recommended on a temporary basis.[11] Nonpharmacologic strategies are emphasized in the protocol.

Outcomes/Evaluation

Expected outcomes or the evaluation of the strategies selected should be based on the results of the assessment. Thus, if the selected strategies were successful, the indicators upon which the individual was determined to have a disturbance in sleep should be minimized or eliminated. For example, if the sleep disturbance was the result of interrupted sleep from a noisy environment, the appropriate strategy would be to reduce the frequency

TABLE 36-3 Nursing Standard of Practice Protocol: Sleep Disturbance in Elderly Patients

ASSESSMENT	INTERVENTION	EVALUATION
Sleep-wake patterns: ■ Inquire about usual times for retiring and rising, time for falling asleep; freq. and duration of night-time awakenings; freq. and duration of daytime naps; daytime physical and social activity ■ Have person provide a subjective evaluation of the quality of sleep **Bedtime routines/rituals:** ■ Inquire about activities performed by the individual before bedtime (e.g., personal hygiene, prayer, reading, watching TV, listening to music, snacks) **Medications:** ■ Obtain information relative to all prescribed and self-selected over-the-counter medications used by person, especially, sleep-aids, diuretics, laxatives ■ Determine types of medications and length of time used by person **Diet effects:** ■ Obtain information about the consumption of caffeinated and alcoholic beverages	**Maintain normal sleep pattern:** ■ Maintain usual bedtime ■ Schedule nighttime activities to provide uninterrupted periods of sleep of at least 2–3 hours ■ Balance daytime activity and rest ■ Discourage daytime naps ■ Promote social interaction **Support bedtime routines/rituals:** ■ Offer a bedtime snack or beverage ■ Enable bedtime reading or listening to music ■ Assist with aspects of personal hygiene at bedtime (e.g., a bath) ■ Encourage prayer or meditation **Avoid/minimize drugs that negatively influence sleep** (see Table 36-4): ■ Pharmacologic treatment of sleep disturbances is treatment of last resort ■ Discontinue or adjust the dose or dosing schedule of any/all offending medications ■ Consider drug-drug potentiation ■ Administer meds to promote sleep; give diuretics at least 4 hours before bedtime **Minimize/avoid foods that negatively influence sleep:** ■ Discourage use of beverages containing stimulants (e.g., coffee, tea, sodas) in afternoon and evening ■ Encourage use of warm milk ■ Provide snacks according to patient preference ■ Generally discourage use of alcoholic beverages ■ Decrease fluid intake 2–4 hours before bedtime	**Objective evidence** ■ Time required to fall asleep; should fall asleep within 30–45 minutes ■ Time for awakening, at usual reported time ■ Behavior, alertness, attention, ability to concentrate, reaction time ■ Observe duration of sleep; patient should remain asleep for at least 4-hour intervals **Subjective evidence:** ■ Verbalizations about the quality and quantity of sleep, e.g., statements of difficulty falling asleep, frequent awakenings; having slept well, feeling well-rested/refreshed; of an increased sense of well-being

Environmental factors:

■ Evaluate noise, light, temperature, ventilation, bedding

Physiologic factors:

■ Evaluate breathing pattern with sleep, with attention to pauses

■ Observe for periodic movement or jerking during sleep

■ Inquire about usual position and the number of pillows used with sleep

■ Note diagnoses of sleep disorders (e.g., sleep apnea or narcolepsy)

■ Note diagnoses of specific health problems that adversely affect sleep (e.g., congestive heart failure)

Illness factors:

■ Inquire about pain, affective disturbances (e.g., depression, anxiety, worry, fatigue, and discomfort)

Create optimal environment for sleep:

■ Keep noise to an absolute minimum

■ Set room temperature according to patient preference

■ Provide blankets as requested

■ Use night light as desired

■ Provide soft music or white noise to mask the noise of hospital activity

Promote physiologic stability:

■ Elevate head of bed as required

■ Provide extra pillows per patient preference

■ Administer bronchodilators, if prescribed, before bedtime

■ Use medical therapeutics (e.g., continuous positive airway pressure machine) as prescribed

Promote comfort:

■ Provide analgesia as needed 30 minutes before bedtime

■ Massage, back or foot, to help patient relax

■ Warm and cool compresses to painful areas as indicated

■ Assist with progressive relaxation or guided imagery

■ Encourage patient to urinate before going to bed

■ Keep path to bathroom clear or provide bedside-commode

Bibliography for development of protocol:

Jenike MA. Geriatric psychiatry and psychopharmacology: a clinical approach. St. Louis: Mosby-Year Book, 1989:272–88.

Johnson JE. Bedtime routines: do they influence the sleep of elderly women? J Appl Gerontol 1988;7:97–110.

National Institutes of Health. Treatment of sleep disorders of older people. Consensus Statement 1990;8(3):1–22.

TABLE 36-4   Drugs and Sleep Disturbances

DRUG TYPE	SPECIFIC DRUG	EFFECT ON SLEEP
CNS Depressants		
Barbiturates	Phenobarbital Nembutal Seconal	Suppresses REM sleep
Narcotics	Demerol	Suppresses REM sleep
Benzodiazepines	Valium Librium Dalmane Restoril Halcion Ativan Serax	Alters REM sleep; reverses normal sleep patterns
Alcohol		Reduces REM sleep and inhibits movement
CNS Stimulants	Caffeine Amphetamine Theophylline	Delays onset of sleep; interferes with REM sleep
Antipsychotics	Mellaril Haldol Thorazine Navane	Causes daytime drowsiness
Autonomic agents	Nasal sprays Cough syrups with dextromethorphan OTCs: Sudafed	Causes daytime sleepiness
Antihypertensives	Methyldopa Reserpine Atenolol Nifedipine	Causes drowsiness
Monoamine oxidase inhibitors	Marplan Nardel Parnate	Improves sleep in depressed persons
Diuretics		Nighttime awakenings caused by nocturia
Steroids		Interferes with sleep

Adapted from Ebersole and Hess[2]

of interruptions to sleep and reduce the noise. Expected outcomes would include subjective verbalizations of having slept better or of feeling more rested. Objectively, there would be evidence of an increased ability to concentrate and a reduction of any previously observed behaviors related to sleep deprivation (e.g., restlessness). Evidence that the strategies are effective would include the observation of appropriate sleep periods (e.g., 6 to 8 hours per night), as well as an alert, attentive patient who is able to concentrate and who follows commands or directions.

Outcomes other than those that are patient specific allow for a more precise evaluation of the quality of the care provided to older patients.

▰ REFERENCES

1. Spenceley SM. Sleep inquiry: a look with fresh eyes. Image J Nurs Sch 1993;25:249–56.
2. Ebersole P, Hess P. Toward healthy aging: human needs and nursing response. 4th ed. St. Louis: Mosby, 1994:64–74.
3. Carskadon MA, Dement WC. Normal human sleep: an overview. In: Kryger MH, Roth T, Dement WC, Eds. Principles and practice of sleep medicine. 2nd ed. Philadelphia: WB Saunders, 1994:16–25.
4. Gottlieb GL. Sleep disorders and their management. Am J Med 1990;88(Suppl 3A):29S–33S.
5. Prinz PN, Vitello MV, Raskind MA, Thorpy MJ. Geriatrics: sleep disorders and aging. N Engl J Med 1990;323:520–6.
6. Bliwise DL. Normal aging. In: Kryger MH, Roth T, Dement WC, eds. Principles and practice of sleep medicine. 2nd ed. Philadelphia: WB Saunders, 1994:26–39.
7. Thorpy MJ. Classification of sleep disorders. In: Kryger MH, Roth T, Dement WC, eds. Principles and practice of sleep medicine. 2nd ed. Philadelphia: WB Saunders, 1994:426–36.
8. Diagnostic Classification Steering Committee (Thorpy MJ, chairman). International classification of sleep disorders: diagnostic and coding manual. Rochester, Minnesota: American Sleep Disorders Association, 1990.
9. Prinz PN, Vitello MV. Sleep loss in aging. Sleep disorders and insomnia in the elderly. Facts and Research in Gerontology 1993;7:55–68.
10. Dudas S, Kim MJ. Sleep pattern disturbance. In: Kim MJ, McFarland GK, McLane AM, eds. Pocket guide to nursing diagnosis. 3rd ed. St. Louis: Mosby, 1989:258–61.
11. Consensus Panel. Drugs and insomnia: the use of medications to promote sleep. JAMA 1984;251:2410–14.

Chapter 37

Mistreatment of Elders: Assessment, Diagnosis, and Intervention

TERRY T. FULMER

Elder abuse and neglect is an unfortunate reality in the United States, and is an important concern to health care providers who work with older adults. Causes of abuse are multifaceted and prevalence figures are elusive; however, this is a major problem that must be addressed. Terry Fulmer presents theoretical constructs that are thought to be the basis of elder mistreatment, including dependence, transgenerational violence, care provider pathology and stress, as well as isolation. Assessment techniques and barriers to assessment are also discussed, along with successful intervention approaches. Team assessment and intervention are recognized as generally the most effective approach. The chapter concludes with a comprehensive table of "Dos and Don'ts" for individuals, families, and communities.

For those afflicted with poverty, disease, and a lack of psychosocial supports, old age brings difficult circumstances. The dramatic increase in average life span of Americans since 1900 is well documented. Although we applaud the advances in medical science that make this possible, there are concomitant problems that can be thought of as resulting from advanced old age.

Physiologically, normal aging is distinct and separate from disease.[14] It is clear, however, that as one advances in age, there is an increased susceptibility and propensity for chronic disorders such as arthritis, decreased visual acuity, hypertension, and orthopedic impairments.[9] Predictably, elderly individuals who are extremely frail, dependent, and perhaps mentally impaired, are at higher risk for elder mistreatment.[5]

▬ OVERVIEW OF THE PHENOMENON

The incidence and prevalence of elder abuse are elusive. Because there are no data bases or universal definitions of mistreatment, the exact frequency of elder mistreatment and its categories are unknown. Estimates suggest that approximately 1.5 million elders are abused or mistreated each

From *Nursing Clinics of North America* 24(3):701–706, 1989. Reprinted with permission.

year, however, and this number is expected to rise as the number of elders increases in this country. An exciting new project under the auspices of the American Public Welfare Association may provide some of the statistics we are looking for in relation to this topic but, to date, none are available.

Hudson and Johnson[6] have provided the best summary of the literature to date. In their paper, research studies on the subject of elder mistreatment are summarized and synthesized relative to the status of knowledge, the evaluation of progress to date, and the identification of future needs for research and practice. This extensive literature review points out the differences in definitions, sample types, and sizes, and describes the major findings and limitations of the studies. It is clear from their work that much progress has been made since the phenomenon of elder abuse came to the forefront in the late 1970s. Their work also reflects momentum that lends optimism for future work.

If definitions are elusive, it seems there is more consensus related to proposed theories of causation for elder mistreatment. Increased dependency and frailty, non-normal care providers, transgenerational violence, stressed caregivers, and isolated elders generally are discussed when theories are posed for when and why elder mistreatment may occur. It is useful to review each of these theoretical variables as a basis for appropriate and effective assessment of elder mistreatment.

▬THEORETICAL VARIABLES
Elder Dependency

Dependency is an important variable that has been debated at length in the elder mistreatment literature. On the one hand, dependency of an adult-child on an older person has been suggested as a high-risk situation for elder mistreatment. Pillemer[11] suggests that it is the adult-child dependent on the elder who is more likely to be aggressive and mistreat the elder. On the other hand, Fulmer and Ashley[5] suggest that elders who are dependent on others for their care in activities of daily living are more likely to be victims of abuse or neglect. The key issue in this category seems to be in the definition of "universes" (Figure 37-1).

When Pillemer discusses dependency,[11] the universe under study relates to all dependent elders with care needs. The subset of mistreated individuals is relatively small. His work would suggest that of all dependent elders who need help with activities of daily living only a small subset are mistreated. Fulmer and Ashley[5] are describing the universe of individuals who are referred for mistreatment. Of those individuals, the majority are multiply impaired, dependent, and frail. When these two research papers are compared, therefore, it would seem that there is disagreement about the role of dependency in elder mistreatment. In fact, the important notion is the group under study. At this point, it is fair to say that each is correct, but the differences need to be clarified for the public in order to teach the content accurately.

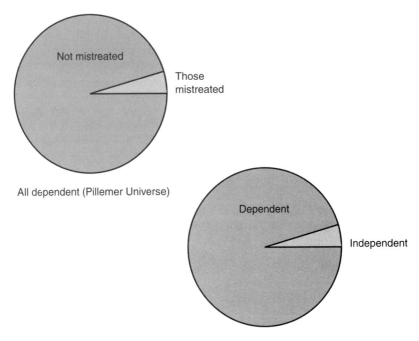

All dependent (Pillemer Universe)

All mistreated (Fulmer Universe)

FIGURE 37-1   A theoretical representation of the different universes of dependency and elder mistreatment.

Transgenerational Violence

This theoretical construct holds that violence is a learned behavior and if a child grows up in a family where violence is accepted and normative, they will learn it and demonstrate aggressive behavior as they age. Another theme often listed under this heading is that of retribution. In this line of thinking, if a child is abused or mistreated, as he grows older, and perhaps becomes responsible for the care of a parent, he will get back at that aged parent through mistreatment. This is an important construct and although no systematic studies have been conducted to date, it will be important to follow families with violent behavior in order to learn more about this.

Non-normal Care Provider (Psychopathology of the Abuser)

The belief inherent in this theoretical variable is that elder mistreatment occurs at the hands of an individual who has some underlying psychopathology. If a person has a psychiatric disease, a drug or alcohol addiction, or perhaps some form of mental retardation, it may be that he is less effective at impulse control and more likely to mistreat elders. This is not to suggest that all individuals with these disorders mistreat elders, but that they may be more likely to do so. Murray Strauss of the University of New Hampshire[15] makes a very poignant point when he says that substance abuse should not be considered an acceptable "excuse or reason" for violent behavior. The example he presents relates to the man who batters his wife. Strauss suggests that the question to ask this batterer is "if you had no impulse control in relation to beating her, why didn't you kill her?" This chilling question is one that makes us wonder whether alcohol releases inhibitions for violent behavior or whether it simply is used as an excuse for intentionally violent acts.

Stressed Caregivers

The notion that underlies the stressed caregiver variable is that an individual who is responsible for providing care to an elderly person has only a limited number of internal resources. If the elderly individual needs a number of supports to stay well and if the caregiver comes under stress from unrelated things such as the loss of a job, a divorce, difficulty with his own child, and so on, then that individual may express his stress through mistreatment of the elder. This theory reminds us of "the straw that breaks the camel's back" and proposes that caregivers who have many demands and who are pulled in several different directions may not be able to cope and may become abusive or neglectful. There are anecdotal reports that individuals who are provided respite or adult day care services seem to be able to avoid mistreating their elders, but more research is needed in order to understand the exact impact of such support services.

Isolated Elders

The exchange theory, proposed by Pillemer,[11] focuses on the relationship between an isolated elderly person and an individual who is abusive. In this relationship, it is believed that mistreatment of elders will occur as long as there is some gain for the abuser. If there no longer is anything to be gained from the situation and, further, if there is some threat of a sanction from the behavior, it is likely that the mistreatment will stop. This may be why the presence of a home health aide or home care attendant can be so effective in halting elder mistreatment. When an outsider is observing the situation, it is less likely that mistreatment will occur because there is a "watchdog" effect. Further, the intermittent visit of a neighbor or visiting nurse may be extremely effective in decreasing the incidence of elder mistreatment because the abuser never knows when he is likely to be under surveillance. Clearly, isolated elders are at extremely high risk for mistreatment under the premises of this theory.

Much more needs to be understood relative to these theoretical variables in order to come to a clearer understanding of why elder mistreatment occurs but, for the time being, these variables and their related theories are extremely important in the understanding of elder mistreatment.

■MISTREATMENT ASSESSMENT TECHNIQUES

During the past decade, a number of assessment instruments, guidelines, and protocols have been developed by a number of different professional groups to assist with the difficult task of assessing elder mistreatment. Ashley and Fulmer[2] have provided a comprehensive discussion of assessment instruments that is helpful to individuals who are interested in the array of approaches currently under use. Both qualitative and quantitative approaches are employed in the available instruments and protocols.

Qualitative instruments and protocols, including those developed by Johnson,[8] Tomita,[17] and Rathbone-McCuan and Voyles,[13] have an open-ended format and ask professionals to use subjective and objective data to determine an elderly person's status and type of maltreatment. Most of these qualitative instruments include a general health assessment section, a home assessment section, and a section that asks the assessor to describe the etiology of the mistreatment. Qualitative approaches give the assessor more leeway in terms of describing the nature of the event and depicting the state of the elderly person.

Quantitative instruments and protocols, in most cases, use a Likert-type scale that guides the assessor to specific areas for consideration. Health status, family situations, living arrangements, and finances may be evaluated on these scales, for example.

▬ PROBLEMS IN ASSESSING ELDERS FOR MISTREATMENT

Elder mistreatment assessment is an extremely complicated, multifactorial process. There is little to be learned from the child abuse literature in the realm of assessment because there are few parallels. Ageism, disease in old age, the impact of multiple factors on decision making, and the autonomy of the elderly person each play a significant role in this complexity.

Ageism

There are no growth and developmental standards for extremely old people. Although we can say with some certainty what a five-year-old child should look like and be physically capable of, it is much more difficult to conjure up the "typical" 89-year-old. "Ageism," a term coined by Butler[3] in the early 1970s, refers to the negative stereotypes attributed to the elderly simply because they are old. This is relevant in the assessment of elder mistreatment because elderly who complain, present with confusion, exhibit bizarre behavior, or have bruises on their skin are overlooked because "they are old." If a child presented with bruised arms, there would be an immediate line of questioning. There needs to be a heightened sensitivity to the possibility of elder mistreatment; for this to occur, the impact of ageism must be overcome. Further, we expect less from home health aide or nursing home aide care and accept poor care when it should be determined as unacceptable. Simply because an elderly person is receiving care from a paraprofessional is an unacceptable reason for any form of mistreatment. The majority of aides who are delivering excellent care suffer from this notion, as do the elderly. When an older person is admitted to the hospital from a nursing home with wrist burns from the inappropriate use of restraints, everyone involved needs to see this as unacceptable.[16] Staffing problems are not a reason for such a presentation, nor is the fear that the elder could fall. There must be a clear threat of harm to oneself or to others to justify restraints. This frequently is not the case. Age should not be considered a reason for physical symptoms, unusual behavior, or complaints of mistreatment.

Disease in Old Age

Aging is a universal phenomenon that is exhibited in extremely individualistic ways. Lifestyle is known to influence health in old age and it has been suggested that regular exercise and prudent dietary habits can modify the negative impact of aging.[14] Aging, however, should not be equated with disease and, in the same light, symptoms of disease should not be accepted as age-related changes. The paper-thin appearance of the skin of a person who is on high-dose steroids is very different from the skin of an older person, which has lost some of its elasticity and underlying adipose layers. Decubiti should not be accepted as inevitable in elderly people. Decubitus ulcers may be the result of inadequate care and should be evaluated carefully for causative factors. They may be considered as elder mistreatment in certain circumstances. Similarly, poor hygiene is not a result of old age. When an elderly person presents in a disheveled, dirty state, something is wrong. The situation warrants immediate follow-up. Elder mistreatment can be overlooked when nurses assume that a particular presentation of an elderly person is related to a disease. It may be that lack of care is responsible.

Decision Making

Phillips and Rempusheski[10] reported a model that identifies three types of decisions (diagnostic, value, and intervention) and the categories that health care providers consider in making those decisions. Their work describes the human side of problem solving and decision making related to cases of elder mistreatment. They describe the factors that are taken into account when elder mistreatment is suspected and conclude that the association between the intervention decision and the diagnostic decision is surprisingly low. Caregiver resources, elder attributes, amount of effort being expended, health care providers' personal values, and the mental health of the caregiver are examples of factors considered in decision making. This author's experience with the Beth Israel Hospital Elder Assessment[4] team reinforces the complex nature of case analysis in elder mistreatment. Factors such as intentionality, knowledge level of the caregiver, and health problems of the elder all impact on the process of evaluating elder mistreatment cases. Hudson[7] recently conducted an in-depth analysis of the way "experts" define elder mistreatment and the variables considered when thinking about the subcategories of mistreatment. More research is needed to describe this decision-making behavior further.

Autonomy of the Elder

Elders have the right to self-determination, even though we may not always agree with or like the decisions they make. An elderly person may choose to remain in an abusive or neglectful environment despite alternatives offered by health care providers and social service workers, for example. When this occurs, questions regarding the elder's mental status and deci- sion-making capacity often are raised. This probably stems from concern about the elder's well-being, but his decisions and choices must be re- spected. Coercion, undue influence, or duress by health care professionals should be thought of as elder mistreatment. Child abuse models are inap- propriate and just as a battered wife may choose to remain in her environ- ment so, too, may the elder. Wetle[18] points out that an elderly person's competence may be variable and exist on a continuum, with fluctuations from day to day. Re-evaluation on a regular basis is required for appro- priate intervention.

▬ INTERVENTION

Teaming

Elder mistreatment is a complex phenomenon that is difficult to assess and requires a wide array of expertise. Those who have the greatest difficulty in case management are individuals who try to solve problems alone. The most successful approach to case assessment is the multidisciplinary team process, which enables an exchange of ideas and a broad base for potential solutions. Procedures, including review of recent and past medical records, patient and family interviews, and an examination of the elderly person, take a great deal of time and expertise. The utilization of a multidisciplinary team facilitates these activities by providing the necessary expertise.[4] In settings in which the multidisciplinary teaming process is less well estab- lished, individuals who identify themselves as gerontological/geriatric spe- cialists can consult with knowledgeable individuals from other fields related to the medical assessment, psychosocial assessment, or available community resources. Guidance usually is available from state agencies on aging and 48 states now have mandatory elder abuse reporting laws. Teaming, no matter how loosely defined, enables an individual to obtain a variety of opinions about the nature of a given case in order to make appropriate decisions and care planning with the elderly person.

Goals of Intervention When Mistreatment Is Suspected

Safety of the elder and breaking the cycle of mistreatment are two goals of intervention. When mistreatment is suspected and all data from the assessment process suggest that it has occurred, a key question to ask relates to the safety of the elderly person. Is there an immediate threat of danger for the elder? Is there anyone else in the environment who may be in danger? Is there a possibility that protective service case workers may be in jeopardy if they should go out to obtain more information about the situation? Elder mistreatment cases can be extremely volatile and potentially dangerous. It is important to make a determination about the extent or degree of danger apparent in the situation before proceeding. Above all, the elderly person and other individuals involved should be kept from any further harm. Inherent in the second goal of intervention, breaking the cycle of mistreatment, are the issues of family as client, mandatory reporting laws, and long-term follow-up of high-risk and mistreated elders.

"Family as client" is an important construct in elder mistreatment. Usually, there is more than one person in the family unit who is in need of some type of psychosocial or health intervention. If the elderly person is being neglected by a daughter who is a severe alcoholic, for example, it is important to enlist the necessary resources to treat both sides of the equation. Seldom is the situation unidimensional.

Some mandatory reporting laws include the category of self-abuse / self-neglect. These cases can be very difficult, in that they frequently relate to issues of autonomy, self-determination, and life-long patterns of behavior. Collaboration with state agencies that can provide protective services and psychosocial support may be most useful in these cases.

Follow-up to assure the well-being of elders over time is extremely important in elder mistreatment cases. The old adage that "the operation was a success but the patient died" is particularly appropriate here. Although an elder mistreatment case may be resolved successfully in a short-term way, it is likely that, over time, the situation may flare again. A mechanism for regular contact with elders who previously have been mistreated or are at high risk for mistreatment is a very effective way of decreasing cases.

All individuals who enter any kind of health care system, whether it be a hospital, a home health care agency, a nursing home, or some other organized system, have a record or chart. In the event that elder mistreatment has been suspected or documented, an unobtrusive symbol that is recognized only by individuals who work in that system can be applied to the record to serve as a reminder that the elder has been at risk in the past. During subsequent evaluations, the health care professional or case worker is reminded by the symbol and can provide the necessary evaluation and follow-up to ensure the continuing well-being of the elderly person.

Empowering the Elderly

Central to effective follow-up are nursing actions that help empower elders who are high risk or victims of mistreatment. Although many elderly individuals will not be able to benefit from such strategies (those who are profoundly demented or those with major psychological impediments), a large number will be able to gain from programs that teach empowerment strategies.

In a recent monograph published by the American Association of Retired Persons,[1] several points are outlined that describe ways in which elders can protect themselves from mistreatment. Highlights of this report are printed in Table 37-1, and the reader is urged to refer to this document when teaching elderly clients about elder mistreatment.

■SUMMARY

Elder mistreatment is a significant elder care issue that demands a concerted, multidisciplinary effort and systematic follow-up in order to provide positive results. As our nation continues to age and the profile of the care

404

TABLE 37-1   Toward Prevention: Some Dos and Don'ts

TOWARD PREVENTION . . . FOR INDIVIDUALS

Dos

— Stay sociable as you age; maintain and increase your network of friends and acquaintances.
— Keep in contact with old friends and neighbors if you move in with a relative or to a new address.
— Develop a "buddy system" with a friend outside the home. Plan for at least a weekly contact and share openly with this person.
— Ask friends to visit you at home; even a brief visit can allow observations of your well-being.
— Accept new opportunities for activities. They can bring new friends.
— Participate in community activities as long as you are able.
— Volunteer or become a member or officer of an organization. Participate regularly.
— Have your own telephone; post and open your own mail. If your mail is being intercepted, discuss the problem with postal authorities.
— Stay organized. Keep your belongings neat and orderly. Make sure others are aware that you know where everything is kept.
— Take care of your personal needs. Keep regular medical, dental, barber, hairdresser, and other personal appointments.
— Arrange to have your Social Security or pension check deposited directly to a bank account.
— Get legal advice about arrangements you can make now for possible future disability, including powers-of-attorney, guardianships, or conservatorships.
— Keep records, accounts, and property available for examination by someone you trust, as well as by the person you or the court has designated to manage your affairs.
— Review your will periodically.
— Give up control of your property or assets only when *you* decide you cannot manage them.
— Ask for help when you need it. Discuss your plans with your attorney, physician, or family members.

Don'ts

— Don't live with a person who has a background of violent behavior or alcohol or drug abuse.
— Don't leave your home unattended. Notify police if you are going to be away for a long period. Don't leave messages on the door while you are away.
— Don't leave cash, jewelry, or prized possessions lying about.
— Don't accept personal care in return for transfer or assignments of your property or assets unless a lawyer, advocate, or another trusted person acts as a witness to the transaction.
— Don't sign a document unless someone you trust has reviewed it.
— Don't allow anyone else to keep details of your finances or property management from you.

TOWARD PREVENTION ... FOR FAMILIES

Dos

— Maintain close ties with aging relatives and friends. Keep abreast of changes in their health and ability to live independently.

— Discuss an older relative's wishes regarding health care, terminal medical care alternatives, home care in the case of incapacitation, and disposition of his or her personal assets.

— Find sources of help and use them. Chore services, housekeeping, home-delivered meals, senior recreation, day care, respite care, and transportation assistance are available in many communities.

— With the older person's consent, become familiar with his/her financial records, bank accounts, will, safe deposit boxes, insurance, debts, and sources of income before he or she becomes incapacitated. Talk and plan together *now* about how these affairs should be handled.

— Anticipate potential incapacitation by planning as a family who will take responsibility, such as power-of-attorney or in-home caregiving if an aging relative becomes incapacitated.

— Closely examine your family's ability to provide long-term, in-home care for a frail and increasingly dependent relative. Consider the family's physical limits.

— Plan how your own needs will be met when your responsibility for the dependent older relative increases.

— Explore alternative sources of care, including nursing homes or other relatives' homes, in case your situation changes.

— Discuss your plans with friends, neighbors, and other sources of support before your responsibilities become a burden. Ask for their understanding and emotional support — you may need them.

— Familiarize family members with emergency response agencies and services available in case of sudden need.

Don'ts

— Don't offer personal home care unless you thoroughly understand and can meet the responsibilities and costs involved.

— Don't wait until a frail older person has moved in with you to examine his or her needs. You'd need to consider access, safety, containment, and special needs. (Do you need a first-floor bathroom, bedroom, or entry ramp? Will carpets or stairs become barriers? Do you need a fenced yard to prevent the loved one from wandering away? Does your kitchen allow you to prepare special diets or store medications properly? Can you move the person safely in case of fire?)

— Don't assume that poor interpersonal relationships between you or other members of the household and the older person involved will disappear.

— Don't expect irritating habits or problems such as alcohol abuse to stop or be controlled once the dependent person moves into your home.

— Don't ignore your limitations and overextend yourself. Passive neglect could result.

— Don't hamper the older person's independence or intrude unnecessarily on his or her privacy. Provide a private telephone if you can and make other changes if possible.

— Don't label your efforts a failure if home care is not possible and you must seek an alternative.

(continued)

TABLE 37-1 Toward Prevention: Some Dos and Don'ts (*continued*)

TOWARD PREVENTION . . . FOR COMMUNITIES

Dos

— Develop new ways to provide direct assistance to caregiving families. Improve crisis response to help families that face the difficult decision to discontinue home care.

— Through public awareness programs, advocate the cause of caregiving families and the needs of victims of mistreatment.

— Ask other community groups to become more involved in aging service programs, including those at nursing homes or senior citizen housing projects. Their involvement can lead to improved facilities and services.

— Encourage both public and private employers to help caregiving families, especially those with caregivers nearing or beyond retirement age, with fixed incomes and increasing health problems.

— Publicize available support services and professionals available to caregivers, such as senior day care centers, chore services, companions, and housekeeping services. Caregivers may not know about them.

— Give public agency employees basic training in responses and case management. They can be trained to recognize some of the causes of neglect or abuse of older persons and can help in support roles.

— Provide training for community "gatekeepers" and service workers — primary care physicians, public health and social workers, law enforcement officers, transportation and utility workers, postal employees, and others — to help them recognize at-risk situations and take appropriate action.

— Expand Neighborhood Watch programs and similar community groups to include training on home care of frail elderly, identification of the signs of mistreatment, and how to provide assistance or initiate preventive actions to reduce such victimization.

— Open your eyes and ears to the possibility that mistreatment is occurring. Become aware of individuals who are at risk. Develop procedures for investigation, public education, and public support of assistance to troubled families.

— Recognize that many forms of mistreatment or abuse are *crimes*. Volunteers can help victims file formal complaints, seek compensation for losses, seek prosecution of guilty parties, and give the victim assistance subsequent to prosecution. Prosecution can result in sentencing, diversion, training, counseling, or other types of family assistance services as alternatives to criminal sanctions. Urge public support of agencies to provide the necessary services.

Don'ts

— Don't ignore family caregivers of dependent elderly. They are significant parts of the community. Community services can try to involve isolated people in appropriate services or self-help programs. Those at risk, or living in isolation, simply may lack knowledge or information and may welcome community outreach.

— Don't assume that gerontology is a study confined to universities and hospitals. Begin to educate the entire community about aging. (This should be as common in public education as information about child care.)

— Don't sensationalize stories of abuse of older persons. Instead, try to arouse public interest in techniques and strategies to prevent abuse.

— Don't start a major intervention just because an older person is alone or is said to be eccentric. The goal is to seek the least intrusive alternative.

Adapted from AARP: Domestic Mistreatment of the Elderly: Towards Prevention — Some Dos and Don'ts (Pamphlet), 1987; with permission.

provider changes with more women in the work force and fewer offspring to provide care, there is a potential for an epidemic of elder mistreatment. Thoughtful planning now can provide the system and personnel to make the difference as more and more people become potential victims.

▬REFERENCES

1. AARP: Domestic Mistreatment of the Elderly: Toward Prevention — Some Dos and Don'ts (Pamphlet), 1987
2. Ashley J, Fulmer T: No simple way to determine elder abuse. Geriatr Nurs 9:286–288, 1988
3. Butler RN: Why Survive? Being Old in America. New York, Harper & Row, 1975
4. Elder abuse assessment team in an acute hospital setting. Gerontologist 26:115–118, 1986
5. Fulmer T, Ashley J: Clinical indicators which signal neglect. Applied Nurs Res, submitted
6. Hudson MF, Johnson TF: Elder neglect and abuse: A review of the literature. Annu Rev Gerontol Geriatr 6:81–134, 1986
7. Hudson M: Analysis of the concepts of elder mistreatment: Abuse and neglect. J Elder Abuse Neglect 1:1, 1989
8. Johnson D: Abuse of the elderly. Nurse Pract 6:29–34, 1982
9. National Center for Health Statistics: Current Estimates from the National Health Interview Survey, United States, 1986: Vital and Health Statistics Series 10, No. 164, October 1987
10. Phillips LR, Rempusheski VR: A decision-making model for diagnosing and intervening in elder abuse and neglect. Nurs Res 34:314–139, 1985
11. Pillemer KA: The dangers of dependency: new findings on domestic violence against the elderly. Durham, New Hampshire, University of New Hampshire Family Research Program, 1984, unpublished paper
12. Pillemer KA: Risk factors in elder abuse: Results from a case-control study. In Pillemer KA, Wolf RA: Elder Abuse: Conflict in the Family. Dover, Massachusetts, Auburn House, 1986, pp 239–263
13. Rathbone-McCuan E, Voyles B: Case detection of abused elderly parents. Am J Psych 139:189–192, 1982
14. Schneider EL, Reed JD: Life Extension. N Engl J Med 312:1159, 1985
15. Strauss M: Presentation at the Third National Family Violence Research Conference, University of New Hampshire, Durham, New Hampshire, July 6–9, 1987
16. Strumpf NE, Evan LK: Physical restraint of the hospitalized elderly: Perceptions of patients and nurses. Nurs Res 37:132–137, 1988
17. Tomita SK: Detection and treatment of elderly abuse and neglect: A protocol for health care professionals. Phys Occup Ther Geriatr 2:37–51, 1982
18. Wetle TT: Ethical aspects of decision making for and with the elderly. In Kapp MB, Pies H, Doudera AE: Legal and Ethical Aspects of Health Care for the Elderly. Ann Arbor, Michigan, Health Administration Press, 1985, pp 258–267

Chapter 38

Assessing Cognitive Function

MARQUIS D. FOREMAN   KATHLEEN FLETCHER

LORRAINE C. MION   LARK SIMON   THE NICHE FACULTY

Elderly in many settings may have signs and symptoms of impaired cognitive functioning, especially during times of illness or hospitalization. Memory impairments can be owing to several causes, such as depression or early dementia. In order to make accurate and comprehensive evaluations of an older individual's cognitive status, it is important to choose the right tool as well as the right time and place to conduct the examination. The authors of this chapter provide a facile comparison of the clinical behaviors of patients with delirium, dementia, and depression, and list the basic components of a thorough cognitive assessment. This chapter also highlights some basic guidelines for performing accurate cognitive assessments.

Cognitive functioning encompasses the processes by which an individual perceives, registers, stores, retrieves, and uses information. In elders cognitive functioning is particularly vulnerable to insult during an episode of illness. Given the importance and precariousness of cognitive functioning in the old, nurses' assessments of these processes are critical. The nurse's assessment of an individual's cognitive status can be instrumental in identifying the presence and monitoring the course of specific pathophysiologic states, for example, dementia, depression, or delirium (Table 38-1); determining the individual's readiness to learn; establishing clinical goals; or evaluating the effectiveness of a treatment regimen. We report on a standard or practice protocol for assessing cognitive functioning (Table 38-2).

Two caveats must be considered when cognitive function is assessed. First, when selecting an instrument to assess cognitive functioning, consider the following questions: What is the purpose of the measurement? Is the assessment for screening, monitoring, diagnosis, or more than one of these purposes? Each of these purposes requires different qualities of an instrument. Screening is conducted to determine whether an impairment is present; as a result, relatively imprecise methods are acceptable. Also, for the purposes of screening, the exact nature and cause of the impairment are considered irrelevant. Therefore screening methods will not determine

From *Geriatric Nursing* 17(5):228–233, 1996. Reprinted with permission.

TABLE 38-1   A Comparison of the Clinical Features of Delirium, Dementia, and Depression

CLINICAL FEATURE	DELIRIUM	DEMENTIA	DEPRESSION
Onset	Acute/subacute, depends on cause, often at twilight or in darkness	Chronic, generally insidious, depends on cause	Coincides with major life changes, often abrupt
Course	Short, diurnal fluctuations in symptoms, worse at night, in darkness, and on awakening	Long, no diurnal effects, symptoms progressive yet relatively stable over time	Diurnal effects, typically worse in the morning, situational fluctuations, but less than with delirium
Progression	Abrupt	Slow but uneven	Variable, rapid or slow but even
Duration	Hours to less than 1 month, seldom longer	Months to years	At least 6 weeks, can be several months to years
Awareness	Reduced	Clear	Clear
Alertness	Fluctuates, lethargic or hypervigilant	Generally normal	Normal
Attention	Impaired, fluctuates	Generally normal	Minimal impairment, but is easily distracted
Orientation	Generally impaired, severity varies	Generally normal	Selective disorientation
Memory	Recent and immediate impaired	Recent and remote impaired	Selective or "patchy" impairment, "islands" of intact memory
Thinking	Disorganized, distorted, fragmented, incoherent speech, either slow or accelerated	Difficulty with abstraction, thoughts impoverished, judgment impaired, words difficult to find	Intact but with themes of hopelessness, helplessness, or self-deprecation
Perception	Distorted illusions, delusions, and hallucinations, difficulty distinguishing between reality and misperceptions	Misperceptions usually absent	Intact, delusions and hallucinations absent except in severe cases
Psychomotor behavior	Variable, hypokinetic, hyperkinetic, and mixed	Normal, may have apraxia	Variable, psychomotor retardation or agitation
Sleep/wake cycle	Disturbed, cycle reversed	Fragmented	Disturbed, usually early morning awakening
Associated features	Variable affective changes, symptoms of autonomic hyperarousal, exaggeration of personality type, associated with acute physical illness	Affect tends to be superficial, inappropriate and labile, attempts to conceal deficits in intellect, personality changes, aphasia, agnosia may be present, lacks insight	Affect depressed, dysphoric mood, exaggerated and detailed complaints, preoccupied with personal thoughts, insight present, verbal elaboration
Assessment	Distracted from task, numerous errors	Failings highlighted by family, frequent "near miss" answers, struggles with test, great effort to find an appropriate reply, frequent requests for feedback on performance	Failings highlighted by individual, frequently answers "don't know," little effort, frequently gives up, indifferent toward test, does not care or attempt to find answer

409

TABLE 38-2 Overview of Cognitive Assessment[3-8]

A. Concepts and categories
   1. Definition: cognitive function: the processes by which an individual perceives, registers, stores, retrieves, and uses information
   2. Categories of cognitive change/decline
      a. The dementias (e.g., Alzheimer's, vascular) are chronic, progressive, insidious, and permanent states of cognitive impairment
      b. Delirium/acute confusion: an acute and sudden impairment of cognition that is considered temporary, generally an identifiable, biophysical cause
      c. Impairment in thought processes
B. Assessment
   1. Methods of assessment
      a. Formal — cognitive testing using standardized instruments
         i. Advantages: standardized; enables comparison across individuals and nurses
         ii. Disadvantages: individual performance influenced by pain, education, fatigue, cultural background, and perceptual and physical abilities
      b. Informal — through structured observations of nurse-individual interactions
         i. Advantages: may have greater meaning about individual's actual cognitive ability/performance
         ii. Disadvantages: difficult to make judgments regarding change in individual condition; variability in interpretation
   2. Other considerations for assessment
      a. Characteristics of the environment for assessment
         i. Physical environment
            — Comfortable ambient temperature
            — Adequate lighting but not glaring
            — Free of distractions, e.g., should be conducted in the absence of others and other activities
            — Position self to maximize individual's sensory abilities
         ii. Interpersonal environment
            — Use individual's self-paced rate for assessment
            — Emotionally nonthreatening
      b. Timing considerations
         i. Timing should reflect the actual cognitive abilities of the individual and not extraneous factors
         ii. Times of the day to generally avoid
            — Immediately on awakening from sleep, wait at least 30 minutes
            — Immediately before or after meals
            — Immediately before or after medical diagnostic or therapeutic procedures
            — When patient has pain or discomfort

410

3. Parameters of assessment
   a. Alertness/level of consciousness: the most rudimentary cognitive function and level of arousal, or responsiveness to stimuli determined by interaction with individual and determination of level made on the basis of the individual's best eye, verbal, and motor response to stimuli
      i. Alertness — able to interact in a meaningful way with the examiner
      ii. Lethargy or somnolence — not fully alert; individual tends to drift to sleep when not stimulated, diminished spontaneous physical movement, loses train of thought, ideas wander
      iii. Obtundation — transitional stage between lethargy and stupor; difficult to arouse, meaningful testing futile, requires constant stimulation to elicit response
      iv. Stupor or semicoma — individual mumbles/groans in response to persistent and vigorous physical stimulation
      v. Coma — completely unable to be aroused, no behavioral response to stimuli
   b. Attention: ability to attend/concentrate on stimuli: can follow through with directions, especially a three-stage command; is easily distracted
   c. Memory: ability to register, retain, and recall information both new and old; does individual remember your name? Is individual able to learn and remember new information?
   d. Orientation to time, place, and person
   e. Thinking: ability to organize and communicate ideas; thoughts should be organized, coherent, and appropriate
   f. Perception: presence/absence of illusions, delusions, or visual or auditory hallucinations
   g. Psychomotor behavior: ability to comprehend and perform simple motor skills. Relative to execution ability ask the individual to perform certain ADLs/IADLs, or to perform a three-step command, and to copy a figure
   h. Insight: ability to understand oneself and the situation in which one finds oneself
   i. Judgment: ability to evaluate a situation (real or hypothetical) and determine an appropriate action
C. Outcomes of assessment
   1. Individual
      a. Detection of deviations will be prompt and early with appropriate care and treatment instituted in a timely manner
      b. Plans of care will appropriately address corrective and supportive cognitive function
   2. Health care provider
      a. Assessment and documentation of cognitive function
      b. Appropriate strategies to address any deviation in cognitive function
      c. Competence in cognitive assessment
      d. Evidence of ability to differentiate among the different types of cognitive change/decline
   3. Institution
      a. Documentation of cognitive function will increase
      b. Referral to appropriate advanced practitioners (e.g., geriatrician, geriatric/gerotological or psychiatric clinical nurse specialist or nurse practitioner, or consultation-liaison service) will increase

---

ADL, Activities of daily living; IADL, Instrumental activities of daily living.

whether the impairment is, for example, dementia, delirium, or depression. Conversely, methods useful for diagnostic purposes provide more precise, detailed, and comprehensive information about an individual's cognitive functioning. Diagnostic methods are used to identify the exact nature and cause of the impairment, as well as an indication of the remaining cognitive abilities of the individual. Monitoring of activities is used to determine cognitive status over time. Such measures generally are useful in documenting an individual's response to treatment.

Closely linked to the purpose of assessment is the question, "How often are the ratings to be made?" Depending on the purpose of the assessment, it may be important to assess the examinee more than once. The first assessment should occur in a well-controlled environment to provide information about the individual's maximal abilities, whereas the second should occur in a more real-world setting to provide an indication of the individual's ability to function relative to performing everyday activities. Monitoring of activities and function typically requires multiple assessments.

■ASSESSMENT

Numerous instruments have been developed to evaluate an individual's cognitive functioning. These instruments range from full-scale batteries that require an exquisitely skilled examiner and place intense demands on the examinee, to instruments that can be used at the bedside and place little demand on the examiner and examinee. Additionally, some of these instruments are constructed to assess a single process (e.g., attention) in great detail versus others that assess the spectrum of cognitive processes, including affect and function.

Each approach has its advantages and disadvantages. An advantage of assessing only a single cognitive process is that it minimizes the demands on the examiner and examinee; however, focusing the assessment on a single process, such as orientation, may overlook an important deficit in another, such as judgment. Conversely, an assessment of all cognitive processes provides a global indication of the individual's cognitive abilities, but it is time-consuming, places intensive demands on the examinee, and may be less sensitive to some aspects of cognition. An extensive review of these instruments is reported elsewhere.[1]

■SELECTING AN INSTRUMENT

What level of impairment is to be assessed? It is important to select an instrument that is adequate for the level of impairment. An instrument may be highly sensitive to a part of the spectrum of impairment; for example, it may be useful for mild to moderate impairment and insensitive to differences at the severe range. For example, many instruments will rate an individual with dementia as having severe cognitive impairment but will be unable to differentiate an individual who is totally dependent for care from an individual who can still walk and feed himself or herself.

For what specific subpopulation is the instrument designed? The answer to this question will assist in determining the general content and level of functioning that is assessed by the instrument. Examples of subpopulations are individuals who are educationally disadvantaged, who speak English as a second language, or who have various physical handicaps. An instrument for cognitive assessment may also be selected on the basis of abilities or handicaps of the examinee. Lezak[2] provides an excellent discussion of features to be considered when selecting an instrument for use with individuals with sensory-motor handicaps or those with severe brain damage. Additional characteristics of the examinee to consider are age, educational level, race, and socioeconomic level.

Should subjective (individual self-reports) and objective (observations or testing by the nurse or some other) ratings be distinguished? Again, the answer to this question will be influenced by many of the previous questions. Subjective and objective evidence is often critical to an accurate diagnosis.

In the use of an instrument, the comfort and privacy of both the examiner and examinee should be considered. The room should be well lit and set at a comfortable ambient temperature, so that neither the examiner nor the examinee is distracted from the cognitive task. Lighting must be balanced to be sufficient for the examinee to see the examination materials adequately, while not being so bright as to create glare. Laminated materials create glare. Positioning is important relative to lighting and glare. Also, the assessment environment should be free from distractions that can result from extraneous noise, assessment materials scattered about, or brightly colored or patterned clothing and flashy jewelry on the examiner.[2]

Performing the assessment in the presence of others should be avoided when possible, because the other individual can be distracting. If the other is a significant intimate relative, additional problems arise. For example, when the examinee fails to respond or responds in error, the significant other has been known to provide the answer, or to say, "Now, you know the answer to that" or "Now, you know that's wrong." In most instances, the presence of another only serves to heighten anxiety.

The assessment environment should be emotionally nonthreatening. For example, older adults are especially sensitive to any insinuation that they may have some "memory problem." Therefore the dilemma for the examiner is to stress the importance of the assessment while taking care not to increase the examinee's anxiety by asking the elder about memory problems; explaining that these often occur with various diseases is useful. It is important to create an environment in which the examinee is motivated to perform and to perform well, while not being overly anxious and thereby perform poorly. It is counterproductive to describe the assessment as consisting of "simple," "silly," or "stupid" questions. Anxiety is heightened after a series of failures on assessment. Lezak[2] suggests altering the order of the presentation of items so that the examinee can have some experience with success.

Various characteristics of the examiner and examinee also should be considered. Many of the instruments to assess cognitive functioning can be perceived by the examinee as intrusive, intimidating, fatiguing, and offensive — characteristics that can seriously and negatively affect performance. Consequently, Lezak[2] recommends a 15- to 20-minute period to establish rapport with the examinee. This period also allows a determination of the examinee's capacity for tolerating the assessment. For example, this period can be used to determine special problems that could influence testing or its interpretation (e.g., sensory decrements). With elderly individuals who may have some decrements in sensory abilities, the examiner can improve the examinee's ability to perform through simple methods. For example, if the examinee has any degree of hearing impairment, taking a position across from the examiner or a little to the side may enhance the examinee's hearing. In this position, the examinee can readily use the examiner's nonverbal communication, as well as read the examiner's lips. Sitting a little to the side of the ear with the better auditory function of the examinee also improves the examinee's hearing.

Cognitive assessment can be fatiguing to both the examiner and examinee. Thus examiners are cautioned to be alert for fatigue, because not all examinees will inform the examiner they are becoming fatigued. Lezak[2] recommends observing for physical evidence of being tired — slurring of speech, motor slowing, and restlessness. When the examinee is fatigued, temporarily terminating the assessment should be considered. Many of the assessment instruments can be administered in sections; however, if the assessment must be terminated in the middle of a section, it would be wise to repeat the entire section.

Clearly, certain times of the day are inappropriate for obtaining reliable and valid assessments of cognitive functioning. Times of the day that generally should be avoided are immediately on awakening from sleep, immediately before and after meals, immediately before and after medical diagnostic and therapeutic procedures, or when the examinee has discomfort or pain. The timing of the assessment should be selected to best reflect the true abilities of the individual and not extraneous factors.

Interpretation of the results of cognitive assessment is not simple and should consist of more than just the score obtained on testing. The following must be considered when the results of the cognitive assessment are interpreted: the nature and pattern of the examinee's responses to testing, the examinee's behavior during testing, the context of the assessment, the examinee's health history, physical examination results, and results of various laboratory and other tests, educational level, occupation, family history, current living situation, and level of social functioning, and presence of sensory or motor deficits.

The nature and pattern of the responses to testing can also provide valuable information about an individual's cognitive status. Noting the examinee's verbatim responses on testing is often valuable in differential diagnosis.

Anecdotal notes of the context of testing, the testing environment, and the appearance of the examinee during testing also are important for better understanding the performance on testing. Supplementary information from the examinee's health history, physical examination result, and laboratory and other test results can provide valuable insight into the individual's performance on testing.

Clearly, the determination of an individual's cognitive status is important in the process and outcomes of illness and its treatment. Being competent in the assessment of cognitive functioning requires the following: (1) knowledge and skill as they relate to the performance of a cognitive assessment, (2) sensitivity to the issues that can negatively bias the results of this assessment, (3) accurate and comprehensive documentation of the assessment, and (4) the incorporation of the results of the assessment in the development of the individual's plan of care.

■REFERENCES

1. Foreman MD. Measuring cognitive status. In: Frank-Stromborg M, Olsen S, eds. Instruments for clinical research in health care. 2nd ed. Wilsonville, Ore.: Jones and Bartlett, 1996.
2. Lezak MD. Neuropsychological assessment. 2nd ed. New York: Oxford University Press, 1983.
3. Abraham IL, Manning CA, Snustad DG, Brashear HR, Newman MC, Wofford AB. Cognitive screening of nursing home residents: factor structures of the Mini-Mental State Examination. J Am Geriatr Soc 1994;42:750–6.
4. Foreman MD, Grabowski R. Diagnostic dilemma: cognitive impairment in the elderly. J Gerontol Nurs 1992;18(9):5–12.
5. Mandell AM, Knoefel JE, Albert ML. Mental status examination in the elderly. In: Albert ML, Knoefel JE, Clinical neurology of aging. 2nd ed. New York: Oxford University Press, 1994:277–313.
6. Smith MJ, Breibart WS, Platt MM. A critique of instruments and methods to detect, diagnose, and rate delirium. J Pain Symptom Manage 1995;10;35–77.
7. Strub RL, Black FW. The mental status examination in neurology. 2nd ed. Philadelphia: Davis, 1985.
8. Tombaugh TN, McIntyre NJ. The mini-mental state examination: a comprehensive review. J Am Geriatr Soc 1992;40:922–35.

SELECTED BIBLIOGRAPHY

Beck, J. C., Freedman, M. L. & Warshaw, G. A. (1994). Geriatric assessment: Focus on function. *Patient Care* 28(4): 19–25.

Campbell, L. A. & Thompson, B. L. (1990). Evaluating elderly patients: A critique of comprehensive functional assessment tools. *Nurse Practitioner* 15(8): 11–18.

Collinsworth, R. (1991). Determining nutritional status of the elderly surgical patient: Steps in the assessment process. *AORN Journal* 54(3): 622–631.

Decker, K. (1989). Theory in action: The geriatric assessment team. *Journal of Gerontological Nursing* 15(10): 15–33.

Dracup, K., Dunbar, S. & Baker, D. (1995, July). Rethinking heart failure. *American Journal of Nursing* 23–27.

Foreman, M. D. (1992). Adverse psychologic responses of the elderly to critical illness. *AACN Clinical Issues in Critical Care Nursing* 3(1): 64–72.

Frost, M. H. & Willite, K. (1994). Risk for abuse/neglect: Documentation of assessment data and diagnoses. *Journal of Gerontological Nursing* 20(8): 37–45.

Fulmer, T. T., Mion, L. C., Bottrell, M. M. & N.I.C.H.E. faculty. (1996). Pain management protocol. *Geriatric Nursing* 17(5): 222–227.

Kravitz, R. L., Reuben, D. B., Davis, J. W., Mitchell, A., Hemmerlling, K., Kington, R. S. & Siu, A. L. (1994). Geriatric home assessment after hospital discharge. *Journal of the American Geriatrics Society* 42(12): 1229–1234.

Lee, M. (1996). Drugs and the elderly: Do you know the risks? *American Journal of Nursing* 96(7): 25–31.

Mion, L. C., McDowell, J. A. & Heaney, L. K. (1994). Nutritional assessment of the elderly in the ambulatory care setting. *Nurse Practitioner Forum* 5(1): 46–51.

Redeker, N. S. & Sadowski, A. V. (1995). Update on cardiovascular drugs and elders. *American Journal of Nursing* 95(9): 34–40.

Soltys, F. G. & Coats, L. (1995). The SolCos Model: Facilitating reminiscence therapy. *Journal of Psychosocial Nursing* 33(11): 21–26.

Wiseman, E. J. & Souder, E. (1996). The older driver: A handy tool to assess competence behind the wheel. *Geriatrics* 51(7): 36–42.

Woolf, S. H., Kamerow, D. B., Lawrence, R. S., Medalie, J. H. & Estes, E. H. (1990). The periodic health examination of older adults: The recommendations of the U.S. preventive services task force. *Journal of the American Geriatric Society* 38(7): 817–823.

Unit 7
Managing Elders With Selected Health Care Issues

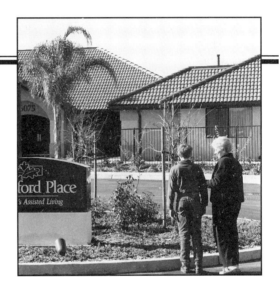

A s we age there are a variety of ills that may befall us. The longer we live there are more years in which problems may occur. If the illnesses or injuries are minor or self-limiting, we can manage them successfully and go on. Sometimes the problems are overwhelming; they may be chronic and change the quality of our life with minor to major adjustments in daily living. They may be acute and need expert management for the short term to have a positive outcome. Unfortunately, some are terminal with years of deterioration, incapacitation, pain, and death. The conditions are emotional, psychological, or physical.

This view does not exaggerate the facts; it is reality. Forty percent of acute care beds are occupied by clients over the age of 65. As we age, most of us will have 20 or more years in which health problems may affect our older years. How one has spent life preparing for old age has great impact on the quality of life in those years, as seen in Unit 2. Similarly, if health care providers become more informed about the latest research and management practices surrounding specific health care issues, this will also influence the quality of life and health related outcomes in the aged.

In this unit, eight chapters are devoted to specific issues related to the health of the elderly. The first two chapters discuss emotional or psychological health related issues; people with controlling personalities and depression. Assessment, diagnosis, and management skills are presented in these chapters in order to give the reader helpful tools when working with these clients.

The remaining six chapters focus on selected altered states of physical health; aged clients with postoperative pain; falls as a preventable crisis; congestive heart failure, the most common acute care admission diagnosis; sundown syndrome; elders with AIDS; and Alzheimer's disease. Because there is limited space in this book and many other timely topics exist, it was necessary to select some of the most pertinent concerns.

The chapters selected represent conditions commonly seen by health care workers; conditions that can be prevented with thorough assessment and teaching; situations that are becoming more prevalent and ones that health care workers will be seeing in their practice settings in greater numbers; and finally, ones whose nursing care and management have been the most influenced by the latest research. The health care issues presented in this unit fit two or more of the preceding characteristics. It is hoped that this overview of selected health care problems will enrich the nursing practice delivered by the reader.

Chapter 39

Care of Elders With Controlling Dispositions

E. J. MATTHIS

Dr. Matthis presents an issue in this chapter that often confounds health care providers who work with elders. The issue of older adults with controlling dispositions often frustrates the efforts of healthcare workers to help them. This excellent chapter includes developmental background to help the reader understand what provokes the need to control, criteria for identifying controlling dispositions, and several care strategies to enhance outcomes. The author also suggests that readers apply and test ideas shared here by conducting clinical practice studies in their areas of practice to add to or correct the perspective she presents.

Attention to the dispositions of clients can enhance outcomes of healthcare services. Disposition refers to the prevailing nature of a client's frame of mind, spirit, and mood. Disregard of clients' dispositions undermines the efficacy of care, even when other aspects of the service are excellent. Older adults are likely to be uncooperative, noncompliant, or resistive if healthcare providers neglect needs stemming from their controlling dispositions. These conclusions are based on qualitative field studies of elder-stage dispositions conducted by the author during the past decade.

This qualitative research yielded conceptualizations of several elder-stage disposition syndromes and disposition-specific care strategies. The label, "controlling disposition," was given to the syndrome identified and defined by the manifestations listed in Table 39-1. Home healthcare providers from all disciplines are encouraged to further test the conceptualization of controlling disposition and the care strategies presented in this article.

▬ BACKGROUND

The study population was composed of convenience samples of disabled older adults (older than 64 years of age). Subjects were living at home, in nursing homes, or in a retirement community. Only those who could

From *Home Healthcare Nurse* 12(4):29–33, 1994. Reproduced with permission.

TABLE 39-1   Criteria to Identify Controlling Dispositions

Associative Factors
    Moderate to severe multiple losses*
    Inadequate capacity/energy to achieve activities of daily living unassisted
    Adherence to habitual behaviors
    Inability/unwillingness to visualize and face entire reality of own situation

Manifestations
    General muscular tenseness
    Definite movements in space
    Avoids sustained eye contact
    Avoids touch and closeness
    Occasional mild confusion
    Denies and attempts to hide confusion
    Denies emotional feelings and their influence
    Disgusted/angered by open expression of emotional feelings by others
    Blames others for adverse happenings
    Possessive of material objects and current realities of this world
    Self-centered in relating to others
    Competitive

---

* Severity may be in terms of degree, number, and/or rapidity of losses.

---

communicate verbally were accepted as subjects. No clients with diagnosed mental illnesses or organic brain disorders were included. Although men were not excluded intentionally, the samples included few.

The author was practicing as a nurse and as a horticultural therapist at different times during the research. Nursing students enrolled in gerontology and community health courses were involved occasionally. They assisted in identifying various dispositions and testing strategies of care.

▬ ELDER STAGE

Four key assumptions undergird the concept of elder-stage human development as used in these studies. First, aging is a normal process that begins at birth and continues throughout the lifespan. Second, psychosocial, spiritual, and physical changes are a part of this normal aging process. Third, the older a given population, the greater the variation is among members, which is attributable to increasing diversity in life experiences and different responses to these experiences. Finally, coping mechanisms that are effective in one stage of life are not always effective in other stages.

Psychosocial–spiritual developmental tasks fuel elder-stage dispositions. A wide range of tasks of elder-stage development are described by theorists,[1-4] including attempts to integrate past and present, solve unresolved psychosocial conflicts, and grasp the meaning of life and death. Role reorganization and goal adjustments are important tasks for all stages, including the elder stage. Erikson[1] emphasizes that achieving elder-stage tasks is essential for ego integrity. He predicts despair for elders who cannot achieve these tasks.

Feil[5] described an elder-stage beyond Erikson's eighth, or late adulthood, stage of human development. She calls it, "Resolution versus Vegetation," and delineates four substages. These include malorientation, time confusion, repetitive movement, and vegetation. Feil addresses issues of loss, control, resolution of life conflicts, and need for acceptance of the expressed real self by another. Her conceptualization was useful in identifying different types of elder-stage dispositions, particularly her description of how malorientation relates to elders with controlling dispositions.

In the culture of the United States, being in control is considered a mark of responsible adulthood. Lack of control in small children is excused. Conversely, adults are expected to be in control of themselves and of their situations. For adults who fail to meet this social expectation, there are negative social consequences. Hence, it is not surprising that some elders struggle to maintain control even when they suffer losses that impair their abilities to control.

▬IDENTIFICATION OF CONTROLLING DISPOSITIONS

Associative factors and manifestations most helpful in recognizing elders with controlling dispositions are presented in Table 39-1. The term "associative factors" is used rather than etiology because no effort has been made to establish causative or contributory relationships.

The data in the table was a consistent syndromic indicator for controlling dispositions when all associative factors and two thirds of the manifestations were present. Elders in the study who met these criteria responded positively to care strategies designed for controlling elders. The responses included more cooperative behaviors and increased expressed satisfaction.

Controlling elders are struggling to maintain control of themselves and their day-to-day situations. They are unable to do so unassisted because of losses that impair their capacities. Although they deny it, they are on retreat from the issues of this world. Their perspectives are narrowed. They are self-centered in their struggles for survival of self and in their fights to maintain control.

Although they are aware of occasional confusion in their thinking, these elders deny it and may confabulate to cover it up. They pride themselves in being rational and intellectual in their approach to problems. They deny the presence or influence of their own feelings. Toward others who are expressing feelings freely, they express disgust and sometimes anger. They tend to blame others for adverse happenings. Possessiveness of current reality, relationships, and material objects is a strong characteristic of elders with controlling dispositions. In relating to others, they are competitive and often resistive to change and ideas initiated by others.

The appearance of a person with a controlling disposition is that of general muscular tenseness. The jaw is usually jutting, and movements are precise, sustained, and definite. Avoidance of sustained eye contact, touch, and closeness is typical behavior.

▄ IMPLICATIONS FOR CARE

Disabled older adults with controlling dispositions endeavor to maintain control to an extent that is counterproductive to their well-being. As they become more physically disabled, they become more verbally controlling. Healthcare workers who attempt to control such clients often find themselves in a war of wills with diminishing desired outcomes. Frustrated care providers label these clients "demanding, uncooperative, or noncompliant." Clients with controlling dispositions express dissatisfaction when they believe their rights to control are being usurped by healthcare providers. In this research, strategies were developed to lessen this impasse. These strategies focused primarily on increasing sense of control or decreasing perception of loss of control.

Involve Elders in Their Care

To the degree that they are willing and able, controlling elders need to be maximally involved in their care decisions and activities. Encourage them to express their perspectives by using open-ended comments and questions. To show your real interest in their views, ask for clarification. To let them know you are really trying to understand, ask them to correct your expressed understanding of their views. Be as nondirective as possible. Avoid using such word as must, should, don't, and can't.

At times, safety and efficacy of care requires staying within certain specifications. Share the specifications and supporting rationale. Explain consequences of not abiding by the specifications. Furthermore, point out good options that are within the specifications. Encourage the client to make choices from the limited list of good options.

When elders are not able to choose from safe an effective options, divert their minds to areas where they are in control of their lives. Engage them in conversations about the decisions they are making for later in the day, next week, or next month. This strategy of focusing away from the present moment decreases the need to vie for control in the situation at hand. However, one must remember that mentally competent adults have a right to refuse care. This right must be respected. When they consider refusing care, they need to have full knowledge of the consequences. Discussing rationale and consequences (positive and negative) of various courses of action is always an integral part of providing services. This facilitates sound judgments from clients.

Psychological Defense Mechanisms

Use of psychological defense mechanisms is a prevailing characteristic of controlling elders. Confronting elders concerning use of mechanisms such as denial, projection, or rationalization increases defensiveness and resistiveness. Respecting elders' needs to use defense mechanisms is the best approach for most healthcare workers. Referral to a psychiatric mental health professional is appropriate if a client is having extraordinary emotional difficulty. Persistent withdrawal and depression are atypical of controlling dispositions and may signal a need for mental health assistance. Controlling elders do experience normal situational depression in response to losses such as death of a spouse or friend.

Psychosocial Needs

Several psychosocial needs were identified as high priorities among elders with controlling dispositions. These include (a) intact personal space, (b) respect of ownership, (c) esteem from self and others, (d) right to express self freely, and (e) sense of belonging. When attainment of these basic psychological needs is blocked, controlling behaviors escalate.

Older adults with controlling dispositions are hypersensitive to incursions into their personal space. Antagonistic episodes may occur, even in friendly situations, when they experience physical closeness or touch. Also, it is unusual for these clients to maintain sustained eye contact. This averting of the eyes is not likely to change when they are confronted about it. Rather, such confrontation just tends to increase resistive and uncooperative behaviors.

Handling the material possessions of controlling elders without expressed permission is liable to bring untoward reactions. Likewise, possessiveness is seen in their social relationships. Jealousy may be expressed when persons whom they consider friends do not maintain the exclusivity they desire. They sometimes act as if healthcare workers are exclusively theirs. An illustration of this occurred in a home health aid service situations. The wife manifested a controlling disposition. An aid was caring for her husband several times a week. Later, the wife's capacities declined and she needed aid services too. However, she did not want "my husband's aid." She wanted "my own home health aid." Accommodating elders' possessiveness whenever feasible lessens their untoward response in occasional situations when accommodation is impossible.

Although controlling elders primarily focus on the present, they sometimes relate stories from the past. This especially occurs when they are having difficulty meeting a psychological need. For instance, if an elder lacks esteem in the current situation, he or she may share a situation from the past that bolsters his or her esteem. Additionally, such an elder may engage in one-upmanship. For any incident described, the elder tells a story about a past event that is one-better (or one-worse). Group activities in which these elders feel a sense of belonging and acceptance can contribute to meeting esteem needs. Antithetically, these needs are further frustrated when they are rejected by members of a group.

Elders with controlling dispositions are fiercely competitive, perversely controlling, and impolite in group activities. Group members who are more adherent to social mores are offended by these behaviors. If controlling elders are in the minority, they are likely to be ostracized; otherwise, those offended are apt to withdraw from the group process to avoid what they feel are disgusting interactions. Others just withdraw to avoid the competitive milieu. Obviously, such a group is not of therapeutic value.

However, group activities designed specifically for elders with controlling dispositions yielded positive benefits. The research groups were limited to seven or fewer members. Clients invited to a specific club (group) were matched for similarity in levels of assertiveness. Physically combative elders were excluded.

Some activities were designed to permit individual creativity and owner-ship of the end product. These individual projects within the group allowed remote competition and met needs for ownership, esteem, and gift-giving. Greater emphasis was placed on projects requiring group consensus, coop-eration, and joint ownership of the end products. Projects requiring close cooperation offered opportunities for the development of group solidarity, sense of belonging, and mutual respect. Debates to achieve group consensus were loud and included exchanges of language unacceptable if judged by usual social standards. Despite (or secondary to) these heated disputes, bonds of friendship emerged among members. Products enjoining shared responsibility brought chronic bickering. For instance,members in one group continually argued about who should remove dead blossoms and water the plants in their raised flower garden. However, heated arguments at group meetings were followed by softening of relations with persons outside the group. Healthcare personnel interacting with members after such meetings commented that the elders were unusually cooperative and compliant. Also, they were noted to be less antagonist toward other clients and relatives after they had vented strong feelings during a club meeting. These selected elders participated fully and expressed much satisfaction with group activities.

■SUMMARY AND DISCUSSION

The qualitative field studies from which this chapter was derived explored ways to mitigate problems emanating from elder-stage dispositions. During the field studies, several different types of elder-stage dispositions were identified. This article focuses only on controlling dispositions in older adults (older than 64 years of age). Because of their dispositions, controlling elders frequently have adversarial relationships with healthcare profession-als and other caregivers. This untowardly affects the outcomes of health services. Understanding controlling disposition can enable home health-care staff to reduce these adverse effects.

Criteria for identifying elders with controlling dispositions are delineated in the table. Care strategies discussed in this article include the following:

1. Increase client's sense of control.
2. Decrease perception of loss of control.
3. Increase satisfaction of basic psychosocial needs and rights, including esteem from self and others, sense of belonging, freedom of expres-sion, intact personal space, jurisdiction over possessions, and freedom of choice.

Results of implementing these strategies include the controlling elders being (a) more cooperative with healthcare providers, (b) less antagonistic toward healthcare workers and others, and (c) more satisfied with the delivery of health services.

The author recommends that this information be used in further clinical practice studies. This will avoid the error of overgeneralization of results based on convenience samples. Publication of further findings by others will add to (or correct) the perspective presented by this author. A clinical practice study can be set up as follows:

1. Identify an older adult client who has a controlling disposition according to the criteria discussed in this article.
2. Hypothesize (plan) that the implementation of selected strategies will be succeeded by specified client changes such as the results listed above.
3. During and after implementation, determine if the strategies were implemented, if the specified changes occurred, or if other changes occurred.
4. After completing the above with a number of controlling elders, analyze your results and publish your findings.

Professional staff, aids, and family caregivers can be involved in clinical practice studies. This type of client outcome study can enhance staff education and quality assurance in an agency.

The degree to which these controlling elders persist in struggling to control is counterproductive to well-being. Care strategies in this research were aimed at increasing sense of control or decreasing perceptions of loss of control. Hence, only some symptomatic relief and reduction of secondary effects were intended. No effort was made to decipher the genesis of controlling dispositions. Insights from researching the genesis could probably benefit controlling elders even more. Further insights also are needed regarding other elder-state dispositions.

■ REFERENCES

1. Erikson EH. *Childhood and Society*. New York: WW Norton, 1964.
2. Abrahams JP. The search for forgiveness: A theme in geriatric psychotherapy. *Gerontologist* 1983; 23:240.
3. Havighurst R. Developmental tasks. In: Maddox GL, ed. *The Encyclopedia of Aging*. New York: Springer, 1987.
4. Newman BM, Newman PR. *Development Through life: A Psychosocial Approach*. Homewood, IL: The Dorsey Press, 1984.
5. Feil N. *Validation: The Feil Method of How to Help Disoriented Old-Old*. Cleveland, OH: Edward Feil Productions, 1982.

Chapter 40

Geriatric Depression

MARYBETH TANK BUSCHMANN   MARGUERITE A. DIXON
ANNA M. TICHY

Among older adults, depression is the most prevalent functional psychiatric disorder. Longevity brings with it a poorer quality of life with multiple disabilities and chronic conditions for some people. There are many causes for depression and clinically it can be quite complex. The authors present a comprehensive overview of depression including the epidemiological aspects, definition, etiology, clinical presentation, and management of depression. Management discussed includes pharmacotherapy, electroconvulsive therapy, and interpersonal therapies. A case study of an 88-year-old woman illustrates for the reader application of material presented in this chapter. A glossary of terms used in this chapter is included.

A dramatic increase in the absolute number and relative proportion of the elderly population has occurred during this century. In 1900, 4% of the population in the United States was 65 years or older; currently the figure is approximately 13%.[1] The enhanced survival rate has resulted inevitably in an increased prevalence of disabilities and chronic conditions. Thus, the elderly person may be surviving longer but also may be experiencing a poorer quality of life.

In addition to general disabilities, the incidence of mental health problems and emotional disorders in the elderly is increasing. The elderly either remain untreated or are seen within the primary care setting where detection and management of mental morbidity by primary care providers are ineffective.[2,3] Several factors are related to the generally ineffectual mental healthcare of the elderly. The barriers include the avoidance of mental healthcare because of the associated stigma; the coexistence of mental and physical morbidity; and a subtle form of "ageism" on the part of some primary healthcare providers who may attribute psychiatric symptoms to expected outcomes of physical conditions or to the "normal" changes associated with aging.[4]

This paper focuses on the interrelationship of depression, a mental health problem, and somatic disorders in the elderly. After a brief review

From *Home Healthcare Nurse* 13(3):47–55, 1995. Reprinted with permission.

of the varied presentations of late-life depression, recommendations for appropriate management interventions for the elderly person will be provided.

EPIDEMIOLOGIC ASPECTS

The most common emotional disorder in the elderly is depression with debilitating and potentially lethal consequences.[5-7] Estimates of the prevalence of depressive symptoms and depression vary considerably according to the definition, assessment techniques, and particular population studied. The risk for depression is two to three times higher among women than men.[8,9] The prevalence of depression increases with age until 80 years, at which time a marked decline occurs.[10] A community survey of elderly persons identified dysphoric symptomatology in the majority studied.[11] Additionally, nearly 4% of the elderly population has been diagnosed with a major affective primary disorder, the most frequent being unipolar affective disorder.[12] Depression is a major public health problem associated with a high risk of mortality and suicidal behavior.[13-15] Although the elderly constitute only 13% of the population, 25% of all suicides occur in persons older than 65 years of age.[16-18]

DEFINITION

The term depression may refer to a mood state, a symptom, or a disease.[19] As an appropriate mood state of healthy persons, depression is characterized by feelings of sadness, discouragement, disappointment, and social withdrawal. Medical diseases, drug effects, and other psychiatric disorders may be associated with depressive mood changes. Symptoms of depressive illnesses reflect disturbances in cognitive, affective, vegetative, and motor areas.[20] The depressive syndrome as a major psychiatric disorder has been defined by the American Psychiatric Association[21] as a dysphoric mood or loss of interest or pleasure in almost all activities for at least a 2-week duration. Additionally, a minimum of four of the following symptoms must be associated with the dysphoria and must occur in the absence of signs or symptoms that suggest schizophrenia: appetite changes with weight loss or weight gain; insomnia or hypersomnia; loss of energy, fatigability, or tiredness; psychomotor agitation or retardation; loss of interest or pleasure in usual activities or a decrease in sexual drive; feelings of self-reproach or excessive or inappropriate guilt; diminished ability to think or concentrate; and recurrent thoughts of death or suicide.[19,21] Whereas bipolar disease is characterized by manic-depressive episodes, the unipolar disease, more common in elderly persons, is manifested solely by single or recurrent episodes of depression.

Since late-life depression is usually amenable to treatment, early diagnosis and appropriate referral are important in ameliorating the associated morbidity and mortality. However, detecting depression in the elderly may be a considerable challenge because the origin may be multicausal and the clinical presentation may be complex.[22] The coexistence of physical illnesses (which may produce symptoms suggestive of depression) and depression (which may be manifested by symptoms indicative of organic disease) is common in aged persons.[10]

ETIOLOGY

Biologic and psychosocial factors have been implicated in the pathogenesis of late-life depression. Physiologic theories of the cause of depression in the elderly rely on laboratory studies that have identified age-related biochemical abnormalities in the norepinephrine system and structural abnormalities in the central nervous system.[23] Deficiencies in the concentrations of neurotransmitters, such as dopamine, norepinephrine, serotonin, and acetylcholine, and elevated cortisol, sodium, and monoamine oxidase levels have been suggested as possible etiologic factors.[23] Genetic vulnerability also has been implicated in depressive disorders. Some subtypes of bipolar affective disorders have been documented in consecutive family generations, suggesting genetic transmission in an autosomal dominant mode. The same genetic pattern is not evident in unipolar affective disorders that are more common in the elderly.[20] Therefore, it is assumed that late-life depression is genetically different from early-life depression. This had led to an increased focus on psychosocial, psychologic, and physiologic precipitants as more significant etiologic factors in the old than in younger persons.

The psychosocial theory of the etiology of late-life depression has two major interacting components: (1) environmental factors that may precipitate a reactive depression; and (2) intrapsychic factors that include the life-long adaptive strategies and coping pattern of the elderly person.[24] Old age is characterized by predictable life events, inside and outside the body, that necessitate continual adaptation and changes in self-concept. Many of these anticipated marker events, such as chronic illness, physical and cognitive decline, functional disability, reduced finances, death of a spouse, retirement, and societal devaluation, require major adaptation and may precipitate a crisis reaction in some persons. However, the majority of elderly persons have developed effective coping strategies that enable them to deal appropriately with multiple real or perceived losses and environmental stresses, particularly if the loss is not unexpected. The response, a natural reaction to loss, is manifested by sadness and mourning, but not by the devastating shattering of a sense of continuity characteristic of clinical depression.[25] Grief, as differentiated from depression, is defined as a time-limited, realistic sadness proportionate to what has been lost. The incompletely delineated gradient between appropriate mood and affective disorder makes the distinction between a normal and a pathologic response to a loss difficult. A number of risk factors for prolonged, morbid grief reaction have been identified. Among these are the presence of a concurrent life crisis, lack of a social support system, traumatic death of a spouse, and an ambivalent marital relationship.[20] Concurrent life crises and an inadequate support system are risk factors commonly associated with depression in the elderly.

Chronic illness becomes more common in old age. A number of neurologic, endocrine, metabolic, and nutritional disorders are frequently characterized by depressive manifestations, which, if treated as such, will be refractory to antidepressant drugs.[10] However, elderly patients who are medically ill often develop a concurrent depression that has been associated with a decreased life expectancy.[10,26] Iatrogenic, drug-induced depression always should be considered in elderly persons using multiple medications for a variety of illnesses. Pharmacologic agents that may precipitate depressive episodes in the elderly include antihypertensives, neuroleptics, minor tranquilizers, digitalis, antiparkinson and anticancer drugs, corticosteroids, and nonsteroidal antiinflammatory agents.[27] Of these, the antihypertensives produce the greatest risk of depression.[28] Alcohol, used to blunt or block feelings, also may precipitate depressive symptoms.[22]

A relationship between depressive disorders and dementia has been noted for some years. Coexistence of depression has been documented in approximately one fourth of the patients in whom senile dementia of the Alzheimer's Type (SDAT) is diagnosed.[29] Cognitive impairment is characteristic of dementia and depression. A differentiating feature is that the cognitive impairment and consciousness level of dementia are constant, whereas they fluctuate in depression.[10] Treatment of depressed patients with SDAT with antidepressant pharmacologic agents or electroconvulsive therapy results in a degree of clinical improvement in cognition, mood, and functional ability.[30] Thus, differential diagnosis and correction of the underlying etiology are imperative in the elderly depressed person.

CLINICAL PRESENTATION

Late-life depression can be manifested by the classic signs and symptoms of depression, such as depressed facies, unkempt appearance, feelings of useless existence, dysphoric mood, loss of interest in activities that were former sources of enjoyment, sleep and appetite disturbances, fatigue, restlessness, low self-esteem, poor concentration or memory failure, and thoughts of death or suicidal ideation. These symptoms may range in severity from mild to incapacitating. More commonly, however, the elderly person has atypical depressive equivalents, such as somatic and cognitive conditions, and vague physiologic decline that may mask an underlying depression. These patients either fail to express or deny emotional afflictions. It is common for the depressed elderly to avoid verbal communication. In the absence of emotional equivalents,[31] the recognition of depression and its subsequent treatment are compromised.[32]

Depression often is masked by somatic ailments. Somatization in elderly people is a problem that recently has been recognized as a psychiatric disorder.[33,34] In this form of presentation, reports of physical symptoms from an older person to the caregiver cannot be verified with accompanying, objective signs. These patients do not report anxiety, depression, or an apparent inability to cope, but rather numerous physical symptoms.[35]

Somatization can be differentiated from normal and abnormal physical aging changes by the lack of signs to confirm the symptoms.[34,36] In a study of somatic symptomatology,[29] patients who were clinically depressed were compared with 124 nondepressed patients. Of six common somatic ailments (fatigue, insomnia, upper gastrointestinal distress, anorexia, lower gastrointestinal complaints, and headaches), 80% of the patients reported at least four of the six ailments.[5] In another investigation, 20 to 50% of the patients with somatic reports of insomnia, anorexia, decreased libido, and constipation also were found to have depressive illness.[37] Therefore, patients who are depressed and have somatic symptoms are even less likely than nonsomatizing patients to appear depressed and to be diagnosed and managed appropriately.

Conversion symptoms may be a feature of somatization. These symptoms conform to the person's inability to deal with and focus on specific problems. Conversion is usually an unconscious process.[35] However, the symptom may be symbolically significant (eg, "blindness" occurs when there is something the patient does not want to look at or see).[33,35] If this symbolism is successful in substituting for the repressed wishes, it is considered a primary gain. The gratification obtained from sympathy and attention from others, as a result of the sick role, is referred to as a secondary gain.[33,38]

The diagnostic dilemma of depression may be complicated additionally by the presence of coexisting medical problems.[39] Vague, multisystem somatic symptoms such as unusual pain, chest pain, gastrointestinal discomfort, musculoskeletal pain, and sensory disturbances are often the presenting symptoms in the depressed elderly person in the absence of a clear physical basis or an obvious mood disorder.[40] Among the pathognomic characteristics of depression that mimic medical illness are a phasic manifestation of somatic signs, diurnal fluctuations, mild cognitive inhibition, dysthymic mood, fatigue, sleep disturbances, anxiety, and nonspecific apprehension.[10] Hypochondriasis, which may mask depression, is another distinct disorder in which normal physiologic sensations are misinterpreted as harbingers or indicators of disease.[31,35] The diagnosis of hypochondriasis applies to persons preoccupied with somatic and depressive symptoms in the absence of depressive illness.[36]

Assessment of depression is problematic when the elderly person has a single symptom, such as insomnia, or cognitive symptoms, such as attentional disturbances, confusion, and memory impairment. In a report of elderly persons referred to a sleep disorder clinic, depression was the most frequent diagnosis.[28] Cognitive dysfunction, common in late-life depression, may mimic dementia and lead to an erroneous diagnosis of organic brain disease. The cognitive impairment of depression is potentially reversible with appropriate therapy; therefore, accurate diagnosis is critical to ensure that treatable problems are not overlooked. In the differential diagnosis, it should be noted that somatic symptoms are characteristic of depression and not of dementia, and that cognitive impairment fluctuates in depression but is constant in dementia.[10,28] Furthermore, depression may coexist in patients with an irreversible, organic dementia, and warrants treatment of possible depression even when a differentiating diagnosis cannot be established clearly. Depression responds to appropriate therapy, although marked improvement in cognitive ability in the patient with dementia and depression is unlikely.[12]

TABLE 40-1 Interventions

PSYCHOTHERAPEUTIC	PSYCHOSOCIAL
Convey hope	Establish a network if living alone
Present optimistic attitude	Arrange for transportation
Empathetic listening	Encourage family involvement
Cognitive therapy	Use the healthcare team
Behavioral therapy	Encourage positive coping patterns
Present alternatives and options	Lower expectations of self
	Compare self to cohort
Use of expressive touch	Discourage negative coping patterns
Restoration of self-esteem	Somatization
Reminiscence	Conversion symptoms

MANAGEMENT

The pain of depression, in the absence of adequate recognition and intervention, heralds a chronicle of deterioration (Table 40-1). The goals of healthcare in the elderly population are the restoration or maintenance of function and the promotion of a vigorous quality of life. Depression is treatable if it is appropriately diagnosed and managed. The underpinnings for effective intervention include overcoming the health caregiver's possible identification with the depressed elderly person's sense of helplessness and hopelessness. Hope and an optimistic attitude must be conveyed if intervention is to be effective.

Therapeutic management of depression includes a thorough assessment to confirm the diagnosis, to evaluate suicide risk, to determine the presence of medical conditions or psychosocial factors contributing to the depression, and to consider the risks and benefits of treatment modalities. The elderly person with depression frequently seeks treatment for a physical discomfort or illness. The treatment plan must include empathetic listening, inclusion of the family, collaborations with members of a multidisciplinary healthcare team, and exploration of a number of alternate courses of action. Hospitalization may be indicated when the depression remains severe, when there is preoccupation with suicidal thoughts, and/or when social support is lacking. In those instances when the depression is treatment resistant, the healthcare professional's role is to support the person and family to cope with a chronic, disabling condition.

Pharmacotherapy

Aggressive therapy, consisting of tricyclic antidepressants, monoamine oxidase inhibitors, lithium, and electroconvulsive therapy, is the mainstay of management of the elderly patient with a major affective depressive disorder. Psychotherapy, alone or in conjunction with pharmacologic agents, is indicated in mild to severe depressive states. Tricyclic antidepressants block the reuptake of norepinephrine by adrenergic nerve terminals. The therapeutic clinical effect of mood elevation occurs approximately 3 to 4 weeks after initiation of the medication. Special precautions in antidepressant drug treatment of the elderly must be exercised in light of age-related alterations in absorption, metabolism, detoxification, and elimination of drugs.[10] Additionally, the presence of concomitant physical illness and the interaction of antidepressant drugs with medications for the treatment of multisystem disease require very low initial doses, careful titration, and gradual increases[20] to achieve therapeutic efficacy. Adverse side effects of tricyclic drug therapy in the elderly include cardiovascular, neurologic, and anticholinergic problems. Among these are dry mouth, sweating, constipation, urinary hesitancy, and delayed ejaculation, effects mediated by the autonomic nervous system.[38] In addition, precipitation of narrow angle glaucoma is rare, whereas tremor occurs frequently at therapeutic doses. Finally, confusional reactions are seen more often in elderly individuals. The cardiovascular side effects (tachyarrhythmias, orthostatic hypotension, and congestive heart failure) are particularly dangerous.[28,41,42] However, new classes of tricyclic secondary amines such as desipramine and nortriptyline have fewer adverse side effects. Also, the development of heterocyclic antidepressants has been beneficial in the treatment of late-life depression.[27]

Monamine oxidase inhibitors are used for the treatment of primary mood disorders and atypical depression, and for patients who do not respond to heterocyclic antidepressant therapy.[23] Monamine oxidase inhibitors increase dopamine, norepinephrine, and serotonin levels in the brain.[24] Therapeutic efficacy is achieved in several days to weeks. Dietary instruction to avoid foods, such as strong or aged cheese, yogurt, bananas, coffee, beer and wine, chicken, and chocolate,[43] that contain the amino acid tyramine is imperative to prevent hypertensive crisis. These dietary proscriptions for noncompliant patients need to be considered carefully.[44] Orthostatic hypotension, a common complication of monoamine oxidase inhibitors in the elderly, requires careful monitoring and appropriate dose reduction.[45]

Lithium is useful in the treatment of bipolar affective disorders and in patients who respond poorly to heterocyclic antidepressants.[23] Lithium dosage must be titrated carefully based on serum levels. Although the pharmacodynamic effects of lithium are not understood completely, the neurochemical changes may be related to the ion fluxes across cell membranes in the central nervous system.[46,47] Therapeutic effects of lithium occur at much lower levels in the elderly because of a prolonged half-life resulting from an age-related decrease in renal glomerular filtration rate.[20] Undesirable side effects of lithium therapy, such as decreased awareness or clouding of sensorium, require dose reduction or discontinuation of the drug.

Electroconvulsive Therapy

Electroconvulsive therapy may be used in patients with major depression after stroke or in those for whom drugs are contraindicated, in those unresponsive to antidepressant therapy, and in those with high risk of suicide.[48] Electronconvulsive therapy may exert its therapeutic effect by "resetting" the cellular receptors for chemical messengers.[49] The efficacy and safety of electroconvulsive therapy for geriatric patients is well accepted.[27,50,52] A history of recent myocardial infarction, decompensated heart failure, and the presence of increased intracranial pressure or a mass lesion in the brain are contraindications for electroconvulsive therapy.[53] Additionally, in elderly persons the treatments should be less frequent and should be discontinued as soon as a clinical response is evident, to be replaced by pharmacologic antidepressant therapy. Possible side effectives of electroconvulsive therapy include worsening of even mild dementia, and confusion and memory loss in the elderly who are nondemented.[23] Unilateral non-dominant electroconvulsive therapy is associated with transient memory loss, though the confusion and memory loss occur less than with bilateral placement or combined unilateral and bilateral stimulation.[51,53]

Interpersonal Therapies

Pharmacologic intervention and electroconvulsive therapy are mechanisms by which the patient becomes more manageable. The best probability for cure is human contact and nurturing relationships (Table 40-1). Touch is considered one of the primary components of comforting and is an integral part of the nurse-patient interaction fundamental to the provision of nursing care. Touch is an important form of nonverbal communication in human interaction and is essential throughout the lifespan. A few studies have related touch to feelings of well-being in an elderly population.[54-58] Persons with less severe depressions may respond well to psychotherapy. Psychotherapy, when applied in psychogeriatrics, has a number of unique characteristics. Although the aged client may have a reduced capacity for insight, because of limited ability to assimilate new experiences, there may be a greater readiness for critical self-reflection. Aims and time for therapy should be limited, with an emphasis on adapting to reality, relieving symptoms, and functioning as independently as possible.[59] A supportive therapeutic relationship, based on empathy and understanding, provides the basis for future social integration and new alternatives to hopelessness and self-negation. In this process, the healthcare professional is used to restore the individual's feelings of security and self-esteem in a trusting, nurturing relationship. The professional aids the elderly person to overcome a sense of helplessness, powerlessness, and ineffectuality. Depression may be resolved in the nurturing relationship in a variety of ways, among which are attainment of a seemingly unreachable goal, modification of a goal allowing for attainment, goal abandonment, restoration of self-esteem irrespective of goal attainment, and creation of a defense against the depressive feeling.[60]

Despite some skepticism regarding the benefits of psychotherapy in advanced age, its effectiveness has been demonstrated in the treatment of elderly depressives.[61,62] Successful psychotherapy frequently results in improved functional ability and involvement in daily life.[16] As the person's mental health status improves, substitute relationships for those that have been lost offer enduring adaptations. If life is to be perceived as meaningful, the elderly person must view in each experienced event some response worth making. The quality of the response, and hence its meaning, is contingent on the person's lifelong commitment of purpose. The multiple losses experienced in old age may disrupt the relationships that incorporated the person's commitment of purpose. The healing process requires reformulation of this purpose by extracting its fundamental meaning and reattaching it to the present. Analogous to grieving, the reformulation process requires an ambivalent testing of past and future, questioning and reaffirming the original commitment, and searching for terms that would give meaning and worth to life.[63]

The healthcare practitioner must be sensitive to losses the elderly person with depression has experienced and suggest alternatives that would minimize their effects. New relationships and activities may provide an avenue for enhanced social integration. Involvement in alternative housing, community centers, volunteer programs and organizations, and surrogate parenting are examples of options that may enhance the person's potential for social participation and a fulfilling, productive life. Likewise, working with plants and animals may provide a sense of peace, pleasure, and comfort that may provide an emotional bridge for subsequent relationships with people.

Reminiscence also can be a valuable intervention.[64,65] For most people, regardless of age, the recalling of life's events to an interested person or group is pleasurable. It is therapeutic in that it validates an elder's life experiences, promotes a sense of commonality with one's peers, combats depression,[37] and, therefore, increases self-esteem. Reminiscence often is called "life review." According to Burnside,[66] reminiscence and life review are different, even though these terms are used interchangeably. Reminiscence is the recalling of a number of past events in one's life that may or may not be connected; life-review therapy must be done by a specially trained individual who has a background in special education, gerontology, and a related discipline (eg, psychiatry, geropsychiatric nursing, pastoral counseling, clinical psychology, or social work). Therefore, in contrast to life review, reminiscence is a psychosocial intervention, not a psychoanalytic one.[66] The effects of reminiscence therapy have not been documented by data-based research studies. Reminiscence therapy may be painful for an elder. The resultant guilt, anger, and pain must be acknowledged by the nurse so that the elder can establish new relationships.[67] In resolving and reintegrating past conflicts, new significance is given to life.[68] Reminiscence therapy gives the elder a feeling of accomplishment, a sense of a job well done, and an opportunity to decide what to do with the time that is left.

Cognitive and behavioral therapies, focused on education and based on an active interchange between the therapist and client, are accepted more readily by older adults than is traditional psychotherapy.[53,69] Cognitive behavior therapy is directed at modifying the depressive thoughts by identifying distortions in cognition and discussing the validity of basic assumptions, beliefs, and attitudes related to the depression.[70,71] Therapy consists of behavioral rehearsal techniques, such as role playing and verbal contracts, to enhance the client's effective regulation of communication, self-esteem, and social reinforcement skills. The elderly can be taught to avoid or change thinking patterns that lead to depression. Additionally, the client is encouraged to participate in activities that are pleasurable or provide a sense of achievement. Cognitive behavior therapy also may be conducted with groups of elderly persons. This latter form is more cost-effective than individual therapy.

Activities that distract from real or imagined problems are frequently therapeutic. Scheduling daily activities to avoid long periods of inactivity may provide a sense of control over external events and minimize rumination that is counter therapeutic.[72] Realistic activities or exercise have been shown to have a therapeutic effect on depression in the elderly.[73,74] Training in social skills and assertiveness, and marital or family therapy may be useful adjuncts to treating persons who manifest chronic low self-esteem and who are coping with tension and resolving conflict.

Home Treatment

Patients with significant medical illnesses and psychiatric disorders treated at home by a collaborative team, consisting of a psychiatrist, appropriate medical colleagues, a nurse, and other mental health professionals, has been demonstrated to be therapeutically effective. Home visits serve to minimize isolation, check withdrawal, interject opportunity, and dampen the cycle of medical illness and depression.[75] Home treatment may include medications, psychotherapy, and behavior modification techniques. As an alternative to hospitalization, home treatment of elderly clients with depression, whether living alone or within a family, has been well accepted by people who feel trapped and lonely and are willing to change behavior but lack the necessary skills. A critical component of effective home treatment requires identifying the person's support system and working within this network of involved, concerned, and caring people. The elderly population is at risk for recurrent episodes of depression and may require ongoing treatment. Home therapy for the elderly is an opportunity for significant team interaction with family members who frequently feel alienated. Family members often respond to intervention with new insight, realization of options, and a change of focus.

■CONCLUSION

In the past decade, significant advances have been made in understanding the etiology, mechanisms, assessment, and treatment of late-life depression. Despite this progress, late-life depression is frequently undiagnosed, misdiagnosed, and undertreated. Although not all depressive episodes in the elderly end in suicide, all depression is characterized by acute psychic pain and dysfunction that not only affects the elderly person with depression, but also adversely affects those who associate with and care for him or her. It is imperative that nurses be cognizant of the varied forms of presentation of depression in the elderly and initiate appropriate management strategies.

To illustrate the above discussion, the following case study is presented.

CASE STUDY

Mrs C, an 88-year-old widowed woman, lived alone in a house she and her husband of 53 years had built 48 years earlier. She has two sons, one of whom lives with his wife and their two adult children in Tucson, Arizona. The younger son lives with his wife in Michigan City, Indiana. Mr C had died 10 years earlier; until 4 months ago, Mrs C had had wonderful social support from her two neighbors on either side of her house in Washington, DC.

There was no family history of psychiatric illness, but Mrs C had reported feeling blue and alone several times in the past 10 years since her husband's death. It never seemed important enough to her to report this to her physician. Mrs C had always been active in her home, garden, and church. Lately, however, joint pain was bothersome, and with the recent move of one and the death of another close neighbor, she was feeling isolated.

The sense of isolation progressed to feelings of hopelessness and despair, so on her next visit to her physician, she discussed her feelings. The physician gave her a prescription for Motrin for the pain in her joints. However, before treating her with an antidepressant, he tried a nonpharmacologic approach. Arrangements were made for a home healthcare nurse to visit Mrs C once a week. The nurse was a very empathetic listener, and while Mrs C talked, she would often hold her hand or place her hand on Mrs C's shoulder. The nurse realized that Mrs C had become isolated and helped to establish a network of caring people from Mrs C's church to visit her several times a week. At least twice a week, a caring visitor would bring an evening meal and share it with Mrs C. During these visits, Mrs C often found herself talking about her past years with her husband and the raising of her two sons. These moments of remembering made Mrs C realize how accomplished she had been in the past. Along with these positive thoughts, Mrs C's affect improved. Her spirits brightened and soon the nurse noticed that Mrs C's self-esteem was returning. With encouragement from the nurse, Mrs C began to call her sons regularly on the phone and spend time talking with their families. Before long, plans were being made for visits to occur between Mrs C and her sons and their families.

Six months later, when Mrs C visited her physician, he noticed a noteworthy change in her. She was more optimistic and had plans for the future. She once again became involved with her hobbies and other people. The physician was confident that Mrs C would not have to have antidepressants or psychotherapy prescribed for her. Both he and Mrs C were pleased with the outcome.

The following glossary contains terms that were used in the article.

GLOSSARY

Behavioral therapy: a form of psychotherapy that deals with modifying problematic behaviors an individual may have with the environment, interpersonal relationships, and daily living.

Cognitive therapy: a form of psychotherapy that helps an individual to alter her or his negative thinking, unrealistic misperceptions, and erroneous attitudes or beliefs.

Conversion disorder: to convert a psychological problem into a physical symptom. This only happens with the special senses or voluntary nervous system, such as becoming blind when there is no physical disorder as an attempt to not see.

Dysphoric mood: a disorder with mild symptoms similar to depression, with lowered self-esteem, poor concentration, difficulty in making decisions, etc.

Dysthymic mood: a disorder with a depressed affect and loss of interest or pleasure in activities that were once enjoyed.

Electroconvulsive therapy: a treatment given with general anesthesia that involves applying a low-voltage current to the nondominant side of the head, producing a convulsion or seizure. Because of muscle relaxants and the anesthesia, no harm comes to the patient. It is used for patients who are suicidal or resistant to other forms of treatment, especially medications.

Hypochondriasis: a disorder in which one is overly concerned with physical symptoms for which there is no biologic basis, but an emotional basis.

Iatrogenic: an abnormal state or condition produced inadvertently by inappropriate or inadequate treatment.

Psychotherapy: therapy that deals with psychological problems, done on an individual, group, or family basis.

Reminiscence: a form of therapy that focuses on the past; usually happy and warm memories are recalled, but painful times also may be remembered; it can be free flowing or structured, and helps the individually recall his or her accomplishments and good times in years past.

Somatization: a disorder identified usually by many and longstanding physical/somatic ailments involving bodily dysfunction, such as back pain and constipation.

▆REFERENCES

1. Grossberg GT, Hassan R, Szwabo PA, et al. Psychiatric problems in the nursing home. *J Am Geriatr Soc* 1990; 38:907–917.
2. German PS, Shapiro S, Skinner EA, et al. Detection and management of mental health problems of older patients by primary care providers. *JAMA* 1987; 257:489–493.
3. Glass RM. Psychiatric megatrends and the elderly. *JAMA* 1987; 257:527–528.
4. Lipowski ZJ. Somatization and depression. *Psychosomatics* 1990; 31:13–21.
5. Chaisson-Stewart GM (ed). *Depression in the Elderly.* New York, J. Wiley & Sons, 1985.
6. Holt S, Alexopouloos GS. Depression and the Aged. In Robinson RG, Rabins PV (eds). *Depression and Co-Existing Disease.* New York, Igaku-Shoin, 1989, pp 10–26.
7. Chiu E, Ames D. Depression in the elderly. *Aust Fam Physician* 1990; 19:1379–1386.
8. Klerman GL, Weissman MM. Increasing rates of depression. *JAMA* 1989; 261:2229–2234.
9. Turner RJ, Avison WR. Gender and depression: Assessing exposure and vulnerability to life events in a chronically strained population. *J Nerv Ment Dis* 1989; 177:443–455.
10. Ban T. Chronic disease and depression in the geriatric population. *J Clin Psychiatry* 1984; 45:18–24.
11. Thompson LW, Gallagher D, Breckenridge JS. Comparative effectiveness of psychotherapies for depressed elders. *J Consult Clin Psychol* 1987; 55:385–390.
12. Reifler BV. Mixed cognitive-affective disturbances in the elderly: A new classification. *J Clin Psychiatry* 1986; 47:354–356.
13. Parmelee PA, Katz IR, Lawton MP. Depression and mortality among institutionalized aged. *J Gerontol: Psychol Sci* 1992; 47:P3–10.
14. Rovner BW, German PS, Brant LJ, et al. Depression and mortality in nursing homes. *JAMA* 1991; 265:993–996.
15. Thomas C, Kelman HR, Kennedy GJ, et al. Depressive symptoms and mortality in elderly persons. *J Gerontol: Soc Sci* 1992; 47:S80–87.
16. Victoroff VM. Depression in the elderly. *Ohio State Med J* 1984; 80:180–183,187.
17. Osgood N. *Suicide in the Elderly.* Rockville, MD: Aspen Systems Corp, 1985.
18. Richardson R, Lowenstein S, Weissberg M. Coping with the suicidal elderly: A physicians guide. *Geriatrics* 1989; 44:43–51.
19. Dreyfus JK. Depression assessment and intervention in the medically ill frail elderly. *J Gerontol Nurs* 1988; 14:27–36.

20. Wasylenki D. Depression in the elderly. *Can Med Assoc J* 1980; 122:525–533.
21. American Psychological Association. *Diagnostic and statistical manual of mental disorders* (DSM-III-R). Washington, DC: American Psychological Association, 1987, pp 222–224.
22. Browning MA. Depression. In MO Hogstel (ed). *Geropsychiatric Nursing.* St Louis: CV Mosby Company, 1990, pp 130–176.
23. Fitten LJ, Morley JE, Gross PL, et al. Depression: UCLA geriatric grand rounds. *J Am Geriatric Soc* 1989; 37:459–472.
24. Willner P. *Depression: A Psychological Synthesis.* New York, John Wiley and Sons, 1985.
25. Neugarten BL. Psychological aspects of aging and illness. *Psychosomatics* 1984; 25:123–125.
26. Goff DC, Jenike MA. Treatment-resistant depression in the elderly. *J Am Geriatr Soc* 1986; 34:63–70.
27. Buckwalter KC. How to unmask depression. *Geriatr Nurs* 1990; 11:179–181.
28. Busse E, Simpson D. Depression and antidepressants and the elderly. *J Clin Psychiatry* 1983; 44:35–39.
29. Reifler BV, Larson E, Teri L, et al. Dementia of the Alzheimer's type and depression. *J Am Geriatr Soc* 1986; 34:855–859.
30. Feinberg T, Goodman B. Affective illness, dementia, and pseudodementia. *J Clin Psychiatry* 1984; 45:99–103.
31. Kramer-Ginsberg E, Greenwald BS, Aisen PS, et al. Hypochondriasis in the elderly depressed. *J Am Geriatr Soc* 1989; 37:507–510.
32. Portnoi VA. Diagnostic dilemma of the aged. *Arch Intern Med* 1981; 141:734–737.
33. Lazare A. Current concepts in psychiatry: Conversion symptoms. *N Engl J Med* 1981; 305:745–748.
34. Smith Jr. GM, Monson RA, Ray DC. Psychiatric consultation in a somatization disorder: A randomized controlled study. *N Engl J Med* 1986;3 14:1407–1413.
35. Quill TE. Somatization disorder: One of medicine's blind spots. *JAMA* 1985; 254:3075–3079.
36. Kellner R. Hypochondriasis and somatization. *JAMA* 1987; 258:2718–2722.
37. Kreitman N, Samsburg P, Pearce D, et al. Hypochondriasis and depression in out-patients in a general hospital. *Br J Psychiatry* 1965; 111:607–615.
38. Breslau LD, Haug MR (eds). *Depression and Aging: Causes, Care, and Consequences.* New York: Springer, 1983.
39. Kukull WA, Koepsell TD, Inui TS, et al. Depression and physical illness among elderly general medical clinic patients. *J Affect Disord* 1986; 10:153–162.
40. Finlayson RE, Martin LM. Recognition and management of depression in the elderly. *Mayo Clin Proc* 1982; 57:115–120.
41. Weiner MF, Fitzpatrick MC. Treating depression in elderly patients. *Compr Ther* 1987; 13:65–70.
42. Davenport J. Cardiovascular effects of antidepressants. *Postgrad Med* 1988; 84:105–115.
43. Haver J, Haskins PP, Luch AM, et al. *Comprehensive Psychiatric Nursing.* New York: McGraw-Hill, 1987, pp 524–526.
44. Judd FK, Norman TR. Current treatment concepts in depression. *Aust Fam Physician* 1990; 19:1347–1354.
45. Raskin DE. Psychiatry and the elderly: Diagnosis, treatment, and medical/ethical dilemmas. *Del Med J* 1988; 60:371–373.
46. Beck CM, Rawlins RP, Williams SR. *Mental health psychiatric nursing: A holistic life-cycle approach.* St Louis: CV Mosby, 1984, pp 1042–1043.
47. Luke Jr. EA, Psychotropic drugs. In MO Hogstel (ed). *Geropsychiatric Nursing.* St Louis: CV Mosby, 1990, pp 110–129.
48. House A. Depression after stroke. *Br Med J* 1987; 294:76–78.
49. Blazer DG. Affective disorders in late life. In Busse EW, Blazer DG (eds). *Geriatric Psychiatry.* Washington, DC: American Psychiatric Press, 1989, pp 389–402.
50. Kramer BA. Electroconvulsive therapy use in geriatric depression. *J Nerv Ment Dis* 1987; 175:233–235.
51. Mielke DH, Winstead DK, Goethe JW, et al. Multiple-monitored electroconvulsive therapy: Safety and efficacy in elderly depressed patients. *J Am Geriatr Soc* 1984; 32:180–182.
52. Raskind M. Electroconvulsive therapy in the elderly. *J Am Geriatr Soc* 1984; 32:177–178.

53. Beck JC. *Geriatrics Review Syllabus: A Core Curriculum in Geriatric Medicine.* New York: American Geriatric Society, 1989, pp 137–144.
54. Copstead L. Effects of touch and self-appraisal and interaction appraisal for permanently institutionalized older adults.*J Gerontol Nurs* 1980; 6:747–752.
55. Eaton M, Mitchell-Bonair I, Friedmann E. The effect of touch on nutritional intake on chronic organic brain syndrome patients. *J Gerontol* 1986; 41:661–616.
56. Hollinger L. Communicating with the elderly. *J Gerontol Nurs* 1986; 12:8–13.
57. Hollinger L, Buschmann MB. Factors influencing the perception of touch by elderly nursing home residents and their health care givers. *Int J Nurs Stud* 1993; 30:445–461.
58. Vortherms R. Clinically improving communication through touch. *J Gerontol Nurs* 1991; 17:6–10.
59. Kockott G. Psychotherapy in advanced age. In Bergener M (ed). *Psychogeriatrics: An International Handbook.* New York: Springer, 1987.
60. Bibring E. *The Mechanism of Depression in Affective Disorers: Psychoanalytic Contribution to Their Study.* New York, International University Press, 1953, p 13.
61. Gallagher DE, Thompson LW. Treatment of major depressive disorder in older adult outpatients with brief psychotherapies. *Psychother: Theory, Res Prac* 1982; 19:482–490.
62. Thompson LW, Gong V, Haskins E, et al. Assessment of depression and dementia during the late years. *Ann Rev Gerontol Geriatr* 1987; 7:295–324.
63. Marris P. *Mourning and the Projection of Ambivalence in Loss and Change.* New York: Pantheon Books, Random House, 1974, p 92.
64. Newbern VB. Sharing the memories: The value of reminiscence as a research tool. *J Gerontol Nurs* 1992; 18:13–18.
65. Wallace JB. Reconsidering the life review: The social construction of talk about the past. *Gerontologist* 1992; 32:120–125.
66. Burnside IM. *Nursing in the Aged: A Self-Care Approach.* Ed 3. New York: McGraw-Hill, 1988.
67. Mattson MA, McConnell ES. Psychosocial problems associated with aging. *Gerontological Nursing: Concepts and Practice.* Philadelphia: WB Saunders, 1988.
68. Butler RN, Lewis MI. *Aging and mental health,* Ed 3. St Louis: CV Mosby, 1982.
69. Blazer D. Depression in the elderly. *N Engl J Med* 1989; 320:164–166.
70. Beck AT, Rush AS, Shaw BF, Emery G. *Cognitive Therapy of Depression.* New York: Guildford Press, 1979.
71. Quality assurance project: A treatment outline for depressive disorders. *Aust N Z J Psychiatry* 1983; 17:129–146.
72. Crook T. Diagnosis and treatment of mixed anxiety-depression in the elderly. *J Clin Psychiatry* 1982; 43:35–43.
73. Verwoerdt A. *Clinical Geropsychiatry.* Baltimore: Williams & Wilkins, 1976.
74. Pappas GP, Golin S, Meyer DL. Reducing symptoms of depression with exercise [letter]. *Psychosomatics* 1990; 31:112–113.
75. Soreff SM. Indications for home treatment. *Psychiatr Clin North Am* 1985; 8:563–575.

Chapter 41

Managing Postoperative Pain in the Elderly

CHRISTINE L. PASERO   MARGO MCCAFFERY

Older Americans are recipients of surgical procedures in increasing numbers. Restorative and corrective surgeries are adding quality to the lives of many people past age 65, even into their 90s. Nurses who work in acute care and outpatient settings see many older patients for surgical services. One goal of nursing care is to provide comfort measures, which include analgesic substances that are well tolerated by the elderly. Christine Pasero and Margo McCaffery, a nursing leader in pain management, present the most current thinking on postoperative pain control. In this chapter they discuss individualized pain management plans, patient teaching, preemptive and balanced analgesia, and planning for discharge. They include useful tables with tips, guidelines, and what to avoid and why, when managing postoperative pain in the elderly.

As you're checking patients during your shift, you come to John Hecht, 70. It's been 12 hours since he underwent knee-replacement surgery. You find him lying in bed with his eyes open, staring at the ceiling. His affect appears strained as you exchange greetings. Touching his arm, you notice that he's tense.

You ask Mr. Hecht if he's in pain. He replies, "Oh, it's okay." At the same time, you note that he's refused his last analgesic dose, according to the bedside flowsheet, yet is rating his pain at 5 (on the 0-to-10 scale).

The elderly, as you know, are the fastest growing segment of the U.S. population. So you can expect to see more patients like Mr. Hecht admitted for surgical procedures and experiencing postoperative pain. Pain tends to be undertreated in all patients, regardless of the clinical setting. But elderly patients present special challenges for acute postoperative pain management.

To help you meet their needs, we'll review the essential elements of an individualized pain management plan for elderly patients. We'll also discuss patient teaching, using preemptive and balanced analgesia, and planning for discharge.

From *American Journal of Nursing* 96(10):38–45, 1996. Reproduced with permission.

■ BARRIERS TO EFFECTIVE PAIN MANAGEMENT

Effective pain relief in the elderly is subject to all of the usual barriers to pain management, such as fear of addiction. With the elderly, however, there are additional problems to be overcome.

For example, opioid analgesics are the cornerstone of postoperative pain management. But some nurses may be reluctant to administer them to older patients, believing that elders can't tolerate these drugs, especially when given intravenously or epidurally.

While it's true that elderly patients can be more sensitive to the effects of opioids, measures such as reducing the initial dose, titrating doses slowly, using combined regimens with nonopioid analgesics, and closely monitoring patient response can ensure safe and effective opioid administration.

Common misconceptions about aging can also complicate postoperative pain management and perpetuate the cycle of undertreatment. These include believing either that pain perception decreases with age or that pain is an inevitable consequence of aging and should be expected after surgery.

In addition, some elderly patients may believe that their nurses know their surgery has caused pain and that everything possible is already being done to relieve it. Some may not tell you of their pain because they're afraid that something has gone wrong. On the other hand, nurses may mistake patients who don't report pain as not experiencing pain.

Often elderly patients' fears of drug addiction and overdose, IV apparatus, and bedside technology can be barriers to effective pain control. Some worry that opioids will cause adverse effects such as constipation, sedation, dizziness, confusion, or lead to a fall. Many elders are hesitant about learning to use unfamiliar equipment, such as patient-controlled analgesia pumps. Others won't press the PCA button because they're afraid of "making a mistake." As a result, they may refuse pain medication and suffer needlessly.

■ USING BALANCED AND PREEMPTIVE ANALGESIA

A continuous multimodal approach to postoperative pain management, commonly called *balanced analgesia,* is indicated for elderly patients because it minimizes potential adverse effects from high doses of any single agent.

The three drug classes commonly used for balanced analgesia are opioids, nonsteroidal anti-inflammatory drugs (NSAIDs), and local anesthetics. Opioids act at opioid receptor sites in the brain and spinal cord to block the transmission of pain. NSAIDs inhibit pain mediators like prostaglandins, bradykinins, and histamines at the site of incision or injury. Local anesthetics block sensory inflow at the dorsal horn. A balanced approach to severe postoperative pain might include an opioid and a local anesthetic, given epidurally, and an oral or parenteral NSAID.

The goals of any postoperative pain management plan are to ensure a positive patient outcome and to minimize the cost of care and the length of stay. To do this, postoperative pain management needs to begin before surgery. A primary aim is to reduce the amount of opioid required for adequate pain relief, thus minimizing potential adverse effects like sedation, respiratory depression, urinary retention, and constipation.

Preoperative — often referred to as *preemptive* — analgesia can combine opioids, NSAIDs, and local anesthetics to treat pain at several levels before it occurs. For example, orthopedic procedures are often particularly painful and may require relatively high opioid doses. But several studies have shown that postoperative opioid doses can be reduced by premedication with opioids, preoperative regional anesthesia by nerve block, or simply single doses of NSAIDs administered preoperatively.

The preoperative period can also be crucial for managing a patient's expectations and compliance with postoperative rehabilitation regimens and pain management plans. For example, patients need to be taught about their responsibilities during recovery, such as ambulating, deep breathing, and eating. For these activities to be effective, the patient must be comfortable. You can explain that PCA or medication administration principles such as around-the-clock (ATC) administration can help accomplish this.

Occasionally, other medications or nondrug alternative therapies can be used in the acute postoperative period. But certain drugs should be used with extreme caution or avoided altogether. For example, benzodiazepines, which don't relieve pain unless it's caused by muscle spasm, are sometimes prescribed to treat anxiety or agitation. But they're an especially poor choice for elderly patients because, as a recent study showed, they can triple the incidence of delirium. And because older patients don't clear drugs as quickly, long-acting agents like diazepam (Valium) are riskier than short-acting ones like midazolam (Versed).

▬ NSAIDS AND ACETAMINOPHEN: OPTIONS OFTEN OVERLOOKED

NSAIDs and acetaminophen are often underutilized to manage postoperative pain. The American Pain Society (APS) and the Agency for Health Care Policy and Research (AHCPR) acute pain management guidelines recommend that every surgical patient should receive NSAIDs or acetaminophen ATC unless contraindicated.

Oral NSAIDs alone may be sufficient for mild postoperative pain. They're also effective and safe in combination with opioids for treating moderate to severe postoperative pain. NSAIDs exhibit opioid dose-sparing capabilities — that is, they provide additional analgesia that allows lower doses of opioid and fewer adverse effects.

However, NSAIDs must be used with caution in the elderly because of the higher prevalence of renal insufficiency in these patients, which may result in decreased drug clearance. For this reason, NSAIDs with long half-lives, such as piroxicam (Feldene) or nabumetone (Relafen), are usually avoided. Gastrointestinal disturbances can also result from NSAIDs, regardless of the route of administration, because they reduce prostaglandin production in the stomach.

Although caution is required, the benefits of reduced opioid use and improved patient outcome from better pain management may outweigh the risk associated with short-term NSAIDs. It may also be possible to guard against the risk of adverse effects from NSAIDs by adding ranitidine (Zantac) or misoprostol (Cytotec), which can help protect against gastric and duodenal ulcers, respectively. Otherwise, NSAIDs that have little or no effect on platelet aggregation, such as choline-magnesium salicylate (Trilisate) or salsalate (Disalcid), or acetaminophen can be used.

Intravenous ketorolac (Toradol) alone may be indicated for moderate postoperative pain and as an addition to opioids for severe pain. Although the manufacturer doesn't recommend using ketorolac preoperatively, it's been used safely and effectively as a preemptive analgesic.

For patients over 65, the recommended adult dose should be decreased by 50%, and may even be further reduced to as little as 10 mg. The total daily dose of ketorolac shouldn't exceed 60 mg; the daily dose can be reduced by administering doses every eight hours instead of every six hours. The intramuscular route isn't recommended because of unreliable absorption. This is especially important in the elderly because they may often have decreased muscle mass. Ketorolac should be used for no more than five days. In elderly postoperative patients, it's often discontinued after 48 hours.

Acetaminophen is an alternative for patients who can't tolerate NSAIDs. It can be given preoperatively or intraoperatively and continued during the postoperative course. Remember, acetaminophen or indomethacin (Indocin) can be given rectally until patients can tolerate oral fluids.

■ OPIOID GUIDELINE: START LOW AND GO SLOW

In the elderly, the effects of opioids are stronger and last longer, so the basic guideline for administration is to start low and go slow. Because elderly patients may experience a higher peak effect and a longer duration of action from an opioid, it's prudent to begin with a dose 25% to 50% of the recommended adult dose and titrate upward slowly, such as in 25% increments, as needed.

Although meperidine (Demerol) is commonly prescribed, it's not desirable, especially for elderly patients. Its active metabolite, normeperidine, can accumulate regardless of the route of administration and can cause central nervous system (CNS) excitatory toxicity. Normeperidine is eliminated by the kidneys, so meperidine is contraindicated in patients with compromised renal function, which can exclude many elderly patients. If meperidine is used in an elderly patient like Mr. Hecht, he'll need to be evaluated every eight to 12 hours for signs of neurotoxicity, specifically tremors and myoclonus.

An early indication of excitatory toxicity may be a tremor that's difficult for the patient to control, especially if it began after meperidine was started. Also, question the patient about any twitching and jerking, which may awaken him several times during the night. If normeperidine is implicated as the cause of these symptoms, the patient should be switched immediately to another morphine-like opioid (such as morphine or hydromorphone).

If this change isn't made, further accumulation of normeperidine can result in seizures and possibly death.

When normeperidine toxicity is found or suspected, remember that it can't be reversed with the opioid antagonist naloxone (Narcan). In fact, naloxone may even exacerbate hyperexcitability by decreasing the level of meperidine, which is a CNS depressant. Recent research also shows that meperidine is much more likely than other opioids to cause delirium postoperatively. In one study, meperidine more than doubled the risk of delirium when given IV or epidurally.

■ IV AND INTRASPINAL ROUTES

The parenteral route is indicated for most postoperative patients with severe pain because of the need for rapid onset. Intravenous, rather than IM, administration should be used in the elderly because they often have muscle wasting and less fatty tissue than younger patients (see Box 41-1).

BOX 41-1   Guidelines for Administering Pain Medication

- Use IV or intraspinal, not IM, analgesia to get severe pain under control quickly.
- Initiate opioid therapy with 25% to 50% lower dose than recommended for adults.
- Titrate doses upward slowly (with 25% increases) because elders experience higher peak effects and longer duration of action.
- Use a multimodal approach including balanced analgesia (opioids, NSAIDs, and local anesthetics) to maximize pain relief and minimize adverse effects from any single agent.
- Consider preemptive analgesia using opioids, NSAIDs, and local anesthetics.
- Use ATC dosing for all routes, but carefully evaluate the interval — it may need to be longer than in younger patients.
- Use NSAIDs to provide pain relief with lower opioid doses, but be cautious. Limit doses of ketorolac (60 mg/day), especially if patient has impaired renal function, weighs less than 50 kg, or serum creatinine is moderately elevated.
- Use acetaminophen as an alternative when NSAIDs are contraindicated.
- Prevent opioid-induced respiratory depression by monitoring sedation levels hourly and decreasing opioid doses when increased sedation is detected. If additional pain relief is needed, add acetaminophen or NSAIDs.
- If naloxone is given for clinically significant respiratory depression, titrate in small doses.
- Return to the oral route of administration as early as possible and evaluate its effectiveness before discharge. Continue IV or spinal analgesics, initially at lowered doses (or maintain access to bolus doses) until safe and effective oral doses have been established.
- Postoperative pain may be more severe and last longer in elderly patients than in younger patients. Consider oral morphine or hydromorphone rather than opioid-acetaminophen combinations.

Intraspinal administration of opioids is indicated for major thoracic, abdominal, and joint surgeries, which are associated with severe postoperative pain. A major benefit of delivering opioids directly to the site of their action in the CNS is that less drug is likely to reach the supraspinal structures, reducing the risk of sedation and respiratory depression.

The intraspinal route can even improve postoperative outcomes. For example, one important goal after a thoracotomy is improved pulmonary function. Studies have shown that not only does thoracic epidural analgesia provide superior pain relief compared to IM and IV routes following thoracotomy, but it also allows the patient to deep-breathe better. This improves pulmonary function and reduces the length of time that patient needs to be on a mechanical ventilator. Continuous epidural analgesia has also been shown to improve pulmonary function and bowel motility after abdominal surgery.

The two opioids most commonly administered epidurally are morphine and fentanyl (Sublimaze). The amount administered epidurally can be reduced by adding low doses of a local anesthetic, such as bupivacaine (Marcaine). The anesthetic acts synergistically with these opioids and has dose-sparing capabilities.

Whenever local epidural anesthetics are administered, institutional protocols should include nursing assessments for lower extremity motor and sensory deficits because partial anesthesia may occur and for orthostatic hypotension due to sympathetic blockade. Enforce precautions, such as the use of side rails and assisted ambulation. Because of altered drug clearance in the elderly, systemic accumulation of the local anesthetic may occur, resulting in cognitive impairment.

Intravenous PCA has been shown to be safe in elderly patients, but practitioners often hesitate to prescribe it because they're concerned about causing confusion. However, when IV or epidural PCA is warranted, elderly patients shouldn't be automatically excluded. Rather, their cognitive and physical abilities should be carefully evaluated on an individual basis.

Adding a continuous infusion to IV or epidural PCA boluses must be done cautiously with elderly patients. Bolus-only PCA can be used initially, and the decision to add a continuous infusion can be made after the patient's responses to boluses are evaluated.

■ KEY PREOPERATIVE TEACHING POINTS

Institutional protocols and physicians' orders must support your role in teaching patients about pain and in assessing and managing it. This is especially critical with regard to titrating opioid doses, adding nonopioid analgesics, and treating adverse effects, including respiratory depression.

The preoperative interview is critical to the success of the pain management plan. In addition to providing essential information, preoperative teaching may decrease the patient's anxiety, reduce analgesic dose requirements, and improve patient outcomes.

Whenever possible, an elderly patient's family members or significant others should participate in the initial teaching session. This is especially true for cognitively impaired elders. Postoperatively, family members can be invaluable in reinforcing important information provided during the preoperative session.

Elderly patients tend to have impaired vision and hearing. Many will be better able to concentrate and hear what you're saying if you can find a private, quiet location for the teaching session. Ask them if they need eyeglasses to see or read. If they normally wear a hearing aid, make sure that it's on and working properly. Speak clearly, slowly, and loudly enough. It may be necessary to repeat information and confirm that the patient understands what's being said by asking for feedback. Allow time for him to answer you fully and to ask questions (see Box 41-2).

Elderly patients often have some chronic pain problem, such as lower back, shoulder, or neck pain, or arthritis. Since pain can interfere with the ability to concentrate, determine if your patient is in pain at the time of the initial interview and, if so, intervene appropriately to relieve it. Also, ensure that the postoperative plan includes managing any preexisting pain.

Provide patients with written materials about the pain management plan and refer to the materials frequently. If patients become familiar with these materials before surgery, they'll be more likely to refer to them postoperatively. If the hospital has an educational video channel, a video-tape may be developed or purchased to reinforce information in the preoperative interview.

◼ USE THE WORDS "PAIN MEDICINE"

Patients and their families often have many fears about pain medication. A national telephone survey of 1,000 Americans conducted in 1993 revealed that 82% were concerned about becoming addicted. They were particularly alarmed by the word "narcotic." And only 41% of them believed that all or almost all acute pain could be relieved. Another study of patients with

---

BOX 41-2   *Tips for Managing Pain in the Elderly*

- Ensure that appropriate aids for hearing and seeing are available.
- Use enlarged visual aids (for example, a pain rating scale).
- Speak slowly, clearly, and loudly enough.
- Assume that surgery will result in pain and that, if untreated, it could have a negative effect on recovery. Prepare an individual pain management plan.
- Involve family members.
- Teach the patient how to use the pain rating scale. Set goals for pain relief, especially during recovery activities.
- Reinforce that pain relief promotes recovery by using tangible examples, such as: "You need enough pain relief to use the incentive spirometer properly. It will help prevent pneumonia."
- Explain unfamiliar equipment. Let the patient hold and push the PCA button.
- Address the patient's and family's concerns about addiction and overdose.

cancer pain showed that reluctance to report pain and use analgesics was associated with concerns about addiction, adverse effects, injections, and tolerance, as well as believing that "good" patients don't complain and that pain is inevitable.

To avoid negative connotations associated with the words "drugs" or "narcotics," use the words "pain medicine" instead. Since fear of addiction is well-documented as a barrier to pain control, it's probably wise to say to all patients in the preoperative interview: "These pain medicines are necessary for your recovery and they won't cause addiction."

To further reinforce that pain medicines are "good," you need to make the link between adequate pain control and the activities necessary to improve outcome very clear during the preoperative interview and throughout the patient's postoperative course. For example, if he'll be using an incentive spirometer postoperatively, teach this technique preoperatively. Emphasize that it's his responsibility to use the spirometer regularly to prevent congestion and possibly pneumonia — and that he must obtain sufficient pain relief to do this.

Many elders grew up as passive recipients of health care. In the 1940s and 1950s, for example, hospital stays were much longer, patients stayed in bed while nurses ministered to their needs, and considerably less information was given to patients about their diagnoses and surgical procedures. Today, your preoperative teaching for elderly patients needs to emphasize their active role in avoiding postoperative complications. The goal of timely discharge and the value of pain medications in achieving this can be your focus.

■PATIENT-DIRECTED GOALS

The best time to familiarize your patients with the pain rating scale is during your preoperative teaching. Many elderly patients may have difficulty seeing it, so give them an enlarged version. As a reference, the patient can keep this at the bedside with a notation of his pain relief goals. Verify that the patient understands the scale by asking him to give you an example of pain he's experienced in the past and how he would rate it.

Next, ask him to set a goal for his postoperative pain relief by selecting a number on the pain rating scale. Ask him to rate the usual and worst intensity of that pain. Explain that you'll work with him to maintain an acceptable level during activities as well as during rest. Reassure him that you're aware that more pain medication is usually necessary during activities. One of the most important points to stress is that he's expected to take action to decrease his pain to that level (by using the PCA pump), or to notify a member of the health care team if his pain increases above the pain relief goal that's been set.

Elderly patients will be less fearful and more likely to be successful in using a PCA pump if they're given information when they're lucid. The immediate postoperative period isn't a good time to teach any patient the fundamentals of PCA. Plan on spending extra time preoperatively teaching your elderly patients if PCA is to be used.

When IV or epidural PCA is planned, give the patient the PCA button and ask him to press it. Explain that this activates the pump. Assure him that safety mechanisms, such as the lockout interval, will help to prevent overdosing.

Plan for the possibility that family members may decide to activate PCA for elderly patients. In a study of respiratory depression in 3,785 patients receiving IV PCA, a total of 14 critical events occurred. Three involved a family member activating the device. Explain to patients and family members the dangers of such an action. As alternatives, encourage them to remind the patient to activate PCA or to contact a staff member if they think their loved one is experiencing unacceptable pain.

Sometimes family-controlled analgesia is useful for patients who are cognitively or physically unable to manage PCA. If so, the designated family member must be present for the entire preoperative interview and demonstrate an understanding of pain assessment, adverse effects, and use of the equipment. For impaired patients who don't have family or significant others, plan to use ATC IV bolusing or nurse-activated dosing with the PCA pump. Appropriate protocols to ensure patient safety and staff responsibilities should be in place when using these methods.

Nondrug methods to manage pain also have a place. But reinforce that these methods are a supplement, not a replacement, for pain medications. Elderly patients often express references for certain types of nondrug methods. For example, at home they may be accustomed to using music or television to distract themselves from a chronic pain condition and may find that the same methods are helpful in coping with postoperative pain as well.

Cold compresses aren't usually a popular choice among the elderly. However, if you describe this measure in terms of providing a cool sensation over the surgical site, it may be much more appealing. Show the patient a lightweight, well wrapped cold pack and ask him to evaluate whether or not it's too cold. If it is, it can be modified until the temperature is right. Although patients may be reluctant to try cold, some research has shown that it relieves pain faster and longer than heat. It also has the beneficial effect of vasoconstriction to reduce bleeding and edema.

▬DANGEROUS SCENARIO TO AVOID

Even before patients recover from anesthesia enough to report their pain, the PACU nurse and physician must assume that pain is present and administer opioids as soon as possible. Intravenous PCA or epidural analgesia should be initiated in the PACU rather than on the nursing unit. This allows the PACU nurse to evaluate the patient's ability to use PCA early in the postoperative course and prevents delays in analgesia on the nursing unit. A particularly dangerous scenario unfolds when patients receive IM opioid injections on the nursing unit while waiting for IV PCA to be initiated, which can result in an inadvertent overdose.

The clinician-administered bolus mode on the infusion pump can be used in the PACU to titrate the dose to ensure patient comfort, eliminating the time-consuming task of signing out, drawing up, and administering opioid boluses from a separate syringe. When patients are cognizant, they can be reminded to use the PCA button and encouraged to manage their own pain.

All opioid-induced adverse effects should be assessed along with pain intensity at least every 15 minutes and before and after every nurse-administered analgesic bolus dose in the PACU. Providing effective pain relief while minimizing opioid-induced adverse effects is a special challenge for the PACU nurse, who must deal with the additional CNS depression caused by the sedative and anesthetic agents administered intraoperatively.

Here again a multimodal approach can help. The simple intervention of administering an NSAID preoperatively may reduce pain rating scores and analgesic requirements in the PACU. If an NSAID wasn't given, it can be started in the PACU or epidural opioids may be combined with a long-acting local anesthetic.

Criteria for discharge from the PACU should include ensuring that patients understand their postoperative pain management plan and have satisfactory pain control with minimal adverse effects. A standard should be set for the level of pain relief to be achieved before patients are discharged to the clinical unit. If safe and effective analgesia is established in the PACU and if patients have been well educated about their role in pain relief, postoperative pain management on the clinical unit is simplified.

Being transferred to a medical-surgical unit from the PACU and getting settled in bed are likely to produce pain. As a result, it may be necessary to reestablish analgesia with opioid boluses.

On the clinical unit, assess postoperative pain in elderly patients using the pain rating scale every one to two hours during the first 24 hours. Compare current pain assessments with the original pain relief goals. More important than pain ratings while a patient is resting is obtaining ratings while they're engaged in recovery activities, such as position changes or deep breathing. Once safe and satisfactory pain relief is established, pain assessment every two to four hours for the remainder of the postoperative course is usually adequate.

Again, ensure that elderly patients' hearing aids are working properly and that eyeglasses are within reach. Also, during every pain assessment, reinforce the active role elderly patients have in preventing postoperative complications — including unrelieved pain.

▬MINIMIZING ADVERSE EFFECTS

The most effective strategy for managing any opioid-induced adverse effect is to decrease the dose of the opioid. If the patient experiences an adverse effect but also has satisfactory pain relief, the opioid dose can be decreased by 25% to 50%, depending on the severity of the adverse effect. Medications to relieve the immediate symptoms of such adverse effects as pruritus or nausea may be indicated while the dose is decreased. But by decreasing the opioid dose, the cause of the adverse effect is being eliminated, which is a better strategy than repeatedly treating symptoms (see Box 41-3).

BOX 41-3   What to Avoid — and Why

- *PRN dosing.* The elderly are especially reluctant to ask for medication. ATC dosing ensures effective analgesic coverage.
- *Benzodiazepines.* They contribute to delirium and aren't analgesic.
- *NSAIDs with long half-lives.* Piroxicam and nabumetone, for example, tend to accumulate, especially when renal function is impaired.
- *Meperidine.* It increases the risk of delirium. Impaired renal function increases the accumulation of its active metabolite, normeperidine.
- *Routine use of antiemetics.* They can cause adverse effects, and nausea and vomiting are less common in elderly patients.
- *Ongoing administration of drugs to treat opioid-induced adverse effects.* Instead, decrease the opioid dose, monitor the patient closely, and add an NSAID.
- IM *route.* It's painful, absorption is unreliable, and the elderly often have muscle wasting.

Also, medications commonly prescribed to treat adverse effects can cause other adverse effects. For example, elderly patients are sensitive to the sedating effects of antihistamines, such as diphenhydramine (Benadryl), which is often prescribed for pruritus. They're also vulnerable to the anticholinergic adverse effects of phenothiazines, such as promethazine (Phenergan), which is often used for nausea. Since nausea and vomiting occur less often in the elderly than in younger patients, routine use of antiemetics isn't recommended.

For patients who have adverse effects but are in pain, consider adding an NSAID, such as ibuprofen or ketorolac. Then the opioid dose can be decreased. This provides additional analgesia without opioid-related adverse effects.

■MONITOR SEDATION LEVELS

Respiratory depression is probably more feared than any other adverse effect, especially in sensitive elderly patients. However, frequent nurse monitoring of sedation levels using a sedation scale (typically from 1 to 4, with 1 indicating full alertness) will help prevent this problem.

Sedation precedes respiratory depression, because more opioid is required to produce respiratory depression than is required to produce sedation. Since the risk of respiratory depression is greatest during the first 24 postoperative hours, check the patient's sedation level and respiratory status (including rate, depth, and quality of respirations) at least every one to two hours. If no problems have occurred after the first 24 hours, the frequency may be decreased to every two to four hours. Mechanical monitoring, such as pulse oximetry, is usually warranted only if patients have preexisting conditions that require it.

If you detect increased sedation, you can still prevent clinically significant respiratory depression (usually less than eight breaths per minute) by promptly reducing opioid doses and monitoring respiratory status and sedation more frequently. If it's necessary to administer naloxone to reverse respiratory depression, titrating it to effect is essential. If too much is given or it's given too quickly, analgesia will also be reversed. Appropriate titration is most easily accomplished by diluting the naloxone. The APS recommends diluting 0.4 mg naloxone in 10 mL saline and administering 0.5 mL iv push every two minutes.

The goal is to prevent rather than treat opioid-induced adverse effects. If attention is given to preemptive analgesia and the addition of acetaminophen or NSAIDs or other nonopioid analgesics postoperatively, the likelihood of adverse effects can be minimized.

■PREPARING FOR DISCHARGE

In preparation for discharge, transition from parenteral or intraspinal analgesia to oral analgesia should be done as soon as the patient is able to retain fluids and pain is well controlled. The duration of postoperative pain tends to be longer in the elderly. Although most patients experience less pain as the days pass after surgery, don't assume that all patients will follow this pattern. It's best to evaluate patients individually and reduce analgesic doses based on their reports of pain and ability to perform recovery activities such as ambulating or deep-breathing.

It's important to administer oral analgesics before discontinuing parenteral or intraspinal analgesia so that patients remain comfortable during the transition. Using opioids complemented with acetaminophen or aspirin limits the total daily doses of both since NSAIDs have a firm upper dose limit. More flexible and potentially more effective oral analgesics, such as hydromorphone 4 to 8 mg or morphine 15 to 30 mg, must be considered. NSAIDs, at recommended doses, can be given separately ATC.

Discharge planning includes establishing that patients are experiencing no adverse effects and can ambulate while taking the analgesics prescribed to control pain at home. Patients will need a thorough explanation of all the medications they're expected to take at home, including the resumption of medications they were taking prior to admission.

Possible overdoses or incompatibilities should be identified. For example, different proprietary names can be confusing. A patient might take too much naproxen sodium if he was taking Aleve prior to hospitalization, receives a prescription for Anaprox on discharge from the hospital, and takes both at home. If patients have been taking agonist-antagonists, such as pentazocine (Talwin) tablets or butorphanol (Stadol) nasal spray, at home prior to surgery, caution them about combining those drugs with a prescription for morphine-like drug, such as oxycodone-acetaminophen, because they may reverse analgesia.

While postoperative pain management poses special challenges in the elderly, a comfortable patient and a successful recovery are compatible goals. In fact, research strongly suggests that desired surgical outcomes are more easily achieved when pain is well managed.

Still, all analgesic regimens to control postoperative pain have both risks and benefits. In elderly patients, concerns about the risks of various methods of analgesia often overshadow the fact that unrelieved pain is also a risk. Research now shows that past attitudes of expecting surgery to hurt and believing that pain never killed anyone are no longer justified. Pain *can* kill in the sense that it delays healing and contributes to complications that can be life-threatening. Unrelieved postoperative pain, in itself, must now be viewed and treated as a serious complication of surgery, not as an acceptable consequence.

▬ SELECTED REFERENCES

American Pain Society. *Principles of Analgesic Use in the Treatment of Acute Pain and Cancer Pain,* 3rd ed. Skokie, IL, The Society, 1992.

Ashburn, M. A., et al. Respiratory-related critical events with intravenous patient-controlled analgesia. *Clin. J. Pain* 10(1):52–56, Mar. 1994.

Egbert, A. M., et al. Randomized trial of postoperative patient-controlled analgesia vs intramuscular narcotics in frail elderly men. *Arch. Intern. Med.* 150:1897–1903, Sept. 1990.

Gordon, D B., and Ward, S. E. Correcting patient misconceptions about pain. *Am. J. Nurs.* 95(7):43–45, July 1995.

Kehler, H. Postoperative pain relief — what is the issue? *Br. J. Anaesth.* 72:375–378, Apr. 1994.

Liu, S., et al. Epidural anesthesia and analgesia: Their role in postoperative outcome. *Anesthesiology* 82:1474–1506, June 1995.

Marcantonio, E. R., et al. The relationship of postoperative delirium with psychoactive medications. *JAMA* 272:1518–1522, Nov. 16, 1994.

The Mayday Fund. *1993 Pain Survey:* New York, The Fund, 1993.

McCaffery, M., and Beebe, A. *Pain: Clinical Manual for Nursing Practice.* St. Louis, MO, Mosby, 1989.

Pasero, C. *Acute Pain Management Service Policy and Procedure Guideline Manual.* Rancho Palos Verdes, CA, American Medical Systems, 1994.

Pasero, C., and McCaffery, M. Postoperative pain management in the elderly. In *Pain in the Elderly,* ed. by B. Ferrell and B. Ferrell. Seattle, WA, International Association for the Study of Pain (IASP) Press, 1996.

Pasero, C., and McCaffery, M. Unconventional PCA: Making it work for your patient. *Am. J. Nurs.* 93(9):38–41, Sept. 1993.

Pasero, C. L., and McCaffery, M. Avoiding opioid-induced respiratory depression. *Am. J. Nurs.* 94(4):25–31, Apr. 1994.

Quinn, A. C., et al. Studies in postoperative sequelae: Nausea and vomiting — still a problem. *Anaesthesia* 49(1):62–65, Jan. 1994.

Swindale, J. E. The nurse's role in giving pre-operative information to reduce anxiety in patients admitted to hospital for elective minor surgery. *J. Adv. Nurs.* 14:899–905, Nov. 1989.

U.S. Agency for Health Care Policy and Research. *Acute Pain Management: Operative or Medical Procedures and Trauma* (AHCPR Pub. No. 92-0032). Rockville, MD, U.S. Department of Health and Human Services, 1992.

Varrassi, G., et al. The effects of perioperative ketorolac infusion on postoperative pain and endocrine-metabolic response. *Anesth. Analg.* 78:514–519, Mar. 1994.

Ward, S. E., et al. Patient-related barriers to management of cancer pain. *Pain* 52:319–324, Mar. 1993.

Woolf, C. J., and Chong, M. S. Preemptive analgesia — treating postoperative pain by preventing the establishment of central sensitization. *Anesth. Analg.* 77:362–379, Aug. 1993.

Chapter 42

Preventing Falls: How to Identify Risk Factors and Reduce Complications

REIN TIDEIKSAAR

> Your client is 86 years old, eats heartily, exercises regularly, follows
> all preventative health practices her health care provider suggests,
> and is experiencing a "healthy old age." A telephone cord carelessly
> draped across the floor, a new accent rug in the hall, or a hasty move
> to see who is at the door has the potential to destroy all she has
> accomplished to be in good health. A fall can be the *one* significant
> event that starts the downward trajectory of health for older adults.
> Thus, preventing falls is of primary importance for everyone,
> especially nurses. The tables and figure in the chapter are useful
> when conducting a home safety assessment, mobility appraisal, or
> identifying health-related risk factors in elders.

Mrs. W, age 89, comes to you for a routine examination. She has a history of hypertension managed with diuretics, hypothyroidism, degenerative joint disease in her knees, and bilateral cataracts. She complains of nocturia over the past 6 months, but her history is otherwise unremarkable.

Her daughter, who has accompanied Mrs. W during the visit, reveals that her mother has fallen several times in the last few months. The daughter is worried about her mother's safety and whether she can continue living alone. Mrs. W denies the significance of these falling episodes, as she has not been injured.

Despite what she may think, the risk of serious injury is very real in patients such as Mrs. W. One objective of the Healthy People 2000 initiative of the U.S. Public Health Service is to reduce hip fractures among persons age 65 and older so that fracture-related hospitalizations are no more than 607 per 100,000 (from a baseline of 714 per 100,000). The government initiative also calls for a reduction in deaths from falls and fall-related injuries.

To help you play a part in achieving these goals, this article uses Mrs. W's case to illustrate the risk factors for falls, the patient workup, and a comprehensive strategy for preventing falls and related injuries.

From *Geriatrics* 51(2):43–53, 1996. Reprinted with permission.

▬ SCOPE OF THE PROBLEM: COMPLICATIONS OF FALLS

Each year, one-fourth of all persons age 65 to 74 and one-third or more of those age 75 and older report having fallen.[1] About two-thirds of older people who fall suffer another fall within the next 6 months.[2] Significant morbid complications are associated with falls:

- Approximately 15% of falls result in physical injury serious enough to warrant medical attention,[3] with about 5 to 10% of these leading to serious injuries (eg, head and soft tissue trauma and musculoskeletal sprains) and the remaining 3 to 5% resulting in bone fractures.[3] Any bone may break following a fall, but hip fractures are the most serious. Only about one-half of older persons able to walk independently prior to fracturing a hip can do so following surgical repair, and they often require a cane or walker or the assistance of another person.
- Inability to get up from the ground unassisted results in a prolonged "lie time," which can lead to dehydration, rhabdomyolysis, and pressure sores. Persons with medical conditions affecting lower extremity function (eg, arthritis, hemiplegia/paresis, parkinsonism) are at greatest risk for long lie times.
- Falls often lead to a fear of falling, which can decrease mobility and independence — particularly if an older person loses confidence in the ability to perform activities. Up to 50% of those who have fallen admit to avoiding activities because of fear of further falls or injury.[4] The risk of developing a fear of falling is greatest in people with underlying gait and balance disorders who experience recurrent falls, an injury, and/or prolonged lie times.
- Falls are distressing for family members, as in the case of Mrs. W. At issue is whether the patient can live at home alone and remain safe or whether she requires the assistance of home attendants or protective nursing home placement.

Mrs. W's initial workup indicates her high risk for several of these complications. Her kyphosis suggests osteoporosis, which increases the risk of significant injury from subsequent falls. At least one of her falls resulted in a long lie on the bathroom floor, so she may be at risk for similar episodes. She also has a fear of falling, which has begun to affect her mobility. Therefore, she requires further evaluation aimed at identifying risk factors for falls and appropriate treatment.

▬ HISTORY: REVIEW RISK FACTORS, FALLING EPISODES

Falls have many different causes, and patients may have several predisposing risk factors (Table 42-1).[1,3,4] Mrs. W's history reveals these medical risk factors:

- visual impairment (cataracts)
- postural hypotension

TABLE 42-1 Medical Risk Factors for Falls

Poor vision*	Bladder dysfunction
Cataracts	Nocturia
Macular degeneration	Incontinence
Glaucoma	Frequency
Cardiovascular	Cognitive dysfunction
Postural hypotension	Dementia*
Syncope	Depression
Arrhythmia	Anxiety
Drop attacks	Medications
Lower extremity dysfunction	Diuretics
Arthritis	Antihypertensives
Muscle weakness*	Sedatives*
Foot problems	Psychotropics*
Peripheral neuropathy	
Gait and balance disorders	
Stroke	
Parkinson's disease	
Myelopathy	
Cerebellar disorders	
Hypothyroidism	

* Associated with risk of fall-related injury

- lower extremity dysfunction (muscle weakness, degenerative joint disease)
- hypothyroidism
- nocturia
- diuretic use
- and osteoporosis (kyphotic posture).

The relative contribution of each risk factor diffuses according to the individual's underlying medical condition, functional level, and environmental circumstances. In general, "vigorous" older people are likely to experience falls because of acute medical or environmental factors that occur in isolation, whereas "frail" individuals fall due to a combination of medical factors — particularly chronic diseases — and environmental factors.

Falling Episodes

Begin by taking a careful history of the circumstances surrounding the fall(s). Ask the patient about all falls over the past 3 months and to recount any symptoms preceding the fall. Document the location of the fall, activity being performed, time of day, and what happened after the fall (ie, physical injury, long lies, or fear of further falls).

To ascertain significant fear of falling, ask patients about their level of confidence in performing certain mobility tasks by themselves (eg, walking outdoors, using the toilet, taking a bath or shower, etc.) or what activities they have begun to avoid as a result of falling. Use the mnemonic device "SPLATT" to remember the components of the fall history:

Symptoms

Previous falls

Location

Activity

Time

Trauma

Remember that older adults may not report falls because of embarrassment or fear of nursing home placement. If the patient fails to tell you about the falls, can't remember, or is unable to remember the events surrounding their fall(s), question family members and home attendants who may have witnessed the event(s).

Mrs. W had experienced three falls over the past month, all under similar circumstances. Each time, she awakened in the middle of the night with an urge to urinate. After getting out of bed, she hurried to the bathroom without her walker (to guard against incontinence). One time, she slipped on a small area rug by her bed and fell.

Both her bedroom and narrow hallway are poorly illuminated. She felt a little dizzy after getting out of bed and used furnishings and walls to support her balance when walking. In the bathroom, she was able to sit down and get up from the toilet, although she needed to hold onto the sink for balance. Another time, her hand slipped off the sink, which caused her to lose her balance and fall. After she fell, she was unable to get up from the bathroom floor.

Because she is afraid of falling again, Mrs. W has begun to restrict her activities. She goes outdoors only when accompanied by another person and recently limited the number of baths she takes, because her bathtub is "too dangerous."

Physical Exam

After obtaining the fall history, conduct a physical exam (Table 42-2) to search for acute and chronic diseases that may precipitate falls. Base your diagnosis on the history, physical findings, and clinical suspicions. A comprehensive battery of laboratory studies rarely yields an underlying cause, although routine chemistries may detect additional risk factors.

▬ EVALUATE MOBILITY

Chronic medical conditions that affect gait and balance increase susceptibility to falls and injury, but their impact is more accurately reflected by their effect on mobility (ie, the ability to walk and transfer safely and independently in the living environment). This relationship becomes significant in light of known environmental hazards.

To evaluate for mobility dysfunction, ask the patient to perform simple gait and balance maneuvers in your office (see Fig. 42-1). Any mobility

---

TABLE 42-2   The Fall-Related Physical Examination: What to Check for

---

Postural blood pressure
  Orthostatic hypotension

Mental status evaluation
  Delirium, dementia, depression

Visual assessment
  Visual acuity, cataracts, glaucoma, macular degeneration

Cardiac evaluation
  Arrhythmias, valvular disorders, bruits

Neurologic evaluation
  Focal deficits, peripheral neuropathy, tremor

Musculoskeletal evaluation
  Muscular weakness, arthritis

Podiatric evaluation
  Nail disorders, toe deformities, condition of footwear

---

impairment is a strong predictor of subsequent falls and injury. Such an assessment will help you determine additional risk factors not discovered by the history/physical exam and to design environmental interventions to improve mobility.

Recall factors from the patient's history that may have contributed to her falls. On mobility evaluation, Mrs. W demonstrated:

- poor seated transfers (her toilet is quite low)
- a positive sternal nudge maneuver (her poor postural response to balance loss made the sliding rug by the bedside doubly dangerous)
- altered gait and balance (noncompliance with her walker further increased her risk)
- inability to get up from the floor (she experienced and is at risk for prolonged lie times).

▬PREVENTION: REDUCING FALLS, INJURIES

Goals of fall prevention are to maximize mobility, reduce the threat of falls and their complications, and maintain autonomy. Potential interventions are based on known risk factors and consist of medical, rehabilitative, environmental, and psychosocial approaches. Medical intervention alone may be sufficient when falls are due to isolated acute medical problems. However, a combination of interventions is often required when falls are multifactorial — as are Mrs. W's.

Medical Interventions

Medical strategies for Mrs. W consist of two approaches:

- treat her immediate medical problems
- attempt to modify each risk factor.

1. **Sit and rise from a chair**

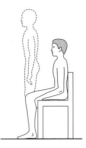

Watch for ability to sit and rise in a smooth, controlled movement without balance loss or use of armrests. Poor performance signifies lower extremity dysfunction.

2. **Stand in place for 10 to 15 seconds after rising from chair**

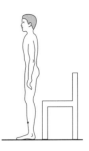

Watch for ability to stand steady unassisted without balance loss or dizziness. Poor performance signifies postural hypotension or vestibular dysfunction.

3. **Stand, with eyes closed, arms at sides, and feet about 3 inches apart**

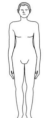

Watch for ability to stand without support and without sway or balance loss. Poor performance signifies proprioceptive loss.

4. **Maintain balance when receiving a light nudge on sternum (sternal nudge maneuver)**

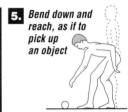

Normal reaction is to stretch out arms forward and away from body and to take a step or two backward to regain balance. Poor performance signifies postural instability.

5. **Bend down and reach, as if to pick up an object**

Watch for ability to maintain balance. Poor performance signifies altered balance, indicating that retrieving hard-to-reach objects may increase fall risk.

6. **Walk in a straight line (about 15 feet), turn around, and walk back**

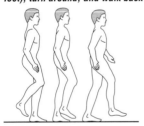

Watch for ability to walk and turn around without hesitation, excessive deviation from side to side, or feet scraping the floor. Poor performance signifies gait/balance dysfunction.

7. **Get up from floor**

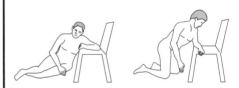

Watch for ability to get up either unassisted or with the help of a chair for support. Poor performance signifies lower extremity dysfunction, indicating risk for long lies.

FIGURE 42-1   Office-based mobility screen: Seven basic steps

As she is at risk for fractures, an evaluation of her osteoporosis is warranted. Consider prescribing nutritional supplements and medications that reduce bone resorption. If her nocturia persists after stopping the diuretic, pursue a more comprehensive evaluation of bladder dysfunction. If poor vision interferes with safe mobility, discuss the possibility of cataract surgery.

Rehabilitation

Patients may benefit from rehabilitative interventions. First, recommend a program of exercises to maintain and increase bone density, improve gait and balance, and improve postural reflexes or the response to balance loss. Many community senior centers offer such programs. If a patient such as Mrs. W hesitates to participate for fear of falling, I would recommend starting with a simple home-based program of strengthening and flexibility exercises that can be done safely while seated. When she becomes stronger and less fearful of falling, she can exercise at a senior center.

Two approaches may be offered to reduce the patient's risk for long lies subsequent to a fall:

- Teach her how to get up by moving along the floor to a chair (or toilet) and, with its support, maneuver into a side-sitting position. With the support of the chair or toilet, she can then kneel and push herself into a seated position.
- In patients who are reluctant to attempt this maneuver, consider recommending a personal emergency response system. This small, light-weight portable call button is worn as a pendant or wrist watch. When activated, it automatically dials an emergency response center for help.

A walker may benefit a patient such as Mrs. W. It can support her gait and balance as well as diminish her fear of falling by providing a visual and physical means of support should she lose her balance. If a walker has been prescribed but is not being used, find out why. Ask whether the device is the wrong size (too tall or short), has a poor or clumsy design (must be "picked up and moved" or small-wheeled), requires a great deal of space in which to maneuver, or carries a psychological stigma (symbolizes frailty and incompetence).

As a last alternative, advise the patient to rearrange her home environment to make walking as safe as possible (eg, clear pathways so that walls, door openings, and stable furnishings can be used for support and stability). A commercially available hip protector (ie, a padded garment worn similar to a girdle) may be worn to help absorb the impact of a fall onto the hip. These garments have been shown to reduce the incidence of hip fractures by up to 50%.[5]

Environment

Environmental interventions include patient education to eliminate fall hazards in the home and the use of durable medical equipment (eg, toilet risers and grab bars, bathtub/shower chairs or benches and grab bars) to maintain safe mobility. Provide the patient and family with a checklist of environmental hazards and modifications (Table 42-3).

In Mrs. W's case, one goal would be to reduce the hazards that have caused her to fall at night on her trips to the bathroom. Modifications could include:

- replacing the bedroom rug with one that is slip-free or placing nonskid matting underneath the existing rug
- removing all hallway clutter and furnishings interfering with safe gait, and install night lights to improve nocturnal vision
- installing indoor-outdoor carpet in the bathroom to help her avoid slipping on wet tiles and provide cushioning to decrease the impact of a fall.

A toilet riser or a toilet safety frame (ie, armrest grab bars that provide hand support when transferring) can be recommended. Wall-mounted grab bars may provide less support than safety frames and are sometimes difficult to install. If the patient's nocturia persists, a portable commode in the bedroom may help to decrease fall risk.

Recommend tub grab bars and a bath transfer bench to allow the patient to resume bathing. Assistive toileting and bathtub equipment can be found in drug stores or through medical device catalogs. Keep several copies of these catalogs in your office to provide a visual aid for patients and family members. Urge patients to check with you before purchasing devices to ensure that they provide proper support and are safe.

Psychosocial Intervention

Mrs. W is afraid of falling, and her daughter is concerned about her mother's safety and living arrangements. Generally, success in decreasing fear of falling depends on your ability to quickly restore the patient's confidence. Modifying risk factors for injuries and falls and encouraging independent mobility will often improve the patient's gait and balance. Family members will probably feel relieved and allow patients to maintain their autonomy.

If a fear of falling persists despite intervention, patients may require a home attendant. With Mrs. W, continued falls at night and heightened fear of falling might cause her to avoid attempts at independent toileting, which may lead to functional urinary incontinence. Suggest either a home attendant at night (to help with toileting) or the use of a bedside commode.

Follow-Up

At subsequent office visits, monitor compliance with the recommended interventions and determine if they are successful in preventing falls and/or modifying fall and injury risk. In case of noncompliance or subsequent falls, interventions may need to be redesigned.

During each visit (or at least annually) it is important to:

- monitor fall and injury risk factors
- review medications (prescription and OTC) that may lead to cognitive dysfunction, postural hypotension, sedation, and other adverse effects
- inquire about recent falls and fear of falling.

TABLE 42-3   Checklist of Common Hazards Linked to Falls in the Home

HAZARDS	MODIFICATIONS
Lighting problems ■ Poor access to switches/lamps ■ Low lighting ■ Lack of night lights ■ Increased lighting glare	Provide ample lighting in rooms and hallways, with switches located at room entrances Provide extra lighting along path from bedroom to bathroom, by one- and two-step elevations, and by top and bottom of stairway landings Use nightlights, 100- to 200-watt bulbs, and 3-way light bulbs to increase lighting levels Eliminate glare from exposed light bulbs by using translucent light shades or frosted light bulbs
Floors and hallway problems ■ Clutter ■ Low-lying objects ■ Limited walking space ■ Waste/wet floors ■ Sliding throw rugs ■ Worn carpets ■ Upended/curled carpet edges ■ Raised door sills	Arrange furnishings so that pathways are not obstructed Removable low-lying objects Provide stable furnishings along pathways for balance support Provide nonskid rugs and carpet runners on slippery floors; use nonskid floor wax Replace sliding area rugs with nonskid rugs or place nonskid tape or pads underneath existing rugs Repair or replace worn carpets Tape down all carpet edges prone to buckling or curling Remove or replace carpeting over threshold to create smooth transition between rooms
Bathroom problems ■ Low toilet seat ■ Inaccessible tub/shower stall ■ Slippery floor tiles ■ Slippery tub/shower floor	Use elevated toilet seat or install toilet safety frame Install wall-mounted or tub-attached grab bar or shower chair/tub transfer bench Apply nonskid strips/decals to bathroom tiled floors Place nonskid rubber mat on tub floor
Stairway problems ■ Lack of handrails ■ Slippery steps ■ Steps in poor repair	Install well-anchored cylindrical handrails (for hand grasp) Apply nonskid treads to steps Repair worn carpet on steps Apply color-contrasted nonskid tape for visibility
Furniture problems ■ Low chair seats ■ Armless chairs ■ Low/high bed	Replace low chairs with those that are easy to get up from/sit down in Provide chairs with armrest support Add a seat cushion to raise seat height Replace existing mattress with one that is thinner (to lower bed height) or thicker (to raise)
Storage problems ■ Shelves too low/high ■ Unstable chairs/step stools ■ Lack of adequate storage space	Keep frequently-used objects at waist level Use reacher device to obtain objects Install shelves and cupboards at accessible height

▬ CONCLUSION

Mrs. W's medical condition and mobility improved as a result of the rehabilitative and environmental interventions outlined here. She experienced no further falls or injury. Her fear of falling subsided enough for her to feel more comfortable being outdoors by herself and bathing She joined a community center for exercises. Her daughter felt more at ease with her mother living by herself at home — an outcome that the patient herself fully embraced.

▬ REFERENCES

1. Tinetti ME, Speechley M, Ginter SF. Risk factors for falls among elderly persons. *N Engl J Med* 1988; 319:1701–7.
2. Perry BC. Falls among the elderly. *J Am Geriatr Soc* 1982; 30:367–71.
3. Tinetti ME, Speechley M. Prevention of falls among the elderly. *N Engl J Med* 1989; 320:1055–9.
4. Nevitt MC, Cummings SR, Kidd S, Black D. Risk factors for recurrent falls: A prospective study. *JAMA* 1989; 261:2663–8.
5. Lauritzen JB, Petersen MM, Lund B. Effect of external hip protectors on hip fractures. *Lancet* 1993; 341:11–3.

Chapter 43

Congestive Heart Failure: Mapping the Way to Quality Outcomes

TRIXIE NEWKIRK　　BARBARA LEEPER

Congestive heart failure (CHF) is the leading reason for admission to acute care settings among clients over the age of 65. The cost of managing CHF is high, in dollars and quality of life. These authors, very concisely, offer that the best approach to managing CHF is through the benefits achieved by teamwork among professionals, clients, and their families. A "care path," with timelines for completion, is developed using the best ideas from all team members. This mapping of care demonstrates how cooperatively team members must work in order to achieve quality client outcomes. Although this short chapter focuses on CHF that is managed in the acute care setting, the idea of a "care path" is appropriate for clients in all care setting with any diagnosis.

In the United States alone, congestive heart failure (CHF) accounts for about $8 billion in health care expenditures each year (1). Managing patients with CHF has become more challenging, as insurance companies demand lower costs and negotiate set rates per procedure and diagnosis. In today's managed care environment, any provider who exceeds the contracted amount won't be reimbursed for the overrun. Consequently, providers are constantly challenged to find more cost-effective ways to care for CHF patients without compromising quality of care.

Patients with CHF are especially problematic because of their high readmission rates (17.2% nationally) to acute care facilities, usually resulting from an exacerbation of their symptoms (2). Indeed, chronic heart failure is the leading cause of hospital admissions in patients older than 65 (3).

A multidisciplinary team of health care professionals at Baylor University Medical Center has tackled the enormous challenge of developing critical paths aimed at reducing such costs while ensuring quality-based outcomes. At Baylor, a Quality Resource Council oversees the development and approval of all care paths. Recently, a group of physicians and nurses at Baylor requested approval from the Quality Resource Council to develop a care

From *AJN/Supplement* 25–27, May 1996. Reprinted with permission.

path for the uncomplicated CHF patient, intending to expand the care path for the complicated heart failure patient after a pilot study. Here we'll present the development process used by the multidisciplinary team that accepted that challenge.

■ RESEARCHING THE LITERATURE

To prepare for developing the care path, all team members researched CHF and brought relevant articles from the literature to the table. We began with a working definition of heart failure from the Agency for Health Care Policy and Research: "Heart failure is a clinical syndrome or condition characterized by signs and symptoms of intravascular and interstitial volume overload, including shortness of breath, rales, and edema or manifestations of inadequate tissue perfusion, such as fatigue or poor exercise tolerance" (4).

Several studies we reviewed focused on lowering readmission rates in elderly patients with CHF. One reported a 45.7% readmission rate within 90 days of discharge with the usual care, which dropped to 33% after a multidisciplinary team intervened with an intensive teaching strategy and close follow-up after discharge (5). Another reported a 40% readmission rate within 90 days of discharge, which was reduced to 23.2% after initiating referrals for home health-care services (6). We incorporated some of the interventions described in these studies into our care path for CHF patients.

Another study highlighted five strategies for effective management of CHF: prevention and early recognition of CHF, close follow-up, patient education, exercise training, and end-of-life decision-making (7). Those researchers consider CHF a public and private burden; they emphasized that nurses play a key role in identifying strategies for effective management of CHF.

Other studies focused on the pathophysiology of CHF, specifically the activation of neurohormonal responses contributing to the severity of the disease, as well as CHF's progression over time (3). Treatment of CHF with beta-adrenergic blockade might help these patients by reducing the activation of the sympathetic nervous system, resulting in better quality of life and long-term survival rates. This pharmacologic intervention is still in clinical trials and can't be generalized to the larger population at this time.

Lastly, we found information on the development and operation of heart failure clinics, where outpatients with refractory heart failure are treated (2,8,9). These clinics provide intermittent IV infusions of inotropic agents to patients with CHF categorized as class III or IV by New York Heart Association guidelines.

Before starting to develop the care path, we had to identify the allotted length of stay (LOS) and average LOS for our facility. Our task force formed two groups: One team assumed the task of finding out the LOS for DRG 127 (CHF), while the other audited charts to identify current practice.

We found that the allotted LOS for DRG 127 is 6.7 days — that is, Medicare reimburses for 6.7 hospital days for CHF diagnosis and treatment. Chart audits identified actual LOS (4.5 days), number of readmissions to the hospital, complications, patient teaching done, comorbidities, use of

ACE inhibitors and diuretics, ICU stay, use of telemetry and duration of telemetry, etiology of heart failure, and noncompliance issues. An average LOS of 4 days was identified as the target benchmark for this care path.

■ HOW THE CARE PATH WAS DRAFTED

Establishing time lines for completion helps ensure progress and discourages procrastination. We began by planning to meet every two weeks until completion. Members were given assignments to complete before the next scheduled meeting. Our target date for initiating the care path was April 1996. The next step was to begin mapping it out.

We used a blank shell of our institution's standard care path, which includes the following categories: assessment/monitoring, procedures/tests, treatments, activity, medications/IVs, nutrition, patient/family education, discharge planning, and psychosocial/emotional/spiritual care. Through the process of group interaction, use of current practice standards, and individual team-member input, the care that should be given each day was "penciled in" to the shell.

The group discussed the cost of various essential tests (SMA-6 versus SMA-20, for example), as well as those that might be nice to have but aren't really necessary for diagnosis and management. We used this process for each day of the care path. We invited a pharmacist to join the group to provide a cost analysis of the drugs used to treat CHF, then the physician group examined the cost-benefit ratio of those drugs. Those they selected were added to the physician order sets then under development.

Next, we discussed postdiuresis potassium replacement. We decided to use the potassium protocol currently in place in the cardiology units. That protocol addresses serum creatinine levels and renal function. It specifies that if the creatinine level is 1.8 or higher, the nurse must first check with the physician before administering potassium.

We invited a dietitian to join the group to provide input on a low-sodium (2 g), low-fat, low-cholesterol diet, and on fluid restriction. We also wanted to explore the availability of nutritional services to facilitate diet teaching with every patient on the care path.

A clinical nurse specialist (CNS) and a physical therapist developed an activity protocol to be included in the plan for all CHF patients. We consulted the cardiac rehabilitation department about any activity programs available to CHF patients after they leave the hospital. We soon found out that Medicare doesn't reimburse for cardiac rehabilitation for these patients. Medicare patients must pay for it out of pocket, unless they carry supplemental insurance that covers it. A CHF patient would have to attend three days per week for six weeks, resulting in a cost of $1,620. And, of course, the literature supports the need for improving exercise tolerance in these patients (7).

■ INPATIENT PROGRAM DEVELOPED

We decided to develop an inpatient program that would be continued at home, with home care nurses following up to ensure compliance. The activity protocol included having patients sit up in a chair for all meals, do basic leg exercises while up, and begin ambulation on hospital day 2. The distance patients walk and the corresponding time frames would be recorded. The protocol also includes checking pulse oximetry after the first walk and prior to discharge.

Each day, patients would be encouraged to increase the distance walked as well as the length of time walking. They would be asked to add two minutes per week to their walk time until they reached 30 minutes. After that, they would exercise two to three times per week. The nursing staff would assess the patient for signs and symptoms of intolerance, such as an increase in shortness of breath or rales after activity, an increase in heart rate of more than 20 beats per minute (bpm) at rest, or a heart rate above 120 bpm.

Finding any of those, the nurse would consult physical therapy for help in designing an individualized program for that patient. Patients would be asked to rate on a scale of 1 to 20 (the Borg rating of perceived exertion) how hard they feel they're working. If the patient chooses a number higher than 12, he would be asked to slow down.

We gave the protocol to the cardiac rehabilitation staff to review, make suggestions, and approve. After their suggestions were incorporated, we brought the protocol to the CHF task force for final approval and for insertion into the care path. We felt strongly that, by improving exercise tolerance, we would increase physical capacity and possibly reduce symptoms.

Having achieved many of our goals, we were ready to address patient/family education. The CNS for cardiovascular services pointed out that the lack of patient/family teaching and a lack of understanding in this patient population are major contributors to hospital readmissions. So the task force decided to include the following into the care path: giving patients copies of the CHF book developed by the hospital's cardiovascular patient education committee; reviewing heart failure with the patients and families; instructing them in the importance of monitoring daily weights and watching for weight gain; reporting any gain of three pounds or more to the physician; and reviewing signs and symptoms of heart failure, drug benefits and adverse effects, dosing schedules, activity protocols, smoking cessation, and alcohol-intake limits.

We developed behavioral objectives and intermediate outcomes for each content area. Some of our other goals in developing this care path were to include a daily chaplain visit if the patient wanted it and to develop a care path for the patient to follow each day while in the hospital.

Discharge planning must begin with the patient's admission and not on the day of discharge. So we included a home health care and social services screening on admission. At that time, the patient's situation would be evaluated and home care services or other community resources brought in as needed then and throughout the hospital stay.

A team member from home care planned to define what information was needed while the patient was hospitalized in order to coordinate a home care path. This would begin where the hospital care path left off, with home care nurses reinforcing what would be taught in the hospital — ideally a seamless delivery of care.

Our last step in developing the care path was to agree on discharge outcomes. We included the following:

- stable vital signs;
- all lab values within normal limits;
- O_2 saturation above 92%;
- patient able to state the importance of activity after discharge;
- patient/family able to state medication benefits, adverse effects, and dosing schedule;
- patient/family able to state examples of a low-sodium (2 g), low-fat, low-cholesterol diet and explain fluid restrictions;
- patient able to state importance of daily weights and reporting a three-pound weight gain to the physician; and
- access to a scale at home.

IMPLEMENTING THE CARE PATH

We brought the completed care path to the Quality Resource Council for final approval (currently pending). Before initiating it, however, we will have to educate the nursing staff and other disciplines on the CHF activity protocol, the potassium protocol, and the patient-teaching content.

The care path will be included in Baylor's documentation systems. A care coordinator for each floor will follow the CHF patients, helping each primary nurse achieve discharge outcomes and identify variances. Currently, another group is investigating the value of an outpatient CHF clinic, which would eventually be linked to the care path as a discharge option. The patient would either attend the CHF clinic or have home care services after discharge.

Care path development is a process that involves many disciplines. The team approach brings a variety of ideas to the group so that the best ideas can be integrated into the care path. As a result, each discipline takes ownership of their role in the process.

After the initial trial of a care path, follow-up data must be retrieved to determine if LOS was affected, costs were reduced, discharge outcomes were met, and readmission rates were reduced. Once developed, the care path becomes a dynamic tool. As we review our data, we will modify the care path accordingly. Once the uncomplicated CHF trial is completed, our CHF task force will reconvene to develop an insert for the more complicated CHF patient who needs admission to the ICU.

REFERENCES

1. Funk, M., and Krumholz, H. Epidemiologic and economic impact of advanced heart failure. *J. Cardiovasc. Nurs.* 10(2):1–10, 1996.
2. Venner, G., and Seelbinder, J. Team management of congestive heart failure across the continuum. *J. Cardiovasc. Nurs.* 10(2):71–84, 1996.
3. Sackner-Bernstein, J. D., and Mancini, D. M. Rationale for treatment of patients with chronic heart failure with adrenergic blockade. *JAMA* 274:1462–1467, Nov. 8, 1995.

4. Konstam, M. A., et al. *Heart Failure Evaluation and Care of Patients With Left-Ventricular Systolic Dysfunction* (AHCPR Pub. No. 94-0612). Rockville, MD, U.S. Department of Health and Human Services, 1995.
5. Rich, M. W., et al. Prevention of readmission in elderly patients with congestive heart failure: Results of a prospective, randomized pilot study. *J. Gen. Intern. Med.* 8:585–590, Nov. 1993.
6. Rich, M., and Freedland, K. E. Effect of DRGs on three-month readmission rate of geriatric patients with congestive heart failure. *Am. J. Publ. Health* 78:680–682, June 1988.
7. English, M. A., and Mastrean, M. B. Congestive heart failure: Public and private burden. *Crit. Care Nurs. Q.* 18(1):1–6, May 1995.
8. Heaney, L., et al. Intermittent inotropic infusions: Critical care in an outpatient setting. *Congestive Heart Failure.* 15–18, July–Aug. 1995.

Chapter 44

Sundown Syndrome: Etiology and Management

MARGARET BURNEY-PUCKETT

Night time may bring with it symptoms of agitation and confusion for elderly patients exhibiting Sundown Syndrome. This can upset family members and pose threats to patient safety and staff morale. This chapter reviews current research on sundowning, and discusses three possible etiologies. What can nurses do to help patients exhibiting these symptoms? Both medication and environmental interventions have been used, but careful patient assessment is needed.

What causes some patients who have dementia to get out of bed at night, put on their clothes, and try to leave their environment? Is darkness a precipitating factor for the increasing agitation in patients with dementia?

For health care professionals who care for patients with dementia, the term sundowning is associated with the phenomenon of increasing agitation that occurs near sunset or evening hours. Two terms, sundowning and sundown syndrome, are used synonomously to describe a variety of behaviors that occur in the evening hours.

▄ LITERATURE REVIEW

There is controversy in the literature about the definition of sundowning and the causes of increased agitation that seems to be associated with darkness. A review of the literature discloses numerous studies that contribute conflicting data about causes and timing of agitation. The physiologic basis for sundowning as cited by Bliwise (1994) includes three hypotheses: rapid eye movement (REM) sleep behavior disorder, sleep apnea, and deterioration of the suprachiasmatic nucleus, which results in the disruption of circadian rhythms and a disturbance in the sleepwake cycle. This article addresses the range of definitions that describe sundowning, prevalence and associated factors, specific hypotheses of its etiology, and management of the phenomenon.

From *Journal of Psychosocial Nursing* 34(5):40–43, 1996. Reproduced with permission.

▬VARIOUS DEFINITIONS

Many references in the literature link sundowning to delirium. Data from the time of Hippocrates describe increasing agitation and confusion in the evening hours experienced by some patients as a nocturnal exacerbation of delirium (Lipowski, 1989).

Delirium

In the *Diagnostic and Statistical Manual of Mental Disorders, 4th ed.* (DSM-IV, American Psychiatric Association, 1994), delirium is described as a psychiatric diagnosis characterized by a state of confusion subject to diurnal variability with various potential medical and physiologic etiologies.

Causes of delirium can include a variety of toxic, metabolic, infectious, nutritional, and substance-induced states that may occur at any age. Delirium may or may not accompany dementia (Lipowski, 1989). Criteria necessary for delirium are disturbance of consciousness and changes in cognition that are not better accounted for by a pre-existing, established, or evolving dementia. Delirium develops over a short period and tends to fluctuate during the day. Sleep-wake cycle disturbances often are associated with delirium, which can be manifested by daytime sleepiness or nighttime agitation and difficulty falling asleep, or a complete reversal of the sleep-wake cycle. The symptoms of delirium may resolve in a few hours or persist for days, and, if the underlying etiologic factor is corrected, recovery can occur.

Dementia

Dementia, based on the definition in the DSM-IV (1994), is characterized by the development of multiple cognitive defects that include memory impairment and a disturbance in executive functioning. Dementia may be progressive, static, or remitting. The DSM-IV (1994) definition is based on the pattern of cognitive deficits and carries no connotation about prognosis. The multiple cognitive impairments of dementia often are associated with anxiety and mood and sleep disturbances.

Sundowning, often observed in patients with dementia, is a description of behavior that seems to worsen in the evening; it is not a psychiatric diagnosis. Various behaviors specific to this phenomenon include wandering, confusion, hyperactivity, restlessness, aggressive behavior, and disorientation. These can be observed either singly or in combination (Bliwise, Carroll, Lee, Nekich, & Dement, 1993). Alterations in sleep architecture patterns, identified by polysomographs, have been found in patients with dementia (Vitiello, Bliwise, & Prinz, 1992).

Various behavioral studies have attempted to categorize agitation that corresponds to time frames. The earliest work, by Cameron (1941), noted that sundowning could be induced by bringing patients with dementia into a darkened room during the daytime. Cohen-Mansfield, Marx, Werner, and Freeman (1992) found that vocalizations, and carphologic (involuntary picking at bed clothes) and physically aggressive behaviors, were likely to occur in the late afternoon and evening (4:30 PM to 11:00 PM) rather than just during the sunset period (4:30 PM to 7:00 PM). Contrary to the above study, Bliwise, Bevier, and Bliwise (1990) determined that sunset may be a vulnerable period for agitation. Jacobs, Ancoli-Israel, Parker, and Krepke (1989) noted apparent wakefulness in the afternoon; however, Bliwise, et al. (1993) found that agitation was no more likely to occur during the afternoon or at night than during the daytime. Bliwise (1994) states that his studies of time-agitation relationships showed that more severe agitation occurred in the winter months rather than autumn, and the time of occurrence was near sunset.

▬PREVALENCE AND ASSOCIATED FACTORS

The DSM-IV (1994) states that in patients older than 65 who are hospitalized for a general medical condition, approximately 10% are reported to exhibit delirium during their hospital stay. Prevalence of dementia in the 65 and older age group is estimated at 2% to 4%; after age 85, prevalence can increase to more than 20%. Sleep disturbance is associated with both delirium and dementia. Little agreement exists about how often disruptive behaviors occur in the specific evening hours; most studies report data that cover the entire period of wakefulness rather than the period of sunset (Bliwise, 1994).

Other factors that affect nursing home residents' behavior include recent room changes, incontinence, and the patients' inability to respond to environmental stimuli, such as light and dark' or day and night. Studies by Cohen-Mansfield, Marx, and Rosenthal (1990) indicated that agitation was found more commonly during the day shift than the evening shift. Environmental factors, such as illumination, nursing staff uniform colors, and invasion of personal space; and patient factors, such as premorbid personality, physical pain, febrile illness, and incontinence; can also affect behavior (Vitiello et al., 1992).

▬HYPOTHESES RELATED TO ETIOLOGY

Bliwise (1994) states that there are specific physiologic conditions that may account for sundowning. These are rapid eye movement (REM) sleep behavior disorder, sleep apnea, and deterioration of the suprachiasmatic nucleus.

REM Sleep Behavior Disorder

The syndrome of REM sleep behavior disorder occurs primarily in elderly males, and has been observed and documented by Schenck, Bundlie, Ettinger, and Mahowald (1986). In this syndrome, lesions have been found within the pontine tegmentum. The patient's behavior consists of complex and bizarre motor activities during sleep that occurs without the individual being cognizant of his or her physical surroundings. Studies of these patients show that not all are demented, and some, in fact, are essentially neurologically normal. Because of these factors and the relatively low prevalence of this condition relative to sundowning, these researchers believe

REM behavior is probably a different disorder from the sundowning seen in patients with dementia (Bliwise, 1994).

Sleep Apnea
Sleep apnea, the second possibility suggested by Bliwise (1994), is defined as cessation of respiration for 10 seconds or longer during sleep. In some patients who are affected by sleep apnea, when awakened subsequent to these episodes, confusion and mental status changes are manifested. This behavior also exists in patients who suffer from nocturnal hypoxemia.

Deterioration of the Suprachiasmatic Nucleus
The suprachiasmatic nucleus of the hypothalamus is the principal pacemaker of the circadian system. The retinohypothalamic tracts link the retina to the suprachiasmatic nucleus, conveying information that mediates the synchronization of the circadian pacemaker. A disruption in the sleep-wake cycle can occur if these rhythms are disrupted. Bliwise (1994) states that this hypothesis is the most logical cause of sundowning. The biologic mechanism of circadian rhythms comes from studies that implicate the suprachiasmatic nucleus as the putative biologic clock.

Recent discoveries have indicated that a deterioration in the hypothalamus in patients with dementia is specific for the suprachiasmatic nucleus. If sundowning was shown to exist and to occur at predictable times of the day, the implication that neurologic involvement of portions of the brain that control regular timing of behaviors (such as sleep-wakefulness) and of the physiologic body temperature cycle were involved would be validated.

Early studies by deMairan in the 1700s showed that nearly all biologic systems have the internal capacity to generate endogenous rhythms that persist even in the presence of constant darkness (Vitiello, et al., 1992). In mammals, the variations in sleep-wakefulness, body temperature, cortisol secretion, red blood cell production, blood pressure, and other physiologic parameters are manifestations of these endogenous rhythms. If sundowning falls into the category of time-specific, regularly occurring behavior that is under total or partial control of this circadian timing system, then it may be subject to manipulation and control variables known to affect these systems (Bliwise, 1994).

▰ MANAGEMENT
Pharmacologic Treatment
Treatment of nocturnal confusion of delirium begins with identifying the underlying causes (toxic, infectious, metabolic, or pharmacologic). In the absence of such reversible conditions, pharmacologic treatment for the nocturnal agitation accompanying dementia involves the use of low dose neuroleptics such as haloperidol (Haldol), or thioridazine hydrochloride (Navane). The rationale for using neuroleptics to control aggressive and disordered behavior relates to the effect of these drugs as dopamine-blocking agents (Jenike, 1989). Although this pharmacologic treatment is

used sometimes in acute situations, long-term pharmacotherapy of this type can be problematic.

Side effects of haloperidol include extrapyramidal symptoms that can lead to tardive dyskinesia; side effects of thioridazine hydrochloride may lead to orthostatic hypotension and anticholinergic symptoms. There is little evidence to favor any single neuroleptic in terms of behavioral effects. Periodic withdrawal is recommended to reconfirm the need for such medications (Lipowski, 1989). Bliwise (1994) states that benzodiazepine hypnotics have minimal effects on sundowning. Exum, Phelps, Nabers, and Osborne's (1993) study suggests that a relationship of as-needed medication used for agitation to environmental stimuli not related to the setting sun have contributed to hip fractures or other broken bones while under the influence of psychotropic medication.

The use of propranolol and pindolol for aggressive behavior is reported by Jenike (1989) and Greendyke and Kanter (1986). Although research studies of these drugs have not been specifically directed to the symptoms of sundowning, and the Food and Drug Administration has not approved beta blockers for treatment of psychiatric illness, these studies support their use.

Nonpharmacologic Treatment

Nonpharmacologic treatment is based on environmental and activity factors. Restriction of daytime sleep has shown to ensure better sleep during the night (Bliwise, Bevier, & Bliwise, 1990). Campbell, Satlin, & Volicer (1991) suggest that minimal exposure to bright light may improve sleep in dementia patients.

Okawa, Mishima, & Hishikawa (1994) found that increased contact between staff and patients with dementia was successful in decreasing sundowning behaviors. This finding indicates that the disturbance in the sleep-wake rhythm and the sundowning behavior might be influenced in part by the lack of social stimulation and physical and mental exercise in the daytime. In this particular study, nurses attended to patients individually by talking to them and engaging the patient in walks outdoors for 2 hours in the early morning and one hour in late afternoon. The patients in this study also were restricted from daytime napping.

▬CONCLUSION

Various and conflicting descriptions of the behavior that is known as sundowning is observed in patients with dementia. Environmental and patient characteristics contribute to the phenomenon. The management of sundowning in dementia patients is a challenge for nurses and for caregivers in the home.

When studying possible etiologies for sundowning, it seems logical that the deterioration of the suprachiasmatic nucleus, the mechanism that controls the sleep-wake cycle, could be responsible for the disturbance of circadian rhythm. The importance of understanding this connection can lead to more effective ways to manage the behavior. Pharmacologic treatment for this behavior has drawbacks for the elderly. Alternative non-pharmacologic interventions, such as restriction of daytime sleep, exposure to bright lights, and mild activity schedules, have been effective.

■REFERENCES

American Psychiatric Association. (1994). *Diagnostic and statistical manual of mental health disorders (4th ed.)*. Washington, DC: Author.

Bliwise, D. L. (1994). Dementia. In M. H. Kryger, T. Roth, & W. C. Dement, (Eds.), *Principles and practice of sleep medicine* (pp. 790–800). Philadelphia: W. B. Saunders.

Bliwise, D. L., Bevier, W. C., & Bliwise, N. G. (1990). Systematic 24 hr behavioral observations of sleep and wakefulness in a skilled care nursing facility. *Psychology & Aging, 5*(1), 16–24.

Bliwise, D. L., Carroll, J. S., Lee, K. A., Nekich, J. C., & Dement, W. C. (1993). Sleep and "sundowning" in nursing home patients with dementia. *Psychiatric Research, 48*, 277–292.

Cameron, D. E. (1941). Studies in senile nocturnal dementia. *Psychiatric Quarterly, 15*, 47–53.

Campbell, S., Satlin, A., & Volicer, L. (1991). Management of behavioral and sleep disturbance in Alzheimer's patients using timed exposure to bright light. *Sleep Research, 20*, 446.

Cohen-Mansfield, J., Marx, M. S., & Rosenthal, A. S. (1990). Dementia and agitation in nursing home residents: How are they related? *Psychology and Aging, 5*, 3–8.

Cohen-Mansfield, J., Marx, M. S., Werner, P., & Freeman, L. (1992). Temporal patterns of agitated nursing home residents. *International Psychogeriatrics, 4*, 197–206.

Exum, M. E., Phelps, B. J., Nabers, K. E., & Osborne, J. G. (1993). Sundown syndrome: Is it reflected in the use of PRN medications for nursing home residents? *Gerontologist, 33*, 756–761.

Greendyke, R. M., & Kanter, D. R. (1986). Therapeutic effects of pindodal on behavioral disturbances associated with organic brain disease: A double blind study. *Journal of Clinical Psychiatry, 47*, 423–426.

Jacobs, D., Ancoli-Israel, S., Parker, L., & Krepke, D. F. (1989). 24-hour sleep/wake patterns in a nursing home population. *Psychology & Aging, 48*, 277–292.

Jenike, M. A. (1989). *Geriatric psychiatry and psychopharmacology*. St. Louis, MO: Mosby Year Book.

Lipowski, Z. J. (1989). Delirium in the elderly patient. *New England Journal of Medicine, 320*, 578–582.

Okawa, M., Mishima, K., & Hishikawa, Y. (1991). Circadian rhythm disorder in sleep-waking and body temperature in elderly patients with dementia and their treatment. *Sleep, 14*, 478–485.

Schenck, C. H., Bundlie, S. R., Ettinger, M. G., & Mahowald, M. W. (1986). Chronic behavioral disorders of human REM sleep: A new category of parasomnia. *Sleep, 9*, 293–308.

Vitiello, M. V., Bliwise, D. L., & Prinz, P. N. (1992). Sleep in Alzheimer's disease and the sundown syndrome. *Neurology, 42*(Suppl 6), 83–94.

Chapter 45

Clinical Concerns: AIDS in the Elderly

DEBRA A. SCHUERMAN

Acquired immunodeficiency syndrome (AIDS) is often thought of as only occurring among younger people. As a result, it can be overlooked or not considered in the elderly. But AIDS in older adults makes up 10% of all AIDS cases. As life-prolonging medication combinations are used more successfully, the population will continue to get older. Debra Schuerman discusses the clinical concerns of AIDS in the elderly, including diagnosis, AIDS dementia, and the course of the disease. A nursing implications section addresses issues raised by practitioners, educators, and researchers. Nursing care considerations are included and deal with the issues of clients who require functional assistance earlier than younger AIDS victims and who have a more limited support system.

Diagnosing AIDS in the elderly is a major problem. AIDS often presents in the form of other illnesses that can be misleading in the elderly population (Weiler, 1989). Most often, AIDS presents in a form of dementia that is sometimes confused with Alzheimer's disease (AD) (Sabin, 1987). Perhaps the biggest problem in diagnosing AIDS in elders is that many clinicians fail to recognize AIDS as a possibility (Scharnhorst, 1992).

The nursing implications concerning AIDS in the elderly are endless. Practitioners, educators, and researchers can have a major impact in combating this problem. The purpose of this article is to review the literature concerning AIDS in the elderly and to consider the nursing implications surrounding the issue.

▬ THE PROBLEM

Many health care workers believe that AIDS is one problem with which elders need not be concerned; however, this is no longer true. The number of elders with AIDS is substantial and on the rise (Ship, 1991).

Moss and Miles (1987), however, noted that AIDS may be underreported in the elderly because clinicians are not recognizing it as a possible diagnosis. In addition, older persons may be more reluctant to disclose previous

From *Journal of Gerontological Nursing* 20(7):11–17, 1994. Reproduced with permission.

sexual behavior or drug abuse to their physicians, which also may hinder accurate identification of cases (Ship, 1991).

▰ TRANSMISSION

Sexual contact with homosexual or bisexual men remains the chief mode of transmission of the human immunodeficiency virus (HIV), which causes AIDS. This is true for all age groups except the over-65 group, for which transfusion acquired infection becomes more prevalent (Ship, 1991).

Transfusion is the second leading cause of HIV transmission in persons over 50. When one considers that 25% of all blood transfusions are given to individuals between 50 and 60, and that 15% are given to individuals over 60, it becomes clear why transfusion acquired infection is so prevalent in this age group (Weiler, 1989).

In the study by Ship and colleagues (1991), the researchers compared younger and older persons who had AIDS. They found that the incidence of transmission through male homosexual/bisexual contact and/or intravenous drug use declined with age. In contrast, the proportion of AIDS cases in which blood transfusion was thought to be the cause increased with age.

Although transfusion-acquired infection is the most likely means of transmission in the elderly, other modes must be considered. Catania and coworkers (1989) identified three major groups within the elderly population thought to be at risk for acquiring HIV infection:

- Pre-1985 blood product recipients;
- Spouses of those recipients; and
- Persons who participate in unprotected anal or vaginal intercourse outside a monogamous relationship.

In our society, sexuality often goes together with youth and physical attractiveness. As one ages, therefore, desirability and sexuality are thought to decrease (Parke, 1991). Health care professionals often believe many of the same stereotypes held by the rest of society, and do not view elders as sexual beings (Steinke, 1986). Persons in their later years often are assumed not to be sexually active (Whipple, 1989).

There are some physiologic changes with age that affect the sexual response for both men and women. In men, the time required to achieve an erection is lengthened, and the force and volume of ejaculate is decreased (Steinke, 1986). In women, there is a thinning of the vaginal mucosa and a shortening of the vaginal length and width. In addition, a decrease in vaginal lubrication also is evident (Steinke, 1986).

Despite these physical changes with aging, the elderly can and do remain sexually active. Diokno and associates (1990) found that although frequency of sexual activity declines with age, a majority of persons over 60 remain sexually active — 66.6% of the men and 31.7% of the women in their study. Whipple and Scura (1989) noted that sexually active elders are not using condoms because pregnancy is no longer a concern.

Heterosexual transmission of HIV in the elderly, therefore, should not be overlooked. Rosenzweig and Fillit (1992) reported a case in which an

88-year-old female contracted HIV infection from her husband. Wallace and colleagues (1993) pointed out that elderly women may be at a higher risk of acquiring HIV from an infected partner than elderly men.

The higher risk may be due in part to the changes in the vaginal tissue that occur with aging, making the potential for disruption of the vaginal mucosa greater. Furthermore, infrequent condom use within this population also puts elderly women at risk (Wallace, 1993).

In addition, Butler (1989) stated that one should not underestimate the sexual activity of older persons. He pointed out older men have been known to frequent prostitutes, a group thought to be at high risk for having AIDS.

Homosexuality is a subject that often is not discussed within the elderly population. Whipple and Scura (1989) noted that older men may have more difficulty disclosing their sexual preference. In addition, the authors reported that elderly gay men may be at an increased risk for exposure to HIV. After the death of a long-term mate, the older gay man may turn to a more available, younger partner — who is more likely to be infected with HIV.

Elders may be at risk for HIV infection simply because of a lack of knowledge regarding its transmission. Allers (1990) noted that most educational efforts concerning HIV/AIDS are aimed at teenagers and young adults. Information on how to protect oneself from AIDS, therefore, may not be reaching the elderly population.

DIAGNOSIS

Perhaps the biggest problem with AIDS in the elderly is making the diagnosis. The presentation of AIDS in this age group often can be misleading (Weiler, 1989). Fillit and co-workers (1989) reported a case in which an 89-year-old man presented with easy bruisability and was found to have a low platelet count. The patient was treated with steroids and the platelet count returned to normal. Later, he traveled outside the US and developed a diarrheal illness that forced him to seek medical attention. It was that country's policy for medical treatment of foreigners to include HIV testing; the patient tested positive. The patient's history revealed a blood transfusion in 1983, with no other risk factors.

Another case in which diagnosis was inaccurate was reported by O'Neil and associates (1988). A 73-year-old bachelor was admitted for confusion and falls. He suffered a cardiac arrest and died a week later, before any diagnosis was made. Later, it was discovered that he was a homosexual, and had tested positive for HIV several days prior to admission.

AIDS DEMENTIA

AIDS in the elderly is now being called the "great imitator," because it also can present as a form of dementia that is often mistaken for other chronic illnesses (Sabin, 1987). In the early stages of AIDS dementia the patient may present with apathy, social withdrawal, forgetfulness, loss of concentration, confusion, slowness of thought, loss of balance, and leg weakness. Later symptoms may include moderate to severe dementia, ataxia, moderate to severe weakness, tremors, and seizures (Navia, 1986).

Sabin (1987) noted that AIDS dementia is often confused with AD, because the symptoms are somewhat similar and there is no definite way of diagnosing AD. Weiler and colleagues (1988) reported a case in which the wife of a 63-year-old man was told that her husband was dying of AD and that nothing could be done for him. He appeared wasted and lethargic. Mental status exam results, however, were inconsistent with the diagnosis of AD. The patient's history was positive for a blood transfusion prior to screening for HIV. He was tested for HIV, and the diagnosis of AIDS followed.

Although AIDS dementia and AD have similar presenting symptoms, Sabin (1987) noted some distinguishing characteristics. In early AD, there are no definite neurologic findings. With AIDS dementia, however, ataxia, leg weakness, tremors, and or signs of peripheral neuropathy may be present. In addition, Sabin reported that the aphasia that often accompanies AD is infrequently seen in AIDS dementia. Further, AIDS dementia has been noted to progress more rapidly than AD (Wallace, 1993).

The frequency of dementia in AIDS patients appears to be high. Navia and associates (1986) studied 70 patients with AIDS after death and found AIDS dementia to be present in two thirds of the patients. Further, in 25% of those patients, dementia was the only presenting symptom. Scharnhorst (1992) stressed that AIDS should be considered as a possible diagnosis in the cognitively impaired older person, because dementia may be the only presenting clinical symptom.

◼COURSE OF AIDS IN THE ELDERLY

Wallace and co-workers (1993) reported that elderly patients in early stages of HIV infection often present with vague symptoms that can be confused with other disease processes, making an accurate diagnosis difficult. For instance, decreased appetite, weight loss, fatigue, and diminished physical and mental capabilities often are seen frequently in early HIV infection. Further, Butler (1993) noted that not only are dementia, malnutrition, and pneumonia characteristics of AIDS patients, but also they are seen in many hospitalized elderly patients.

In elders, the course of the disease from initial infection with HIV to development of AIDS appears to be more rapid than in younger individuals. Blaxhult and colleagues (1990) followed cases in HIV infection acquired through blood transfusion and found that increased age at the time of infection shortened the latency period to the development of AIDS. Ship and co-workers (1991) concluded that disease progression and clinical deterioration may be more rapid in the elderly. Further, older adults were more likely to die in the same month as diagnosed with AIDS than younger persons.

Rapid disease progression may be because the diagnosis of HIV infection can be difficult to make in the elderly population. Scharnhorst (1992) noted that late diagnosis also may be attributed to a patient's delay in admitting exposure to HIV, or to clinician's failure to identify HIV/AIDS as a possibility in elders.

■ NURSING IMPLICATIONS

Practitioners

The nursing implications concerning AIDS in the elderly seem endless. Whipple and Scura (1989) stressed the importance of universal precautions to geriatric nurses: wearing gloves, aprons, and protective eye wear when coming in contact with blood or bodily fluids of elderly patients. Again, it is generally thought that the elderly are not at risk for HIV/AIDS, and many nurses are not protecting themselves.

Nurses, as primary caregivers, have more contact with the patient who has, or might have, HIV/AIDS than any other health care provider. Therefore, they must be informed regarding all aspects of care concerning elderly patients with HIV/AIDS in order to protect themselves (Scura, 1990). Especially because AIDS can present in many different ways, the geriatric nurse practitioner or clinician must recognize AIDS as a possible diagnosis in elderly patients.

In addition, the importance of accurate histories is essential. The history should include previous surgical procedures that may have entailed a blood transfusion, previous IV drug use, and current and past sexual practices. This history is important in order to avoid misdiagnosis of AIDS dementia (Scharnhorst, 1992).

Educators

Tichy and Talashek (1992) noted that it is imperative that schools of nursing address HIV/AIDS across the life span. It is important for students to understand that AIDS is not necessarily a disease of the young.

Further, Hinkle (1991) stressed that nurses have an important role in educating their colleagues and the public regarding the transmission and prevention of AIDS in elders. Hinkle (1991) went on to note that AIDS has not yet become endemic to this population; thus, nurses have a window of time in which to act with educational measures to help curtail the spread of AIDS in the elderly.

Researchers

Whipple and Scura (1989) reported that there is a "paucity" of literature available concerning HIV/AIDS in the elderly. In doing this review, little nursing literature nursing literature was found. The biggest gap lies in the area of elders' knowledge concerning HIV/AIDS transmission and perceptions of risk level. In order to target educational efforts, further research must be done to assess the knowledge base of elders' regarding HIV/AIDS transmission.

In addition, several sources speculated that condom use within this population is low. Tichy and Talashek (1992) noted that there is limited data available on condom use within the elderly population. Clearly, more research in this area is necessary.

▬NURSING CARE

In considering nursing care of the elder with HIV infection, it is important to remember that an older person is more likely to present with AIDS at the time of diagnosis (Ferro, 1992). Keeping this in mind, actual nursing care of the elderly patient with AIDS does not differ greatly from a younger patient with AIDS (Fillit, 1989).

However, Kendig and Adler (1990) pointed out that elders with AIDS often require functional assistance sooner, and may not have the family support system in place for care at home. Consequently, AIDS patients of all age groups are beginning to be cared for in long-term care facilities.

Nurses can play a significant role in providing comfort to the elderly patient with AIDS. Frequently seen problems, such as pain, gastrointestinal symptoms, fevers, potential for skin breakdown, falls and drug reactions, can be particularly distressing to the elder with AIDS. The following sections represent specific comfort measures in providing nursing care to the elderly patient with AIDS.

Pain

Pain is not uncommon to the person with AIDS. The goal of pain management is to allow the patient to be pain free, or to decrease the pain to a tolerable level. This usually is done in the form of narcotic analgesia, titrated to individual patient response (Nelson, 1991).

Malaise and generalized body discomfort commonly are seen in the bedridden AIDS patient. Non-narcotic pain medications, such as aspirin, acetaminophen, and nonsteroidal anti-inflammatory drugs, may be helpful in relieving discomfort. Massage therapy also may be of great benefit — physically and emotionally (Abrams, 1989).

Neurogenic pain often can be the most distressing and difficult to relieve. Peripheral neuropathy is common as the HIV infection invades the neural pathways. Narcotics may have limited benefits in such cases. Other classifications of drugs may be ordered by the physician. Antidepressants (specifically tricyclics) and anticonvulsants have been used with some success (Abrams, 1989).

Common oral lesions seen in AIDS patients also can cause significant discomfort. Oral candidiasis is a fungal infection that frequently is present. Its appearance resembles that of cottage cheese; it adheres to the mucosa of the mouth and/or the esophagus. These lesions often are painful; in the presence of esophageal involvement, dysphagia, chest pain, substernal burning, and nausea also may be present (Abrams, 1989).

Treatment of oral candidiasis is done with oral antifungal medications. In addition, meticulous oral care is important. Abrams and associates (1989) suggested using a soft toothbrush to gently scrub the teeth, gums and tongue, and then rinsing with salt or lemon water, or mouthwash, before meals and antifungal treatments.

In the presence of painful oral lesions, a soft diet also may be necessary to decrease discomfort (Abrams, 1989). A soft diet may be of particular importance to the elderly patient who is unable to wear dentures due to painful oral lesions.

Viscous solution of lidocaine 2% may be of benefit before meals if swallowing is painful (O'Brien, 1993). In order to prevent injury, however, patients should be cautioned against consuming extremely hot foods or liquids when using oral lidocaine in this manner (Abrams, 1989).

Gastrointestinal Symptoms

Diarrhea is a problem frequently seen in AIDS patients. A number of different parasites and bacteria can cause diarrhea. Some microorganisms respond to treatment and others do not, causing distress to both patient and nurse. Nelson (1991) pointed out that the goals in cases of persistent diarrhea include providing adequate nutrition and maintaining hydration, in order to keep the patient hemodynamically stable.

Specific measures include watching intake and output, keeping calorie counts, monitoring electrolytes, and observing for signs of dehydration (Nelson, 1991). Other helpful suggestions include avoiding foods or medications that may aggravate diarrhea, such as antacids that contain magnesium, stool softeners, milk products, and commercially prepared nutritional supplements (eg, Ensure). Liberal intake of clear fluids should be encouraged. Fresh fruits and vegetables should be replaced with canned products, and foods high in potassium also should be encouraged (Abrams, 1989).

Nausea and vomiting (N&V) also are a problem in patients with AIDS. A variety of factors, ranging from infection to medication side effects, can produce symptoms. In treating N&V, Abrams and co-workers (1989) suggested holding food, as well as fluids, for 1 to 2 hours. Fluids then can be restarted in the form of ice chips or clear liquids in small amounts (30 mL/hr) for 2 to 3 hours. Fluids then can be increased gradually to normal intake during the next several hours.

Food can be reintroduced once the cause of N&V has been established or antiemetics have been started. Other helpful measures to decrease N&V include application of a cool compress to the forehead, providing fresh air to the patient's room, and giving frequent oral care (Abrams, 1989).

Fevers

One of the most common problems encountered by AIDS patients is fever followed by profuse sweating. Fevers can be a result of infection or medication, or be idiopathic in nature. Nursing goals are to monitor and report fevers to the physician and provide patient comfort. Common comfort measures include administering acetaminophen, encouraging fluids, and giving a tepid or alcohol bath. A cooling mattress may be necessary when other measures are unsuccessful in lowering body temperature (Nelson, 1991).

Skin Breakdown

Skin breakdown is of major concern to the patient with AIDS. It is of special importance to the bedridden elderly patient with AIDS. With the aging process, muscle mass and subcutaneous fat are decreased, increasing the chance for skin breakdown.

Initial steps to prevent skin breakdown include performing a complete assessment, noting any reddened areas that require attention. Frequent changing of position, with massaging of pressure areas, can greatly help to reduce the potential for skin breakdown. In addition, the use of special mattresses, flotation pads, fleeces, and alternating pressure mattresses may prevent pressure sores (Nelson, 1989).

In the presence of diarrhea, frequent skin care to the perineal area is essential. After each loose stool, the skin should be washed with warm soapy water and dried, and a skin barrier cream should be applied (Abrams, 1989).

Falls

Falls are known to be a problem among the elderly (Costa, 1991). To the elderly patient with AIDS, falls may be of special concern. Such conditions are malaise, fatigue and pain, which are common to AIDS patients, can impair mobility and increase the likelihood of falls. Altered mental status, as seen with AIDS dementia, also may increase the potential for the risk for falls within this population (Nelson, 1991).

Identifying whether a patient is at risk for falls is an important goal in caring for the elderly patient with AIDS. It is important to note the patient's mental status, ability to perform activities of daily living, and gait. If the patient is at risk for falls, instructing him or her to call for assistance when getting up may be necessary. If the patient cannot be relied on to call for assistance, restraints or constant supervision may be required (Nelson, 1991).

Drug Reactions

Currently, the only way to slow progression of HIV infection is by using antiviral drugs, such as zidovudine (AZT). The elderly are a population known to have adverse reactions to many drugs. Kendig and Adler (1990) noted that the side effects with use of antiviral agents within this population are not widely known. Wallace and colleagues (1993) stressed that monitoring for adverse reactions is extremely important when using HIV/AIDS-related medications in elderly patients.

■ CONCLUSION

AIDS in the elderly is a growing concern. Nursing will have a major role in beginning to recognize AIDS within the elderly population, and in formalizing educational efforts to combat this deadly disease. Further, as more elders with AIDS enter hospitals and extended care facilities, nurses will have a greater impact in providing treatment and comfort to them.

■ REFERENCES

Abrams, D. I., Martin, J., Unger, K. W. AIDS: Caring for the dying patient. *Patient Care* 1989;23:22–36.

Allers, C. T. AIDS and the older adult. *Gerontologist* 1990;30(3):405–407.

Blaxhult, A., Granath, F., Lindman, K., Giesecke, J. The influence of age on the latency period to AIDS in people infected by HIV through blood transfusion. *AIDS* 1990;4(2):125–129.

Butler, R. N. Geriatric AIDS is a growing concern. *Geriatrics* 1989;44(7):21.

Butler, R. N. AIDS: Older patients aren't immune. *Geriatrics* 1993;48(3):9–10.

Catania, J. A., Turner, H., Kegeles, S. M., Stall, R., Pollack, L., Coates, T. J. Older Americans and AIDS: Transmission risks and primary prevention research needs. *Gerontologist* 1989;29(3):373–381.

Centers for Disease Control. *HIV/AIDS Surveillance Report,* 1993;5(2):8.

Costa, A. J. Preventing falls in your elderly patients. *Postgrad Med* 1991;89(1):139–142.

Diokno, A. C., Brown, M. B., Herzog, A. R. Sexual function in the elderly. *Arch Intern Med* 1990;150:197–200.

Ferro, S., Salit, I. E. HIV infection in patients over 55 years of age. *J Acquir Immune Defic Syndr* 1992;5(4):348–355.

Fillit, H., Fruchtman, S., Sell, L., Rosen, N. AIDS in the elderly: A case and its implications. *Geriatrics* 1989;44(7):65–70.

Hinkle, K. L. A literature review: HIV seropositivity in the elderly. *Journal of Gerontological Nursing* 1991;17(10):12–17.

Kendig, N. E., Adler, W. H. The implications of the acquired immunodeficiency syndrome for gerontology research and geriatric medicine. *J Gerontol* 1990;45(3):77–80.

Moss, R. J., Miles, J. H. AIDS and the geriatrician. *J Am Geriatr Soc* 1987;35(5):460–464.

Navia, B. A., Jordan, B. D., Price, R. W. The AIDS dementia complex: I. Clinical features. *Ann Neurol* 1986;19(6):517–524.

Nelson, W. J. Nursing care of acutely ill persons with AIDS. In J. Durham, F. Cohen (Eds.), *The person with AIDS: Nursing perspectives.* New York: Springer, 1991, pp. 206–225.

O'Brien, M. E., Pheifer, W. G. Physical and psychosocial nursing care for patients with HIV infection. *Nurs Clin North Am* 1993;28(2):303–315.

O'Neil, D., Coakley, D., Walsh, J. B., O'Neil, J. HIV seropositivity in a geriatric medical unit [Letter to the editor]. *Postgrad Med J* 1988;64:832–834.

Parke, F. Sexuality in later life. *Nursing Times* 1991;87(50):40–42.

Rosenzweig, R., Fillit, H. Probable heterosexual transmission of AIDS in an aged woman. *J Am Geriatr Soc* 1992;40(12):61–70.

Sabin, T. D. AIDS: The new "great imitator." *J Am Geriatr Soc* 1987;35(5):467–468.

Scharnhorst, S. AIDS dementia complex in the elderly. *Nurse Pract* 1992;17(8):37–43.

Scura, K. W., Whipple, B. Older adults as an HIV-positive risk group. *Journal of Gerontological Nursing* 1990;16(2):6–10.

Ship, J. A., Wolff, A., Selik, R. M. Epidemiology of acquired immune deficiency syndrome in persons aged 50 years or older. *J Acquir Immune Defic Syndr* 1991;4(1):84–88.

Steinke, E. E., Bergen, M. B. Sexuality and aging. *Journal of Gerontological Nursing* 1986;12(6):6–10.

Tichy, A. M., Talashek, M. L. Older women: sexually transmitted diseases and acquired immunodeficiency syndrome. *Nurs Clin North Am* 1992;27(4):937–947.

Wallace, J. I., Paauw, D. S., Spach, D. H. HIV infection in older patients: When to expect the unexpected. *Geriatrics* 1993;48(6):61–70.

Weiler, P. G. Why AIDS is becoming a geriatric problem. *Geriatrics* 1989;44(7):81–87.

Weiler, P. G., Mungas, D., Pomerantz, S. AIDS as a cause of dementia in the elderly. *J Am Geriatr Soc* 1988;36(2):139–141.

Whipple, B., Scura, K. W. HIV and the older adult: Taking the necessary precautions. *Journal of Gerontological Nursing* 1989;15(9):15–19.

Chapter 46

Alzheimer's Disease, a Hopeful Note for the Closing of a Century: Challenges for the New Millennium

LINDA J. HEWETT   FEN-LEI CHANG

The incidence of Alzheimer's disease (AD) increases as people age. As more of us live into our 80s and beyond, the issue of AD becomes more significant. AD diagnosis and successful case management is important for those involved; the aging person, caregivers, health care providers, and families. Diagnosis and management are discussed in this chapter, which was written expressly for this edition by two experts in the field of Alzheimer's disease. Linda Hewett and Fen-Lei Chang give an overview of the latest research and management modalities within the complexities of this disease. Specifics are shared about the interprofessional collaborative approach to research, diagnosis, and the services for clients, caregivers, and students of AD, who are part of the program at the UCSF Alzheimer's Disease Center in Fresno, CA; a model program for replication elsewhere.

■ INTRODUCTION

Alzheimer's disease (AD) has risen from relative obscurity over the past two decades. Once considered a rare disorder, it is now recognized as a major public health problem having a severe impact on millions of Americans and their families. Clinicians accept that the illness seen in a relatively young woman (age 55) and described by Dr. Alois Alzheimer in a German medical journal in 1907 is the same illness that produces the majority of cases of progressive dementia in the elderly today.

The giving of a name to this illness is important. Until quite recently physicians and families accepted vague diagnostic labels such as "atherosclerosis" or "organic brain syndrome" as suitable explanations for the slow and inexorable brain failure noted in many elderly patients. Acceptance of a name that encompasses recognizable signs and symptoms implies a need for diagnosis and a rationale for management that extends beyond the excuse of "old age" or willfulness.

This chapter is original for this book.

The concentrated work of academic Alzheimer's Disease Research Centers (ADRCs) and Diagnostic Centers (ADCs) around the United States and the growing political power and support of such groups as the Alzheimer's Association (AA) and the American Association of Retired Persons (AARP) have kept the spotlight on Alzheimer's disease and forced the tremendous progress that has been witnessed in the latter decade of this century.

Without the articulation of a diagnosis, patients and families are left in limbo as to the reasons for the patient's symptoms, and are unable to access and utilize available treatments and support resources. Ten years ago those with early signs of dementia might have been ignored or swept into the broad and poorly defined category of senile dementia. With the recognition of Alzheimer's disease as a distinct and common disease, progress in diagnosing it has been rapid. Although development of a simple, reliable, inexpensive, and specific early marker is still some way off, it is now possible to diagnose AD with 85 to 90 percent accuracy.

▰PUBLIC HEALTH IMPACT: PREVALENCE AND COSTS

Currently, it is estimated that AD affects 4 million Americans, with slightly more than half being cared for at home. However, because AD is not routinely reported on death certificates, estimates of prevalence vary. AD is an age-associated disease, with the risk increasing exponentially with each decade of late life. Thus, at age 65 one's risk is about 5 percent for developing the disease. By age 75 the risk has increased to about 18 percent, and by age 85 the risk is substantial and may be as high as 47 percent among the "oldest-old" (those aged 85 and older) (Evans, 1990; Jorm, Corten, Henderson, 1987).

Life expectancy has been increasing since the turn of the century and there are now approximately 33 million people aged 65 and older, accounting for about 13 percent of the total population of the United States. According to the Bureau of the Census (1995), this percentage will increase to 20 percent by the year 2030. In addition, this number and the proportion of the "oldest-old," who are often most in need of care, will increase dramatically. Currently 3.5 million, the number of Americans aged 85 and older, will total nearly 9 million by the year 2030.

It is conservatively estimated that as many as 3.1 million spouses, relatives, and friends provide care to people with AD. This informal network of caregivers forms the backbone of the long-term care system for AD patients. AD has been estimated to cost the nation $80–90 billion a year. This figure includes both direct outlays, such as for nursing care, as well as indirect costs, such as lost productivity on the part of patients and the family members who care for them (Ernst & Hay, 1994). Caring for a patient with AD costs more than $47,000 a year whether the person lives at home or in a nursing home, according to a recent study in northern California (Ernst & Hay, 1994). This study found that families of AD patients living at home spent about $12,000 annually per family for formal services, such as physician and home health care services. However, when the researchers added the estimated cost of unpaid, informal care provided by family members, the total annual cost was comparable to the cost of nursing home care.

▰ NEW APPROACHES TO CAUSE, DIAGNOSIS, TREATMENT AND CARE

Alzheimer's disease is a progressive neurodegenerative disease marked by changes in behavior and personality and by a decline in thinking abilities that cannot be reversed. AD is the most common of the irreversible dementias, accounting for about 60 percent of these disorders. As AD progresses it gradually destroys memory, reason, judgment, language, and eventually the ability to carry out even the simplest of tasks. Although AD can now be diagnosed with great accuracy, definitive diagnosis is still only possible when an autopsy confirms the hallmark presence of amyloid plaques and neurofibrillary tangles in the cerebral cortical areas.

Located outside and around neurons, plaques are dense deposits of amyloid protein and other associated proteins. Neurofibrillary tangles are abnormal collections of twisted threads inside the nerve cell bodies. These tangles are the remains of the neuron's microtubules, the cells internal support structures, composed of a protein called tau (Khachaturian & Radebaugh, 1995).

AD begins in the entorrhinal cortex and spreads to the hippocampus, eventually involving the association cortices of the brain and disrupting all higher cognitive processes. The hippocampus is a way station essential to memory formation and storage. As hippocampal neurons degenerate, short-term memory falters and performance of other routine tasks begins to deteriorate as well. As the disease spreads through the cortex it affects language, first with word finding difficulty, but gradually affecting all aspects of expressive and receptive language. Judgment and problem-solving ability declines, so that a person must have supervision at all times, and safety becomes the highest priority.

Disturbing behaviors, such as wandering and agitation, are common as the disease progresses. In its final stages AD extinguishes the ability to recognize even close family members, and all sense of self seems to vanish. Patients often live for years in a completely dependent state, exhausting their funds and their caregivers, eventually to die of pneumonia or some other infection. The duration of AD may be 20 years or more, with the average length of time from diagnosis to death being about 4 to 8 years (Khachaturian & Radebaugh, 1995; Reisburg, 1996).

The Search for Causes

There is a great deal of variability between patients in age of onset, cognitive function, behavioral features, rate of progression, associated motor deficits, and so on, reflecting the heterogeneous nature and multiple etiologies of AD. In the past two decades, neuroscientists have concentrated on the search for defects that might explain what goes wrong in AD. Promising leads involve the role of neurotransmitters, proteins, genes, metabolism, and environmental suspects.

The messaging system of the brain is complex. When a neurotransmitter binds to a receptor, it triggers a cascade of biochemical interactions that relay the message to the neuron's nucleus or to the end of the axon and to the next neuron. In this process, a number of genes may be activated, various proteins are implicated, and metabolism must be intact.

Neuroscientists are finding new clues to AD in postsynaptic receptors, which are coil-shaped proteins embedded in the neuron membrane. The protein molecules have bonds with phospholipids, that lie next to them in the postsynaptic membrane. Several studies have detected phospholipid abnormalities in neurons affected by AD. It is possible that these abnormalities change the behavior of neighboring receptors, garbling the message as it passes from neuron to neuron.

Neurotransmitters

Neurotransmitters are released into the synapse when electrical impulses pass along the axon. They pass across the synapse and bind to a receptor molecule in the membrane of the next neuron. The neurotransmitter then either breaks down or uptakes back into the first neuron, whereas other substances in the second neuron pick up and relay the message.

Acetylcholine is a critical neurotransmitter in the process of reasoning and the formation of memories. Levels of acetylcholine fall drastically in the hippocampus and cerebral cortex of persons with AD, areas that are known to be devastated in the disease. It is known that levels of acetylcholine fall in normal aging but, in those with AD, levels drop by about 90 percent. Other neurotransmitters have also been implicated in AD. Serotonin, somatostatin, and noradrenaline levels have been found to be diminished in AD and may be a cause of aggressive behavior and sensory disturbances in some persons (Geula & Mesulam, 1994).

Proteins

Plaques, the neuropathological hallmark of AD, are composed of a protein fragment called beta amyloid mixed with other proteins. Beta amyloid is a string of about 40 amino acids formed from a larger protein called amyloid precursor protein (APP). What happens to the beta amyloid once it is processed from the APP is unclear. However, research suggests: (1) it may be toxic to neurons; (2) it may cause the release of free radicals that attack neurons; (3) it may attack channel function in neuron membranes that allow calcium levels to rise within the neuron — excess calcium can be lethal to any cell; (4) it may disrupt potassium homeostasis, also known to affect calcium levels; or (5) it may reduce choline levels in the neuron, disrupting the cell's ability to synthesize acetylcholine.

Chronic inflammatory processes may be involved in events leading to the deposition of beta amyloid and/or steps linking beta amyloid to neuronal degeneration. Anti-inflammatory drugs have been proposed as protective against AD (McGreer, Schulzer, & McGreer, 1996).

The neuron's internal structure, or microtubule, carries nutrients from the body of the cell to the axon ends. Tau protein forms cross bars between the microtubules giving strength and stability to the structure. In cells

affected by AD, the microtubule collapses when the abnormally phosphory-
lated tau in the crosspieces degenerates into paired helical filaments and
forms tangles, another neuropathological marker.

Having identified beta amyloid and tau, researchers are now working
to find out what they do in the brain and in AD. The study of certain genes
known to be linked to AD may lead to new information about the functions
of these proteins (Cotman & Pike, 1994; Kosik & Greenberg, 1994).

Genes

All genes function by transcribing their codes into proteins. Apolipoprotein
E (apoE) is a carrier of cholesterol in blood, but has been found to bind
quickly and tightly to beta amyloid. The gene apoE, which produces the
protein, is found on chromosome 19 and one version of it is now known
to be much more common among Alzheimer's patients than among the
general population. Like other genes, apoE comes in three different forms
or alleles, apoE2, apoE3, and apoE4, ApoE3 is the most common in the
general population. However, apoE4 occurs in approximately 40 percent
of all late-onset AD patients, including those so-called "sporadic" cases
with no known family history of the disease. Dozens of studies have now
confirmed that the apoE4 allele increases the risk of developing AD. Those
inheriting two apoE4 genes are at least eight times more likely to develop
AD than those inheriting two copies of the apoE3 gene. The least common
apoE2 gene seems to lower the risk. This research promises to increase
our understanding of the role of these genes and their proteins and, in
particular, apoE4's role in causing beta amyloid to become insoluble and
the tau infrastructure of the microtubule to disassemble. However, apoE4
is not a consistent marker for AD and apoE4 testing is not recommended
for screening.

AD strikes early and often in certain families identified around the world.
This early-onset form of the disease is called "Familial" AD (FAD). A
mutation on chromosome 21 is common to some of these families, but a
larger group of families have a marker on chromosome 14 associated with
an abnormality in a membrane protein so-called presenilin 1. The chromosome 21 gene carries the code for a mutated form of the amyloid precursor
protein, APP, the parent protein for beta amyloid, supporting the theory
that beta amyloid plays a role in AD. However, this mutation only occurs
in about 5 percent of early-onset FAD. Recently a mutation on chromosome
1, another protein abnormality called presenilin 2, has been implicated in
the form of FAD that affects Volga Germans (Levy-Lahad, Wijsman, &
Nemens, 1995). Researchers believe that several other genes are involved
in AD and that other conditions, such as a problem with glucose metabolism, must be present for AD to develop (St. George-Hyslop, 1994).

Metabolism

The mechanism of glucose metabolism is complex, but simply put, transporter molecules carry glucose molecules through the blood-brain barrier
into the neurons. Transporter molecules come in several forms, but two
of them (GLUT1 and GLUT3) have been found to be in short supply in

the brains of AD patients. Other studies have found that enzymes important in glucose metabolism are also produced at lower levels in AD. Neurons are wholly dependent on glucose for their sustenance. When glucose metabolism falters, they cannot manufacture acetylcholine at the normal rate and they affect glutamate metabolism, allowing calcium to flood into the cells causing neuronal death (Beal, 1994).

Environmental Suspects

While the role of genetics is not disputed, many researchers believe that environmental factors may contribute to the development of AD. Aluminum, zinc, foodborne toxins, and viruses have been the most studied.

Aluminum is the most controversial of the environmental suspects in AD. It has been found in abnormally high levels in the brains of AD patients at autopsy. It is also found in many common household and personal products, such as cooking pans, antacids, and deodorants. Although some studies have found an association between aluminum exposure and AD, others have found no association at all. What has been found is that the presence of abnormally high aluminum levels at autopsy may have more to do with a particular staining technique than premorbid exposure, that aluminum from vegetables such as potatoes is not well-absorbed by the body, and that the aluminum from cooking utensils is not in a form that is absorbed by the body (Markesbery & Ehmann, 1994).

Zinc is another element surrounded by ambiguous information. Some reports have suggested that low levels of zinc observed at autopsy might have contributed to the development of AD. Conversely, one recent experiment found that zinc caused soluble beta amyloid from the cerebrospinal fluid to clump in a similar form to the plaques associated with AD (Markesbery & Ehmann, 1994).

Foodborne poisons have come under scrutiny because some cases of dementia, reportedly caused by vegetable amino acids acting as glutamate antagonists, have been observed in Africa, India, and Guam. Similarly, dementia was reported among people who had eaten mussels contaminated with demoic acid. Study of these rare types of dementia may illuminate underlying mechanisms of neuronal degeneration (Gatz, Lowe, Berg, et al., 1994).

The discovery of a link between a viral agent, or more properly, a virus particle called a prion, and the infectious Creutzfeld-Jakob disease and other diseases has spurred researchers to look for a similar viral, or infectious, link to AD. Prion disease is relatively rare in humans but infection is thought to occur many years prior to the actual onset of the dementing process (Ironside, 1996).

Risk Factors

Thus far, only two risk factors have been solidly linked to AD, although several epidemiologic studies are under way. Age is a risk factor for AD, with the numbers of affected people doubling in each decade after age 65. Family history is the other known risk factor. Those with a relative who has developed AD have a genetic predisposition that may increase their own risk by an estimated 5 percent (Khatchaturian & Radebaugh, 1995).

Other minor risk factors are prior head injury, gender, and educational level. Even decreased idea density in early life has been considered as a potential risk factor (Snowden, Kemper, Mortimer, et al., 1996). Some studies have suggested that AD occurs with greater frequency among those who suffered traumatic head injuries earlier in life. Women also may have a higher risk of developing AD, although their rates may really only reflect the fact that women live longer than men on the average. Lower education levels are also implicated as a risk factor for the development of AD, since some studies have suggested that the greater number of years of formal education a person has the less likely he or she is to develop AD (Khatachurian & Radebaugh, 1994; Paschalis, Polychronopoulos, & Lekka, 1990).

Other Forms of Neurodegenerative Dementia

The advent of specialized diagnostic and research centers for AD has led to greater accuracy in diagnosis. Experience with the many presentations of dementia has facilitated description of several subtypes of dementia that are now seen as something other than AD.

Lewy Body Dementia (LBD), also referred to as Diffuse Lewy Body Disease and Lewy Body variant of AD, has clinical and pathological features that are distinct from AD. Cognitive impairment may fluctuate, and the disease may progress rapidly to an end stage of severe dementia. Parkinsonian features such as bradykinesia, cogwheel rigidity, or postural instability are common, whereas tremor is rare (McKeith, Fairbairn, & Perry, et al., 1992). Visual hallucinations are common, occurring in perhaps 80 percent of patients with LBD, whereas they are less common in classic AD and occur later in the disease process. Hallucinations in LBD typically feature complex scenes with animals, children, or supernatural creatures often visualized in miniature (Cummings & Miller, 1987). Treatment of hallucinations with neuroleptics may cause severe Parkinsonian symptoms in patients with LBD owing to loss of dopaminergic neurons in the substantia nigra. Careful medication dosage adjustment is required. Pathologically Lewy bodies are seen in the substantia nigra and cortex, staining positively with ubiquitin. Plaques are less common than in AD and tangles are rare (McKeith, Fairbairn, Bothwell, et al., 1994).

Frontal Lobe Dementia (FLD) is a neurodegenerative process characterized by prominent behavioral and personality changes early in the course of the disease. In contrast to AD, memory, spatial, and praxis problems are not among the first presenting symptoms. FLD often has its onset prior to age 65, may be associated with motor neuron disease in some cases, and for a subgroup, has a familial component that is associated with chromosome 17 (Wilhelmsen, Lynch, & Pavlou, 1994). Once considered rare, and indistinguishable prior to death, FLD may account for 25 percent of all presenile dementias. Disinhibition, apathy, social withdrawal, hyperorality, and ritualistic compulsive behaviors are common presenting behavioral manifestations of FLD (Miller, Cummings, Villanueva-Meyer, et al., 1991). Patients with FLD demonstrate decreased speech with verbal stereotypies early on.

Executive functions such as planning, organization and completion of complex activities are also lost early in FLD. In contrast, comprehension, geographic orientation, copying skills, and memory are relatively spared. This pattern of deficits is related to neuronal loss in the prefrontal and temporal areas of the cortex with a resulting serotonergic defect (Miller, Datby, Swartz, et al., 1995). Functional imaging with positron emission tomography (PET) and single photon emission computed tomography (SPECT) will increase the diagnostic accuracy of FLD (Read, Miller, Mena, et al., 1995).

Lobar atrophies are much rarer forms of disease causing asymmetrical or focal cortical degenerative syndromes. Three syndromes in this category are progressive nonfluent aphasia, progressive frontal lobe syndrome, and perceptual-motor impairment. Perceptual-motor impairment is characterized by the presence of dementia with early, prominent visuospatial dysfunction, apraxia and prominent parieto-occipital atrophy (Casselli, Jack, Petersen, et al., 1992; Victoroff, Ross, Benson, et al., 1994).

■ DIAGNOSIS AND TREATMENT: A MULTIDISCIPLINARY MODEL

Lacking a clear direction for cure or prevention, the immediate challenge is to ensure comprehensive and specific diagnosis and treatments that address quality of life issues presented by the behaviors and symptoms of each individual. Early diagnosis will become even more critical in the future as more effective treatments become available to slow down progression of the disease, and ultimately to halt it. Eventually it is to be hoped that those at risk can be identified before the earliest symptoms of the disease have started so that treatment to prevent onset may be initiated.

The UCSF Fresno/Alzheimer's Disease Center (ADC) is one of the nine multidisciplinary Alzheimer's Disease Diagnostic and Treatment Centers (ADDTCs) funded in part by the State of California Alzheimer's Disease Program. Affiliated with the UCSF School of Medicine, the ADC maintains an academic program for medical students and residents in varying disciplines (e.g., family medicine, internal medicine, and psychiatry). Close educational ties are also maintained with the Gerontology, Nursing, and Social Work programs of California State University, Fresno (CSUF). It is the ADDTCs' firm philosophy that patients deserve as full an evaluation of their cognitive problems as they would receive for any other disease process. Having received a diagnosis, an explanation of it is ethically warranted, and implies a responsibility to direct patients and their families to the available medical and community resources that will facilitate coping and symptom management (Post & Whitehouse, 1995).

A comprehensive state-of-the-art diagnostic work-up by our multidisciplinary team is the primary objective for all patients and their families who come to the Center. The multidisciplinary team is composed of a family practitioner, geriatric psychiatrist, neurologist, neuropsychologist, clinical psychologist, nurse educator, and social worker. Clarification of the diagnosis leads to a full treatment plan which includes recommendations for medical management, treatment of psychiatric symptoms, legal and financial planning, management of 24-hour supervision, and placement, with care taken to provide resources and recommendations that are culturally sensitive and appropriate. Clinical drug trials are available and opportunities for participation are offered to qualified patients.

AD cannot be determined through computerized tomography (CT), electroencephalography (EEG), or other laboratory tests alone, although specific causes of dementia may be identified by these means (National Institute on Aging, 1995). Dementia is caused by many conditions; some conditions can be reversed, others cannot. Further, many different medical conditions may cause symptoms that seem like Alzheimer's disease, but are not. Some of these medical conditions may be treatable. Reversible conditions causing dementia include infections, dehydration, vitamin B_{12} or folate deficiencies and poor nutrition, medication side effects and polypharmacy, hypothyroidism, or normal pressure hydrocephalus.

A thorough diagnostic work-up will uncover such conditions, and allow treatment of these potentially reversible causes (NIH Consensus Conference, 1987). However, it is clear that a high proportion of patients with apparently "reversible" causes for their dementia have an underlying concurrent neurodegenerative process; thus the dementia is not truly reversible but will progress despite the treatment.

Dementia patients are at high risk for delirium, which can produce irreversible damage if allowed to go untreated. It is especially important to differentiate AD from toxic-metabolic encephalopathy, vascular dementia (VaD), Lewy Body dementia, and frontal lobe dementia (Cummings & Benson, 1992) because of the differing treatment/management implications.

Although it is critical to attempt to distinguish between dementia caused by depression and degenerative dementias such as AD, accurate diagnosis must take into account that they often coexist. Depression occurs in 25 to 30 percent of patients diagnosed with AD, and isolated depressive symptoms are more common than major depression (Teri, Robins, & Whitehouse, et al., 1992).

Clinicians diagnose "possible AD" and "probable AD" using criteria established in 1984 by the National Institute of Neurological and Communicative Disorders and Stroke and the Alzheimer's Disease and Related Disease Association (NINCDS/ADRDA Guidelines; see Table 46-1).

A comprehensive multidisciplinary, diagnostic workup includes a full patient history, physical examination, and laboratory tests, usually including a brain scan, and neuropsychological testing. A multidisciplinary team approach has the advantage of several professionals evaluating the patient on multiple occasions and from different professional perspectives. This may be of critical importance in the early stages of AD, since patients are able to preserve a "normal" facade in response to conventional inquiries as to health and particular problems during the course of a short office visit. Evaluation by a nurse or social worker provides critical information regarding the needed resources for continued home care, as well as an assessment of the impact of the caregiving role on family members.

It is critical to interview collateral informants when gathering a detailed description of how and when symptoms developed, the patient's and fam-

---

TABLE 46-1 NINCDS-ADRDA* Diagnostic Criteria for Alzheimer's Disease (AD) (McKhann et al., 1984)

Definite AD
  Clinical criteria for probable AD
  Histopathological evidence of AD (autopsy or biopsy)

Probable AD
  Dementia established by clinical examination and documented by mental status question-
    naire
  Dementia confirmed by neuropsychological testing
  Deficits in two or more areas of cognition
  Progressive worsening of memory and other cognitive functions
  No disturbance of consciousness
  Onset between ages 40 and 90
  Absence of systemic or other brain diseases capable of producing a dementia syndrome

Possible AD
  Atypical onset, presentation, or progression of a dementia syndrome without a known eti-
    ology
  A systemic or other brain disease capable of producing dementia but not thought to be
    the cause of dementia is present
  There is a gradually progressive decline in a single intellectual function in the absence of
    any other identifiable cause

Unlikely AD
  Sudden onset
  Focal signs
  Seizures or gait disturbance early in the course of the illness

---

Note. From "Clinical diagnosis of Alzheimer's disease: Report of the NINCDS-ADRDA Work Group under the auspices of Department of Health and Human Services Task Force on Alzheimer's Disease." by
McKhann, G., Drachman, D., Folstein, M., Katzman, R., Price, D., & Stadlan, E. M., 1984, *Neurology*
*34:*939–944. Copyright American Academy of Neurology, with permission.
* NINCDS-ADRDA = National Institute of Neurological and Communicative Disorders and Stroke and
the Alzheimer's Disease and Related Disorders Association.

ily's medical history, and an assessment of the patient's emotional and functional status and living environment. A multidisciplinary team approach usually incorporates a home visit that may be crucial in the assessment of safety hazards within the home, the accuracy of family estimates of independent function, and the availability of convenient and attainable community resources. A physical examination and standard medical tests help identify comorbid conditions and other possible causes of dementia.

A thorough neurological examination is essential for reaching the differential diagnosis of the various categories of neurodegenerative dementia. For example, positive extrapyramidal symptoms would be consistent with Lewy Body dementia, whereas different combinations of motor neuron disease, myopathy, cerebellar dysfunction, autonomic failure, or extrapyramidal signs would suggest different disease entities. Focal neurological findings such as deep tendon reflex or sensory deficits, in the presence of a normal head CT scan, may be the only sign of a past stroke. Such subtle findings might serve as the basis for a diagnosis of ischemic vascular dementia.

A CT or magnetic resonance imaging (MRI) scan detects strokes or tumors that could be causing the dementia symptoms and are potentially treatable. Researchers are increasingly using PET and SPECT scans, and magnetic resonance spectroscopy imaging (MRSI) to study brain metabolism and blood flow in AD. These imaging techniques may one day provide an early and cost-effective diagnostic tool for AD (Budinger, 1994).

Neuropsychological testing measures memory, language skills, ability to do simple math, abstract reasoning, judgment, executive functions, and other abilities related to brain functioning. Mental status and neuropsychological testing may be critical to differentiating subtypes of degenerative dementias, but is also useful in determining the severity of disease and identifying strengths and weaknesses, information that can in turn be utilized in treatment planning. Research has shown that those who develop AD begin to lose immediate visual memory sooner than is expected in normal aging and long before other markers of dementia appear (Zonderman, Giambra, & Kawas, 1996). Decline in verbal memory may also be an early marker, and the loss of the familiar visual pattern of a clock may help to differentiate AD from other types of dementia (Bondi, Salmon, & Butters, 1994). There is also some evidence that two facets of personality may change early in AD. Ordinarily personality does not change with age, but in AD "conscientiousness" seems to decline, so that a patient may lose the "critical eye" necessary to maintain sanitary conditions in their home, whereas "vulnerability to stress" increases leaving the person at risk for "catastrophic reactions" to relatively benign circumstances (Siegler, Welsh, Dawson, et al., 1991).

A Model for Treatment and Management of AD

Treatment goals for AD are not unlike those for any other incurable, progressive illness: namely, relief of suffering, preservation of function, avoidance of iatrogenic problems, treatment of coincidental illnesses and sources of excess disability, and patient and family education.

AD is a complex condition that affects both the patient and the family support system. A comprehensive, flexible treatment plan, individualized to meet the patient's physical, psychological, and social needs can only be developed as a result of thorough assessment of the patient and his or her environment and with the involvement of the family (Bennett & Knopman, 1994; Jarvik & Wiseman, 1991; Post & Whitehouse, 1995). Disease management should cover the following domains: on-going primary care, psychiatric care, behavioral management, long-term care planning and community resource referral, and caregiver support.

At the ADC an exit interview includes the patient wherever possible, and is accompanied by a written summary of the team's findings in easily understandable language. Follow up is provided in 6 weeks and then yearly following initial evaluations. A full and very detailed report is furnished to the primary care physician, and other professionals crucial to the patient's welfare. Medical recommendations are reviewed with the patient and family as well as communicated to the primary care physician. Family caregivers are encouraged to assume a greater part in the management of the patient's health care, and educated in the expected progression and potential effects of AD (Cohen, 1994; Friss, 1993).

Early diagnosis has the advantage of allowing the patient to deal with the emotional concomitants of such a diagnosis in individual or group psychotherapy while he or she still can. Care is taken to provide an opportunity to discuss the diagnosis and its implications with the patient and his or her family. It has been our experience that the diagnosis can be presented in an understandable and nonthreatening way.

Persons in the very early stages of a dementing disorder usually retain a great deal of insight into their difficulties and respond well to opportunities to ask questions, clarify their understanding of the disease, and be involved in discussions with family regarding their future care. Focusing on treatment and resources to increase or preserve a good quality of life rather than the diagnosis per se engenders the exit meeting with a sense of hope for the near term if not for the long term.

Moderately impaired patients usually have some sense of what is happening to them, even in the absence of clear insight, and are often afraid. There is a deep sense of shame attached to a fear of being ''crazy.'' Identification of a disease process as the cause of memory problems seems to relieve some of the shame and anxiety, and is worthwhile, even if it requires frequent repetition. A team of two staff members facilitate the exit interview. They take advantage of opportunities to model effective communication with the patient, and to gently initiate discussion between the patient and family members regarding disease-related problems and preferences for care.

Support groups for early-stage patients are a fairly new concept but increasingly available as a treatment option. Experience at the ADC has shown that such groups provide an important therapeutic resource for patients that may alleviate depressive symptoms and anxiety and provide an avenue for socialization in a supportive and nonthreatening environment. A currently active couples group for early-stage patients and their spouses has fostered open discussion of disease process, brainstorming about future needs and potential resource referrals, and direct acknowledgment of the stresses involved for both patients and their caregivers. Although not measured scientifically, participation in this group appears to have facilitated major decisions for lifestyle change and smooth transitions. Members have appreciated the support of others in the same position, and actively maintain an interest in each others lives at a time when friends are not always supportive.

The progression of AD is associated with an increasing prevalence of psychiatric symptoms and disturbances in behavior. Effective pharmacological and behavioral management of agitation, anxiety, hallucinations, and paranoia allows caregivers to maintain the patient at home, potentially deferring or avoiding institutionalization (Teri, Rabins, Whitehouse, et al., 1992; Whitehouse, 1993). Nurses, especially nurse practitioners and those in home health, may be the first to identify these treatable psychiatric symptoms and bring them to the attention of the primary care physician.

Depression and its evaluation occupies a great deal of energy throughout the diagnostic process. Behavioral interventions for depression are addressed in some detail with family members, with care taken that all understand the complicating nature of a depressive syndrome on an underlying dementia. Increased socialization in a sensitive environment, such as adult day care, has been found useful in the treatment of depression in dementia patients.

Behavioral symptoms are a hallmark of dementing illnesses that often lead to crises or emergency interventions, increased caregiver burden and premature placement. Behavioral interventions directed towards health maintenance and compensation for self-care deficits can minimize excess disability. The provision of appropriate psychosocial and environmental support in the form of 24-hour supervision and guidance, and direct help with activities of daily living greatly improves quality of life, reduces comorbidity in terms of behavior disturbance, and potentially reduces community impact in the form of emergency calls, repeated emergency room visits, and other such calls. Making families aware of these needs and helping them identify options for accessing services is a critical aspect of disease management (Stewart, 1991; Whitehouse, 1993).

An integral part of the treatment plan is the education, guidance, and support of family caregivers and others who provide the informal 24-hour supervision mandated by AD and other dementing conditions, recognizing the family caregiver as the instrument of the plan. Caregivers need a range of support services depending on their individual family resources and requirements. Adult day care, respite care, and placement information and referral, legal and financial planning resources, and case management are some of the components of long-term care planning that should be made available to caregivers.

The goals of treatment planning should be to promote independence to the fullest extent possible. The provision of structured activities, whether at home or in a day care setting, is a key component in promoting independence and emotional stability and deferring placement. When caregivers turn to formal support services they commonly seek help in improving their coping skills, meeting the patient's needs, responding to family issues, handling relationship concerns, eliciting formal and informal support, and resolving feelings of inadequacy and guilt. Besides their usefulness as an educational source, support groups may provide a useful forum in which caregivers may address feelings of grief and loss that accompany the progressive decline of AD patients.

Centers for such as the ADC and chapters of the Alzheimer's Association are now providing caregiver education and skills training. Professionally led psychoeducational support groups have been shown to reduce anger and depression in caregivers, leading to improved caregiver well-being and reduced mood swings and difficult behaviors in the patient (Gallagher, 1993). Caregiver training in behavior management, geared toward eliminating catastrophic reactions that may lead to crisis/emergency interventions, has been shown to reduce excessive medical care and premature institutionalization (Alzheimer's Association, 1994; Bennett & Knopman, 1994; Mittelman, Ferris, Steinberg, et al., 1993; Post, 1995).

In addition to the UCSF School of Medicine and Residency programs, the ADC has linkages with other academic centers and community service agencies, and provides a wide range of educational and training resources for an area incorporating 10 counties in the Central Valley area of California and serving a population of about 2 million. The varied research and collaborative nature of the ADC, and other Centers like it in California and around the United States, continues to facilitate a high level of knowledge about the diagnosis, care, and management of AD. This in turn has changed the approach to care in the community beyond all recognition from what was readily available even 10 years ago.

A wide range of educational programs include a six session family caregiver training course that also qualifies for continuing education units for certified nursing assistants, a 3-unit Dementia Care Certificate course taught at CSUF for nurses, social workers, and other professional caregivers, and in-service programs for staff at special care AD units (skilled) as well as residential care facilities. Collaborative interdisciplinary team functioning is demonstrated to students in all aspects of the diagnostic workup, with the weekly team conference serving as a teaching forum available to any community agency personnel.

■CONCLUSION

As we turn to the next millennium the challenge of AD will sharpen. Answers to the questions of cause will continue to be high on the research priority list. Development of effective treatments and interventions to truly halt the progression of the dementias and reliable identification of persons at risk for development of neurodegenerative conditions will move forward with speed. A holistic view of the dementing disorders and wider recognition of the need for inclusion of family members in diagnosis and treatment planning will ease the burden for caregivers and facilitate interventions that maximize function and quality of life.

■REFERENCES

American Psychiatric Association. (1994). *Diagnostic and Statistical Manual of Mental Disorders, IV.* Washington, DC: Author.

Beal, M. F. (1994). Energy, oxidative damage, and Alzheimer's disease. *Neurobiology of Aging* 15(Suppl. 2):S171–S174.

Bennett, D. A., & Knopman, D. S. (1994). Alzheimer's disease: A comprehensive approach to patients' management. *Geriatrics* 49(8):20–26.

Bondi, M. W., Salmon, D. P., & Butters, N. M. (1994). Neuropsychological features of memory disorders in Alzheimer's disease. In Terry, R. D., Katzman, R., & Bick, K. L. (Eds.). *Alzheimer Disease.* New York: Raven Press; pp. 41–64.

Budinger, T. F. (1994). Future research in Alzheimer's disease using imaging techniques. *Neurobiology of Aging* 15(suppl. 2):S41–S48.

Caselli, R. J., Jack, Jr., C. R., Petersen, R. C., Wahner, H. W., & Tanagihara, T. (1992). Asymmetric cortical degenerative syndromes: Clinical and radiological correlations. *Neurology* 42:1462–1468.

Cohen, D. (1994). A primary care checklist for effective family management. *Medical Clinics of North America* 78(4):795–809.

Cotman, C. W., & Pike, C. J. (1994). Beta-amyloid and its contributions to neurodegeneration in Alzheimer disease. In Terry, R. D., Katzman, R., & Bick, K. L. (Eds.). *Alzheimer Disease.* New York: Raven Press; pp. 305–316.

Cummings, J. L., & Benson, D. F. (1992). *Dementia: A clinical approach.* Butterworth-Heinemann: Boston, MA.

Cummings, J. L., & Miller, B. L. (1987). Visual hallucinations: An overview. *Western Journal of Medicine* 146:46–51.

Ernst, R. L., & Hay, J. W. (1994). The U.S. economic and social costs of Alzheimer's disease revisited. *American Journal of Public Health* 84(8):1261–1264.

Evans, D. A. (1990). Estimated prevalence of Alzheimer's disease in the United States. *The Millbank Quarterly* 68(2):267–289.

Friss, L. (1993). Family caregivers as case managers: A statewide model for enhancing consumer choice. *Journal of Case Management* 2(2):53–58.

Gallagher, D. (1993). Clinical intervention strategies for distressed family care givers: Rationale and development of psychoeducational approaches. In Light, E., Niederehe, G., & Lebowitz, B. (Eds.). *Caregiving and Mental Health.* New York: Springer.

Gatz, M., Lowe, B., & Berg, S., et al. (1994). Dementia: Not just a search for the gene. *The Gerontologist* 34:251–255.

Geula, C., & Mesulam, M. (1994). Cholinergic systems and related neuropathological predilection patterns in Alzheimer disease. In Terry, R. D., Katzman, R., & Bick, K. L. (Eds.). *Alzheimer's Disease.* New York: Raven Press; pp. 263–292.

Ironside, J. W. (1996). Review: Creutzfeld-Jakob disease. *Brain Pathology* 6:379–388.

Jorm, A. F., Korten, A. E., & Henderson, A. S. (1987). The prevalence of dementia: a quantitative integration of the literature. *Acta Psychiatr Scand* 76:464–479.

Khatchaturian, Z. S., & Radebaugh, T. S. (1995). *Alzheimer's Disease: Progress toward Untangling the Mystery.* Encyclopaedia Britannica: Medical and Health Annual, Chicago: Encyclopaedia Britannica, Inc., 222–228.

Kosik, K., & Greenberg, S. M. (1994). Tau protein and Alzheimer disease. In Terry, R. D., Katzman, R., & Bick, K. L. (Eds.). *Alzheimer's Disease.* New York: Raven Press; pp. 335–344.

Levy-Lahad, E., Wijsman, E. M., & Nemens, E. (1995). A familial Alzheimer's disease locus on chromosome 1. *Science* 269:970–973.

Markesbery, W. R., & Ehmann, W. D. (1994). Brain trace elements in Alzheimer's disease. In Terry, R. D., Katzman, R., & Bick, K. L. (Eds.). *Alzheimer's Disease.* New York: Raven Press, pp. 353–369.

McGreer, P. L., Schulzer, M., & McGreer, E. G. (1996). Arthritis and anti-inflammatory agents as possible protective factors for Alzheimer's disease: A review of 17 epidemiological studies. *Neurology* 47:425–432.

McKhann, G., Drachman, D., Folstein, M., Katzman, R., Price, D., & Stadlan, E. M. (1984). Clinical diagnosis of Alzheimer's disease: Report of the NINCDS-ADRDA Work Group under the auspices of Department of Health and Human Services Task Force on Alzheimer's Disease. *Neurology* 34:939–944.

McKeith, I., Fairbairn, A., Perry, R., et al. (1992). Neuroleptic sensitivity in patients with senile dementia of Lewy body type. *British Medical Journal* 305:673–678.

McKeith, I. G., Fairbairn, A. F., Bothwell, R. A., et al. (1994). An evaluation of the predictive validity and inter-rater reliability of clinical diagnostic criteria for senile dementia of Lewy body type. *Neurology* 44:872–877.

Miller, B. L., Cummings, J. L., Villanueva-Meyer, J., et al. (1991). Frontal lobe degeneration: Clinical, neuropsychological, and SPECT characteristics. *Neurology* 41:1374–1382.

Miller, B. L., Darby, A. L., Swartz, J. R., Yener, G. G., & Mena, I. (1995). Dietary changes, compulsions and sexual behavior in fronto-temporal degeneration. *Dementia* 6:195–199.

Mittelman, M. S., Ferris, S. H., Steinberg, G., Shulman, E., Mackell, J. A., Ambinder, A., & Kohen, J. (1993). An intervention that delays institutionalization of Alzheimer's disease patients: Treatment of spousal care givers. *Gerontologist* 33(6): 730–740.

National Institutes on Aging (1995). *Alzheimer's Disease Fact Sheet.* Silver Springs, MD: Alzheimer's Disease Education & Referral Center.

NIH Consensus Conference (1987). Differential diagnosis of dementing diseases. *JAMA* 258(23):3411–3416.

Paschalis, C., Polychronopoulos, P., & Lekka, N. P. (1990). The role of head injury, surgical anaesthesia and family history as etiological factors in dementia of the Alzheimer's type. *Dementia* 1:52–55.

Perry, E. K., Kerwin, J. M., Perry, R. H., et al. (1990). Cerebral cholinergic activity is related to the incidence of visual hallucinations in senile dementia of Lewy body type. *Journal Neurol Sci* 95:119–139.

Post, S. G., & Whitehouse, P. J. (1995). The Fairhill Guidelines. In S. G. Post, *The ethics of Alzheimer's Care*. Baltimore: Johns Hopkins University Press.

Read, S., Miller, B. L., Mena, I., et al. (1995). SPECT in dementia: Clinical and pathological correlation. *Journal of the American Geriatric Society* 43:1243–1247.

Reisberg, B. (1996). Alzheimer's Disease. In *Comprehensive Review of Geriatric psychiatry-II*. Sadavoy, J., Lazarus, L. W., Jarvik, L., et al. (Eds.). Washington, DC: American Psychiatric Press.

Siegler, I. C., Welsh, K. A., Dawson, D. V., et al. (1991). Ratings of personality change in patients being evaluated for memory disorders. *Alzheimer's Disease and Associated Disorders: An International Journal* 5:240–250.

Snowden, D. A., Kemper, S. J., et Al., Mortimer, J. A., et al. (1996). Linguistic ability in early life and cognitive function and Alzheimer's disease in late life. Findings from the Nun study. *JAMA* 275:528–532.

St. George-Hyslop, P. H. (1994). The molecular genetics of Alzheimer disease. In Terry, R. D., Katzman, R., & Bick, K. L. (Eds.). *Alzheimer's Disease*. New York: Raven Press, pp. 335–344.

Teri, L., Rabins, P., Whitehouse, P., Berg, L., Reisberg, B., Sunderland, T., Eichelman, B., & Phelps, C. (1992). Management of behavior disturbance in Alzheimer's disease: Current knowledge and future directions. *Alzheimer's Disease and Associated Disorders* 6(2):77–88.

United States Bureau of the Census. (1995). *Sixty-Five Plus in the United States*. Statistical Brief, Economics and Statistics Administration, U.S. Department of Commerce.

Victoroff, J., Ross, G. W., Benson, D. F., Verity, M. A., & Vinters, H. V. (1994). Posterior cortical atrophy: Neuropathological correlations. *Archives of Neurology* 51:269–274.

Whitehouse, P. J. (Ed.). (1993). *Dementia*. Philadelphia: F.A. Davis Company.

Wilhelmsen, K., Lynch, T., & Pavlou, E. (1994). Localization of disinhibition-dementia-parkinsonism-amyotrophy complex to 17q21-22. *American Journal of Human Genetics* 55:1150–1165.

Zonderman, A. B., Giambra, L. M., Kawas, C. H. (In press). Changes in immediate visual memory predicts cognitive impairment. *Archives of Clinical Neuropsychology*.

SELECTED BIBLIOGRAPHY

Bove, L. A. (1995). Now! Surgery for heart failure. *RN* 58(5):26–30.

Bultema, J. K., Mailliard, L., Getzfrid, M. K., Lerner, R. D., & Colone, M. (1996). Geriatric patients with depression. *Journal of Nursing Administration* 26(1):31–38.

D'Arrigo, T. (February 1994). Aim for the heart: Taking control of cardiovascular care. *CARING Magazine* 14–21.

Deakins, D. A. (1994). Teaching elderly patients about diabetes. *American Journal of Nursing* 94(4):38–42.

Devons, C. A. J. (1996). Suicide in the elderly: How to identify and treat patients at risk. *Geriatrics* 51(3):67–73.

Forbes, S. B. (1994). Hope: An essential human need in the elderly. *Journal of Gerontological Nursing* 20(6):5–10.

Kanacki, L. S., Jones, P. S., & Galbraith, M. E. (1996). Social support and depression in widows and widowers. *Journal of Gerontological Nursing* 22(2):39–45.

Kelly, M. (1995). Surgery, anesthesia, and the geriatric patient. *Geriatric Nursing* 16(5):213–216.

Letvak, S., & Schoder, D. (1996). Sexually transmitted diseases in the elderly: What you need to know. *Geriatric Nursing* 17(4):156–160.

Leventhal, E. A., Hansell, S., Diefenbach, M., Leventhal, H., & Glass, D. C. (1996). Negative affect and self-report of physical symptoms: Two longitudinal studies of older adults. *Health Psychology* 15(3):193–199.

McMahon, A. L. (1993). Substance abuse among the elderly. *Nurse Practitioner Forum* 4(4):231–238.

Nazon, M., & Levine-Perkell, J. (1996). AIDS and aging. *Journal of Gerontological Social Work* 25(1/2):21–31.

Resnick, B. (1996). Motivation in geriatric rehabilitation. *Image: Journal Nursing Scholarship* 28(1):41–45.

Singh, P. (1995). Managing chronic congestive heart failure in the home. *Home Healthcare Nurse* 13(2):11–13.

Sullivan-Marx, E. M. (1994). Delirium and physical restraint in the hospitalized elderly. *Image: Journal of Nursing Scholarship* 26(4):295–300.

Tempkin, T., Tempkin, A., & Goodman, H. (1995). Geriatric rehabilitation. *Nurse Practitioner Forum* 6(3):173–177.

Tibbits, G. M. (1996). Patients who fall: How to predict and prevent injuries. *Geriatrics* 51(9):24–31.

Unit 8

Older Adults and Caregivers: Changing Needs and Settings

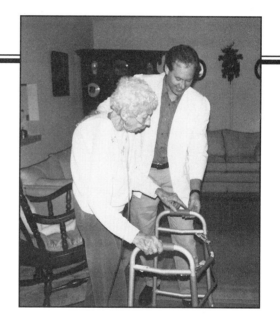

I n this final unit we look at the changing needs of the aging adult and the oldest-old among us. With advanced age comes increasing frailty and dependence
for most. Even those who have lived a hearty life and enter old age in good
health with robust energy and strong reserves, begin to slow down and need assistance or perhaps a change in living setting.

Included in this unit are a selection of readings that highlight family, caregiver,
and caregiving issues related to the increasing needs of older adults with debilitating chronic illnesses. How aging affects family relationships as members age and
roles change is also addressed. Care settings for the most dependent clients have
specific caregiving challenges that are unique to long-term care settings. And finally, improving the quality of life for the most dependent in our society, the con-

fused and the terminally ill elder, suitably end the readings chosen for this unit of the text.

The multiplicity of setting choices and services available for the dependent elder will only increase as our nation ages. It is important for today's health care provider to have an understanding of these changing needs, the bevy of choices available, and what will be needed in the future. With this understanding comes a responsibility to be a role model and nursing leader by providing quality care to all clients. Some will take up the challenge to be a change agent. They will be ones who motivate others, bring about needed changes, establish new services, and insure that quality care exists now and will exist in the future for those to come.

The healthy independent older adult has needs well represented in other units in this text. However, our greatest national challenge comes when we look at the care we give the most frail and needy in our society. It is a measure of the quality of our country some would rather not address and find easy to put aside. We can make it something to be proud of and be in the forefront of the health care delivery system. Nurses can make a difference. We have the skills needed. We have the essence of caring, the formal education, and we are at the bedside and know what is needed. The time is now!

Chapter 47

Daughters Caring for Their Aging Mothers: A Midlife Developmental Process

JANE W. ECKERT   SUSAN C. SHULMAN

Developmental crises punctuate our lives. There is one midlife developmental crisis for women that is discussed by these authors in this chapter. It is the process of adult daughters caring for their aging mothers. The chapter is a result of research conducted by the authors through their clinical experiences in outpatient settings. They found that although family situations differ, there were parameters and major themes that were central to work with this population. Examples are presented to illustrate common challenges which are experienced by daughters as they care for their mothers. It is presented through the process of the treatment relationship and giving the daughters an opportunity to grieve parental shortcomings and achieve more comfortable adaptation.

▬ INTRODUCTION

"I need some information on retirement homes for my mother." "I went to visit my parents and I'm concerned about how poorly my father is doing, yet my mother won't let me help." "My mother needs to go to the doctor but she refuses. I need some names of doctors who might be good for her." "I think my mother needs some more help at home, but she refuses to accept it."

These are the initial concerns one hears from adult children, typically daughters and typically in midlife. For a midlife individual, caring for a parent can represent a developmental opportunity which can be facilitated by an appropriately focused treatment relationship. This paper uses clinical examples and findings from research to illustrate this point and to identify the parameters and major themes which we have found to be central to work with this population. The nature of the problems and their presentation makes this a population whose treatment can be enhanced by therapeutic intervention informed by social work principles.

From *Journal of Gerontological Social Work* 25(3/4):17–32, 1996. Reprinted with permission.

The central thesis is that caregiving for a parent respresents a crisis in an adult child's life which offers the opportunity for working on internal issues or, conversely, for stagnating and even regressing. The caregiving crisis is accompanied by the realization that life and time are finite and that what occurs in the present between parent and child is all that will be (Neugarten, 1968). It is a last chance for rapprochement or resolution of earlier life issues, including fantasies of restitution for earlier disappointments. Examples from clinical practice will be used here to illustrate this thesis and highlight the common challenges which such treatment relationships present. The journey a midlife woman traverses toward filial maturity and the achievement of a mature caregiving stance towards her parent will be explicated.

Background

The authors' interest in this topic is based on their own research and clinical practices. Both have long held a strong interest in older people and their families and have worked with a broad social spectrum of this population in various settings including medical and psychiatric hospitals, outpatient clinics, mental health centers and private practice. This paper is based particularly on our experiences with white, middle-class clients seen in an outpatient context. It is a descriptive empirical work, rather than a quantitative research report, and reflects our ongoing conceptualizations of our work. Therefore, our conclusions are working hypotheses which need to be tested with other ethnic and income groups.

Another impetus for this paper was one of the authors' dissertation research which described a sample of twenty midlife daughters providing or managing care for their aging mothers (Shulman, 1988). The study's conclusions were that the differential quality of caregiving provided for an aging parent and the burden or stress experienced by the provider could be strongly correlated with the midlife daughter's level of object relations maturity. This appraisal included an individual's levels of altruism and self-care, degree of separation-individuation, idealization and devaluation, and narcissistic vulnerability. This conclusion has been empirically reflected in our clinical practices, in which the practitioner is known as having an expertise with older people. Women come for help with the kinds of opening requests already cited. However, this focus on concrete services represents only a fraction of the story.

One client who exemplifies this population was an attractive, upper middle-class woman in her early 40s who appeared in great distress about her caregiving role with her parents. The client described that her father had impaired memory and judgment–Alzheimer's disease, she thought. To her he seemed to be getting worse. She hoped the clinician would help her insure that her father was getting what he needed. The client focused on the concrete aspects of care for her father. How could she get a diagnosis? How could she get more involved in his care? How was she to understand what was going on? As she continued to speak, however, it became apparent that these presenting problems masked the client's longstanding underlying difficulties with her own self-esteem. Her lovability had constantly been in question in a family situation in which her mother had been unable to affirm her daughter's worth. In fact, her mother had been undermining her daughter due to her own limitations and her competition with her. The client's father's illness and her difficulty and conflict over her role as an adult wanting to care for her father presented a new stage upon which these issues could be replayed and reworked.

Issues of parent-caring as exemplified by this client have not been addressed in the literature as a distinctive clinical phenomenon. The parameters of parent-caring have been considered from descriptive, demographic, and sociological perspectives (Archbold, 1983; Shanas, 1979; Treas, 1977). It is rare to find anyone taking a careful look at the unique intrapsychic concomitants of becoming reengaged with one's parents in midlife. Nonetheless, this is an area of great interest to those working with older people and their families. This paper is hence based upon the sociological and developmental literature and enhances this with a theoretical formulation of individual psychodynamic processes.

▬REVIEW OF THE LITERATURE

One of the best known writers in this area, the social work researcher Elaine Brody (Brody, 1985), was the earliest to study what has been termed the "sandwich generation"–a phrase which is now part of the vernacular (D. Miller, 1981). Her work describes the various roles caretakers of aging parents assume and the stressors this places on the caretaker. This family member is described as a daughter and caretaker, as well as a wife and a mother herself, often of adolescents (and these days, more often, of younger children). Further studies have shown that most of the caregiving of the frail aged population is done by family members, most particularly women (Brody, 1988; Shanas, 1979; Treas, 1977). Coupled with this has been a huge body of research about the "burden" of caregiving, which has concluded that the caregiver can deal better with an acute crisis and an intense period of caregiving, but that chronic caregiving wears one down (Zarit, 1985). This research has also attempted to characterize "burden" in particular ways using broad, descriptive terms or quantitative measures. In addition, stimulated by the increasing numbers of women in the workplace, industry has focused attention on the toll that caregiving takes on the employee and the need for employers to attend to this stress to enhance productivity (Anastas, Gibeau, & Larson, 1990). All of these studies provide a demographic overview of individuals in caregiving situations.

Concurrent with this descriptive research which defines caregiving as both a critical social problem and an important opportunity, developmental psychologists have begun to focus on the unique aspects of personality development in midlife and the changes which are possible at this time. Erikson, in his classic stages of development, views the crisis of midlife as conflict between a stance of generativity and one of stagnation (Erikson, 1950). While Erikson means by generativity the capacity to give and care particularly for those in the younger generation, by extension it is assumed here that his ideas can include the ability to nurture preceding generations as well. Erikson posits that resolving the crisis which occurs in midlife leads to the capacity to master the next life stage, old age, by recognizing and coming to terms with one's life course as the only life one has to live. Reconciliation with the parental generation is certainly a part of this process.

Other social psychologists such as Havighurst (1973) and Neugarten (1968) and, more recently, psychoanalysts such as Oldham (1987) and Kernberg (1985) have suggested that events in midlife can lead to the achievement of new perspectives on the self and on one's parents. These include enhanced awareness of mortality and finitude which can be prompted by a parent's terminal illness or death, and the increasing assumption of the adult role in the extended family. This process has also been conceptualized developmentally as a third separation-individuation process in which more realistic internalizations of oneself and one's parents can evolve.

Increasingly, moreover, personality theory has been influenced by models which are more fluid than the earlier deterministic developmental ideas which posited that the foundations of personality were fixed during the early years. Object relations theory, self-psychology, and adult developmental theories allow for the notion of personality development and shifts in later life. These changes result from the impact of adult relationships and the modification of personality which the internal and external events of later life can stimulate. Thus, some attention has been given in the theoretical literature to the intrapsychic maturational possibilities which midlife can bring for individuals (Colarusso & Nemiroff, 1981).

The only theorist to actually identify the parent-caring experience as a developmental milestone in itself was Margaret Blenkner (1965), a sociologist. She conceptualized parent-caring as offering a particular impetus for personal growth, linking this social event with an intrapsychic phenomenon. She described this developmental achievement as "filial maturity," a process which results from an adult's realization that a parent has become frail and is in need of a different kind of relationship with her offspring. This process involves the child's growing past earlier struggles with a parent and her assuming an objective, mutually respectful stance in midlife. This developmental achievement can be reflected in the quality of the child's caregiving for her parent. There has been some debate in the literature as to whether this is a normative developmental crisis, since the trajectories of individuals' lives vary so widely (Brody, 1988). Nonetheless, the concept of filial maturity is a useful way to identify an individual's specific midlife achievements in relation to (her/his) family of origin.

Optimally, caring for an aging parent can offer some restitution for previous limitations in the parent-child relationship as well as allow an individual to assume the full role of adult in her own mind as well as in her family of origin. It is an opportunity to attain a new mutuality with one's parents in which the parent accepts increasing dependency and the child embraces new, adult responsibilities (Greenberg, 1994). This concept is central in the clinical work to be described.

▰ PROCESS OF THE TREATMENT RELATIONSHIP

The population of women seeking help around parent-caring needs is characterized by striking differences. However, the recognition of the many shared characteristics among this group provides a useful framework for practice. These similarities include: the client presenting in what looks like a crisis situation; framing the request as meeting a concrete need; and relating to the practitioner in a distant or somewhat tentative manner which reflects ambivalence about dependency. It is the experience of the authors that most of these women seek help in response to an underlying concern around early unmet self-esteem needs reflected in problematic identifications and a vulnerable sense of self. This concern remains latent throughout the treatment rather than an overt focus of the work.

Initial Presentation

As suggested by the beginning quotes, midlife women often present their issues in terms of concrete requests for help for themselves as the caregivers of frail and aging parents. They do not see themselves as looking for a "therapist" or for "therapy," if that is defined as a process of personal self-examination and growth. Rather, they see themselves as looking for advice, information, and, in a less manifest way, relief from their parents' needs and demands. These women characterize themselves as caretakers who are too burdened or overwhelmed to do any more and who need help with the caretaking. Skilled practitioners recognize that these requests are sometimes symptomatic of more complex concerns.

For these clients, the request for help is in response to a crisis situation. One client felt her father needed immediate transfer to a new nursing home because she was upset by what was objectively an expectable decline in his functioning which she was having difficulty accepting and mourning. Another became enraged when her mother physically blockaded her from intervening with her father's care. And a third wondered if she should give up her life and job in order to move across the country to be with her parent who had just had a medical emergency. These people feel they must do something immediately and they communicate this sense of urgency and a strong wish for action. The clinician's challenge is to reframe the current crisis in a way which will lead to enhanced ongoing functioning.

Consider Mrs. J. This woman came stating that she needed some help deciding on living alternatives for her mother. As she related her story, Mrs. J. revealed that in the prior two months, her eighty-seven-year-old widowed mother had become more ill and more demanding. The current crisis was that Mrs. J.'s mother was asking her daughter where she should live. Whenever Mrs. J. tried to answer her mother's questions directly, her mother would disagree with her. Mrs. J. soon realized she could never give her mother the right response. She came to the practitioner looking for the "expert's" answer. Fortunately, the practitioner didn't have it! As the clinician explored further, it became clear that Mrs. J. was extremely anxious and filled with shame. She was ashamed at her anger at her mother's 3 a.m. phone calls; ashamed of her inability to fulfill her mother's wishes to be driven to a million doctor's appointments; and mostly ashamed at her inability to be the model "good daughter." Although she would never phrase her concerns this way, Mrs. J. was struggling with her own failure to live up to internalized idealizations and to acknowledge her feelings in relation to the provocations presented by her mother's increasingly regressive and dependent demands.

Mrs. J.'s intensity suggests that the request for concrete information masked a more subtle and complex concern. Merely responding to this request is to deny the actual ongoing crisis, which has to do with her self-esteem vulnerabilities. In this instance, the crisis was Mrs. J.'s desperate wish to be an ideal daughter, providing ideal care to a mother, who (in Mrs. J.'s fantasy) would then validate her. Mrs. J. had always wanted a mother who could be demonstrative in her show of love towards her daughter. Instead of affection, Mrs. J. received insistent demands to be taken to the doctor, multiple requests to run errands, and "emergency" telephone calls in the middle of the night for nonemergency situations—requests which she could not lovingly meet.

Time was running out for her mother to be transformed into a generous, affirmative individual. Her age and illness precluded any such imagined metamorphosis. The gap between Mrs. J.'s wishes and reality reflected Mrs. J.'s inability to let go of an idealized image of the mother–daughter relationship. The therapeutic task is to help Mrs. J. hear her mother's requests symbolically, as emotional expressions of increased dependency rather than as concrete demands to which she needs to respond immediately. The therapist must also enable Mrs. J. to mourn for her wishes to attain an idealized restitution for the disappointments she experienced with her mother and to accept what is realistically possible. Helping her discover how she can be helpful in a limited manner is the only way the resolution of the crisis can lead to a better adaptation.

In this client population, asking for help by defining a problem in concrete terms is not indicative of either lack of insight or lack of capacity to relate. It more clearly reflects the client's life stage concerns and is normative. As midlife adults, members of what Robert Havighurst (1973) called the "command generation," this group of women is invested in seeing themselves as being competent and adult. Whether or not these feelings of competence are well integrated, these women struggle to preserve their sense of integrity in the face of demands from both their parents and their children. These are often conflicting demands which test the core sense of self. At the same time, repressed infantile or childlike vulnerabilities and feelings may reemerge in the face of these demands.

Dynamic Understanding of the Crisis
The authors have found that most of the women who present for help are those whose early relationships with their parents lacked sufficient emotional responsiveness and availability to enable them to internalize a strong, positive sense of self. Their narcissistic vulnerabilities resemble those of the population which Alice Miller (1981) describes in her work. They are psychologically needy individuals whose sense of self is vulnerable. The stimulation of being engaged in a caregiving situation may precipitate

unresolved needs in this midlife adult. Faced with the challenges of rekindled needs for dependency, nurture and soothing, it is often necessary for the client to defend herself by focusing on the here and now of "what can be done" rather than on the sense of personal deficiency which emerges in the caregiving situation. A sense of deficiency is evident in the shame with which these women present. Not only do they describe themselves as inadequate caregivers, but they also feel deeply remorseful about this. They present a veneer of pseudo-competency or pseudo-self-sufficiency and assume high functioning roles despite their own neediness. However, beneath this facade are feelings of emptiness and rage. The essence of the midlife crisis for these women is an unconscious and unspoken choice. Either they may regress to a more dependent, less adaptive way of coping which results from holding on to childlike wishes and feelings; or they may move to a newly defined sense of self with a higher level of adaptation which results from relinquishing earlier ideals, grieving, and reintegrating the self. Individuals are able to resolve this crisis depending on their affective and defensive resources and the accuracy of a clinician's intervention.

The following comparison is an example of the differential ways in which clients may present their problems and utilize help. Two clients expressed (but to different degrees) their concerns as their parents' problems rather than as their own threatened sense of self. The first, Mrs. J., who was discussed earlier, was anxious and ashamed at her failure to meet her high standards of providing for her mother. However, as she engaged in a treatment relationship, she was able to be somewhat reflective about her situation and to express some awareness that the impact of her past relationship with her mother was influencing her current distress. Thus, she could situate the problem within herself and her feelings, not just in the situation. This enabled her to address ways in which she could change her adaptation.

In contrast to her is Mrs. S. This woman described her father's impaired memory and judgement and her fervent wish to be helpful to him within the context of unremitting rage at her mother. She resisted directly discussing the relationship with her mother with the clinician. Instead, she felt compelled to be involved with her parents by precipitously taking over tasks in a manner which was not helpful to anyone, but which she felt expressed her efforts to be the perfect caregiver. She would complain to the therapist about ways in which these efforts were thwarted. Her impulses to action rather than to reflection typified her inability to tolerate affect or ambivalence. She had to keep a distance from the clinician to preserve a very shaky ego; this was reflected in her ability to utilize insight less than Mrs. J. Mrs. S.'s adaptation was more brittle than Mrs. J.'s, despite a similarity in their presentations.

Treatment Relationship

The nature of the treatment relationship which ensues in these situations often consists of a continuous focus on building an alliance. Since the clients we are describing do not usually turn to a professional looking for psychotherapy per se, it is critical that the clinician "meet the person where she is," and respect the "person in the situation," two cardinal tenets of clinical social work practice. This sometimes means responding to the concrete request as if it were the presenting problem, while maintaining enough ambiguity to develop a therapeutic relationship to address the underlying concerns. For example, a psychiatrist colleague had seen a woman who was asking for help with her aged mother. It was clear to him that the mother did not need help. Rather, he felt the daughter needed help with her caretaking role but that she would not accept his involvement in examining her intrapsychic issues. He referred the daughter to a social work practitioner with the awareness that a beginning involvement with her around the mother's concrete needs would be an acceptable bridge to a more encompassing relationship.

In alliance building, the clinician must understand the function of the tentative forays of the client who appears to be "resistant" or undermining of therapy, and tolerate these with awareness of their meaning. For example, one client called once every six months to inquire about resources and to describe her situation with her mother. This went on for a year and one half before the woman was able to make an appointment and meet with the clinician face-to-face. She followed her initial interview with a lengthy telephone contact–then vanished again. It is certain that she will call when another crisis surfaces. These episodic contacts, similar to visits to an emergency or outpatient mental health service, often serve the function of helping the client to maintain control of the treatment process, to act from a position of strength, and to test the reliability and constancy of the clinician. Such an approach to seeking help is consistent with theories of adult development, which emphasize the importance of respecting the strengths and autonomy of the client, and allowing the client to "regroup" and utilize her usual milieu and supports to do so. This is not therapy oriented towards regression in the service of further development; rather, it is therapy which recognizes and respects the client's strong underlying ambivalence about dependency. Some of this ambivalence may relate to the client's personality dynamics, and some to her place in the life cycle.

Without a flexible treatment stance, the client's underlying deficits and vulnerabilities cannot be addressed, because the client will become even more defensive or flee altogether. For example, one client came for help after a previous clinician had told her that she had to "resolve" her conflictual relationship with her mother. While she wanted a place to bring her uncomfortable feelings, this clinician's direct approach, which was based on an accurate diagnostic assessment of the situation, frightened the woman, and threatened her almost symbiotic tie to her parent.

Another example is the client Mrs. S., who was described earlier. As has been indicated, this woman's rage at her mother was restimulated by her father's illness. In her treatment, the client and worker needed to focus on the concrete aspects of Mrs. S.'s father's care for a very long time. This approach enabled her to bind her rage, absorb some positive enhancement and acceptance from her therapist, and diminish her anxiety. The clinician could not explore the relationship with the mother, and surely could not intrepret the client's anger and fear about discussing this relationship. She could only infer its nature from the quality of the client's transference to her. When the initial acute crisis passed (in part because of the work she and the therapist had done), Mrs. S. wanted to leave treatment. There was no way to interpret her motivations for this to the client, who was well defended against her fears of examining her own feelings. Therefore, the clinician concurred with the client's decision to end, laying the ground for further work with this woman by describing the notion of "chapters" in which people return at different times to work on different issues. The client did return several times over the next five years for involvements of varying lengths of three to twenty sessions. Each reengagement was prompted by both changes in her father's status and also her increasing perception of the clinician as a constant and enhancing object–different from her experience of her mother. She was gradually able to let go of her need to intervene as aggressively between her parents. She could increasingly move from a rigidly idealized view of her mother, which denied the mother's limitations, to a more balanced view which acknowledged her deficits as well as her strengths. Her terms for describing this were that her caretaking wishes had been "like rolling a heavy boulder up a hill." She had finally decided that she needed to "stop rolling the boulder."

Treatment as a Grief Process

This case example illustrates what the authors feel is the crux of the treatment process with this population: providing a context in which grief can be addressed, particularly grief over the loss of the idealized parental object or introject and, concurrently, of the idealized self. This is a core midlife developmental task which has been derailed in these clients because of earlier deficits. They have needed to hold onto rigid idealizations as compensation for their failure to experience adequately empathic parenting. The medical or caretaking crisis threatens these individual's brittle adaptations.

There is some recognition by the client that this is the last chance she will have to address and learn to live with the limitations she has experienced. The effort to get nurturance from her parent in the present fails, as does the vicarious wish to get nurturance from giving it. Thus, the client turns to the therapist for the care she needs in the guise of seeking assistance in becoming an even more perfect cargiver, through finding the "right" solutions to concrete requests. If this symbolic request is not recognized and understood, the opportunity for the client's growth is jeopardized. The normative grief process and the process of filial maturity of midlife becomes blocked and may not be able to be attained because of the rage and disappointment felt about earlier lacks.

An example of a successful therapeutic contact addressing these concerns was Ms. G., who sought help when her mother became ill. She came seeking advice about whether or not to give up her work, her house and her friends in order to move across the country to be with her parent. Her idealizations of her mother were quite rigid; and her regrets about not having been the perfect daughter during her mother's earlier illness were intense and debilitating. After a brief encounter with the therapist, in which she decided to visit her mother more often but stay "in her own life," Ms.

G. left therapy. She returned six months later and began a piece of work over the course of several years in which she moved from perceiving her mother as beautiful, graceful and unattainable to also acknowledging the ways in which her mother had been emotionally unavailable to her. Finally, the intense anger which she carried and which had led her to very self-defeating involvements with others began to diminish. She was able to relate to friends and family in a more assertive and enhancing manner and to appreciate them with less rancor or personalization of their slights. In a phrase, Ms. G. summarized what the work meant to her. . . . "No one has ever listened to me as you have." She continued, "I also now realize that when people don't get what they need, they become angry and self-involved."

This therapy provided Ms. G. with a new, enhancing object to internalize, diminishing her negative introjects, enabling her to integrate her ambivalence towards others and to bear the sadness of her losses. Her enhanced self-esteem enabled her to finally move on with her life and to take social risks which she had never attempted. This more positive internalization indicates the developmental strides which can be taken when a client is enabled to grieve. Another way of conceptualizing this is that the client's defensive stance of altruistic surrender is transformed into her ability for "good-enough" self-care and hence more appropriate "other" care.

As described earlier, research by one of the authors (Shulman, 1988) established the parameters for what has been described in this paper. This study had suggested that caregiving may have a variety of meanings to individuals. For some individuals in the study, caregiving involved a reciprocal process which mirrored the kind of care given to the child by her parent, and enabled her to exercise her adult capacities and sense of self. These parent-child relationships were characterized by mutual respect and understanding of one another's strengths and limitations, as well as clarity around issues of differentiation of self and over which had either been ongoing or had been achieved over time. This group empirically defines and meets the theoretical definition of "filial maturity."

A second group of adults was more conflicted about the caregiving process. Old wounds were easily opened, there was more enduring awareness of the adult daughters' earlier unmet needs, and more difficulty moderating idealizations and devaluations of parental figures and personal expectations. This group has been the focus of the authors' clinical practices, since these women are the ones who most frequently seek help. The examples described herein are drawn from this group.

Finally, a third group described in the research was characterized by more brittle, "stuck" attitudes and behavior. These women tend to extreme solutions in parent-caring, either being devoted in a self-abnegating, self-restrictive manner, or experiencing constant rage and resentment and at times acting on these feelings by berating their mothers or, in extreme cases, abusing them. These are the people who rarely come to clinicians on their own accord. If they are referred to a social worker by another concerned professional, e.g., nurse or physician, these clients have difficulty sitting with that clinician long enough to negotiate the crisis and to learn a better adaptation for the future. Individuals from this group appear for help in medical crises and present problems for discharge planning in hospital settings.

In conclusion, the normative developmental task of midlife may be understood as a "third separation-individuation" process (Oldham, 1987), in which individuals are able to achieve a further sense of separation and autonomy from parental objects and an increasing sense of their own adulthood, or effectiveness as caregivers. This is the trajectory which allows for the passage to filial maturity. The concept of filial maturity is central. It acknowledges the interdependence of family members which persists throughout the life course and which is modified by developmental challenges. Difficulties which emerge during earlier separation-individuation processes are brought to the forefront in the parent-caregiving situation. At this juncture, people become overwhelmed with anxiety or entrenched in self-defeating behavior patterns because their relationships with their parents do not have enough positive reserves. This impedes their being able to provide care without severe conflict or self-abnegation. In addition, their incapacity to provide care represents a blow to self-esteem and to the sense of personal integrity which is such an essential achievement at this time of life. Treatment with those who are "stuck" in this process provides a context in which object constancy and enhancement of strengths allow developmental progress. The reliable therapist provides a milieu in which the client can bear her grief about her losses, endure the separation from childhood needs and wishes, and move on to a new integration of the self.

The final word is what a patient said as she was sorting through her caregiving role and attempting to achieve some adaptation and resolution. "Since you can't divorce your parents, you have to find a way to make it work."

▬REFERENCES

Anastas, J., Gibeau, J., & Larson, P. J. (1990). Working families and eldercare: A national perspective. *Social Work, 35*(5), 385–480.

Archbold, P. (1983). Impact of parent-caring on women. *Family Relations, 32,* 39–45.

Blenkner, M. (1965). Social work and family relationships in later life with some thoughts on filial maturity. In E. Shanas & G. Streib (Eds.), *Social Structure and the Family: Generational Relations.* New Jersey: Prentice Hall, Inc.

Brody, E. M. (1988). *Women in the middle: Their parent-care years.* New York: Springer Publishing Company.

Brody, E. M. (1985). Parent care as a normative family stress. *Gerontologist, 25,* 19–29.

Colarusso, C. A., & Nemiroff, R. A. (1981). *Adult development: A new dimension in psychodynamic theory and practice.* New York: Plenum Press.

Erikson, E. (1950). *Childhood and society.* New York: Norton.

Greenberg, S. (1994). Mutuality in families: A framework for continued growth in late life. *Journal of Geriatric Psychiatry, 26*(1), 79–96.

Havighurst, R. (1973). History of developmental psychology: Socialization and personality development. In P. B. Baltes & K. W. Schaie (Eds.), *Life-span developmental psychology* (pp. 3–24). New York: Academic Press.

Kernberg, O. (1985). *Internal world and external reality.* New York: Jason Aronson.

Miller, A. (1981). *The Drama of the Gifted Child.* New York: Basic Books.

Miller, D. A. (1981). The 'sandwich' generation: Adult children of the aging. *Social Work, 26,* 419–423.

Neugarten, B. L. (1968). *Middle-age and aging.* Chicago: University of Chicago Press.

Oldham, J. M. (1987, March). *The third individuation: The middle aged child and his or her parents.* Paper presented at the meeting for the Association for Psychoanalytic Medicine, New York, NY.

Shanas, E. (1979). The family as a social support system in old age. *Gerontologist, 19,* 169–174.

Shulman, S. C. (1988). *Adult daughters: The psychological impact of their aging mothers' need for care.* Unpublished doctoral dissertation: Smith College School for Social Work, Northampton, MA.

Treas, J. (1977). Family support systems for the aged: Some social and demographic considerations. *Gerontologist, 17,* 486–491.

Zarit, S. H., Orr, N., & Zarit, J. (1985). *The hidden victims of Alzheimer's disease: Families under stress.* New York: New York University Press.

Chapter 48

Caring for Caregivers:
Home Care Nursing's Challenge

LUANNE BROGNA

> Families bear the burden of caregiving the majority of the time. Often caregivers are frail and elderly themselves. In fact, 20 percent of children who care for parents are over 65 years old. Others who are younger often work outside the home. These caregivers have needs that may not be met. In this chapter home care nurses meet this challenge as they provide care for the caregiver as well as the client. The stress that caregivers may feel can be anticipated and reduced with good discharge planning. Assessment of the caregiver's perception of what stresses them gives the home care nurse a place to start, and followup can be provided by assisting the family to find the support they need. A case study illustrates the home care nurse's challenge.

Home care nurses frequently encounter elderly or disabled persons who receive a substantial amount of physical care at home from a lay caregiver. With the trend toward health care reform, hospitals are eager to further shorten lengths of stay. Earlier discharges have resulted in an ever-increasing number of patients being cared for at home. Because of this trend, patients are being discharged "quicker and sicker," increasing the demands on caregivers in the home.

In addition to legislative influence, the greater demand for home care services has been affected by the "graying of America." In the United States, more than 30 million people are 65 years old or older, comprising more than 12% of the total population.[1] Persons older than 85 years are the fastest-growing group, and "aging carries with it the likelihood of chronic disease."[2] Approximately 4.6 million noninstitutionalized, elderly persons have physical conditions that render them dependent on a caregiver for assistance with activities of daily living. Consequently, the demand for lay caregivers is enormous. Current estimates indicate that 85% of elderly persons (aged 65 years or older) live in the community by themselves or with spouses, family, or friends.[1] Their families bear the burden of

From *JWOCN* 23(1):10–14, 1996. Reprinted with permission.

providing care at home 80% of the time,[4] and in 72% of cases the burden falls on the shoulders of women.[1]

Because many of these caregivers are themselves frail and elderly, it becomes a challenge for the home care nurse to ensure that the patient receives quality care. Specialty nurses are in an ideal position to assist both the primary home care nurse and the lay caregiver in managing complex health problems associated with early hospital discharge. This article reviews the characteristics of the lay caregiver, the stressors involved in performing the caregiver role, and nursing interventions to assist the caregiver in maintaining the patient at home.

■ CHARACTERISTICS OF THE LAY CAREGIVER

The typical family caregiver is a woman older than 55 years. Other family members, friends, and neighbors assume secondary roles. Because of cultural beliefs and women's longer life expectancies, elderly men are typically cared for by their spouses, whereas elderly women are usually cared for by their daughters. When spouses and children are not available, siblings, grandchildren, nieces, and nephews may assume the caregiver's role.[5]

A sense of moral duty may motivate an adult child to assume the role of lay caregiver, but more often the role is related to proximity and necessity rather than choice.[5] The extended family living together in close proximity rarely exists today. Marital discord and global mobility have resulted in dispersal of families and fragmentation of households, many headed by single-parent, working women.[6] The caregiver role creates an additional stressor for the 44% of caregiving daughters who already work outside the home.[1] Given and Given[5] reported that three basic factors are involved in deciding to take on the role of primary caregiver: demographics, (for example, the case of the only child), proximity, and situational events (for example, the child with the least commitments).

■ STRESSORS OF CAREGIVING

Caregiving for the person with a chronic disease is undoubtedly a stressful experience. Responsibilities increase as the patient's physical condition deteriorates. In their review of the literature, "Family Caregiving for the Elderly," Given and Given[5] reported, "Caregivers who spend time and energy with direct physical and personal care may find tasks restrictive and confining." These increased demands disrupt their regular routines, resulting in decreased time for personal, social, and recreational activities. Caregiving frequently creates a great psychologic burden for the caregiver, manifested by depression, decreased life satisfaction, and lowered sense of well-being.

In their longitudinal study examining the health of family members caring for elderly persons, Baumgarten and associates[7] studied 181 subjects during a 1-year period, focusing on both depression and physical symptoms. Through interviews, they found that for both depression and physical symptoms the deterioration was greatest among caregivers of patients who required admittance to an institution during the study period. In addition, caregiver health was most affected by patients who manifested behavioral disturbances.

Stevens and associates' reviewed the literature and concurred that providing care to elderly persons is stressful and often leads to emotional, physical, interpersonal, and occupational problems. They estimated the incidence of depression among family caregivers to be 40% to 50%.[1] Feelings of anger, hostility, and guilt were often reported.

Parks and Pilisuk[4] confirmed that the caregiver population feels anxiety, depression, resentment, and guilt, and that these emotions exact an enormous personal toll. Women were found to be the predominant caregivers, and significant differences in coping patterns were found between the genders. Women were more likely to cope through fantasizing, whereas men typically handled stress by withdrawing. In addition, although the women were able to verbalize more stress and anxiety related to the caregiver role, the incidence of depression in the two genders was consistent.

Wagnild and Grupp[8] investigated the major stressors for elderly patients and their caregivers after discharge from the hospital. Rather than interviewing patients or caregivers, these investigators questioned Medicare-certified home health agencies. A sample comprising professionals from 105 agencies identified four primary stressors and emphasized the need to assist patients and caregivers in coping with these stressors. First, early discharge from the hospital often caused inadequate patient teaching and discharge planning. The acuteness of the illness at the time of discharge from the hospital also led to distress, particularly when complex, technology-driven treatments were required at home. In addition, the home environment was identified as a stressor when it was unsafe or unsuitable for the recovering patient. Finally, inadequate resources, including lack of caregivers, inadequate finances, or lack of equipment, acted as a significant stressor. This stress often led to feelings of being overwhelmed, rendering both patient and caregiver unable to comprehend or accomplish treatment goals and increasing the risk of rehospitalization. A clearer understanding of these potential stressors allows the home health nurse to intervene more appropriately on behalf of the patient and caregiver and thus to reduce the risk of complications and rehospitalization.

▬INTERVENTIONS

Before the home care nurse can intervene, it is necessary to complete an assessment to identify problems and establish priorities. In addition to completing demographic data, medical history, and a physical assessment, Wagnild and Grupp[8] suggest asking additional questions on the admission visit to identify major stressors. These questions include the following:

1. Do the patient and caregiver understand the discharge plan?
2. Were discharge instructions reviewed more than once?
3. Did the caregiver get an opportunity for hands-on practice?
4. Do the patient and caregiver have written materials describing any treatments to be performed in the home?

5. Have referral agencies followed through?
6. Are friends and family available to help?

In addition, the home health care nurse should evaluate whether potential caregivers are available, capable, and reliable, and whether the home environment is adequate and safe for the patient's needs during recovery. Such an assessment helps to identify specific problems that can be addressed by home health services, but it is also important to consider the patient's and caregiver's perspectives. For a successful outcome, the goals for care must be agreed on by the agency, patient, and caregiver. To determine the patient's and caregiver's perspectives, the following questions may prove helpful:

1. What do you see as the major problem after your hospitalization?
2. Do you feel capable of handling this problem?
3. What are your strengths and weaknesses?
4. Do you feel alone or isolated?
5. What are your plans and hopes for the future?
6. How do you view the role of the home health care nurse?

It is important that caregivers know from the outset what is expected of them and the extent of the services that can be provided.[9] Both formal and informal services can be used to assist the caregiver to cope with multiple stressors. Formal services include nursing, social work, home health aides, respite care, day care, meals-on-wheels, home delivery of groceries, and chore services. Informal services consist of a mixture of family, friends, neighbors, church groups, and volunteer community support services. Enabling the patient and caregiver to mobilize as many services as may be necessary enables a smooth transition into home care. The case report in Box 48-1 illustrates several sources of assistance for the home caregiver.

A major part of the intervention phase involves education, which is a primary role of the professional nurse. Cognitive and perceptual alterations may make teaching the lay caregiver challenging.[2] Keen observation and interviewing skills can make the physical examination an excellent opportunity to evaluate the capabilities of both the patient and the caregiver.

After the level of knowledge of the caregiver has been determined, teaching strategies are developed and implemented. Although it would be desirable to provide detailed instruction to the caregiver and patient, it is more important to identify what they "need to know" than what would be "nice to know."[10] Because of significant stressors associated with providing home care, simple, straightforward instruction concerning treatments or other procedures is most helpful.

Principles of teaching-learning can promote more effective outcomes. The environment should be conducive to learning: clean, quiet, private, and well lit. Instruction begins with simple tasks and moves on to more complex concepts as the caregiver gains confidence. The nurse provides clear and simple directions, in terms that the caregiver can understand, while the procedure is demonstrated. Time is allowed for questions and

BOX 48-1   Case report

Mr. J. C.,* an 84-year-old man, lives with his 80-year-old wife in a private home. He has a long-standing history of Parkinson's disease, with increasing disability as the years have passed. He has been dependent on his wife for assistance with activities of daily living for some time. When he became bedbound, his primary physician made a referral to a home health agency. On admission, the primary nurse assessed Mr. C.'s needs as including incontinence management, pressure ulcer prevention and treatment, nutritional support, and personal care. A stage II pressure ulcer found on the sacral area measured 4 × 3 cm, with a clean granular wound bed.

The home care nurse determined that the patient's elderly caregiver, Mrs. C., was overwhelmed by her spouse's multiple problems. She was unable to manage his care, primarily because of a lack of knowledge and understanding. The couple's two adult children are married and live in other parts of the country. The neighborhood primarily comprises elderly couples and widows. Mrs. C., however, remains on active member of her religious community, and her financial position is good.

The primary home health nurse addressed the patient's and caregiver's concerns. She then placed a home health aide in the home 5 days a week to assist Mrs. C. with Mr. C.'s personal care. She obtained an order from the physician to use a hydrocolloid dressing on the wound and a condom catheter for containment of urinary incontinence. An alternating-air mattress overlay was ordered to prevent further tissue necrosis. Daily visits were made for the first week to instruct the caregiver on turning and positioning, use of a condom catheter and diapers, skin care, range-of-motion exercises, nutritional intake and supplements, rationale for use of hydrocolloid, and signs and symptoms of wound infection. Mrs. C. was also provided with written instructions and a videotape on preventing pressure ulcers. As Mrs. C. showed signs of reduced anxiety and increased control, the visits were decreased to twice a week for wound monitoring and dressing changes.

During the course of 1 month, the wound showed gradual improvement. Healing was slow because of difficulty with feeding the patient. His facial rigidity made chewing impossible, so he was limited to pureed foods. Feeding was a long, tedious process, but Mrs. C. was patient and supplemented his diet with milkshakes.

As the primary home health nurse began to prepare Mrs. C. for Mr. C.'s discharge from home care services, Mr. C.'s condition worsened. His rigidity and his mood swings increased. He refused both turning and food. On the next scheduled visit, the nurse found an eschar in the sacral area measuring 6 × 2 cm. At that time, the primary home health nurse informed the physician and obtained an ET nursing consultation.

Because the patient was still afebrile, an enzymatic debriding agent and low-air loss bed were recommended. Because repositioning the patient was now impossible, the selected mattress replacement unit included a turning mode. Visits were again scheduled daily, and it was suggested that Mrs. C. hire some private help to supplement the Medicare benefit. A social work referral was made for future planning and counseling.

(continued)

> ### BOX 48-1   *Case report* (continued)
>
> Within 2 weeks, the patient became febrile and was admitted to the hospital for treatment of dehydration, pneumonia, and wound infection. During his 10-day stay, Mr. C. was given a course of intravenous antibiotics, was rehydrated, and underwent surgical debridement. A Foley catheter was placed, but the family refused placement of a feeding tube. After Mr. C.'s discharge from hospital, the surgeon ordered normal saline wet-to-damp dressing changes twice a day.
>
> The ET nurse then reevaluated the wound and found it to be 80% granular with 20% slough. It measured 6 × 6 cm and was 1.5 cm deep, with a 2 cm area of undermining from the 9 to 3 o'clock positions. A copious amount of serosanguineous drainage soaked through the dressing within 12 hours. Mrs. C.'s slight frame and Mr. C.'s poor physical condition made it impossible for her to change the dressing. The physician was contacted, and he agreed to the use of a calcium alginate packing to absorb drainage and thereby decrease the frequency of changes.
>
> At this time, the wound is clean and Mr. C. remains afebrile. Mrs. C. is happy to have her husband at home, and she has hired additional help for the weekend. She feeds him as much as she can and understands the importance of good nutrition to wound healing, but she prefers to keep routines as normal as possible. She has her groceries delivered and receives friendly, supportive visits from members of her church. The goal at the home health agency has been altered from wound healing to maintaining the patient at home.
>
> *A pseudonym.

answers. Positive reinforcement is provided when the caregiver shows evidence of understanding concepts, and patient and caregiver are given simple written instructions in bold type.[2,10]

The instruction process is started as early as possible to allow time for the lay caregiver to assimilate the skills required to complete complex tasks. When the caregiver has observed a procedure several times and demonstrates a readiness to progress, he or she can move on to handling equipment. Bold labels on product boxes that correspond to numbered, written instructions are helpful when teaching procedures that require multiple steps. Videotapes and audiotapes are left with the caregiver to allow multiple reviews in an unpressured setting until the knowledge has been acquired. Ample time is allowed for hands-on practice with supervision. In addition, caregivers are encouraged to use calendars and notepads for record keeping if they have trouble recalling when procedures should be performed or when pertinent data are required for ongoing assessments.

Once teaching has been completed, an evaluation of its effectiveness should be performed. Feedback is obtained both verbally and by return demonstration. Caregivers who prove that they can provide adequate care to ensure the prevention of complications should be given plenty of praise and reinforcement. If there is evidence of substandard care, teaching strategies should be reevaluated with consideration of either an alternative treatment or a more capable caregiver. Box 48-1 illustrates changes in treatment in response to a caregiver's physical limitations.

In addition to physical skills, caregivers should be taught interventions to manage behavioral symptoms related to chronic conditions and interventions that support the caregiver's own coping resources.[1] Older women may need to be taught how to be more assertive to enable them to enlist help from family and friends. They may need encouragement to get involved in support groups, or to seek counseling when stressors become overwhelming. Guilt may be the overriding emotion that prevents a caregiver from seeking outside help. Attentive listening and encouragement of verbalization may be enough to allow the caregiver to seek assistance when needed.

Caregivers who are reluctant to obtain support through the community may find comfort and assistance from a church group. Kaye and Robinson[11] found that caregivers identified spirituality as an important resource that helped to provide perspective, support, and strength. Support through religious faith was associated with positive outcomes. Services provided through the church, such as support groups and respite care, may be more acceptable than community-based services to caregivers with a strong spiritual perspective.

Malett[12] outlined three strategies important to assisting caregivers in the home: education, support and referral. When communication problems and confusion arise despite attention to the management of stressors, an outside referral is indicated. Meetings of the primary and secondary caregivers with the home care nurse and social worker allow open, problem-focused discussions. Unresolved, unaddressed family issues can create an environment that leads to neglect or abuse. The family and home health agency may need to establish a written contract or acceptable behaviors. If mutual ground cannot be found, families need guidance to explore other options. Families should be encouraged to discuss options both among themselves and with their outside support systems.

▬ SUMMARY

Today, family caregivers find themselves providing personal care and skilled home health care — tasks at which they have little or no previous experience — in ever-increasing numbers. The home health care nurse is uniquely qualified to assist these lay caregivers with support, education, and referral, enabling them to maintain patients in the comfort of their own home.

▬ REFERENCES

1. Stevens GL, Walsh RA, Baldwin BA. Family caregivers of institutionalized and noninstitutionalized elderly individuals. Nurs Clin North Am 1993;28:349–52.
2. Jubeck ME. Are you sensitive to the cognitive needs of the elderly? Home Health Nurse 1992;10(5):20–5.
3. Steel K. Home care for the elderly: the new institution. Arch Intern Med 1991;81:223–5.

4. Parks SH, Pilisuk M. Caregiver Burden: Gender and the psychological costs of caregiving. Am J Orthopsychiatry 1991;61:501–9.
5. Given BA, Given OW. Family caregiving for the elderly. Annu Rev Nurs Res 1991;9:77–101.
6. Gordon M. Community care for the elderly: is it really better? Can Med Assoc J 1993;148:393–6.
7. Baumgarten M, Hanley JA, Infante-Rirard C, Battista RN, Becker R, Gauthier S. Health of family members caring for elderly persons with dementia: a longitudinal study. Ann Intern Med 1994;120:126–32.
8. Wagnild G, Grupp K. Major stressors among elderly home care clients. Home Health Nurse 1991;9(4):15–21.
9. Papantino CT. Home health care management of chronic wounds. In: Krasner D, ed. Chronic wound care: a clinical sourcebook for healthcare professionals. King of Prussia, Pennsylvania: Health Management Publications, 1990:318–26.
10. Krasner D. The ET nurse's role in educating patients with open or draining wounds. J Enterostom Ther 1986;13:17–9.
11. Kaye J, Robinson K. Spirituality among caregivers. Image J Nurs Sch 1994;26:218–21.
12. Malett J. Caring for the caretakers: the patient's family. J ET Nurs 1993;20:78–81.

Chapter 49

Restraint-Free Care: How Does a Nurse Decide?

EILEEN M. SULLIVAN-MARX

> Caregiving decisions that involve physical restraint is a complex process that involves comprehensive, individualized assessment and creative problem solving. There are increasing institutional and social policy decisions that support physical restraint elimination in the caregiving and management of older adults. At times, these decisions are at odds with nurses' concerns for safety and behavior control, causing conflict in caregiving. As a result, it is important to explore nurses' knowledge, autonomy, and accountability in the decision-making process regarding nursing care. In addition, exploring the elder's feelings of dependence and powerlessness gives credence to policy changes that must be supported by nurses. Eileen Sullivan-Marx explores these issues in depth and suggests a team approach to developing restraint-free care.

As noted by Evans, Strumpf, & Williams (1991) fundamental issues regarding use of physical restraints in older adults are concerned with deleterious effects of restraints, ethical questions of human dignity, and individuals' legal rights. Nurses' concerns for safety and control of behavior form a foundation of belief for restraint use that stands in contrast to the efficacy and ethical arguments against such use. Despite legislative and other efforts to reduce use of physical restraints, the prevalence of physical restraint use in nursing homes in the United States exceeds that in other Western countries (Strumpf & Evans, 1992).

Staff attitude regarding restraint use has come under focus in research to better understand resistance to restraint reduction and to design interventions aimed at reduction of restraints (Schott-Baer, Lusis, & Beauregard, 1995; Sundel, Garrett, & Horn, 1994; Werner, Koroknay, Braun, & Cohen-Mansfield, 1994). Nurses' and other staff's attitudes, defined as a tendency or disposition to use physical restraints in older adults, is a critical component of nurses' decision-making regarding restraint use. To understand nurses' decisions to use restraints despite the limited efficacy and negative

From *Journal of Gerontological Nursing* 22(9):7–14, 1996. Reprinted with permission.

effects of restraint use, contributing factors such as accountability, knowledge, autonomy, and authority need to be considered. Characterizing decision-making about restraint use can facilitate improved problem-solving leading to restraint-free care of older adults.

The purpose of this article is to characterize factors influencing nurses' decision-making regarding physical restraint use with older adults. Discussion includes presentation of a framework, adapted from Baer (1993), for understanding decisions regarding restraint use in older adults and implications for practice and research.

▬ FRAMEWORK

Decisions regarding restraint use or avoidance are highly complex, requiring consideration of a myriad of clinical and environmental factors (Evans, Strumpf, & Williams, 1991; McHutchion & Morse, 1989). Decision-making in clinical practice occurs within a context of professional authority, competence, and autonomy. According to Baer (1993), society ". . . requires from its practitioners independence and autonomous decision-making based on professional knowledge" (p. 104).

The ensuing discussion and Fig. 49-1 are adapted from Baer (1986). The Figure presents a schema which is useful to explain the context of nurses' decision-making regarding physical restraint use in older adults. In this schema, knowledge and accountability contribute to a professional's authority to act. Autonomy, the freedom to independently act, is derived from authority and exists along a continuum which theoretically ranges from no autonomy to full autonomy. In the reality of any practice discipline, however, no clinician functions completely autonomously. Baer (1993) notes that "independent, autonomous practice rests on the assumption that the agent of such a practice has the expertise from which that agent derives the authority to act" (p. 105). In deciding to use or not use restraints, nurses employ their authority that is simultaneously influenced by nurses'

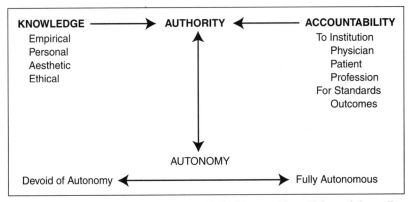

FIGURE 49-1   Schema of the context of decision-making (Adapted from Baer, 1986).

knowledge regarding restraint use and their accountability to patients, colleagues, and professional standards of practice.

Knowledge

Knowledge, including empirical, aesthetic, ethical, and personal knowledge, undergirds authority to practice. Level of education of nursing staff (Ramprogus & Gibson, 1991), empirical knowledge (Scherer, Janelli, Wu, & Kuhn, 1993; Yarmesch & Sheafor, 1984), ethical knowledge (Moss & La Puma, 1991; Strumpf & Evans, 1991), and personal knowledge of the patient (Chinn & Kramer, 1991) contribute to decisions to avoid restraint use.

To make appropriate decisions about interventions with patients, it is essential for nurses to understand how one knows what to practice, research, and teach. The four patterns of knowing in nursing identified by Carper (1978) are "a) empirics, the science of knowing; b) aesthetics, the art of nursing; c) the component of a personal knowledge in nursing; and d) ethics, the component of moral knowledge in nursing" (p. 13).

Empirically, it is clear that use of physical restraints has harmful physical and psychological effects and limited efficacy (Capezuti, Strumpf, Evans, Grisso, & Maislin, 1995; Evans & Strumpf, 1990). Ethical considerations to any use of physical restraints requires exploration of antecedents to behavior, as well as avoiding harm caused by restraint use, particularly in the absence of informed consent. Personal and aesthetic knowledge invite the therapeutic use of self and empathy in the nurse-patient interaction. Exploring the sense of powerlessness a patient feels when restrained dictates that the nurse avoid gaining control of the patient through promotion of dependency. By realizing the meaning of the restraint experience for the confused older adult, a nurse should resolve to adapt an individualized plan of care as opposed to routinely restraining a patient.

Ramprogus and Gibson (1991) surveyed professional nurses' and nursing assistants' reasons for restraint use, knowledge of alternatives, and awareness of effects of retraint use. Professional nurses were more likely than nursing assistants to: 1) associate restraints with loss of freedom, 2) identify more alternatives to restraint use, and 3) list more negative effects of restraint use. In a survey of acute care and intensive care unit nurses, attendance at gerontological continuing education sessions influenced knowledge of alternative measures to restraint use (Yarmesch & Sheafor, 1984).

The expert professional nurse is arguably the most able to synthesize knowledge and experience when addressing multifaceted problems of frail older adults. Benner's (1984) work demonstrates that the expert nurse seems to effortlessly reach conclusions and take action in complex situations. Restraint reduction programs that have incorporated the use of expert, advanced practice nurses (clinical specialists and nurse practitioners) have been the most successful in reducing restraint use, supporting Benner's theory (Evans, Strumpf, Taylor, & Jacobsen, 1990–1992; Sundel, Garrett, & Horn, 1994; Werner, Koroknay, Braun, & Cohen-Mansfield, 1994).

In a study contrasting nursing interventions aimed at restraint reduction in nursing homes, education of staff plus consultation with a gerontological clinical nurse specialist (GNCS) was significantly associated with greater restraint reduction than either an intervention of education alone or a control group (Reducing restraints, 1993). Following initiation of a restraint reduction program in another nursing home study, only 10% of residents were no longer restrained. Subsequently, a GNCS implemented individualized care measures that ultimately resulted in discontinuance of restraints in 90% ($N=52$) of restrained residents ($N=57$) (Werner, Koroknay, Braun, & Cohen-Mansfield, 1994).

Licensed nursing personnel (predominantly licensed practical nurses) were more likely than nonlicensed nursing personnel to initiate new physical restraint use in a study examining predictors of continued and new restraint use. New restraint use was lower, however, on units in which there was a gerontological nursing consultation (Sullivan-Marx, Strumpf, Evans, Baumgarten, & Maislin, 1995).

Clearly, expert nursing knowledge and competence is a significant component of decisions regarding restraint elimination. Restraint studies in nursing homes to date have only defined the expert nurse as an advanced practice nurse. Given the dearth of professional registered nurses in nursing homes, the contribution of the expert generalist nurse needs to be more clearly discerned.

Joel & Patterson (1990) point out that re-direction of professional registered nurses in nursing homes for clinical care is cost-effective and increases quality of care. Professional registered nurses in hospital settings, however, do not easily identify alternatives to restraint use (Strumpf & Evans, 1988). Further study is needed to clearly define the expertise and level of professional practice most germane to restraint avoidance.

Accountability

Authority can be demonstrated through accountability. Professional nurses are concurrently accountable to patients, organized systems of care, professional colleagues, and professional standards of care (Baer, 1986). Decisions regarding physical restraints may create a dilemma of accountability for the nurse (Conely & Campbell, 1991; McHutchion & Morse, 1989). Baer (1986) notes that "nursing finds itself in situations of conflict of accountability quite frequently" (p. 19). To appreciate complexities of these potential conflicts, nurses need to understand how each of these components influence care decisions regarding restraint use.

Organized Systems of Care

The decision-making process regarding restraint use is influenced by social and institutional policies. The enactment in 1990 of the Nursing Home Reform Law, part of the Omnibus Budget Reconciliation Act of 1987 (OBRA), and efforts by public and professional advocates sought to improve quality of care for older adults in nursing homes by encouraging reduction in use of physical and chemical restraints. Policy mandates led to increased activity related to restraint reduction by organizational systems, particularly nursing homes, however, two years following enactment of the Nursing Home Reform Law, prevalence of restraint use still exceeded rates for comparable residents in other Western countries (Strumpf & Evans, 1992). As part of a longitudinal clinical trial aimed at restraint reduction in nursing homes, effects of OBRA legislation were evaluated. Six months following OBRA implementation, there was no significant change in patterns of restraint use with the nursing home residents (Evans, Strumpf, Capezuti, Taylor, & Jacobsen, 1992).

Myths about restraint use in an organizational environment, such as fear of litigation (Evans & Strumpf, 1990; Quinn, 1991) and concern about the need to increase staff (Scherer, Janelli, Wu, & Kuhn, 1993), may influence nurses to routinely use physical restraints in efforts to avoid litigation or costly staff increases. Staff nurses are isolated in an organization in which there is minimal interdisciplinary collaboration, increasing the likelihood that physical restraints are used to control behaviors (Frengley & Mion, 1986; MacPherson, Lofgren, Granieri, & Myllenbeck, 1990; Strumpf & Evans, 1988).

Prevention of harm to self and others, responding to family requests and physician orders, obliging nursing peers, and protection of the hospital from lawsuits were identified as reasons for restraint use in a study of nurses' perceptions of restraint use (Quinn, 1993). In this study, nurses felt a moral dilemma between the patient's right to freedom and the decision to apply restraint. Nurses overcame this dilemma by distancing themselves from the action of restraint and subsequent effects for patients (Quinn, 1993).

Organized systems of care, and nurses who practice within systems, are held accountable to current policies that discourage restraint use. Kapp (1992) notes that "the relative risks for indiscriminate, inappropriate use of physical restraints place them [long-term-care providers] at much greater tort and regulatory jeopardy than does a reduced reliance on restraints" (p. 31).

Staffing concerns have been reported as reasons for physical restraint use (Evans & Strumpf, 1990). Sloane and colleagues (1991) reported that a ratio of greater patients-to-staff was an independent predictor of restraint use in nursing home dementia units. Other studies suggest that restrained individuals require more time to care for, not less (Morse & McHutchion, 1991; Phillips, Hawes, & Fries, 1993; What is the law?, 1989).

To implement a restraint-free policy in nursing homes, the Kendal Corporation (Blakeslee, Goldman, Papougenis, & Torell, 1991) recommended targeting the board of directors, administration, physicians, nursing home staff, residents, and family and friends. Case reports (Kallman, Denine-Flynn, & Blackburn, 1992; Martin & Hughes, 1993; Powell, Mitchell-Pedersen, Fingerote, & Edmund, 1989; Suprock, 1990) and one long-term study (Dunbar, 1993) suggest that an institutional philosophy and program of restraint-free care can be successful. Institutional and social policies, staffing patterns, obligation to institutions, peers, and families influence decision-making regarding restraint use although the degree of influence is subject for further study.

Professional Colleagues

Collaboration among multiple disciplines is a premise of restraint reduction (Evans, Strumpf, & Williams, 1991). Cooperative decision-making between nurses and physicians produces positive outcomes including lower mortality (Aiken, Smith, & Lake, 1994), lower costs, and greater patient satisfaction (Baggs & Schmitt, 1988). Although a physician order is required for a restraint, nurses are given great deference in decisions to use restraints (MacPherson, Lofgren, Granieri, & Myllenbeck, 1990). Efforts mandating a physician signature to initiate restraints forces some level of communication between nurses and physicians but does not specifically encourage collaboration.

In a study of physical restraint use on acute medical units, Frengley and Mion (1986) concluded that nursing staff first perceived a need to restrain a patient and then sought an order from a physician; thus, opportunities to discuss alternatives to restraint use were limited. A survey of nurses and physicians caring for restrained hospitalized patients revealed that nurses initiated restraints in 75% of the cases, 15% of physicians were unaware that their patients were restrained, and more physicians than nurses could identify alternatives to restraints (MacPherson, Lofgren, Granieri, & Myllenbeck, 1990).

Strumpf and Evans (1988) noted that 19 of 20 decisions to restrain a hospitalized patient were made solely by the nurse. Hardin and colleagues (1994) concluded, in contrast, that nurses do use collaboration in decision-making for restraint use. A specific description of interdisciplinary collaboration in these studies would help to clarify differences in findings.

Decision-making by nurses in isolation diminishes discussion of creative approaches to care. Collaborative planning using a team approach would reduce nurses' isolation in care decisions and potentially lead to elimination of restraints.

Patients

Lack of nurse-patient interaction has been found among nurses caring for confused older adults (Armstrong-Esther & Browne, 1986; Liukkonen, 1992). Interactions with patients that are poor in quality may contribute to the perception of the older adult as an object, creating an environment in which the nurse finds it easier to apply restraints. Morse & McHutchion (1991) found that nursing interactions with patients increased after restraints were removed, although actual time with the patient decreased. If nurses have little interaction with confused elderly patients, interaction may decline even further once restraints are applied and thus perpetuate prolonged, unwarranted restraint use.

Accountability to the older adult requires an individualized approach to care leading to assessment of behavior and implementation of interventions other than restraints.

Standards of Care

A movement of non-restraint use espoused by consumers, aging advocates, and professionals took hold in the mid-to-late 1980s and led to legislation, policy change, and a revised standard of care in nursing homes (Evans,

Strumpf, & Williams, 1991; Strumpf & Tomes, 1993). This revision in standards has been felt by acute care hospitals as well, where policies on use of physical restraints are beginning to change. The 1991 restraint and seclusion guidelines of the Joint Commission on Accreditation of Healthcare Organizations (1991) requires hospital policies to specify time frames for medical orders and use of restraints, periodic observations, and re-evaluation and new orders if restraints are to be continued. In addition, the U.S. Food and Drug Administration (FDA), in response to reports of restraint-related deaths and other known risks of physical restraints, mandates that all devices carry a warning label concerning potential hazards (Department of Health & Human Services, 1992).

Restraint-free care, as contrasted with restraint reduction, is currently emerging as the standard of care for older adults (Kapp, 1992). Increasingly nurses are being held accountable to these professional standards and social policies.

Autonomy

Autonomous practices are based on an assumption of knowledge and expertise (Baer, 1993). In making decisions to intervene with patients, nurses need to have autonomy to act with authority. In a study of autonomy in performing nursing activities, autonomy was noted in: 1) nurses with a master's degree in nursing, 2) advanced practice nurses, 3) public health nurses, and 4) psychiatric nurses (Schutzenhofer & Musser, 1994). Development of autonomy in registered nursing staff is key to creating alternatives to restraints (Joel & Patterson, 1990). Increasing autonomy of professional nurses or using advanced practice nurses would increase the likelihood that care decisions other than restraint use would be developed.

■PRACTICE AND RESEARCH IMPLICATIONS
Practice

Need for control of behavior (Evans & Strumpf, 1990), lack of knowledge of alternatives (Evans, Strumpf, & Williams, 1991), limited assessment of behavior (Francis, 1989), belief in a principle of safety above all (Evans & Strumpf, 1990; Yarmesch & Sheafor, 1984), and lack of awareness of negative consequences associated with restraint use (Evans & Strumpf, 1990; MacPherson, Lofgren, Granieri, & Myllenbeck, 1990; Yarmesch & Sheafor, 1984) create a cultural-psychosocial attitude in which restraint use is either tolerated or avoided. Nurses' attitudes and beliefs about restraint use contribute to a context of decision-making in which knowledge, accountability, autonomy, and authority is framed. To improve the quality of care, decisions about care for older adults in which restraints are eliminated require increasing nurses' knowledge through education, accountability through enactment of standards and team approach to care, autonomy to act in ways that they can make decisions without fear of litigation, and authority to initiate creative problem-solving.

To establish restraint-free care, nurses need to focus on environmental designs which facilitate restraint function, provide security, and promote freedom. Implementation of individualized approaches to care promotes restraint elimination and is based on the following principles: 1) all behavior has meaning, 2) systematic approaches are required to assess behavior, and 3) once behavior is understood, underlying needs can be addressed (Strumpf, Wagner, Evans, & Patterson, 1992).

Research

In the last decade, there has been great effort by nurse researchers and others that has led to increased knowledge about restraint-free care with older adults. Further work to enhance current understanding about decision-making regarding restraint-free care includes studies that: 1) evaluate responses to the restraint experience, 2) define levels of professional nursing expertise needed to facilitate restraint-free care, and 3) investigate restraint-free care in acute care facilities.

Conclusion

The multi-faceted and complex needs of the frail older adult in an institutional environment present challenges for the professional nurse. Current transitions in standards regarding use of physical restraints find nurses struggling with convictions of protectionism versus belief in the individual rights of their patients. Decision-making regarding restraint use or avoidance is influenced by the context of institutional and social policies and the nurses' professional personae. It has been argued in this article that knowledge, accountability, and autonomy contribute to decisions that avoid restraint use. Further work is needed to qualify and quantify these efforts.

▬REFERENCES

Aiken, L.H., Smith, H.L., & Lake, E.T. (1994). Lower Medicare mortality among a set of hospitals known for good nursing care. *Medical Care, 32,* 771–787.

Armstrong-Esther, C.A., & Browne, K.D. (1986). The influence of elderly patients' mental impairment on nurse-patient interaction. *Journal of Advanced Nursing, 11,* 379–387.

Baer, E.D. (1986). A philosophical argument supporting primary care nursing. In M.D. Mezey & D.O. McGivern (Eds.), *Nurses, Nurse Practitioners* (pp. 15–28). Boston, MA: Little, Brown and Company.

Baer, E.D. (1993). Philosophical and historical bases of primary care nursing. In M.D. Mezey & D.O. McGivern (Eds.), *Nurses, Nurse Practitioners: Evolution to advanced practice* (pp. 102–116). New York, NY: Springer.

Baggs, J.G., & Schmitt, M.H. (1988). Collaboration between nurses and physicians. *Image: The Journal of Nursing Scholarship, 20,* 145–149.

Benner, P. (1984). *From novice to expert.* Menlo Park, CA: Addison-Wesley.

Blakeslee, J.A., Goldman, B.D., Papougenis, D., & Torell, C.A. (1991). Debunking the myths. *Geriatric Nursing, 11,* 290.

Capezuti, E., Strumpf, N., Evans, L., Grisso, J., & Maislin, G. (1995). *The relationship between physical restraint removal and fall-related incidencts and injuries among nursing home residents.* Paper presented at the 48th Annual Scientific Meeting of the Gerontological Society of America, November, 1995, Los Angeles, CA.

Carper, B.A. (1978). Fundamental patterns of knowing in nursing. *Advances in Nursing Science, 1,* 13–23.

Chinn, P.L., & Kramer, M.K. (1991). *Theory and nursing. A systematic approach* (3rd ed.). St. Louis, MO: Mosby-Year Book.

Conely, L.G., & Campbell, L.A. (1991). The use of restraints in caring for the elderly: Realities, consequences and alternatives. *Nurse Practitioner, 16*(12), 48–52.

Department of Health and Human Services, Food and Drug Administration. (1992). Medical Devices; Protective Restraints; Revocation of Exemptions from 510 (K) Premarket Notification Procedures and Current Manufacturing Resolutions. 21 CFR 880, 890 [Docket No. 91N-0487]. *Federal Register, 7*(119): 27397.

Dunbar, J. (1993, November). *Restraint review.* (Available from Joan Dunbar, The Jewish Home and Hospital for the Aged, 120 West 106th Street, NY, NY 10025.)

Evans, L.K., & Strumpf, N.E. (1990). Myths about elder restraint. *Image: The Journal of Nursing Scholarship, 22,* 124–128.

Evans, L.K., Strumpf, N.E., Capezuti, E., Taylor, L., & Jacobsen, B. (1992, November). *Short-term effects of regulatory change on nursing home practice: The case of physical restraint.* Paper presented at the Annual Meeting of the Gerontological Society of America, New Orleans, LA.

Evans, L.K. Strumpf, N.E., Taylor, L., & Jacobsen, B. (1990–1992). Reducing restraints in nursing homes: A clinical trial. (Grant No. 1, RO1-AGO8324). Washington, D.C.: National Institute of Aging.

Evans, L.K., Strumpf, N.E., & Williams, C. (1991). Redefining a standard of care for frail older people: Alternatives to routine physical restraint. In P. Katz, R. Kane, & M. Mezey (Eds.), *Advances in long term care,* Vol. 1. New York, NY: Springer.

Francis, J. (1989). Using restraints in elderly because of fear of litigation [Letter to the editor]. *The New England Journal of Medicine, 320,* 870.

Frengley, J.D., & Mion, L.C. (1986). Incidence of physical restraints on acute general medical wards. *Journal of the American Geriatrics Society, 34,* 565–568.

Hardin, S.B., Magee, R., Stratman, D., Vinson, M.H., Owen, M., & Hyatt, E.C. (1994). Extended care and nursing home staff attitudes toward restraints. *Journal of Gerontological Nursing, 20*(3), 23–31.

Joel, L.A., & Patterson, J.E. (1990, April). Nursing homes can't afford cheap nursing care. *RN,* 57–60.

Joint Commission on Accreditation of Healthcare Organizations. (1991, January/February). Restraint and seclusion guidelines. *Joint Commission Perspectives.* Insert. D1-5.

Kallman, S.L., Denine-Flynn, M., & Blackburn, D.M. (1992). Comfort, safety, and independence: Restraint release and its challenges. *Geriatric Nursing, 13*(3), 142–148.

Kapp, M.B. (1992). Nursing home restraints and legal liability. *The Journal of Legal Medicine, 13,* 1–32.

Liukkonen, A. (1992). Quality of care on a psychogeriatric nursing unit in Finland: Focus on interaction skills. *Geriatric Nursing, 13,* 167–169.

MacPherson, D.S., Lofgren, R.P., Granieri, R., & Myllenbeck, S. (1990). Deciding to restrain medical patients. *Journal of the American Geriatrics Society, 38,* 516–520.

Martin, L.S., & Hughes, S.R. (1993). Using the mission statement to craft a least-restraint policy. *Nursing Management, 24*(3), 65–66.

McHutchion, E., & Morse, J.M. (1989). Releasing restraints: A nursing dilemma. *Journal of Gerontological Nursing, 15*(2), 16–21.

Morse, J.M., & McHutchion, E. (1991). Releasing restraints: Providing safe care for the elderly. *Research in Nursing and Health, 14,* 187–196.

Moss, R.J., & LaPuma, J. (1991, January/February). The ethics of mechanical restraints. *Hastings Center Report,* 22–25.

Phillips, C.D., Hawes, C., & Fries, B.E. (1993). Reducing the use of physical restraints in nursing homes: Will it increase costs? *American Journal of Public Health, 83,* 342–348.

Powell, C., Mitchell-Pedersen, L., Fingerote, E., & Edmund, L. (1989). Freedom from restraint: Consequences of reducing physical restraints in the management of the elderly. *Canadian Medical Association Journal,* 561–563.

Quinn, C.A. (1991). *Nurses' perception of factors involved in the use of physical restraints with elderly patients in an acute care hospital.* Indiana University: Unpublished dissertation.

Quinn, C.A. (1993). Nurses' perception about physical restraints. *Western Journal of Nursing Research, 15,* 148–162.

Ramprogus, V., & Gibson, J. (1991). Assessing restraints. *Nursing Times, 87*(26), 45–47.

Scherer, Y.K., Janelli, L.M., Wu, Y.B., & Kuhn, M.M. (1993). Restrained patients: An important issue for critical care nursing. *Heart and Lung, 22*(1), 77–83.

Schott-Baer, D., Lusis, S., & Beauregard, K. (1995). Use of restraints: Changes in nurses' attitudes. *Journal of Gerontological Nursing, 21*(2), 39–44.

Schutzenhofer, K.K., & Musser, D.B. (1994). Nurse characteristics and professional autonomy. *Image: The Journal of Nursing Scholarship, 26,* 201–205.

Sloane, P.D., Mathew, L.J., Scarborough, M., Desai, J.R., Koch, G.G., & Tangen, C. (1991). Physical and pharmacologic restraint of nursing home patients with dementia. *Journal of the American Medical Association, 265,* 1278–1282.

Strumpf, N.E., & Evans, L.K. (1988). Physical restraint of the hospitalized elderly: Perceptions of patients and nurses. *Nursing Research, 37,* 132–137.

Strumpf, N.E., & Evans, L.K. (1991). The ethical problems of prolonged physical restraint. *Journal of Gerontological Nursing, 17*(2), 27–30.

Strumpf, N.E., & Evans, L.K. (1992). Alternatives to physical restraints. *Journal of Gerontological Nursing, 18*(2), 4.

Strumpf, N.E., & Tomes, N. (1993). Restraining the troublesome patient: A historical perspective on the contemporary debate. *Nursing History Review, 1,* 3–24.

Strumpf, N.E., Wagner, J., Evans, L.K., & Patterson, J. (1992). Reducing physical restraints: Developing an educational program. *Journal of Gerontological Nursing, 18*(11), 21–27.

Sullivan-Marx, E.M., Strumpf, N.E., Evans, L.K., Baumgarten, M., & Maislin, G. (1995). *Predictors of continued restraint use in nursing home residents.* Paper presented at the 48th Annual Scientific Meeting of the Gerontological Society of America, November, 1995, Los Angeles, CA.

Sundel, M., Garrett, R.M., & Horn, R.D. (1994). Restraint reduction in a nursing home and its impact on employee attitudes. *Journal of the American Geriatrics Society, 42,* 381–387.

Suprock, L.A. (1990). Changing the rules. *Geriatric Nursing, 11,* 288.

Werner, P., Koroknay, V., Braun, J., & Cohen-Mansfield, J. (1994). Individualized care alternatives used in the process of removing physical restraints in the nursing home. *Journal of the American Geriatrics Society, 42,* 321–325.

What is the law? (1989, June). *Untie the elderly, 1*(1), 1.

Yarmesch, M., & Sheafor, M. (1984). The decision to restrain. *Geriatric Nursing, 5,* 242–244.

Chapter 50

A Quality-Oriented Approach to Pressure Ulcer Management in a Nursing Facility

JEFFREY M. LEVINE   ELIZABETH TOTOLOS

Pressure ulcer management is a major concern of nurses in long-term care settings and other settings where clients are prone to this preventable condition. In this chapter the authors present a strategy for pressure ulcer management that relies on documentation, data flow, and feedback. The system was developed at the Jewish Home and Hospital for Aged in the Bronx, NY, and incorporates principles of quality improvement. It has resulted in a remarkable, low nosocomial ulcer prevalence rate in this institution. The details of their system are presented here, along with the organizational structure and tools used. The chapter concludes with a discussion of benefits and costs of the system.

In pursuit of quality health care delivery, our Department of Nursing has developed an effective system for dealing with the pervasive problem of pressure ulcers. The Agency for Health Care Policy and Research states that the prevalence of pressure ulcers among nursing home populations is 23% (Panel for the Prediction and Prevention of Pressure Ulcers in Adults, 1992). Our facility maintains a prevalence of 5%. After excluding residents with ulcers acquired outside the institution, prevalence drops even further to 3.1%. Our system is based on sound standards of nursing and medical management, and incorporates principles of Quality Improvement (QI). Suitable for a large institution, this system may serve as a model for other facilities with a similar philosophy and goals.

The Jewish Home and Hospital for Aged, Bronx Division, is an 816-bed not-for-profit nursing facility. We have 13 full-time primary care physicians and nearly 600 nursing staff including supervisors, registered nurses, licensed practical nurses, nurse's aides, and orderlies. We are an academic affiliate of the Mount Sinai Medical Center Department of Geriatrics, and host ongoing teaching activities for medical students, geriatric fellows,

From *The Gerontologist* 34(3):413–417, 1994. Reproduced with permission.

nurses, nurse practitioners, nursing assistants, and physicians. Average resident age is 85, and 86% are Medicaid-reimbursed. We have roughly 275 admissions and 50 readmissions per year, and the average length of stay is slightly longer than 2 years. According to standard New York state criteria, we have a relatively high illness acuity level.

The backbone of our strategy relies on documentation, data flow, and feedback, and essentially constitutes a supplement to the AHCPR Clinical Practice Guidelines for Prediction and Prevention of Pressure Ulcers (Panel for the Prediction and Prevention of Pressure Ulcers in Adults, 1992). Goals stated in the AHCPR manual include: (1) identifying at-risk individuals; (2) maintaining and improving tissue tolerance; (3) protecting against adverse effects of mechanical forces; and (4) reducing ulcers through educational programs. These guidelines are basic to our system, which supplements them by outlining an institutional management plan which continually reinforces awareness of good skin care as well as application of policy.

■ A QUALITY ORIENTED APPROACH TO PRESSURE ULCERS

Improvement of service to customers is a major challenge for health care in the 1990s. Quality Improvement is a management tool which promotes excellence through continuous system change (Batalden & Buchanan, 1989). This concept had its origin in the 1930s and 1940s, when the exigencies of wartime demanded large quantities of inexpensively produced supplies and goods. These principles, later embraced by Japanese industry, were in large part responsible for remarkable postwar economic success (Ishikawa, 1985). Many experts now advocate introduction of Quality Improvement practices into the health care industry as a replacement for Quality Assurance (QA) (Kritchevsky & Simmons, 1991).

QI is considered an evolutionary advance because it focuses on examining the entire system of care to make protocol changes and improve outcomes (Berwick, 1989). QI ideally encompasses all caregivers, fostering empowerment of team members in joining efforts to improve care, while Quality Assurance is delegated only to members of the QA committee. Quality Improvement focuses on actual ongoing processes of health care, while Quality Assurance works only toward specific endpoints. QI concentrates on careful system analysis to ensure that all functions contributing to a specified outcome are performing well. The analysis fostered by Quality Improvement leads to modification of future results, rather than simple analysis of past performance (Levenson, 1992).

Although Quality Improvement has proven dramatically effective in industries such as manufacturing, fewer successful examples are available in health care settings. The reasons lie in profound structural and cultural differences between organizations which care for the sick and those which produce consumer goods. The complexity of medical illness provides a level of uncertainty not have an equivalent in manufacturing, where goods and services are easily measured in an objective manner (Eddy, 1984). Also, in an era of fundamental changes in medical care, where spending and reimbursement are coming under increased governmental regulation, most organizations are rightfully hesitant to embark on new and costly projects. Implementation of QI requires an organizational commitment which may require consultant fees, learning of new skills by staff, and allocation of time for meetings.

Quality, however, is an increasingly important component of health care systems. Principles of QI can be implemented provided that attention is directed toward carefully defining quality indicators, then developig a plan for systems change. None of this is possible without the commitment of management to support such a project, as implementation involves strategic planning and budgeting to allow for appropriate human and financial resources to ensure success (American Hospital Association, 1992).

Pressure ulcers are an ideal clinical entity for application of QI principles. First, because of the multidisciplinary nature of prevention and treatment, ulcer prevalence can serve as an indicator reflecting the efficiency of the entire system. Second, there are multiple therapeutic modalities available, and each provider brings unique treatment experiences, making efforts to coordinate pressure ulcer management amenable to a facility-wide, systematic approach. Third, although current literature suggests that pressure ulcers may never be entirely eliminated, a new pressure ulcer is generally considered a poor outcome (Smith, Winsemius, & Besdine, 1991). Efforts to minimize pressure ulcers therefore implicitly address two critical dimensions of quality: (1) the achievement of optimal outcomes, and (2) the perception by the patient and family that health needs are being met (Franks, Nutting, & Clancy, 1993).

An efficient organizational strategy will provide for continuous audits of new ulcers, old ulcers, and ulcers present on admission, while monitoring lesions of unequal stages and different phases of healing. When considering ulcer prevalence as a quality indicator, one must remember that substandard quality may be attributable to causes external to the system (Kritchevsky & Simmons, 1991). In nursing homes, residents with pre-existing ulcers are a constant source of new lesions, and as such should not be considered evidence of quality deficiency. When implementing a system for documentation, the distinction between nosocomial ulcers and those imported into the facility is therefore important.

▄ DOCUMENTATION, DATA FLOW, AND FEEDBACK

As a Quality Improvement program cannot exist without accurate data, a strict information gathering and tracking system must be present (Curtis & Simpson, 1985). In our system, data collection is ongoing in order to follow trends, and is integrated into the daily work routine of staff. Written documentation of all aspects of ulcer care provide the basis for a flow of information through a system which comprises the QI infrastructure.

Prevention begins with a "Pressure Ulcer Risk Assessment," completed by the head nurse on all residents within 5 days of admission or return from hospital, and when the resident's physical condition has improved or deteriorated. This tool has been validated and is one of several currently available (Abruzzese, 1985; Towey & Erland, 1988). Any resident scoring equal to or greater than 12, and any resident on bedrest longer than 48 hours, is placed on a mandatory pressure ulcer prevention protocol, which includes alternating pressure air mattress, heel pads, turning and positioning every 2 hours, and gel cushion when positioned in a chair. Other measures include hygiene, hydration, local skin care, and nutritional follow-up. The risk-assessment score is documented in the care plan and forwarded to the rehabilitation nursing clinician.

The nurse's aide plays a critical role in implementation and documentation of prevention and treatment protocols. First, the aide ensures that all aspects of the protocol are in place and functioning properly, and documents this on a shift-by-shift basis using an assistive-device checkoff form. Turning and positioning every 2 hours is performed and documented on a separate flow sheet. In addition, the aide examines skin, reports changes to the nurse, and provides other skin care as needed.

The rehabilitation nursing clinician coordinates follow-up and generation of statistics. Residents on prevention protocols as well as those with ongoing ulcer treatment are followed weekly by a rehabilitation nurse assistant who ensures that required modalities are in place. Monthly statistics list number of residents on prevention protocols grouped by unit, the total of which is usually over 500 residents.

Whenever a new pressure ulcer is detected, or if a pre-existing ulcer begins deteriorating, a physician is contacted immediately for evaluation and update of the treatment plan. The clinical supervisor assesses the plan with the head nurse at regular intervals, and the rehabilitation nurse provides consultation on issues regarding prevention or treatment modalities. Nutritional assessment is mandatory on new and deteriorating ulcers, and recommendations are made regarding fluids, caloric intake, and supplements. Reinforcing this multidisciplinary collaboration is the Comprehensive Care Plan meeting, which is held 2 weeks after admission, then quarterly, with all disciplines — including nursing, medicine, nutrition, recreation, and social service — participating.

Specific documentation standards are followed for residents with pressure ulcers using uniform staging criteria (Shea, 1975). A Pressure Ulcer Report is completed by the head nurse for ulcers greater than stage one, and a copy is sent to rehabilitation nursing. A report is required for new ulcers, for any change in size, depth, or stage of a pre-existing ulcer, and for ulcers which are healed. A report is also generated monthy for existing ulcers which have undergone no change. Each report identifies location, stage, infection, current treatment, and where the ulcer originally developed (hospital or nursing facility). Photographs are taken of new pressure ulcers and are placed in the clinical record. A weekly nursing progress note is required for all pressure ulcers, and must include detailed description of the lesion as well as ongoing treatment and prevention measures.

The organizational structure for information flow is shown in Fig. 50-1. Copies of pressure ulcer reports are forwarded to the rehabilitation nurse clinician, who examines reports for accuracy in completion and checks for compliance with established treatment standards. Reports are logged

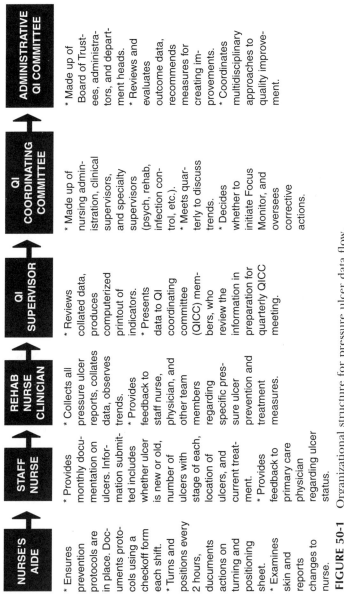

NURSE'S AIDE	STAFF NURSE	REHAB NURSE CLINICIAN	QI SUPERVISOR	QI COORDINATING COMMITTEE	ADMINISTRATIVE QI COMMITTEE
* Ensures prevention protocols are in place. Documents protocols using a checkoff form each shift. * Turns and positions every 2 hours, documents actions on turning and positioning sheet. * Examines skin and reports changes to nurse.	* Provides monthly documentation on ulcers. Information submitted includes whether ulcer is new or old, number of ulcers with stage of each, location of ulcers, and current treatment. * Provides feedback to primary care physician regarding ulcer status.	* Collects all pressure ulcer reports, collates data, observes trends. * Provides feedback to staff nurse, physician, and other team members regarding specific pressure ulcer prevention and treatment measures.	* Reviews collated data, produces computerized printout of indicators. * Presents data to QI coordinating committee (QICC) members, who review the information in preparation for quarterly QICC meeting.	* Made up of nursing administration, clinical supervisors, and specialty supervisors (psych, rehab, infection control, etc.). * Meets quarterly to discuss trends. * Decides whether to initiate Focus Monitor, and oversees corrective actions.	* Made up of Board of Trustees, administrators, and department heads. * Reviews and evaluates outcome data, recommends measures for creating improvements. * Coordinates multidisciplinary approaches to quality improvement.

FIGURE 50-1 Organizational structure for pressure ulcer data flow.

systematically by unit, and specific indicators are determined on a monthly basis. Indicators derived from ulcer reports include: (1) number of hospital-acquired ulcers; (2) number of nosocomial ulcers; (3) number of infected ulcers; (4) number of healed ulcers; (5) breakdown of pressure ulcers by stage; and (6) number of residents on ulcer prevention protocols. These data are submitted the first week of each month to the nursing Quality Assurance clinician who reviews collated data and produces a computerized printout of indicators. Data are shared with supervisors and head nurses and passed on to the Quality Improvement Coordinating Committee (QICC), the central mechanism for monitoring quality indicators.

The QICC is made up of nursing administration, clinical supervisors, and nursing subspecialty supervisors (psychiatry, rehabilitation, infection control, etc.), and meets quarterly to discuss trends. This committee decides how and when to investigate substandard results, oversees corrective actions, and reports to the administrative Quality Improvement committee, made up of the Board of Trustees, administrators, and department heads. This group reviews and evaluates outcome data, recommends measures for creating improvements, and coordinates multidisciplinary approaches to quality management.

If a trend is detected toward increased pressure ulcer prevalence, this is investigated and a plan of corrective action is recommended. If further information is required before a plan of correction can be devised, the Focus Monitor is undertaken. The Focus Monitor (Fig. 50-2) is an indicator-specific audit instrument developed from institutional guidelines for pressure ulcer care. Composed of record review and observation sections which examine risk factor evaluation, prevention, and treatment, audits are completed at random on units where deviation from the norm has been identified. This tool is designed to audit not only written documentation, but also the physical reality of patient care. Corrective action is shared with staff at the unit level, and clinical supervisors are responsible for monitoring changes in outcome. Positive reinforcement is given to staff if improvement is noted.

Several concepts of QI are incorporated into our system. First, all caregivers have clearly defined roles in ulcer prevention and treatment, and several mechanisms provide ongoing examination of the system's efficiency and efficacy. Data collection and analysis do not stop; results are continuously compiled and scrutinized for improvement or deterioration. Unit trends are followed using a "run chart," a Quality Improvement tool recommended for tracking indicators and detecting system problems (Joint Commission on Accreditation of Healthcare Organizations, 1992; Leebov & Ersoz, 1991). Use of the Focus Monitor provides a structured diagnostic step not present in traditional Quality Assurance. Finally, our organizational structure promotes several feedback channels which continually refine the process of care for pressure ulcers, in order to improve outcome.

▄CHALLENGE AND COST

To approach the challenge of improving quality, one must be prepared to accept the cost, which includes a commitment to prevention as well as treatment. The costs, however, must be weighed against increased expense,

Part I: Record Review	Standard met	Not met	n/a
1. Pressure ulcer did not develop while resident was in this facility.			
2. Pressure Ulcer Risk Assessment form was complete within 5 days of admission.			
3. If Pressure Ulcer Risk Assessment score is 12 or higher, there is evidence that preventive measures were taken.			
4. Pressure Ulcer Risk Assessment score is entered onto Nursing Care Plan.			
5. Initial Pressure Ulcer Report form includes documentation of location, size, depth, drainage, level, and origin of decubitus.			
6. Weekly pressure ulcer notes must have complete description of pressure sore; location, size, depth, type, amount of color of drainage, skin or tissue involvement, stage, and intervention.			
7. Monthly Pressure Ulcer Report includes description and level of ulcer, intervention, and plan.			
8. Problem is addressed on Nursing Care Plan with appropriate treatment plan and goals.			
9. There is documented evidence that therapeutic dietitian is involved in planning nutritional intervention.			
10. If purulent drainage is present, wound culture had been done.			
11. There is documentation that the treatment plan ordered by M.D. was carried out.			
12. Turning/positioning sheet is signed and complete.			

Part II: Observation	Standard met	Not met	n/a
1. Resident's position agrees with position indicated on Turning Sheet.			
2. Resident has special mattress.			
3. Resident has special cushion on wheelchair.			
4. Positioning pillows, heel pads, or other devices are in place as indicated on Nursing Care Plan.			
5. Padding is appropriately placed between knees or other skin surfaces.			

Comments _____

FIGURE 50-2 Focus monitor for pressure ulcer care.

pain, mortality, and morbidity incurred through pressure ulcers, not to mention undue hospitalization and unhappy family members. It has been stated that the organizational climate of nursing facilities is the most critical element in enhancing total patient care (Sheridan, White, & Fairchild, 1992). Upgrading to a comprehensive multidisciplinary skin care program will not only help an institution fulfill regulatory requirements, but will benefit the entire health care environment, justifying additional administrative, labor, and materials charges.

Costs incurred by our system can be measured in terms of increased time for monitoring, documentation, data analysis, and meetings. Three rehabilitation nurses spend 25% of their time following residents with pressure ulcer prevention or treatment protocols in place. Monitoring of protocols is incorporated into the duties of every nurse's aide as well as four rehabilitation nurse assistants. To complete the data analysis and generate quality indicators, one rehabilitation nurse devotes one day per month collating pressure ulcer reports. The Quality Improvement committee meets quarterly for 4 hours, and reviews additional indicators including physical restraints, accidents, psychotropic medications, and infections. Finally, no ulcer prevention program is complete without an educational component (Moody et al., 1988). Mandatory pressure sore programs are held twice a year for nursing, medicine, and dietary personnel, with sessions for day, evening, and night shifts. In addition to formal training, unit-based reinforcement of protocol is implemented as required.

In conclusion, pressure ulcers are an ideal indicator to which QI principles can be applied, provided there exists strong administrative leadership with a realistic view of additional costs involved. Institutions desirous of facing the challenge to lower pressure ulcer prevalence can, using readily available guidelines for prevention and treatment, implement a system of documentation, data management, and feedback. A comprehensive system which incorporates principles of Quality Improvement will result in favorable changes in ulcer epidemiology, narrowing the gap between the care actually provided and the best care theoretically possible.

▬REFERENCES

Abruzzese, R. (1985). Early assessment and prevention of pressure sores. In B. Y. Lee (Ed.), *Chronic ulcers of the skin* (pp. 1–19). New York: McGraw-Hill.

American Hospital Association. (1992). *The role of hospital leadership in the continuous improvement of patient care: A technical briefing prepared by the Division of Quality Resources.*

Batalden, P. B., & Buchanan, E. D. (1989). Industrial models of quality improvement. In N. Goldfield & D. B. Nash (Eds.), *Providing quality care: The challenge to clinicians* (pp. 133–155). Philadelphia: American College of Physicians.

Berwick, D. M. (1989). Continuous improvement as an ideal in health care. *New England Journal of Medicine, 320,* 53–56.

Curtis, B. J., & Simpson, L. J. (1985). Auditing: A method for evaluating quality of care. *Journal of Nursing Administration, 15,* 14–21.

Eddy, D. M. (1984). Variations in physician practice: The role of uncertainty. *Health Affairs, 3,* 74–89.

Franks, P., Nutting, P. A., & Clancy, C. M. (1993). Health care reform, primary care, and the need for research. *Journal of the American Medical Association, 270,* 1449–1453.

Ishikawa, J. (1985). *What is total quality control?* Englewood Cliffs, NJ: Prentice Hall.

Joint Commission on Accreditation of Healthcare Organizations. (1992). *Quality improvement in long term care.* Oakbrook Terrace, IL: Author.

Kritchevsky, S. B., & Simmons, B. P. (1991). Continuous quality improvement: Concepts and applications for physician care. *Journal of the American Medical Association, 266,* 1817–1823.

Leebov, W., & Ersoz, C. J. (1991). *The health care manager's guide to continuous quality improvement.* Chicago: American Hospital Publishing.

Levenson, S. A. (1992). The medical director and continuous quality improvement. *Journal of Medical Direction, 2,* 67–75.

Moody, B., Fanale, J., Thompson, M., Vaillancourt, D., Symonds, G., & Bonasoro, C. (1988). Impact of staff education on pressure sore development in elderly hospitalized patients. *Archives of Internal Medicine, 148,* 2241–2243.

Panel for the Prediction and Prevention of Pressure Ulcers in Adults. (1992). *Pressure ulcers in adults: Prediction and prevention.* AHCPR Publication No. 92-0047. Rockville, MD: U.S. Department of Health and Human Services.

Shea, J. D. (1975). Pressure sores: Classification and management. *Clinics in Orthopedics, 112,* 89–100.

Sheridan, J. E., White, J., & Fairchild, J. (1992). Ineffective staff, ineffective supervision, or ineffective administration? Why some nursing homes fail to provide adequate care. *The Gerontologist, 32,* 334–341.

Smith, D. M., Winsemius, D. K., & Besdine, R. W. (1991). Pressure sores in the elderly: Can this outcome be improved? *Journal of General Internal Medicine, 6,* 81–93.

Towey, A. P., & Erland, S. M. (1988). Validity and reliability of an assessment tool for pressure ulcer risk. *Decubitus, 1,* 40–48.

Chapter 51

Validation: Techniques for Communicating With Confused Old-Old Persons and Improving Their Quality of Life

NAOMI FEIL

Communicating with confused older adults can be frustrating and may anger caregivers because of the inability to relate in a meaningful or helpful way. This occurs because they use their familiar ways of communicating. In this chapter Naomi Feil presents validation therapy as a specific communication process for the old-old adult who is disoriented and confused, based on behaviors of respect and empathy. A table, describing the four stages of resolution in the old-old adult, helps the reader understand the specific behavior changes observed in the various stages. The use of validation leads to significant changes in behavior encouraging people to continue to communicate outwardly, thus thwarting progression toward the stage of vegetation. Basic validation beliefs and values, along with useful techniques for implementation, are clearly presented.

Very old age is relatively new. With very old age comes an increased incidence of mental confusion and deterioration. Validation theory arose from the need to communicate empathetically with old-old people to help restore dignity, reduce anxiety, and prevent withdrawal to vegetation. Validation therapy is not just facilitative to patients; it also empowers caregivers and helps them prevent depression and exhaustion. This article describes the psychopathology present in old-old persons with dementia and then outlines how to communicate with them using validation.

■ THE CONFUSED OLD-OLD PERSON

The most crucial characteristic of very old age is that developmental history and physical changes are inseparable. A holistic approach to viewing people reveals that behavior at every age is marked by physical, psychologic, emo-

From *Topics in Geriatric Rehabilitation* 11(4):34–42, 1996. Reprinted with permission.

tional, spiritual, and social development. As advances in health care increase our life span, caregivers are pressed to understand the complex interactions that shape the behavior of very old people. Ultimately, to empathize with old-old people, one must acknowledge the intricate relationship between physical deterioration and developmental needs.

■ THE CONSEQUENCES OF NEGATIVE RESOLUTIONS OF DEVELOPMENTAL LIFE TASKS

Many developmental psychologists believe that at different stages of life, different life tasks need to be accomplished. Failure to resolve a life task successfully can lead to psychologic problems and difficulty resolving the next life task successfully. Trust is learned in infancy. If trust is not mastered, the child is not able to examine himself or herself to explain problems. The child learns to place the blame on others for life's hardships. In childhood, the primary task is to learn control. Rules are fun to follow. However, if the parents require perfection of the child, the child feels the need to keep tight control of his or her feelings. In adolescence, rebellion should occur. If parents do not give unconditional love, rebellion is not acted out for fear of rejection. Therefore, the child hesitates to look inside to discover his or her own identity. In adulthood, the primary task is to get close to another human being. However, if the tasks of earlier stages are not accomplished, intimacy is not reached. Lack of trust, embarrassment, fear of failure, and rejection isolate this person.

In middle age, people learn to adapt to the problems life offers. If the person feels that perfection is expected, the person does not have the capabilities of coping with the changes relating to age, occupation, and relationships. In old age, the task is to justify what has been done throughout life. It is time for reflection, to enjoy one's achievements, and to come to terms with one's failures and mistakes. However, if we cannot accept who we are, feelings of despair result. More important, if despair is ignored, it can evolve into severe depression.

A logical consequence to people living longer lives is that the number of old-old people with unresolved life tasks has greatly increased. Unresolved life tasks become a heavy emotional burden that follows the victim throughout life, finally reemerging and seeking resolution. Old-old people reach a resolution stage of their lives, often struggling to complete unfinished tasks in order to complete their life in peace. Validation is an interpersonal communication strategy founded on the premise that specific techniques can be utilized to communicate and assist the old-old person in resolving past issues.[1]

Social researcher Bernice Neugarten[2] considers "old-old" people to be 75 years and over while "young-old" people are defined as being between 55 and 74 years of age. According to Neugarten, these two groups have significantly different social and psychologic needs, and they should be considered separately. In old-old people, muscle strength often decreases along with bladder control. In addition, arthritis, osteoporosis, and circulatory problems are common. These physical changes many times are coupled with a deterioration of the mind. For this age group, Alzheimer's disease is the prevalent cause of dementia.

The relationship between the biologic aspects of Alzheimer's disease and the behavioral, psychologic, and physical remains to be clarified. Many people over age 80 overcome the limitations of old age, avoid succumbing to chronic organic brain disease, and remain oriented. They still have the ability to communicate, are aware of time and place, and are capable of making appropriate judgments. Obviously, oriented old-old people do not require validation.

However, those who did not resolve important developmental tasks earlier in life have issues that return and affect their mental and emotional well-being. These old-old people no longer have the ability to confront the burden produced by the aging process and the deteriorating brain. Often, the end result is the choice to retreat. Validating these people can assist them in restoring their personal dignity. Often they respond with improved speech, better eye contact, steadier gait, and rediscovered social skills. Once caregivers and health care professionals recognize that disoriented old-old people are struggling with a legitimate life task, the chance of mistreatment is greatly reduced.

THE NEEDS OF DISORIENTED OLD-OLD PEOPLE

People who are diagnosed with early onset Alzheimer's disease are usually between 40 to 60 years of age; they sometimes do not successfully respond to validation. The underlying psychologic and social reasons behind this disoriented behavior are unknown. Unlike the old-old person who is confused, these people often do not respond to the caregiver's eye contact or touch. Validation only momentarily improves the quality of life and does not slow the progression of the disease.

On the other hand, old-old people who are disoriented often respond to validation. By understanding why they behave in a certain manner, the caregiver can communicate with the old-old person. The caregiver can correctly comprehend the person's behavior only after considering the person's age and social and psychologic needs. Common psychologic and social needs of the old-old person who is disoriented include the need to:

- Express feelings that have been locked up inside throughout their lives.
- Restore a sense of equilibrium and relieve loneliness when eyesight, hearing, mobility, and recent memory fail.
- Restore their former social roles. (They often use people in present time to represent significant loved ones from the past.)
- Resolve unsatisfactory relationships from the past before they die.
- Resolve unfinished life tasks in order to die in peace.

When the psychologic and social needs of old-old people who are disoriented are met, often they do not regress to a state of vegetation.

VALIDATION

Validation developed from direct experience with old-old people who are disoriented. It is based on communicating with respect and empathy. Validation provides a way of classifying behaviors and suggests practical techniques that help to restore dignity and avoid further mental deterioration of these persons. Caregivers using validation techniques become nonjudgmental, empathetic listeners. Anxiety is reduced as well as the need for restraints, and a sense of self-worth is restored in the person.

Validation is based on the belief that all behavior is performed for a reason. They key to validation is to understand why the person who is disoriented behaves the way he or she does and then to accept the behavior. Understanding a person's behavior depends on knowing his or her physical strengths and social and psychologic needs. Until these factors are understood, no behavior can be judged appropriate or inappropriate.

The validating caregiver provides a nurturing and trusting atmosphere for the old-old person utilizing genuine touching, nurturing, caring, and empathy. Experience with this technique has shown that increased feelings of self-worth result. These feelings lead to significant changes in behavior wherein people do not withdraw inwardly, but continue to communicate outwardly.

Validation is based on the following 10 underlying beliefs and values:

1. All people are unique and must be treated as individuals.
2. All people are valuable no matter how disoriented they are.
3. There are understandable reasons behind the behavior of disoriented old-old people.
4. Behavior in old-old age is not merely a function of anatomic changes in the brain, but reflects a combination of physical, social, and psychologic changes that take place over the life span.
5. Old-old people cannot be forced to change their behaviors. Behaviors can be changed only if the person wants to change them.
6. Old-old people must be accepted nonjudgmentally.
7. Particular life tasks are associated with each stage of life. Failure to complete a task at the appropriate stage of life may lead to psychologic problems.
8. When more recent memory fails, older adults try to restore balance to their lives by retrieving earlier memories. When eyesight fails, they use the mind's eye to see. When hearing goes, they listen to sounds from the past.
9. Painful feelings that are expressed, acknowledged, and validated by a trusted listener will diminish. Painful feelings that are ignored or suppressed will gain strength.
10. Empathy builds trust, reduces anxiety, and restores dignity.

STAGES OF RESOLUTION — COPING WITH DENIED LIFE TASKS

Ignored or denied life tasks require resolution in the very old. The four stages of resolution are: malorientation, time confusion, repetitive motion, and vegetation. The stages are detailed in Table 51-1. Physical deterioration

TABLE 51-1   Detailed Behavior of the Four Stages of Resolution in the Old-Old Person

	STAGE 1: MALORIENTATION	STAGE 2: TIME CONFUSION	STAGE 3: REPETITIVE MOTION	STAGE 4: VEGETATION
Basic helping clues	Use who, what, where, and when questions Use minimal touch Maintain social distance	Use "feeling" words Use touch and eye contact	Use touch and eye contact Pace to person's movements	Mirror movements Use sensory stimulation
Orientation	Keeps time Holds onto present Realizes and is threatened by own disorientation	Does not keep track of clock time Forgets facts, names, and places Has increasing difficulty with nouns	Shuts out most stimulation from the outside world Has own sense of time	Will not recognize family, visitors, old friends, or staff Has no time sense
Body patterns Muscles	Tense, tight muscles Usually continent Quick, direct movements Purposeful gait	Upright but relaxed Aware of incontinence Slow, smooth movements	Slumped forward Unaware of incontinence Restless, pacing	Flaccid Little movement No effort to control continence Frequent finger movement
Vocal tone	Harsh, accusatory, and often whining	Low, rarely harsh Sings readily	Slow, steady	Usually closed
Eyes	Clear and bright Focused, good eye contact	Clear, unfocused Downcast, eye contact triggers recognition	Eyes shut (face closed, lacks expression) Self-stimulation is minimal	Difficult to assess
Emotions	Denies feelings	Substitutes memories and feelings from past to present situations	Demonstrates sexual feelings openly	Responds to tone and touch
Personal care	Can do basic care Seeks personal reminders	Misplaces personal items often Creates own rules of behavior	Has few commonly used words Does not listen or talk to others	None readily apparent
Communication	Responds positively to recognized roles and persons Responds negatively to those less oriented	Responds to nurturing tone and touch Smiles when greeted	Is not motivated to read or write	
Memory and intellect rules	Can read and write unless blind Sticks to rules and conventions	Can read but can no longer write legibly	Is not motivated to read or write	Difficult to assess
Humor	Some humor retained	Will not play games Humor not evident	Laughs easily, often unprompted	Difficult to assess

parallels these stages. Systematic classification of people into these categories is difficult because each person is unique, and some people fluctuate between stages. Very old people who are not validated will pass through these stages; however, with validation, many of these people can avoid the progression to vegetation. Caregivers should learn to recognize the physical and psychologic characteristics of each of the stages of resolution and adapt to the various stages that the old-old person who is disoriented moves through.

▬ THE TECHNIQUES OF VALIDATION

Caregivers use validation by carrying out 14 simple techniques. First and foremost, however, caregivers must have the ability to accept and empathize with the old-old person. Family members should be taught these techniques because they can improve the lives of both the person receiving care and the caregiver.

Technique 1: Centering

The centering technique makes possible a release of emotion from the caregiver that might bias his or her actions. One concentrates on breathing so that distractions such as anger and frustration are vented. After centering, the caregiver can more readily receive the feelings of his or her patient. The centered caregiver is able to listen more empathetically; therefore, this technique should be done at the beginning of every validation session.

Centering requires only a few minutes, and it is a relaxing exercise. One simply inhales through the nose and exhales through the mouth, removing any other thoughts from the mind and concentrating only on breathing. The procedure is repeated eight times.

Technique 2: Using Nonthreatening, Factual Words to Build Trust

In order to communicate with people in the resolution phase (see Table 51-1), the caregiver should not force a confrontation of emotions. Patients do not want to comprehend their behavior and often retreat when they have to face their feelings. A caregiver can prevent this retreat by avoiding questioning the old-old person about why something occurred or why he or she acted in a certain way. The best approach is to encourage the patient's conversation and avoid pressing him or her with accusations. It is useful to focus conversation on factual information about the topic by questioning about who, what, where, when, and how. If the patient feels comfortable discussing the incident from this approach, often his or her hidden or obscure needs can be met and validation can occur.

Technique 3: Rephrasing

It is often reassuring for a patient to hear his or her own words repeated. In rephrasing, the caregiver responds with the main ideas and key words of the patient, using the same rhythm and expression. Rather than being confronted, the older person hears only a rephrasing of his or her own statements. Rephrasing provides both reassurance and validation.

Technique 4: Using Polarity

Asking a person complaining about food. "Is that the worst chicken you have ever eaten?" invites the person to express his or her feelings more freely, therefore finding relief. The complaint may focus on the food, but there may be a deeper anxiety over, for example, poorly fitting dentures.

The patient simply needs a listening ear to release his or her anger. The concentration on the extreme can serve as a catharsis for the person, who is then given permission to discuss the issue more elaborately and ends up being validated by the caregiver in the process. The simple act of listening creates a release for the person, easing his or her anger and tension.

Technique 5: Imagining the Opposite

Once there is an element of trust in the relationship between a caregiver and an older person, the caregiver can help the patient get through an anxious time by imagining the opposite solution. Through subtle questioning, or possibly rephrasing, the person concentrates more carefully on his or her problem. To validate a person with anxiety complaining about "that man came back last night," the caregiver asks, "Are there nights he does not come?" Many times this approach results in the recollection of a solution that was effective in the past in coping with being left alone. The validating caregiver can reintroduce the patient to forgotten problem-solving abilities.

Technique 6: Reminiscing

When a person reaches old-old age, learning new coping mechanisms is extremely difficult. By reminiscing, the person can recall and then use familiar coping strategies. Words such as "always" and "never" can help trigger the disoriented person's earlier memories. Techniques 5 and 6 are used together to help the old-old person restore familiar ways of overcoming stress.

Technique 7: Maintaining Genuine, Close Eye Contact

This technique is best used with people in the stages of time confusion and repetitive motion (see Table 51-1). Maintaining close eye contact relays a genuine expression of affection to the disoriented old-old person. When the person returns the maintained eye contact, his or her anxiety is reduced. The calmness introduced by the nurturing caregiver allows the person to feel safe and loved.

Technique 8: Using Ambiguity

Very old people in the time confusion stage (see Table 51-1) often create their own special language. This language holds no meaning for anyone but the person who is disoriented. By using ambiguity, the validating caregiver responds to the person by replacing the unknown words with pronouns. The caregiver responds to "The catawalks are hurting me!" with, "Where do *they* hurt?'' Similarly, ''I wild with the woomets'' might bring the reply, ''Was *it* fun? Did *they* say anything?'' Frequently, the disoriented person will reply with more gibberish language. However, if communication can be maintained, progression to the vegetation stage is prevented. This response to the person's unique language validates him or her.

Technique 9: Using a Clear, Low, Loving Tone of Voice

The validating caregiver uses a clear, low, nurturing tone of voice when speaking to the person who is disoriented. Harsh tones may cause the person to become angry or withdrawn, while high-pitched, soft tones are difficult for old-old people to hear. The nurturing tone calms the person, thus reducing his or her anxiety. Often, the nurturing tone triggers loving memories and reduces stress.

Technique 10: Observing and Matching the Person's Motions and Emotions (Mirroring)

This technique works well with people in the stages of time confusion and repetitive motion (see Table 51-1) who often express their emotions without inhibition. The validating caregiver communicates by mirroring movements, postures, facial expressions, and breathing patterns. By mirroring the old-old person, the validating caregiver enters this person's world and demonstrates a willingness to develop a trusting relationship that is both verbal and nonverbal. When the person rocks, the caregiver rocks; when the person paces, the caregiver paces. It takes a certain humility on the part of the caregiver to mirror what may appear to be bizarre behavior with the intention of support and connection.

Technique 11: Linking the Behavior with the Unmet Human Need

Most people need to be loved and nurtured, to be active and employed, and to express their deep emotions to someone who will listen with empathy. An old-old person who is disoriented will often perform a specific behavior repeatedly, such as folding and refolding a napkin. This behavior most likely symbolizes a basic human need of this person. By observing the person's behavior, the validating caregiver can relate the behavior to one of three human needs: love, the need to be useful, or the need to express raw emotions. Folding the napkin may have become a symbol of the need for love. Once the correct interpretation is made, the caregiver can enter the person's world and be an empathetic listener for the person.

Technique 12: Identifying and Using the Preferred Sense

Identifying a person's preferred sense — vision, smell, or touch — is the first step in using this technique. The preferred sense can be determined by carefully listening to the person's word choices. When the person is asked to describe a past experience, the validating caregiver listens for words that describe seeing, smelling, or touching. The first sense used is probably the preferred sense. For example, a resident may describe a trip to the mountains by focusing on being able to see the tips of the trees.

Vision is likely the preferred sense. Once the preferred sense is determined, the caregiver can better speak in the person's terminology, thus helping to build a relationship of trust between the caregiver and the person who is disoriented.

Technique 13: Touching

People who are disoriented often do not respond well to touch, but touching is a way to communicate with a person in the stage of time confusion (see Table 51-1). Cut off from visual and auditory stimuli, these people are often in their own world, unaware of their surroundings. However, in the time confusion stage, people are still willing to incorporate strangers into their world. Once trust is established, the validating caregiver can use touch to enter the person's world and establish a nurturing relationship. To incorporate touch appropriately, the following techniques are the most effective:

- Approach from the front. Approaching from the back or the side may startle the person.
- Use the fingertips in a light, circular motion on the upper cheek.
- Use the fingertips in a circular motion with a moderate amount of pressure on the back of the head.
- Use the outside of the hand, placing the little finger on the ear lobe, curving along the chin with both hands, and make a soft stroking motion downward along the neck.
- Use cupped fingers on the back of the neck with both hands in a small circular motion.
- Use both hands to rub the shoulders and upper back.
- Touch the back of the calf with the fingertips.

Touch must be used very carefully. Always remember that any sign of resistance to contact shows that touch is not appropriate for this person.

Technique 14: Using Music

When a person is in the repetitive motion stage (see Table 51-1), he or she no longer retains the ability to speak and often does not recognize familiar faces. The person can, however, sing words to songs that were meaningful earlier in life. People in the repetitive motion stage often verbally communicate a few words after singing along to music.

▬SUMMARY

This article presents the critical social and psychologic needs of old-old people who are disoriented and briefly describes the theory and specific techniques of validation developed to help restore dignity in each of the stages of resolution — malorientation, time confusion, repetitive motion, and vegetation. Validation therapy has proven to be a more effective approach for the old-old person with dementia than with those whose dementia begins before the age of 70. People with early-onset Alzheimer's disease deteriorate despite validation.

The old-old person who is disoriented presents a great challenge in caregiving. Caregivers left to their own familiar ways of communicating soon become frustrated and angry with the inability to relate in a meaningful or helpful way. Validation teaches a specific communication process for the old-old person that is based on the behaviors of respect and empathy. Experience with this technique reveals that old-old people who are disoriented can respond in positive ways that thwart a natural progression toward the stage of vegetation.

▬ REFERENCES

1. Feil N. *The Validation Breakthrough.* Baltimore, Md: Health Professions Press: 1993.
2. Neugarten B. Dynamics of transition of middle age to old age adaptation and the life cycle. *J Geriatr Psychiatry.* 1970;1.

▬ SUGGESTED READINGS

Feil N. Validation: an empathic approach to the care of dementia. *Clin Gerontol.* 1989;8:89–94.
Feil N. Validation therapy. In: Kim PKH, ed. *Serving the Elderly.* New York, NY: Aldine de Gruyter; 1991.
Feil N, Flynn J. Meaning behind movements of the disoriented old-old. *Somatics.* 1983;4:4–10.

Chapter 52

The Truth-Tellers: How Hospice Nurses Help Patients Confront Death

JOYCE ZERWEKH

> Joyce Zerwekh is a prolific writer focusing on family and community
> health issues. In this chapter, she provides support for nurses who
> work with dying clients to teach them to bring important issues out
> into the open before it's too late. Hospice nurses help clients confront
> death by being truth-tellers; talking openly about what is happening,
> how clients are feeling, and what is normal at this time. For some
> nurses it is "comfortable" for them to avoid talking about death and
> the reality of the dying process. This approach does not meet the
> client's needs and holistic care is not accomplished because of the
> nurse's discomfort or misconceptions. Three hospice nurses describe
> how they interact with clients, thus giving readers a place to begin as
> they think about *really* being there for their clients at the time of
> death.

Hospice home care nurses form deep, long-term relationships with patients
and their families. Those close connections serve them well. Working in
the home, caring for the dying, they learn how to talk about death.

I've collected stories from 32 hospice nurses, who averaged 17 years in
nursing and seven in hospice. As I analyzed their stories, it became evident
that these nurses were particularly adept at two important skills — telling
the truth and encouraging patient autonomy. The "success stories" I've
gathered here offer expert insights into what to say to dying patients and
their families, and when to say it, to help them through their final days.

■ WHAT IS THE "TRUTH?"

During the dying process, the truth is never fully known. Remember the
story about the blind men and the elephant? Depending on the part of
the animal he touched, each man described a different reality: One thought
the elephant's leg was a tree trunk; another thought the tail was a rope.
Similarly, the "truth" will be viewed differently by the patient, his family,
and each health care professional.

From *American Journal of Nursing* 31–34, February 1994. Reprinted with permission.

The hospice nurse's perspective and ability to speak honestly with patients are framed by extensive experience with the common courses of end-stage diseases. These experts have learned to recognize the physiological and psychosocial signs that death is near, and to acknowledge this reality with the patient and his family. Instead of rote treatment plans — "Everyone's treatable, no one's terminal" — they've retrained themselves to see the final stage of life for what it is and to speak openly about it. Three hospice nurses describe how this affects the way they interact with patients:

> *I keep talking to her about what's real and what's honest. She's going to need help. She's getting weaker and weaker. I want to make it work for her at home. We talk to each other. We speak the truth. We say what's happening.*
> *People are getting in touch with what's really going on and we're there to help them with that. . . .*

These anecdotes reveal three vital communication skills: asking the difficult questions, speaking the truth when the truth is in transition, and facing avoidance. Let's take a look at how hospice nurses use these skills. Then consider how you might strengthen your own truth-telling abilities wherever you practice.

◼ASKING DIFFICULT QUESTIONS

Hospice nurses make deliberate decisions to speak about sensitive matters that are customarily avoided. When the difficult questions are left unasked, there's no acknowledgment of dying and no way for the patient to take control of his life. As one nurse put it: "A patient wonders, 'Are you really going to talk to me and tell me what's happening? To tell me the truth?'" But how can you find the right words — at the right time? There is no one right question, one of the nurses I talked to suggested. Instead:

> *It's whatever you say that tends to trigger them. I ask, "What did the doctor really tell you about your illness?" That's the same as asking whether they're aware of how sick they are. We need to ask the question and put it out there for them to be honest. . . .*

Timing the questions takes experience. If you're new at asking such difficult questions, watch for verbal and nonverbal cues (such as staying with or changing the subject, or remaining silent) that may tell you to continue or to back off and try again later. Truth can only be discussed openly when people give permission.

When the timing is right, the truth can be an extraordinary relief:

> *They were going to the theater and symphony and having bridge parties. And they were wondering why she was so tired. I said, "The reason you're so tired is because you're sick and you're not acting like you're sick. You can't be sick and do the things you were doing before." It was like a shade was lifted. They were flabbergasted. They were trying to live as they had before, denying the fact that she had a terminal illness. . . .*

Here's another example of questions working as triggers that free patients to talk about their true concerns and free families to communicate:

I kept going over in my mind how I was going to handle this. I walked into the room and sat down. "I hear you had a bad night?" I began. "Yes." And I asked, "How much did the doctor tell you about how serious your illness was?"

She said, "Well, I do recall him saying something about six months or less." I said, "Yes, I think we are in the 'less' time." She replied, "I kind of had an idea about that. I'd just as soon it be over with."

Her husband was sitting at the end of the bed and he started to sob. When he stopped, we were able to have a marvelous talk about what death meant to her and to him. . . .

▬ A CHANGING REALITY

The condition of a dying person is everchanging. That's why speaking the truth when the truth is in transition is an essential nursing skill. While bearing in mind the uncertainties of prediction, the hospice nurse seeks to help people live with a life expectancy measured in months rather than years. Each loss of function signals a changing truth about what remains.

"The opportunity for the patient to talk to someone who doesn't need to encourage him to look for improvement is a unique part of hospice nursing," one nurse told me. The following anecdote illustrates this point:

She was making a transition from hope for chemotherapy to hope for good days at the end. She needed someone comfortable dealing with the fears. In my time there I tried to normalize her reality that she didn't want to get up in the chair or to try to gain strength. She needed to hear that it was normal to nap in the afternoon and to not want to eat much. . . .

▬ DEALING WITH AVOIDANCE

Again, each participant in the dying person's life may have quite a different take on what's happening. As the nurse, you may have to balance what you know to be true about the patient's condition with what the patient is ready to accept. This can be particularly difficult when a patient has a trusting relationship with a physician who's reluctant to confront the prospect of death: "The doctor . . . just wants to talk about positive things, how we are going to get better. And she's not going to get better."

Rather than disappoint such a physician, some patients may struggle to meet his needs: "I just don't want to let my doctor down." In such cases, respect that strong physician-patient bond with encouraging the patient to recognize his own needs as having the highest priority.

Families who want to speak only about life continuing can also pose great challenges. Try to balance respect for their choices with a commitment to truth-telling:

The patient was alert and needed to sign consent papers that said something about expected death. I got this stern look from the family, who said they wanted to go into the other room to discuss it. After we left the bedside, I got holy heck from them about who did I think I was coming into the house and talking like that. "We don't talk like that in this house. We have a positive attitude."

I made it real clear that I was not going to lie to the patient. I told them, "If she asks me if she's going to die, my comment would be, 'It looks like that but we never really know what's going to happen.'"

That was all right with them. They had worried I might come in like the black angel of death. . . .

People use many strategies to avoid facing death, which nurses need to identify. You want to move around these roadblocks to invite discussion of the truth:

They were all scientists, real head people. Both sides of the family came from an upbringing where facts and figures provided answers to questions, and it was difficult for them to approach a situation where there were no answers. As they would move totally into their head, I would talk about how an experience made them feel. I tried to help them move from their head to their heart. It was a challenge to keep centered and not get sucked into the facts and figures. . . .

It's common for patients as well as families and professional caregivers to become so preoccupied by medical procedures that all conversation and efforts at control are focused on them. When you build a trusting relationship, you can often break this pattern by gently but persistently asking difficult questions and saying the words that need to be said.

Sometimes, the truth won't ever be fully acknowledged. Never use a sledgehammer to impose reality, but remain committed to telling the truth when invited:

I don't know if I've ever seen denial work so well. I was impressed with their zest for life. I told them I would answer their questions honestly, always tell the truth. We rarely discussed death and dying. We talked about the moment-to-moment things that were happening. Whenever I visited they would take a couple of minutes out of each visit to focus on reality. We had to talk gently around it. . . .

▄ENCOURAGING CHOICE

When the truth is being told, people can make informed decisions about how they will live and die. All people, not just the dying, have this right to determine their own lives without being coerced by medical expectations.

How can you encourage choice for your own patients? The hospice nurses' stories describe the skills of assessing patient choice, facilitating choice-making, respecting those choices, and advocating for choice when the medical or social system resists.

Assessing choice involves being attentive to people and asking straightforward questions about their preferences. They are the experts in managing their own lives. Nurses don't push decisions when the family isn't ready, but continue to bring up the possibility of choice. Some people have had limited power in their lives and finally achieve a sense of control in their dying. Others are "never strong enough to make a stand," as one hospice nurse put it.

Becoming actively involved in facilitating choice-making means, as another nurse explained, "opening people up to choices about treatment and how they want to live the rest of their lives." Translate medical information into human terms. Keep reminding patients and families that they have a choice in all the decisions being made. Question the patient regularly to discern his wishes and clarify his options.

Here's an example of the ongoing process of fostering choices by a patient who wants to retain a high degree of control:

> *Everything became a decision. He couldn't swallow. Should he have TPN? We spent our time talking about what that meant. He decided to have it. He wanted to finish his PhD. We had to organize the bedroom so he could set up his computer. He went on to thinking about whether he wanted to kill himself, but he decided he had some more to do. He was hesitant to take pain meds. That was a big discussion too. That's the way it went, trying to give him total control. When he needed several dressing changes, I gave him one dressing that he was in charge of and I was in charge of the other. . . .*

Additional choice-making strategies include what one hospice nurse called "playing out the patient's worst fears and walking through the whole future scenario." Propose a trial to see if a choice is acceptable. For instance, a patient may need to experience the consequence of a proposed method of symptom management:

> *She was vomiting fecal material and her fistula was like a volcano. I suggested that the TPN was causing fluid overload and maybe if we cut it back, she wouldn't have so much vomiting. She wasn't ready to decide. A day later she agreed to slow it and the third day we stopped it. Then the vomiting stopped and she felt so much better that she chose to go back on it. We started it again, and sure enough, the vomiting started and the fistula erupted. You have to give people freedom to make these decisions and see for themselves. . . .*

▬ FOSTERING COMMUNICATION

Helping people make choices may mean first helping the family to communicate with each other. Again, you need to be sensitive to timing and resist pushing: "When they were ready," a nurse told me, "I helped them to make their decision instead of making it for them."

Frequently family members and patients have conflicting choices, which they must work to reconcile. In one case, for instance, a husband wanted hospice and "no code" while his wife wanted everything done to keep him alive. The nurse brought the conflict into the open and encouraged them to talk to each other about it. Over time, "we went through this delicate negotiation so her husband could let her define what her goals and priorities were."

Ironically, helping patients make choices also means recognizing that some people aren't in a position to make choices. For instance, women who are members of patriarchal religions or cultures may not be allowed to express an opinion or make a decision regarding their own future. (In such cases, the nurse tries to negotiate with the family decision-maker on behalf of the woman.)

Some choices have to be limited for active drug and alcohol abusers and those who have been or are becoming cognitively impaired. You may have to make a difficult judgment call to remove choice from a patient's hands when that choice is causing harm:

> *He was so confused and out of control and having everyone around him running in circles. I rarely am very directive with patient and families, but in this situation I held up a figurative mirror for him. I said what was happening to his mother and friends. I said that he didn't need to be in charge of his care anymore. He needed to let other people do that now. He sobbed with relief. . . .*

Respecting choices requires that you let go of any personal agenda about what the patient should do. "I put aside my own wants, try to subordinate them or figure out how to modify them," said one hospice nurse.

It's a given in home hospice care that the nurse respects the patient's choice to receive care at home, which can be a huge challenge, with minimal resources and maximum physical debilitation. During her first visit, one nurse made this commitment to a dying young mother: "I will do everything I can to keep you at home, holding your children next to you." Likewise, the home hospice nurse lets go of the home care agenda when the family chooses to change directions: "Hospitalization was their choice and it felt right."

Respecting choices also means supporting a wide range of decisions. Some affirm the values of the individual and family but may contradict traditional medical practice, mainstream societal values, or what appears to be "common sense." The stories I gathered show patients and families refusing IVs, chemotherapy, tube feeding, transfusions, antibiotics, diuretics, hospitalization, and resuscitation. These nurses have honored nontraditional and perhaps risky end-of-life choices, like going out for pizza, getting in the bathtub despite multiple bleeding wounds, taking final journeys, and participating in memorable events. A vivid example:

> *His goal was their 50th wedding anniversary in April. "I will do anything you tell me to make it to 50 years." So we encouraged activity and eating and regular medications. He would go to the mall and walk with his friends. We made a pain cocktail for his bone pain; I got him on Trilisate 1,500 mg, which really helped. Just prior to the anniversary, he started to fail. We used a Duragesic patch and he perked up. We put him on prednisone for his appetite. He was able to get himself back to the point that he went to the celebration in a wheelchair. . . .*

Sometimes patient and family choices unsettle even the most broadminded nurse, and pose extreme hazards to the dying person or family. Those most troubling to the hospice nurses were choices of suicide or active euthanasia, decisions to go through extraordinary painful and unproven therapies, to suffer rather than control pain, or to reject help.

When you encounter such circumstances, you need to balance respect for individual choices with your responsibility to protect the suffering and do no harm. Ask for help in your own decision-making from nursing colleagues and supervisors, interdisciplinary team members, and even ethics committees.

■ TAKING ON THE SYSTEM

Finally, the hospice nurses advocate for choice when systems resist. When the truth has been spoken and the patient has made his decision, he'll often need help to assert that choice.

You'll find yourself running interference with often resistant medical or social systems, explaining the patient's preferences and mediating as necessary with hospitals, community programs, reimbursement sources, and physicians. "I called the doctor," said one hospice nurse, "and told him that the patient was saying no."

A common dilemma for home hospice nurses is stopping the ball from rolling — like preventing CPR after families have called 911. When your power to speak the truth about patients' choices is constrained by the system in which you practice, this advocacy role requires careful strategy.

Document the patient's choice by recording it and by speaking out. Assuming this responsibility on your own may not be as effective as bringing in other health care professionals and family members who know what the patient wants, and together figuring out how to ensure that his choice — whatever it may be — is respected.

Truth and choice are important to everyone, but particularly to the person who must rely on others for the critical information needed to make difficult decisions. These hospice nurses show us how thoughtful, undaunted, unrelenting insistence on the right to self-determination can help the dying patient live life to the fullest.

■ SELECTED REFERENCES

Amenta, M. O., and Bohnet, N. L. *Nursing Care of the Terminally Ill.* Philadelphia, J. B. Lippincott Co., 1986.

Beauchamp, T. L., and Childress, J. F. *Principles of Biomedical Ethics.* 3rd ed. New York, Oxford University Press, 1989.

Blues, A. G., and Zerwekh, J. V. *Hospice and Palliative Nursing Care.* New York, Grune and Stratton, 1984.

Jonsen, A. R., et al. *Clinical Ethics.* 3rd ed. New York, Macmillan Publishing Co., 1992.

Zerwekh, J. V. *A Family Caregiving Model for Hospice Nursing.* (to be published)

SELECTED BIBLIOGRAPHY

Ballard, T. M. (1995). The need for well-prepared nurse administrators in long-term care. *Image: Journal of Nursing Scholarship* 27(2): 153–154.

Boland, D. L. & Sims, S. L. (1996). Family care giving at home as a solitary journey. *Image: Journal of Nursing Scholarship* 28(1): 55–58.

Chappell, N. L. & Penning, M. (1996). Behavioural problems and distress among caregivers of people with dementia. *Ageing and Society* 16: 57–73.

Dellasega, C., Dansky, K., King, L., & Stricklin, M. L. (1994). Use of home health services by elderly persons with cognitive impairment. *Journal of Nursing Administration* 24(6): 20–25.

Fraser, C. (1996). This dementia patient can be helped. *RN* 59(1): 38–39, 41–42, 44.

Guberman, N., Maheu, P., & Maille, C. (1992). Women as family caregivers: Why do they care? *The Gerontologist* 32(5): 607–617.

Hibbard, J., Neufeld, A., & Harrison, M. J. (1996). Gender differences in the support networks of caregivers. *Journal of Gerontological Nursing* 22(9): 15–23.

Jacob, S. R. (1996). The grief experience of older women whose husbands had hospice care. *Journal of Advanced Nursing* 24(2): 280–286.

Kane, R. A. (Winter 1995–1996). Transforming care institutions for the frail elderly: Out of one shall be many. *Generations* 62–68.

Kelley, S. J. (1993). Caregiver stress in grandparents raising grandchildren. *Image: Journal of Nursing Scholarship* 35(4): 331–337.

Kresevic, D. M. & Naylor, M. (1995). Preventing pressure ulcers through use of protocols in a mentored nursing model. *Geriatric Nursing* 16(5): 225–229.

Mahoney, D. F. (1995). Analysis of restraint-free nursing homes. *Image: Journal of Nursing Scholarship* 27(2): 155–160.

Matteson, M. A. & Linton, A. (1996). Wandering behaviors in institutionalized persons with dementia. *Journal of Gerontological Nursing* 22(9): 39–46.

Morris, R. I. & Branon Christie, K. M. (1995). Initiating hospice care why, when, and how. *Home Healthcare Nurse* 13(5): 21–29.

Smith, C. E. (1994). A model of caregiving effectiveness for technologically dependent adults residing at home. *Advances in Nursing Science* 17(2): 27–40.

Stanford, E. P. & Schmidt, M. G. (Winter 1995–1996). The changing face of nursing home residents: Meeting their diverse needs. *Generations* 20–23.

Walker, A. (1996). The cost-effectiveness of home health: A case presentation. *Geriatric Nursing* 17(1): 37–40.

York, N. (April 1995). Coping with caregiving: Supporting the informal caregiver. *CARING Magazine* 44–47.

Index

Page numbers followed by f indicate figures; those followed by t indicate tables.